Food Science, Health and Nutrition

Food Science, Health and Nutrition

Editor: Logan Bowman

www.callistoreference.com

Callisto Reference,
118-35 Queens Blvd., Suite 400,
Forest Hills, NY 11375, USA

Visit us on the World Wide Web at:
www.callistoreference.com

ISBN: 978-1-63239-843-7 (Hardback)

Printed in the United States of America.

Cataloging-in-publication Data

Food science, health and nutrition / edited by Logan Bowman.
p. cm.
Includes bibliographical references and index.
ISBN 978-1-63239-843-7
1. Food. 2. Nutrition. 3. Health. 4. Food animals. 5. Food preferences. I. Bowman, Logan.
TX357 .F66 2017
641.3--dc23

Table of Contents

Preface

Food science is the science dedicated to the study of food and its characteristics. Nutrition is the science that exemplifies the interaction of nutrients and other substances in food. The aim of this book is to present researches that have transformed this discipline and aided its advancement. This book highlights the relationship between food science, health and nutrition with special emphasis on the importance of nutrients in food and their impact on health. The text covers a broad spectrum of topics under food science including its sub-disciplines such as food engineering, food chemistry, etc. For someone with an interest and eye for detail, this book covers the most significant topics in the field of food science and nutrition. With state-of-the-art inputs by acclaimed experts of this field, this book targets students and professionals alike.

This book aims to highlight the current researches and provides a platform to further the scope of innovations in this area. This book is a product of the combined efforts of many researchers and scientists from different parts of the world. The objective of this book is to provide the readers with the latest information in the field.

I would like to express my sincere thanks to the authors for their dedicated efforts in the completion of this book. I acknowledge the efforts of the publisher for providing constant support. Lastly, I would like to thank my family for their support in all academic endeavors.

Editor

1

Measuring Motivation for Appetitive Behaviour: Food-Restricted Broiler Breeder Chickens Cross a Water Barrier to Forage in an Area of Wood Shavings without Food

Laura M. Dixon[1]*, Sarah Brocklehurst[2], Vicky Sandilands[1], Melissa Bateson[3], Bert J. Tolkamp[1], Rick B. D'Eath[1]

1 Animal and Veterinary Science, SRUC, Edinburgh, United Kingdom, **2** Biomathematics and Statistics Scotland, Edinburgh, United Kingdom, **3** Center for Behaviour and Evolution, Institute of Neuroscience, Newcastle University, United Kingdom

Abstract

Broiler breeders (parents of meat chickens) are selected for fast growth and become obese if fed ad libitum. To avoid this and maintain good health and reproductive ability, they are feed restricted to about 1/3 of what they would eat ad libitum. As a result, they experience chronic hunger and exhibit abnormal behaviour patterns that may indicate stress and frustration. One approach to measuring hunger is to observe how much birds will work, such as pecking a key, for access to more or different types of food. However, the sight, smell, and feedback from consumption of the feed reward changes the context and may artificially raise feeding motivation. To avoid this, we tested broiler breeders in an apparatus in which they could work for access to a wooden platform covered in wood shavings by crossing a water runway which increased in length and depth in 8 successive tests. In the wood shavings area, they could perform exploratory and foraging behaviour (the appetitive phase of feeding) but were never rewarded with feed. Sixty birds were divided into three feed quantity treatments: commercial restriction (R), and twice (2R) or three times (3R) this amount. Overall, birds fed R worked harder to reach the wood shavings area (reached it in a larger number of tests) than 2R and 3R birds ($P<0.001$). More restricted birds took less time to reach the area ($P<0.001$, $R<2R<3R$) and spent more time foraging while there ($P<0.001$, $R>2R>3R$). This indicates that restricted-fed birds were hungry and willing to work for the opportunity to forage even though food was never provided, suggesting that their motivation to perform the appetitive component of feeding behaviour (foraging/food searching) was sufficient to sustain their response. Thus food restriction in broiler breeders is a welfare concern. However these methods could be used to test alternative feeding regimes to attempt to find ways of alleviating hunger while still maintaining healthy growth and reproduction in these birds.

Editor: Claudia Mettke-Hofmann, Liverpool John Moores University, United Kingdom

Funding: This study was funded by the UK Department for Environment, Food, and Rural Affairs (Defra) as part of a larger project (AW1141) investigating the subjective state of food restricted broiler chickens using behavioural and neurochemical measures. The funders had no role in study design, data collection and analysis, decision to publish, or preparation of the manuscript.

Competing Interests: The authors have declared that no competing interests exist.

* Email: laura.dixon@sruc.ac.uk

Introduction

Ethical concerns over animal welfare arise because of the belief that animals can experience and suffer from negative mental states [1,2]. Although we cannot be sure whether animals consciously experience emotions, we can nonetheless investigate the physical and behavioural outward signs of emotion in animals [1,3–6]. Emotional states accompany situations that are rewarding (positive emotions) or punishing (negative emotions), so investigation of animal motivation is an important behavioural approach in animal welfare science [1,7]. Typical methods to measure motivation require animals to overcome a cost to gain access to a resource: for example, the animal is asked to work by e.g. repeatedly pressing a lever or pushing through a weighted door to obtain an immediate reward (operant or consumer demand tests, e.g. [1,8–12]). Animals that are willing to work hard to obtain a resource are said to be motivated to access that resource. Therefore, they would have improved welfare if provided with, and decreased welfare if denied, that resource.

There are some difficulties involved in measuring motivation for a resource (e.g. [13,14]). As most motivation tests provide the resource either as part of the test or as the reward for completing the task (e.g. [8,15,16]), sights and smells and feedback from the resource may initially be artificially raising the animal's motivation for that resource while without these cues motivation may remain low (e.g., out of sight is out of mind, [17]).

The present study focuses on motivation for food in broiler breeders. Broiler breeders (the parents of broiler chickens) grow rapidly, become overweight, and suffer from a number of health problems associated with obesity resulting in high mortality if they are fed to appetite [18]. To prevent this, they are ration-fed, resulting in food restriction which can be as severe as 33% of what they would eat *ad libitum* [19,20]. This gives rise to the welfare concern that they may be suffering from chronic hunger (reviewed by [21,22]). The 'broiler breeder paradox' [23] is that it is difficult to feed them so that they are both 'healthy' and 'have what they want', which Dawkins [24] has proposed as the key determinants of good animal welfare.

Food restricted broiler breeders show increased general activity and in particular foraging activity such as scratching and pecking. This increased foraging activity can also be expressed in abnormal ways, such as through spot pecking and polydipsia or water spillage [25–29].

In addition to these observations, feeding motivation in broiler breeders has also been tested by presenting extra food, for example in a preference or operant conditioning task [30,31] or a relatively short rate of eating task using familiar or novel food [29,32], or in a longer-term compensatory feeding task which assesses the extent of previous food restriction by measuring *ad libitum* food intake over 22 days [33,34]. Taken together, this evidence indicates that food restricted birds will be chronically hungry and experiencing stress, which has a negative impact on bird welfare [19,21,25,27,28]. The use of food in these feeding motivation tests raises a number of difficulties (see [35] for a detailed critique). The presentation of additional food in these tasks changes the context for the animal from having to cope because it has no access to food to being aware that additional food is available (even if they must work to get it). Thus, (i) the potential to obtain the resource is in itself likely to increase motivation and (ii) once the resource has been used motivation may be increased as a result of positive feedback [36], until at least a state of satiety is reached. When birds on different feed treatments are compared, there are additional difficulties of interpretation, and this raises the question of whether the usual treatment food, or a single food type common to all treatments should be used in the test situation.

In the present study, we propose to avoid the difficulties with food-based tests by measuring motivation to access a location where exploratory and food-searching (foraging) behaviour is possible but in the absence of a food reward. Many behaviours, including feeding, contain an appetitive phase which involves the searching phase of a behaviour sequence (exploration, and searching for food; foraging) and indicates the need or motivation to achieve a certain goal. Consummatory behaviour (e.g. eating) follows appetitive behaviour and is the achievement ('consummation') of the goal or behaviour needed to help satisfy the motivation [37,38]. The appetitive phase of behaviour continues until the goal is reached but unless the motivation is fulfilled, performance of the appetitive behaviour should persist (unless it continues to a point where other motivations become more important) [39,40]. Thus feeding motivation could be estimated by measuring motivation to perform the appetitive phase of feeding behaviour, i.e. foraging.

Another difficulty with tasks to measure feeding motivation concerns the nature of the cost imposed. Animals may find it easier to associate a task involving pecking with access to food, rather than with another non-food resource [1,11]. Key pecking at increasing schedules (i.e. more pecks per reward) were used by Savory et al [41] and Savory & Lariviere [42] to show that food-restricted broiler breeders were 3.6 times more motivated for food than *ad libitum* fed birds which had been food deprived for 72 hrs. This striking demonstration of the high feeding motivation resulting from chronic food restriction is nonetheless open to the criticism that hungry birds increase their pecking anyway, so is increased pecking really a cost, or just an expression of this? More 'natural' costs such as squeezing through a narrow gap [43], or pushing through a weighted door [9,10] or walking a long way [44] overcome this difficulty and also have the advantage that they require little or no learning [43]. In the present experiment we chose to use the natural cost of walking through water, which hens find aversive [45–47]. Water also has the advantage that the cost can be varied by increasing the length and depth of the water.

In earlier experiments we had found that broiler breeders were motivated to forage in areas to which they had intermittent access [14]. In the present study we designed a task in which broiler breeder female chickens were tested for their motivation to access a platform covered in wood shavings which was only accessible during the tests and never (at any stage of training or testing) contained a food reward. We imposed a 'natural' cost on access to the wood shavings area using a water runway which increased in length and water depth with each test. Birds were allowed 10 minutes from the start of the test to reach the wood shavings area and given a further 5 minutes in the apparatus if they did reach it. Birds (n = 20 per treatment) were given one of three feed treatments that differed in food quantity: the industry recommended restriction level (R), or two (2R) or three (3R) times this amount. It was predicted that birds fed smaller food portions would be more motivated to reach the wood shavings area, as indicated by i) a higher proportion of birds crossing the water at each cost. In the language of 'animal economics' which can be applied to these types of experiment, this would result in a greater 'maximum price paid' (reservation price [9,10]) to reach the wood shavings area. We also predicted that more food restricted birds would show ii) a less rapid decline in birds crossing the water as it gets longer and deeper; iii) a shorter average time taken to cross the water and iv) a longer average time spent foraging once they reach the wood shavings area.

Materials and Methods

Ethical Considerations

Birds never had their water intake restricted and were housed on a bedding of wood shavings to provide comfort, insulation and allow for dustbathing behaviour. Food restriction is likely to result in hunger, but research into animal welfare problems often faces the difficulty that the problem must be recreated in the laboratory in order to study it. At any one time there are an estimated 7.5 million broiler breeder chickens in the UK alone [32,49] all of which are restricted-fed (R) during rearing. The levels of food restriction we imposed were similar to or less severe than that used routinely in the poultry industry, with birds receiving at least the industry recommended level (R) of food or some multiple of this (2R or 3R). *Ad libitum* fed broiler breeders can suffer from health problems and mortality [18], and the ration of 3R birds in our study was close to *ad libitum* [50]. However, the experiment was ended when birds were 11 weeks old, at which age they were still active and healthy. All procedures in this experiment were carried out under Home Office Licence and with the SRUC Animal Experiment Committee's approval; birds were checked on a minimum of three times per day.

Animals and Housing

Sixty non-beak trimmed Ross308 broiler breeder female chickens were received from Aviagen (Stratford, UK) as day old chicks, and were reared according to the commercial recommendations for housing, lighting, temperature and nutrition for this genotype: the Ross308 parent stock guidelines [48]. They were housed in floor pens (1.0×2.0 m) covered in wood shavings until 4 weeks of age. The lighting schedule for the first day was 23.5L:0.5D hours light:dark, which was then gradually reduced to 8L:16D over 10 days. Temperature decreased from around 30°C at bird level at one day old to around 20°C by four weeks of age. Chicks were given *ad libitum* water from bell drinkers and were fed chick starter crumbs for the first three weeks, chick starter pellets for the following three weeks and then grower pellets (all ABN, Cupar Mills, Fife) from the beginning of six weeks of age to the end of the trial. The feed was formulated in line with commercial broiler breeder standards. Food was provided *ad libitum* for the first 7 days and then in restricted amounts given at 9:00 am each day that were gradually increased from 26 to 44 g per bird per day by the beginning of the 5th week, as per the Ross308 parent stock guidelines [48].

At 4 weeks of age, all birds were weighed, wing tagged (10 mm×10 mm padlock-style tags, Roxan Developments Ltd., UK) and housed in groups of three in twenty-one floor pens (1.5×2.0 m) according to matched body weight. However for three of the pens only two birds were used for the trial, giving a total of twenty birds per feed treatment. Two birds of each group were randomly selected to be the 'marked' birds (marked with either blue or purple livestock spray before testing), while the other was unmarked during testing. Each pen was bedded with wood shavings and provided with water through cup drinkers. To minimise food competition, food was presented in four small (90 mm width ×75 mm height ×55 mm depth) semi-circular food cups, two on the left side of the pen and two on the right. Starting in the 5th week of age, birds began to receive the commercially recommended food quantity (R), or two (2R) or three (3R) times this amount, depending on their feed treatment (see below). All birds were weighed approximately weekly from age 2 weeks to the end of the trial (age 11 weeks) (Fig 1). Although it is difficult to make an exact comparison because of differences in feed, genotype and rearing method, the 3R treatment achieved food intake and growth rate close to that of ad libitum fed birds [41]. However, where an *ad libitum* fed bird would have constant access to feed, the 3R birds generally finished their meals within the light periods (8 hours). The R birds finished their rations in 15 minutes or less and the 2R birds finished in 40 minutes or less.

Apparatus

Two identical sets of apparatus were used. Each apparatus was 6.0 m in length and was constructed with a wooden frame and wire mesh walls (Fig 2). Within this frame, the floor and sides to a depth of 130 mm of the apparatus were covered with a water proof tarp to allow for water to be added to the apparatus. At each test, birds began on a wooden start platform (0.5×0.5 m, height 0.14 m) at one end of the apparatus and they could progress to another wooden platform at the other end which constituted the wood shavings area (0.75×0.5 m, height 0.14 m). A 2 cm layer of wood shavings covered the wooden platform (retained at the front edge by a 10 mm high wooden batten) during training and testing but not habituation. The wood shavings area could be moved along the apparatus, allowing the runway length to vary. Ramps led from the start platform to the runway and from the runway to the wood shavings area (0.4 m each). This prevented the birds from having to jump into and out of the runway, in case they slipped in the water. Ramps were fitted with three lateral wooden battens 20 mmx20 mm in cross section and 0.15 m long, and placed at 0.08 m intervals to improve grip for the birds' feet. The ramps were always placed with a 25 mm overhang on the platforms to ensure ramp length stayed consistent throughout tests. Taking the ramps into account, the length of the runway between the two ramps that the birds needed to cross to reach the wood shavings area could range from 0 to 4 m.

A removable mesh lid that lowered the ceiling for the birds to just above head height was attached to the apparatus at the start platform and extended over the runway area to prevent birds from attempting to fly from the start platform to the wood shavings area. (Birds need extra height to lift off for flight and the lid prevented this). The lid was raised gradually from 0.15 to 0.25 m above the height of the start platform and wood shavings area as the birds grew so that they were always able to stand upright in the apparatus.

Habituation

The chickens were housed in groups of three but were tested in the apparatus singly. Therefore the birds had to be comfortable enough on their own in the apparatus to perform the task. To help to achieve this, at 5 weeks of age, groups of three birds were placed in the apparatus (no water and no wood shavings) for 15 minutes to explore. This was repeated two more times for a total of three group habituation sessions to the apparatus. Next, each bird was placed individually in the apparatus to explore for 15 minutes and this training continued until the individual bird was walking around the apparatus and not making alarm calls: this took about three individual sessions.

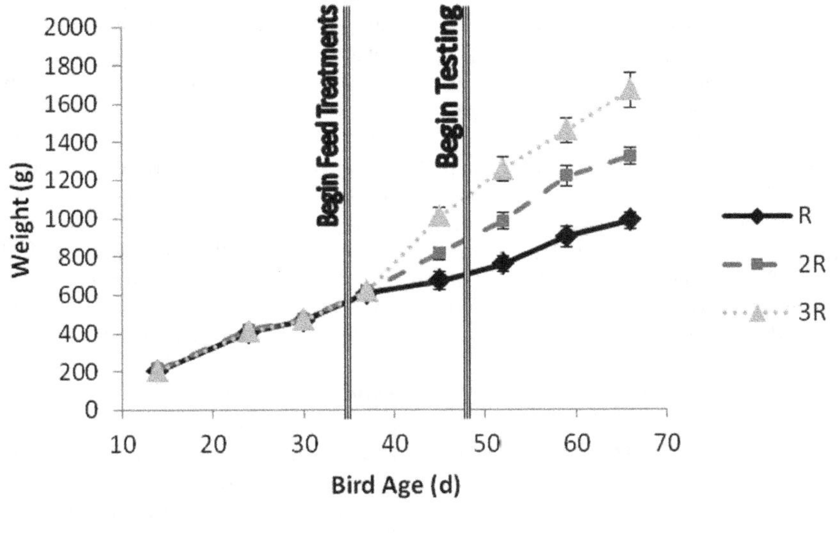

Figure 1. Bird weights for the 3 feed treatments (mean ± SD) from 14 days of age to the end of the trial. Birds began different feed treatments at 35 days of age and testing began at 50 days of age.

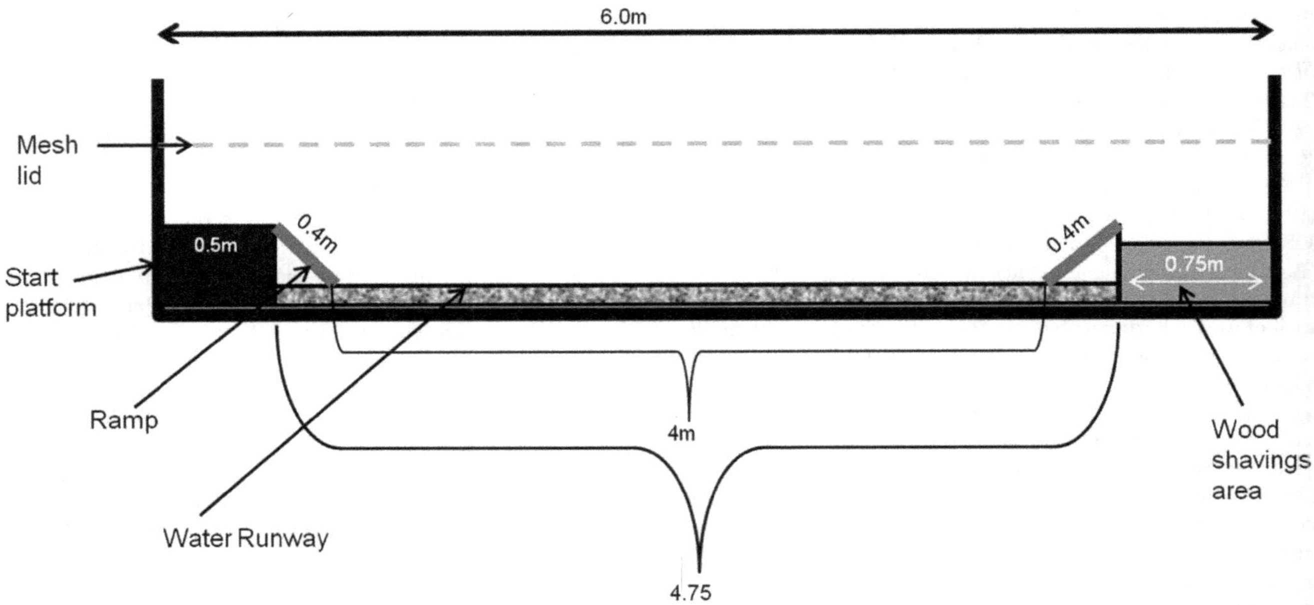

Figure 2. Diagram of the water runway apparatus. Birds were placed on the start platform and could chose to walk down the ramp into the water runway, up the second ramp and go onto the wood shavings area. The wood shavings area could be moved along the runway so that the distance travelled through the water could be increased up to a maximum of 4 m. An adjustable mesh lid covered the apparatus to prevent birds from flying from the start platform to the wood shavings area.

Training

Training began at 6 weeks of age. To begin, the apparatus did not have any water and wood shavings were spread on the wooden platform in the wood shavings area. There was *no* gap between the start platform and the wood shavings area (ramps were removed). Birds were left to explore the apparatus and to find the wood shavings. Once the birds reached the wood shavings area, they were allowed a further 5 minutes in the apparatus before the training session ended. The birds were given 10 minutes to find the wood shavings area. If they did not reach it in the 10 minutes given, they were placed in the wood shavings area for 5 minutes. Birds would not have progressed from this step until they reached the wood shavings area without assistance. However, in practice all birds were successful in their first training session with this apparatus set up.

Next the wood shavings area was moved 0.95 m from the start platform and the ramps were added, with a 20 cm gap between the bottom of the ramps. No water was in the runway and again birds were given 10 minutes to reach the wood shavings area and were left for a further 5 minutes after they did. Birds all reached the wood shavings on the first attempt, otherwise this training step would have been repeated until they did. Finally, this step was repeated but with enough water in the runway to just cover the birds feet (about 20 mm), as pilot studies suggested that birds found the initial appearance of the water aversive and began to alarm call when first exposed to the water. After all birds were successful in reaching the wood shavings area with 20 mm water in the runway, testing began. For this apparatus set up, all but 3 birds were successful in reaching the wood shavings area and the remaining 3 were given another training session the following day in which they all succeeded in reaching the wood shavings area.

Testing

Testing began when the birds were 7 weeks of age and lasted 24 days. Each bird was tested on eight occasions in total, 3 days apart. For the first test, the wood shavings area was moved 1.25 m from the start platform, with 0.5 m between the bottom of the ramps and water was added to the runway. The room was heated to a constant 20–20°C, and the water was at 'ambient temperature' i.e. it was not heated separately. The same source of mains water was used to fill and refill the apparatuses. Because birds on the different feed treatments grew at different rates over the test, the water depth was proportional to mean leg length. To do this, the length of the birds' legs was measured from the ground to the top of the hock before each test for R, 2R and 3R fed birds. Over subsequent tests, the 'cost' of accessing the wood shavings area, in terms of water depth and length was increased in a stepwise manner: water was increased in increments relative to the average length of the birds' legs (Table 1). This resulted in water depth levels that ranged from 8 mm to 110–112 mm by the end of the eight tests. As the water depth increased with each test, the length of the runway was also increased by 0.5 m each time up to a maximum length of 4 m (measured from ramp end to ramp end; Table 1). The environment for the apparatuses was the same for all tests (between 20–22°C) and the water used to increase water depth came from the same source throughout the trial.

Each test lasted up to 15 minutes. A bird was placed on the start platform and given 10 minutes to get to the wood shavings area. Once a bird had reached the wood shavings area, she was allowed 5 minutes before the test was ended. If she did not reach it in the first 10 minutes, she was removed from the apparatus. These time limits were set for practical reasons (to reduce the time taken to test multiple birds) and to reduce the chances of extinction occurring.

Experimental Design

The three different feed treatments (R, 2R and 3R) were allocated at the pen level in a randomized block design. The 21 home pens were divided into sets of three adjacent pens (7 spatial blocks), to which the three treatments were randomly allocated. Six of the blocks contained pens with 3 birds and the remaining block contained pens with 2 experimental birds resulting in 7 pens and 20 birds in each feed treatment. Three of the blocks of pens

Table 1. Cost increases (runway length between the two ramps and water depth) with increasing test number for the 3 feed treatments.

	Test Number							
	1	**2**	**3**	**4**	**5**	**6**	**7**	**8**
Runway Length (m)	0.5	1.0	1.5	2.0	2.5	3.0	3.5	4.0
Water Depth (percentage of leg length)	17%	33%	50%	67%	83%	100%	117%	133%

Water depth is based on percentage of the mean length of the birds' legs, from the ground to top of the hock, for each food treatment. The initial water depth was 1/6th of the average leg length and increments of 1/6th were then made at successive tests so that in the last two tests the water was deeper than the birds' legs were long, meaning that her body was getting wet.

with 3 birds (selected at random) were tested on one set of apparatus, while the other three blocks were tested with the other set of apparatus. For the three pens with only two experimental birds one bird in each pen was tested on each apparatus. Birds within pens were allocated to one of two scheduling groups for which tests were staggered by one day in such a way that each scheduling group contained half of the birds. These two scheduling groups and the use of the two sets of apparatus were balanced with each other and as much as possible with spatial blocks and feed treatments.

Measurements

For all tests, we recorded whether the bird reached the wood shavings area (defined by the bird having both feet on the platform) and the latency to reach the wood shavings area in cases where the bird was successful. For birds that reached the wood shavings area, their behaviour in the wood shavings area was also recorded to allow determination of whether the birds were using the wood shavings area for foraging. In detail, total durations that the birds spent in the wood shavings area standing and foraging (scratching and/or pecking), sitting and foraging (scratching and/or pecking), standing, sitting, walking or preening were measured over the 5 minutes from when they first reached the wood shavings area. Sitting was rare and so this was combined with standing for analyses and the behaviours preening and walking occurred at very low levels throughout all treatments so were not analysed further. Additionally, in the 5 minutes from when birds first reached the wood shavings area, birds were also able to leave the area and their movement was recorded so that the total time spent in the wood shavings area could be measured. Behaviours performed in the wood shavings area were analysed as a proportion of the total time spent there.

All birds were tested with all platform distances and water depths, even if they gave up crossing the water in earlier tests. This allowed statistical analyses of a full complement of longitudinal data which is likely to be more powerful than analyses of summary measures such as the maximum cost paid (distance/depth overcome) to get to the wood shavings area.

Statistical Analysis

All measures were analysed by fitting Linear Mixed Models (LMMs) or Generalized Linear Mixed Models (GLMMs) using Residual Maximum Likelihood (REML) in Genstat (14th edition 2011). Fixed effects included in all models were feed treatment (R, 2R, 3R), scheduling group (1,2) and apparatus (1,2), and for longitudinal data, test number (1,…,8) and 2 way interactions between test number and each of the other 3 factors. Random effects included in all models were pen (1,…,21) (i.e. bird triplet or pair), and bird (1,…,60) and, for longitudinal data, interactions of these with test number (1,…,8). There was little or no variation due to the 7 spatial blocks of 3 pens so this was not included in the random effects. All effects were fitted as factors (i.e. categorical classifications). As well as fitting models with feed treatment as a single factor with 3 levels, alternative models were investigated with a single contrast between each pair of feed treatments fitted before the feed treatment factor, in order to test specifically for differences between each pair of feed treatments.

The proportion of birds that reached the wood shavings area was investigated by fitting a GLMM with logit link function and binomially distributed errors [51,52] to the binary outcome of whether the bird reached the wood shavings area or not. The highest cost each bird paid was analysed by fitting LMMs to the test number of the last test when a bird reached the wood shavings area. It was not possible to analyse the latency to reach the wood shavings area for all tests due to the large proportion (60%) of censored values. Latency to reach the wood shavings area for tests for which the bird did reach the wood shavings area only was analysed by fitting LMMs to natural log transformed data. The proportion of time spent in the wood shavings area (of 300 seconds opportunity to do so) for tests for which the bird did reach the wood shavings area only was analysed by fitting LMMs. The proportion of time spent foraging (scratching and pecking) while standing or sitting of the time spent in the wood shavings area was analysed by fitting LMMs to data transformed using the angular transformation [51]. Apart from the highest cost each bird paid, all of these analyses are of longitudinal data in which the effect of test number is included.

Statistical tests, with significance at the 5% level, were based on approximate F tests when these were available, referencing observed F statistics to the F distribution, but otherwise Wald tests were used in which the Wald statistic was compared to the χ^2-distribution. In approximate F tests, denominator degrees of freedom are estimated and may not be whole numbers when fitted factors are not perfectly balanced/and or when effects are estimated from more than one level of the random hierarchy in the model. Test results given are based on sequential tests and factors are tested in different orders as appropriate to any imbalances between them in order to ensure that the results given are robust against test order, reporting results of each factor when tested last. For example, when analysing measurements from successful tests only, imbalances between feed treatment and test number occur due to loss of more data from feed treatment 3R and least from feed treatment R as test number increases. Therefore, tests for feed treatment are reported adjusting for test number, and for test number adjusting for feed treatment.

Estimated means and standard errors (SEs) from the LMMs and GLMMs are reported for the interaction between feed treatment and test number (averaged over the other fixed effects) and for main effects of feed treatment and test number when significant. In addition, in order to aid interpretation, back transformed means are reported for LMMs when applied to transformed data and for GLMMs. The dataset can be acquired from the PlosOne website as File S1.

Results

Reaching the wood shavings area

The highest cost each bird paid ('Reservation price' or 'Maximum Price Paid') was on average 2–3 times higher ($F_{2,17} = 11.28$, $P<0.001$) for R birds (mean ± SE test number = 6.30±0.64) than for 2R (mean ± SE test number = 2.28±0.65) and 3R (mean ± SE test number = 2.96±0.65) birds.

There was an effect of feed treatment, with a larger proportion of birds fed R reaching the wood shavings area than birds fed 2R and 3R ($\chi^2_2 = 20.25$, $P<0.001$, Fig 3) and there was a decrease in the proportion of birds from all feed treatments that reached the wood shavings area as test number increased ($\chi^2_7 = 25.45$, $P< 0.001$, Fig 3). There was no statistically significant interaction between test number and feed treatment.

For tests in which birds reached the wood shavings area only, on average, birds fed R were quickest to reach the wood shavings area, followed by birds fed 2R and then birds fed 3R ($F_{2,37} = 11.55$, $P<0.001$, Fig 4) and tests of specific contrasts suggested statistically significant differences in mean between all 3 feed treatments (R versus 2R $F_{1,33} = 8.70$, $P = 0.006$, R versus 3R $F_{1,37} = 23.05$, $P<0.001$, 2R vs 3R $F_{1,41} = 5.02$, $P = 0.031$). Test number was only marginally significant ($F_{7,49} = 2.53$, $P = 0.027$) and there was no statistically significant interaction between test number and feed treatment (Fig 4).

Behaviour in the wood shavings area

For tests in which birds reached the wood shavings area, there was no statistically significant effect of test number or feed treatment on the mean time spent in the wood shavings area; birds on average generally spent over 50% of the five minutes available there, ranging from 145±15 sec at the first test to 238±42 sec at the last test (mean ± SE estimated from LMM). However, when birds were in the wood shavings area, birds fed R spent the most time foraging whilst birds fed 3R spent the least time foraging ($F_{2,30} = 18.54$, $P<0.001$; Fig 5) and tests of specific contrasts suggested statistically significant differences in proportions between all 3 feed treatments (R versus 2R $F_{1,26} = 14.95$, $P<0.001$, R versus 3R $F_{1,30} = 37.04$, $P<0.001$, 2R vs 3R $F_{1,35} = 7.12$, $P = 0.011$). Overall, the proportion of time spent foraging (of the time spent in the wood shavings area) increased with test number and peaked at 0.49 at test number 5 and then decreased again ($F_{7,46} = 7.56$, $P<0.001$), with individual feed treatments peaking at 0.87 for R, 0.64 for 2R and 0.11 for 3R (back-transformed values; Fig 5). There was no statistically significant interaction between test number and feed treatment affecting the proportion of time spent foraging.

Discussion

As expected, broiler breeders fed the commercially restricted food allowances (R) accessed the wood shavings area more at all levels of cost than the 2R and 3R birds, resulting in on average a higher Maximum Price Paid (Reservation Price) for access to the wood shavings area. Rate of decline in the proportion of birds reaching the wood shavings area appeared to be less steep for R birds but this effect was not statistically significant (no feed treatment by test interaction). The rate of change of consumption of a resource in response to increasing cost has been highlighted by some authors as a key measure of motivation [1,53]. In this experiment, variation between birds, and the large treatment differences which already meant that a relatively low proportion of 2R and 3R birds visited the wood shavings area even at low cost made it difficult to detect this interaction. Unexpectedly, there was little difference between 2R and 3R birds in these measures, which might suggest that the welfare benefits in terms of reduced hunger of increasing rations from 2R to 3R are limited, in contrast to the welfare benefits of reducing hunger in R birds. Of birds that reached the wood shavings area, on average, restricted birds took less time to reach it and spent a greater proportion of their time there foraging; these behaviours were different between R and 2R, but also between 2R and 3R birds, so were more discriminatory of feeding level.

The low numbers of birds willing to cross the water in the 2R and 3R treatments is a potential weakness for using this technique in future studies when analysing measures that are only defined for birds that reach the wood shavings area. However, the range of treatments chosen here was large, and experimental diets designed to improve satiety which will be of relevance to the poultry industry are likely to be much closer to the R diet tested here. Comparison with this initial validation study will enable any improvements to be put into context.

All of these behavioural differences indicate that birds fed R were highly motivated to reach the wood shavings area in order to perform the food-searching (appetitive) component of foraging behaviour (pecking and scratching) even though they were never rewarded with food (allowed to progress to consummatory

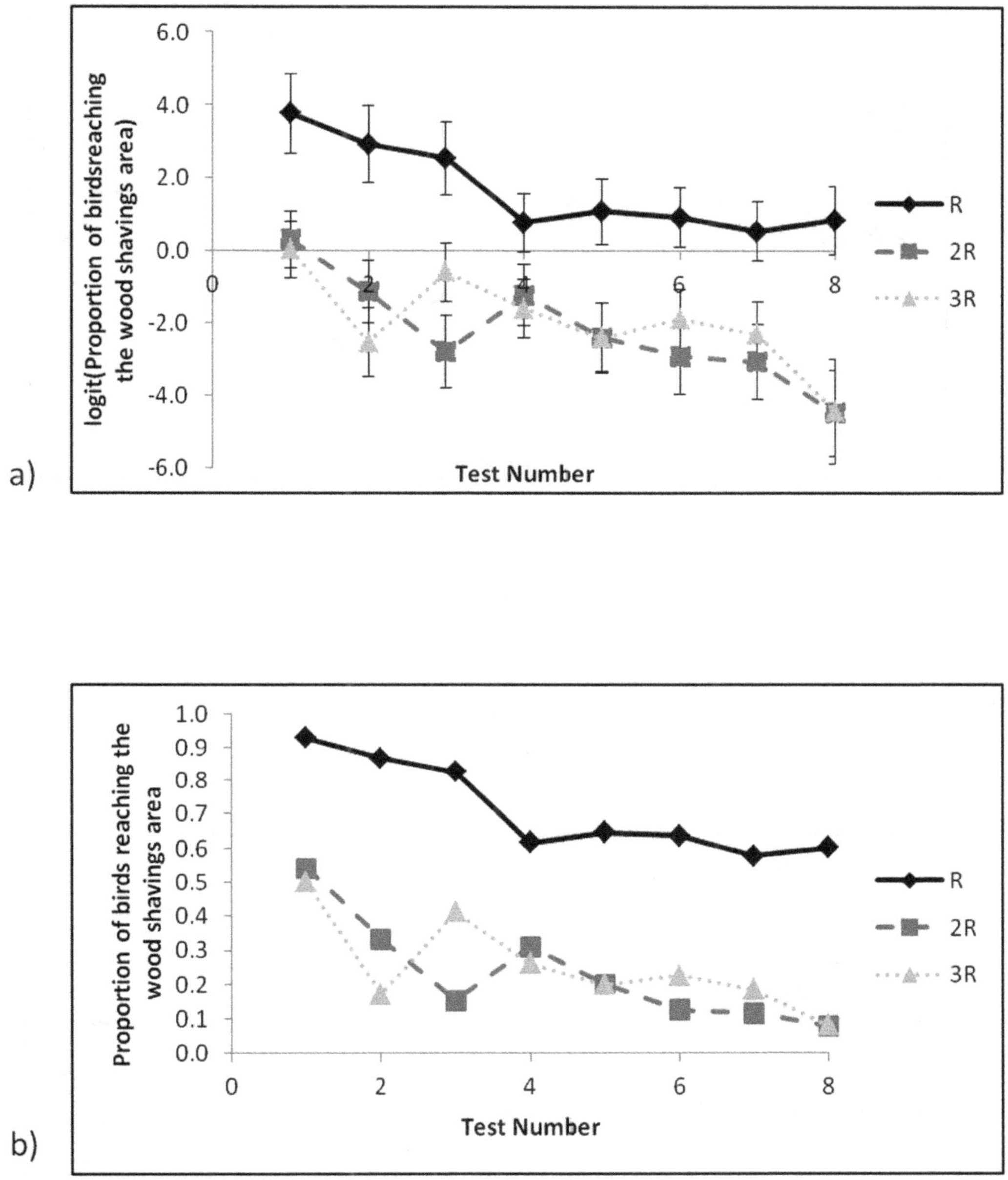

Figure 3. Proportion of birds reaching the wood shavings area across eight tests with increasing water runway length and depth for the three food treatments for a) means (±SE) estimated from GLMM on logit scale and b) back transformed to the proportion of birds reaching the wood shavings area.

behaviour). Repeatedly failing to reward foraging behaviour in this location with a food reward might have been expected to result in extinction of the response [37]. In fact, R birds continued to access the wood shavings area, and on average the performance of foraging behaviour by R (and 2R) birds initially increased over successive tests, before eventually declining. In our study, cost increased over successive tests, so it is not possible to know whether this eventual decline was a result of extinction learning (i.e. that there was never any food), or because of the increasing cost of access. Interpretation of the time spent foraging is made more difficult by the fact that fewer birds reached the wood shavings area in later tests. However, for R birds, there were consistently ~60–65% of them reaching the wood shavings area between tests 4 and 8, so the decline for these may indeed indicate extinction (although it was not statistically significant). In future studies, fewer tests could be used to reduce the possibility of extinction. There are different methods that can be used to present costs for access to a resource – we chose to progressively increase the cost over successive tests. However, costs can be presented, for example, in randomly determined orders or by progressively increasing then decreasing the cost of access. Different methods have their own advantages and disadvantages, for example, cost increases over time may become confounded with fatigue or boredom but random cost presentations may limit the Maximum Price that is tested, i.e. animals may be willing to work harder than the 'highest cost' given but additional 'harder' costs cannot be added to the end of the test [54]; how costs are presented to the animals should be carefully considered when designing a study to ensure questions of interest will be answered.

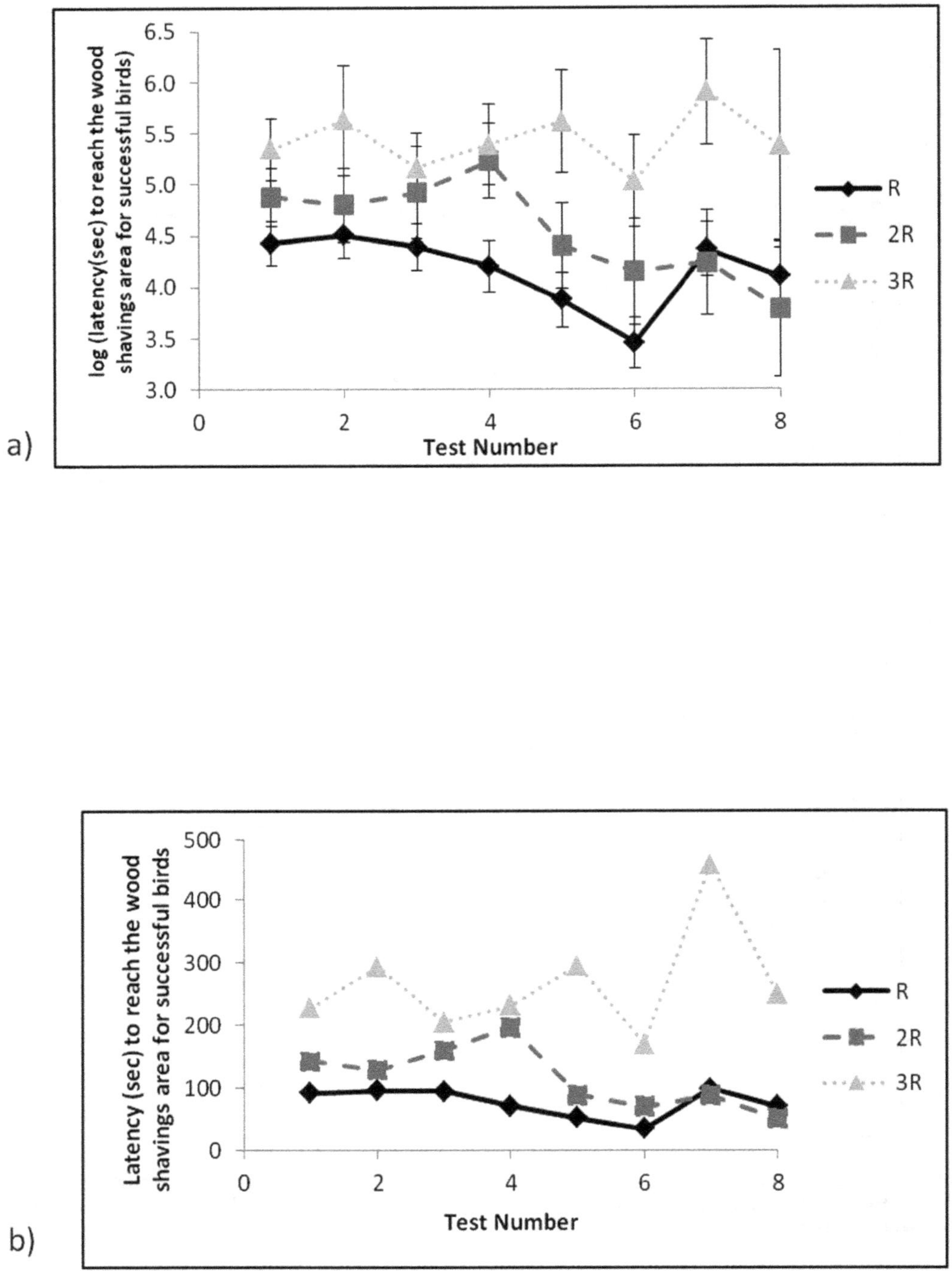

Figure 4. Latency to reach the wood shavings area for tests for which birds were successful across eight tests with increasing water runway length and depth for the three food treatments for a) means (±SE) estimated from LMM on log scale and b) back transformed to the latency to reach the wood shavings area.

Our use of a non-food rewarded task adds to the evidence that commercial restriction levels result in chronic hunger in broiler breeders. Existing data that these birds have high feeding motivation (e.g. [41]) is open to the criticism that offering extra food changes the situation, and increases food motivation. High levels of foraging motivation, even in the absence of food, suggest that food is not 'out of sight, out of mind' for broiler breeders at commercial levels of food restriction [17].

Broilers (offspring of broiler breeders) which are fed *ad libitum* throughout their lives may have gait and movement problems due to their fast growth rates [55,56]; however none of our broiler breeders exhibited any difficulties walking. This is most likely because all birds were reared on the recommended, restricted diets until 5 weeks of age, allowing for a slow, healthy growth until this point [21]. While birds fed 2R and 3R did grow faster than birds fed R, they were still more active than typical broilers in their home pens (L.M. Dixon, Pers. Obs.) throughout the trial which may also have helped prevent some fast growth related issues [55]. Therefore, the slower latencies for 2R and 3R birds to reach the wood shavings area cannot simply be due to difficulties walking in

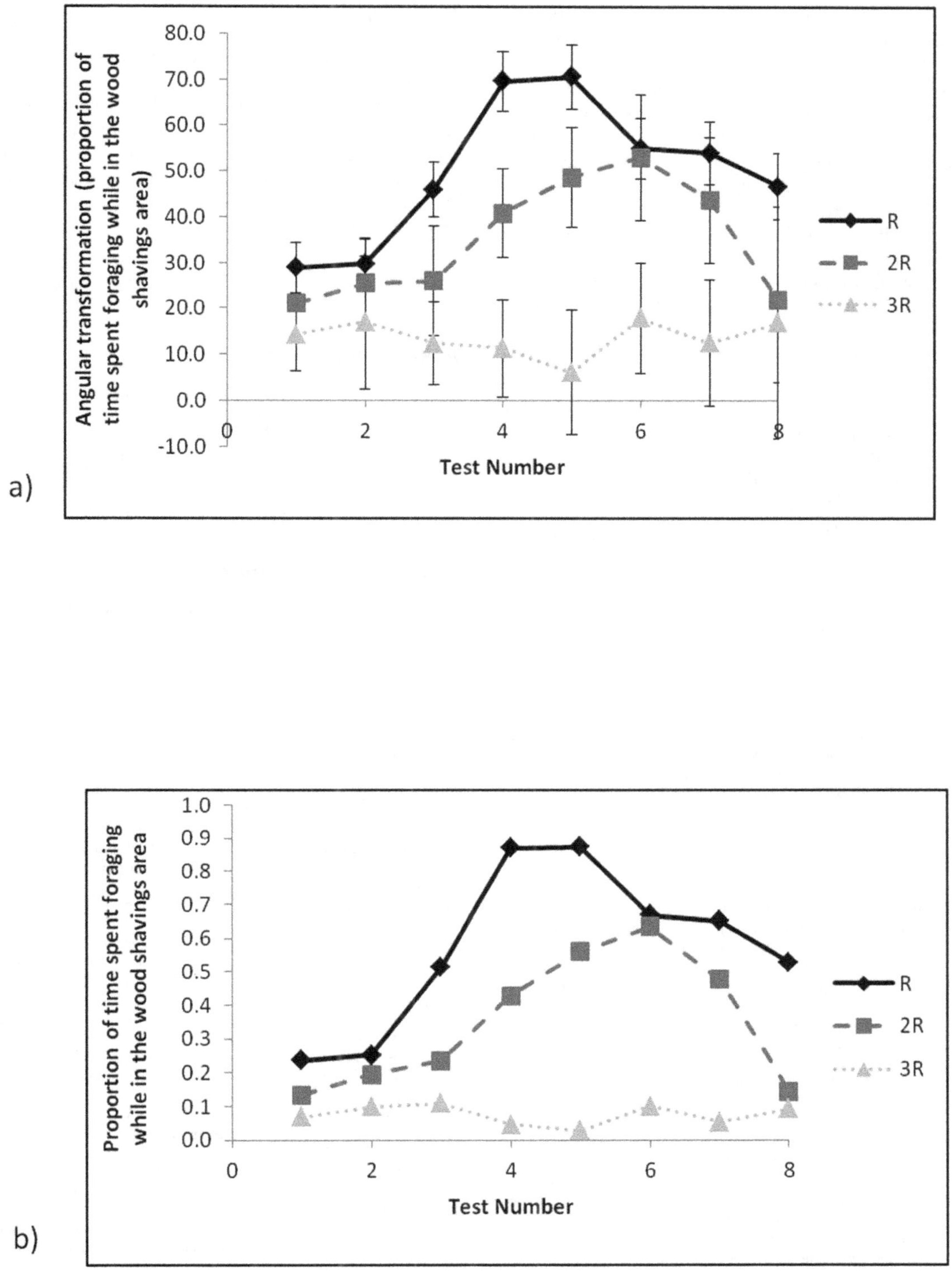

Figure 5. Proportion of time spent foraging while in the wood shavings area for tests for which birds were successful across eight tests with increasing water runway length and depth for the three food treatments for a) means (±SE) estimated from LMM on angular scale and b) back transformed to the proportion of time spent foraging while in the wood shavings area.

heavier birds. It is well established that broiler breeders which are restricted (R) are more active than those which are more generously fed [25–29]. Anecdotally, R birds in our study appeared more active in the apparatus, and it is possible that this explains some aspects of the behavioural differences between the treatments. However, the increased foraging behaviour, and tolerance of deeper water in R birds suggests that as well as being more active, they were also highly motivated to forage.

In future studies, we hope to apply the water runway method to novel diets designed to improve satiety. It will be interesting to compare this method to more conventional home pen behavioural measures, such as time spent resting, foraging and performing abnormal or stereotypic behaviour patterns [27,29]. Additionally comparing these results to tests in which food rewards are offered [29,30,31,32] may help to quantify the changes in motivation that occur due to feedback from the food and may help present a complete picture of hunger in broiler breeders. Various physiological measures of the welfare consequences of hunger have been proposed (e.g. [33]), although the question of validation and comparison between food types remain problematic (see discussion in [35]). Recent work to develop measures that relate directly to the neural circuits in the basal hypothalamus that control food intake [57] shows promise.

In the present study, we validated a test using a natural, variable cost to measure the motivation to perform appetitive behaviour by comparing different feed treatments. There are a number of practices in the broiler breeder industry that have been proposed as ways of reducing the hunger experienced due to restricted feeding. These include modifications of feeding methods; such as adding fibre to the diet [29,32], scatter feeding to increase feeding time and encourage foraging [58], feeding multiple small meals [58] and skip-a-day feeding [59]; and genetic changes, for example by using slow growing or dwarf strains [60,61], or by genetic selection to change the shape of the growth curve [62]. The foraging motivation test used here has potential to be applied alongside other behavioural and physiological measures to determine whether any of these practices result in reduced foraging motivation and thus in reduced hunger and improved welfare.

Conclusions

In conclusion, broiler breeders fed commercially restricted food allowances are more motivated to access an area of wood shavings where they can forage than birds fed twice or three times that amount. This indicates that these birds are hungry and as a result have decreased welfare. In future, the methods described here can be used to assess different broiler breeder practices and strains to attempt to decrease hunger and improve welfare in the broiler breeder industry.

Acknowledgments

SRUC and BioSS facilities and expertise have been developed through their role as Main Research Providers to the Rural and Environment Science and Analytical Services Division of the Scottish Government. Thanks to staff at the Avian Science Research Centre at SRUC Auchincruive for help with day to day care of the birds.

Author Contributions

Conceived and designed the experiments: LMD SB VS MB BJT RBD. Performed the experiments: LMD. Analyzed the data: SB. Wrote the paper: LMD SB RBD.

References

1. Dawkins MS (1990) From an animal's point of view: motivation, fitness and animal welfare. Behaviour and Brain Science 13: 1–61.
2. Duncan IJH (1996) Animal welfare defined in terms of feelings. Acta Agriculturae Scandinavica Section A-Animal Science S27: 29–35.
3. Duncan IJH (2005) Science-based assessment of animal welfare: farm animals. Revue Scientifique et Technique-Office International des Epizooties 24: 483–492.
4. Dawkins MS (2006) Through animal eyes: What behaviour tells us. Applied Animal Behaviour Science 100: 4–10. doi: 10.1016/j.applanim.2006.04.010.
5. Dawkins MS (2008) The science of animal suffering. Ethology 114: 937–945.
6. Mendl M, Burman OHP, Paul ES (2010) An integrative and functional framework for the study of animal emotion and mood. Proceedings of the Royal Society of London B: Biological Sciences 277: 2895–2904.
7. Duncan IJH (1992) Measuring preferences and the strength of preference. Poultry Science 71: 658–663.
8. Dawkins MS (1983) Battery hens name their price: Consumer demand theory and the measurement of ethological 'needs'. Animal Behaviour 31: 1195–1205. doi: 10.1016/S0003-3472(83)80026-8.
9. Mason GJ, Cooper JJ, Clarebourgh C (2001) Frustrations of fur-farmed mink. Nature 410: 35–36.
10. Seaman S, Waran NK, Mason GJ, D'Eath RB (2008) Animal economics: assessing the motivation of female laboratory rabbits to reach a platform, social contact or food. Animal Behaviour 75: 31–42.
11. Kirkden RD, Pajor EA (2006) Using preference, motivation and aversion tests to ask scientific questions about animals' feelings. Applied Animal Behaviour Science 100: 29–47. doi: 10.1016/j.applanim.2006.04.009.
12. Jensen MB, Pedersen LJ (2008) Using motivation tests to assess ethological needs and preferences. Applied Animal Behaviour Science 113: 340–356. doi: 10.1016/j.applanim.2008.02.001.
13. Fraser D, Matthews LR (1997) Preference and motivational testing. In: Appleby MC, Hughes BO, editors. Animal Welfare. Wallingford: CAB International. pp. 159–173.
14. Dixon LM, Sandilands V, Bateson M, Brocklehurst S, Tolkamp BJ, et al. (2013) Conditioned place preference or aversion as animal welfare assessment tools: Limitations in their application. Applied Animal Behaviour Science 148: 164–176.
15. Faure JM, Lagadic H (1994) Elasticity of demand for food and sand in laying hens subjected to variable wind speed. Applied Animal Behaviour Science 42: 49–59. doi: 10.1016/0168-1591(94)90006-X.
16. Olsson IAS, Keeling LJ (2002) The push-door for measuring motivation in hens: laying hens are motivated to perch at night. Animal Welfare 11: 11–19.
17. Warburton H, Mason G (2003) Is out of sight out of mind? The effects of resource cues on motivation in mink, *Mustela vison*. Animal Behaviour 65: 755–762.
18. Renema RA, Robinson FE (2004) Defining normal: comparison of feed restriction and full feeding of female broiler breeders. World's Poultry Science Journal 60: 508–522.
19. Savory CJ, Hocking PM, Mann JS, Maxwell MH (1996) Is broiler breeder welfare improved by using qualitative rather than quantitative food restriction ti limit growth rate? Animal Behaviour 5: 105–127.
20. de Jong IC, van Voorst S, Ehlhardt DA, Blokhuis HJ (2002) Effects of restricted feeding on physiological stress parameters in growing broiler breeders. British Poultry Science 43: 157–168.
21. Mench JA (2002) Broiler breeders: feed restriction and welfare. World's Poultry Science Association 58: 23–29.
22. D'Eath RB, Tolkamp BJ, Kyriazakis I, Lawrence AB (2009) "Freedom from hunger" and preventing obesity: the animal welfare implications of reducing food quantity or quality. Animal Behaviour 77: 275–288. doi: 10.1016/j.anbehav.2008.10.028.
23. Decuypere E, Bruggeman V, Everaert N, Li Y, Boonen R, et al. (2010) The Broiler Breeder Paradox: ethical, genetic and physiological perspectives, and suggestions for solutions. British Poultry Science 51: 569–579.
24. Dawkins MS (2004) Using behaviour to assess animal welfare. Animal Welfare 13: S3–7.
25. Hocking PM, Maxwell MH, Robertson GW, Mitchell MA (2001) Welfare assessment of modified rearing programmes for broiler breeders. British Poultry Science 42: 424–432.
26. Savory CJ, Seawright E, Watson A (1992) Stereotyped behavior in broiler breeders in relation to husbandry and opioid receptor blockade. Applied Animal Behaviour Science 32: 349–360.
27. Savory CJ, Maros K (1993) Influence of degree of food restriction, age and time of day on behavior of broiler breeder chickens. Behavioural Processes 29: 179–190.
28. Hocking PM, Maxwell MH, Mitchell MA (1996) Relationships between the degree of food restriction and welfare indices in broiler breeder females. British Poultry Science 37: 263–278.
29. Sandilands V, Tolkamp BJ, Kyriazakis I (2005) Behaviour of food restricted broilers during rearing and lay: effects of an alternative feeding method. Physiology and Behaviour 85: 115–123.
30. Savory CJ, Maros K, Rutter SM (1993) Assessment of hunger in growing broiler breeders in relation to a commercial restricted feeding programme. Animal Welfare 2: 131–152.
31. Savory CJ, Lariviere JM (2000) Effects of qualitative and quantitative food restriction treatments on feeding motivational state and general activity level of growing broiler breeders. Applied Animal Behaviour Science 69: 135–147.
32. Sandilands V, Tolkamp BJ, Savory CJ, Kyriazakis I (2006) Behaviour and welfare of broiler breeders fed qualitatively restricted diets during rearing: are there viable alternatives to quantitative restriction? Applied Animal Behaviour Science 96: 53–67.

33. de Jong IC, van Voorst S, Blokhuis HJ (2003) Parameters for quantification of hunger in broiler breeders. Physiology and Behaviour 78: 773–783.
34. de Jong IC, Enting H, van Voorst S, Ruesink EW, Blokhuis HJ (2005) Do low density diets improve broiler breeder welfare during rearing and laying? Poultry Science 84: 194–203.
35. D'Eath RB, Tolkamp BJ, Kyriazakis I, Lawrence AB (2009) Freedom from hunger and preventing obesity: the animal welfare implications of reducing food quantity or quality. Animal Behaviour 77: 275–288. doi: 10.1016/j.anbehav.2008.10.028.
36. Day JEL, Kyriazakis I, Lawrence AB (1996) The use of a second-order schedule to measure feeding motivation in the pig. Applied Animal Behaviour Science 50: 15–31.
37. Mills DS, Marchant-Forde JN, McGreevy PD, Morton DB, Nicol CJ, et al. (2010) Encyclopedia of Applied Animal Behaviour Wallingford: CAB International.
38. Berridge KC (2004) Motivation concepts in behavioral neuroscience. Physiology and Behaviour 81: 179–209.
39. Toates FM (1998) Motivation. In: Toates FM, editor. Control of Behaviour. Singapore: Springer-Verlag. pp. 15–45.
40. McFarland DJ (1974) Time sharing as a behavioural phenomenon. Advances in the Study of Behaviour 5: 201–225.
41. Savory CJ, Maros K, Rutter SM (1993) Assessment of hunger in growing broiler breeders in relation to a commercial restricted feeding programme. Animal Welfare 2: 131–152.
42. Savory CJ, Lariviere JM (2000) Effects of qualitative and quantitative food restriction treatments on feeding motivational state and general activity level of growing broiler breeders. Applied Animal Behaviour Science 69: 135–147.
43. Cooper JJ, Appleby MC (1995) Nesting behaviour of hens: Effects of experience on motivation. Applied Animal Behaviour Science 42: 283–295. doi: 10.1016/0168-1591(94)00543-N.
44. Verbeek E, Waas JR, McLeay L, Matthews LR (2011) Measurement of feeding motivation in sheep and the effects of food restriction. Applied Animal Behaviour Science 132: 121–130. doi: 10.1016/j.applanim.2011.03.014.
45. Cooper JJ, Appleby MC (1994) The use of aversive barriers to quantify nesting motivation in domestic hens. Proc Symp Modified Cages 11–24.
46. Weeks CA (2001) Development of a newmethod for quantitatively assessing lameness in broilers. British Poultry Science 42: S79–S80.
47. Weeks CA, Knowles TG, Gordon RG, Kerr AE, Peyton ST, et al. (2002) New method for objectively assessing lameness in broiler chickens. Veterinary Record 151: 762–764.
48. Aviagen (2013) Ross 308 Parentstock Management Handbook 2013. Available: http://en.aviagen.com/assets/Tech_Center/Ross_PS/Ross_PS_Handbook_2013_i-r1.pdf. Accessed 2014 Jul 8.
49. DEFRA (2006) The structure of the United Kingdom poultry industry: Commercial Poultry Sector. Available: http://labourproviders.org.uk/wp-content/uploads/2012/11/Poultry_sector.pdf. Accessed 2014 Jul 8.
50. Buckley LA, Sandilands V, Tolkamp BJ, D'Eath RB (2011) Quantifying hungry broiler breeder dietary preferences using a closed economy T-maze task. Applied Animal Behaviour Science 133: 216–227. doi: 10.1016/j.applanim.2011.06.003.
51. Collett D (1999) Modelling Binary Data. London: Chapman & Hall.
52. Brown H, Prescott R (1999) Applied Mixed Models in Medicine. New York: J. Wiley & Sons.
53. Matthews LR, Ladewig J (1994) Environmental requirements of pigs measured by behavioural demand functions. Animal Behaviour 47: 713–719.
54. Asher L, Kirkden RD, Bateson M (2009) An empirical investigation of two assumptions of motivation testing in captive starlings (Sturnus vulgaris): Do animals have an energy budget to 'spend'? and does cost reduce demand? Applied Animal Behaviour Science 118: 152–160. doi: 10.1016/j.applanim.2009.02.029.
55. Bessei W (2006) Welfare of broilers: a review. World's Poultry Science Journal 62: 455–466.
56. Kestin SC, Knowles TG, Tinch AE, Gregory NG (1992) Prevalence of leg weakness in broiler chickens and its relationship with genotype. Veterinary Record 131: 190–194.
57. Dunn IC, Wilson PW, Smulders TV, Sandilands V, D'Eath RB, et al. (2013) Hypothalamic agouti-related protein expression is affected by both acute and chronic experience of food restriction and re-feeding in chickens. Journal of Neuroendocrinology 25: 920–928.
58. de Jong IC, Fillerup M, Blokhuis HJ (2005) Effect of scattered feeding and feeding twice a day during rearing on indicators of hunger and frustration in broiler breeders. Applied Animal Behaviour Science 92: 61–76.
59. Mench JA (1991) Research note: Feed restriction in broiler breeders causes a persistent elevation in corticosterone secretion that is modulated by dietary tryptophan. Poultry Science 70: 2547–2550.
60. Proudfoot FG, Hulan HA, McRae KB (1984) Effects of photoperiod, light intensity and feed restriction on the performance of dwarf and normal poultry meat genotypes. Canadian Journal of Animal Science 64: 759–768.
61. Jones EKM, Zaczek V, MacLeod M, Hocking PM (2004) Genotype, dietary manipulation and food allocation affect indices of welfare in broiler breeders. British Poultry Science 45: 725–737.
62. Dawkins MS, Layton R (2012) Breeding for better welfare: genetic goals for broiler chickens and their parents. Animal Welfare 21: 147–155.

2

Impact of Chronic Neonicotinoid Exposure on Honeybee Colony Performance and Queen Supersedure

Christoph Sandrock[1]*, Matteo Tanadini[2], Lorenzo G. Tanadini[3], Aline Fauser-Misslin[1,4], Simon G. Potts[5], Peter Neumann[1,4]

1 Agroscope, Swiss Bee Research Centre, Berne, Switzerland, **2** Seminar for Statistics, ETH Zurich, Zurich, Switzerland, **3** Division of Biostatistics, Institute for Social and Preventive Medicine, University of Zurich, Zurich, Switzerland, **4** Institute of Bee Health, Vetsuisse Faculty, University of Berne, Berne, Switzerland, **5** School of Agriculture, Policy and Development, University of Reading, Reading, United Kingdom

Abstract

Background: Honeybees provide economically and ecologically vital pollination services to crops and wild plants. During the last decade elevated colony losses have been documented in Europe and North America. Despite growing consensus on the involvement of multiple causal factors, the underlying interactions impacting on honeybee health and colony failure are not fully resolved. Parasites and pathogens are among the main candidates, but sublethal exposure to widespread agricultural pesticides may also affect bees.

Methodology/Principal Findings: To investigate effects of sublethal dietary neonicotinoid exposure on honeybee colony performance, a fully crossed experimental design was implemented using 24 colonies, including sister-queens from two different strains, and experimental in-hive pollen feeding with or without environmentally relevant concentrations of thiamethoxam and clothianidin. Honeybee colonies chronically exposed to both neonicotinoids over two brood cycles exhibited decreased performance in the short-term resulting in declining numbers of adult bees (−28%) and brood (−13%), as well as a reduction in honey production (−29%) and pollen collections (−19%), but colonies recovered in the medium-term and overwintered successfully. However, significantly decelerated growth of neonicotinoid-exposed colonies during the following spring was associated with queen failure, revealing previously undocumented long-term impacts of neonicotinoids: queen supersedure was observed for 60% of the neonicotinoid-exposed colonies within a one year period, but not for control colonies. Linked to this, neonicotinoid exposure was significantly associated with a reduced propensity to swarm during the next spring. Both short-term and long-term effects of neonicotinoids on colony performance were significantly influenced by the honeybees' genetic background.

Conclusions/Significance: Sublethal neonicotinoid exposure did not provoke increased winter losses. Yet, significant detrimental short and long-term impacts on colony performance and queen fate suggest that neonicotinoids may contribute to colony weakening in a complex manner. Further, we highlight the importance of the genetic basis of neonicotinoid susceptibility in honeybees which can vary substantially.

Editor: Nicolas Desneux, French National Institute for Agricultural Research (INRA), France

Funding: This research received funding from the European Union Framework 7 under grant agreement no. 244090 (CP-FP) STEP (Status and Trends in European Pollinators, www.STEP-project.net). The funders had no role in study design, data collection and analysis, decision to publish, or preparation of the manuscript.

Competing Interests: The authors have declared that no competing interests exist.

* Email: ch.sandrock@gmail.com

Introduction

Ecosystem services provided by pollinating insects are vital for the maintenance of biodiversity [1,2] and food security through agricultural productivity [3,4,5,6]. Recent evidence for globally paralleling declines of various pollinators [7,8,9,10], however, stands in contrast to prospects of continuously increasing demands for pollination services [4,11,12].

The Western honeybee, *Apis mellifera*, is the predominant managed pollinator worldwide [4,8]. Although global stocks of domestic honeybees have increased during the last half century (except in Europe [13] and in the USA [14]), present and predicted agricultural demands for insect pollination far exceed currently available capacities [15]. Repeated, massive declines of managed honeybee colonies during the last decade in North America, Europe and the middle East [8,16,17,18,19,20,21,22] raised substantial concerns about safeguarding future honeybee pollination services. Despite comprehensive recent research, conclusive evidence for common causal drivers is lacking, which points at multiple interacting factors [8,23,24]. The invasive ectoparasitic mite *Varroa destructor* represents a severe problem for honeybees almost worldwide [25,26,27], in particular due to its vital role as a virus vector [28,29]. Some observations of elevated colony losses were also influenced by the widespread gut parasites *Nosema ceranae* [30,31,32]. Microbes and *V. destructor*-associated viruses are prevalent almost globally and commonly co-occurring, yet there is no uniform evidence so far that even the interactions between some of these pathogenic stressors necessarily result in colony failure [33,34,35,36]. Instead, it appears as if more complex interactions with additional environmental stressors and at multiple levels are of key importance [8,24]. Likely candidates, commonly encountered by honeybees, are routinely applied agricultural pesticides [37,38]. For instance, the use of systemic neonicotinoid insecticides has strongly increased on a global scale during the last decade [39,40,41,42]. Mainly acting as specific agonists of the insect acetylcholine receptors, neonicotinoids disrupt neuromuscular signalling pathways and are thus efficiently used for controlling insect pests [39,43]. Systemic compounds like neonicotinoids can be particularly problematic for pollinating insects through exposure to residues in nectar and pollen of treated crops [41,44,45]. Although field-realistic neonicotinoid residue levels in pollen and nectar are generally assumed to result in sublethal dietary exposure [46], sublethal effects on honeybees include various negative impacts, such as impairment of physiology, cognitive abilities like memory and learning, and foraging and homing behaviour [45,47,48,49,50,51,52,53,54,55,56,57,58,59]. In addition, combined exposure to multiple pesticides can have additive or synergistic adverse effects in bees [60,61,62,63] with eventually underestimated consequences [64]. Similarly, multifactorial impact arising through combined chronic exposure to pathogens and pesticides may trigger detrimental feedbacks of supposedly sublethal individual stressors at the colony level that could explain otherwise enigmatic negative impacts [65]. In this regard, an important but yet poorly understood aspect represents the adverse influence of neonicotinoids on the honeybee's immune system [66,67]. There is growing evidence for detrimental interactions and compromised immunity in honeybees upon combined exposure to neonicotinoids and pathogens, including the prevalent gut-parasite *Nosema* spp. [36,68,69,70,71] and near-ubiquitous viruses, such as the typically *V. destructor*-associated deformed wing virus [72] or the black queen cell virus [36]. To date it remains unclear to what extent these findings can be extrapolated to field settings where, for example, immunity-related patterns in honeybees may be strongly influenced by many more environmental factors, such as the overall nutritional status [24,73,74,75,76]. While several unplanned field exposures resulted in massive effects of neonicotinoids under certain circumstances [41,77,78], there is no compelling evidence so far that field-realistic neonicotinoid exposure resulting from standard agronomic implementations of neonicotinoids pose a serious threat to whole colonies [79,80,81,82,83]. Nevertheless, some regulatory bodies reacted recently [84,85] in order to clarify whether the overall contrasting results may have been influenced by: overestimating individual predictors while dynamics at multiple levels were neglected [65]; by the lack of statistical power for individual studies [44]; or by the possibility that especially sensitive endpoints have simply been missed. For instance, the long-term impacts of neonicotinoids, which might only become evident during sensitive phases like overwintering, have received little attention to date. Moreover, information on how neonicotinoids could impact on queens is virtually lacking [64]. It is unknown whether queens are relatively protected from agricultural pesticides through receiving processed food from hive bees only, or whether trophallactic interactions with the usually most long-lived honeybee in a hive could indeed represent a sink for trace residues of such systemic compounds. Sublethal pesticide exposure could have important consequences for colony fate through compromising the queen's cognitive abilities or immune system and thereby reducing her performance. For instance, it is known that replacement of failing queens by the worker bees, i.e. queen supersedure, can be triggered by reduced oviposition of old or insufficiently mated queens [86,87]. Colony fitness is another sensitive but largely neglected aspect of honeybee colony performance. In bumblebees, for example, it has repeatedly been shown that the negative impact of chronic neonicotinoid exposure on individuals and colony performance was less pronounced compared to queen production [88,89,90]. Similarly alarming fitness effects upon chronic sublethal neonicotinoid exposure are indicated in solitary bees [91]. Reproductive success, however, is vital for inferring long-term population level consequences. Compared to the assessment of much more general traits of colony performance and productivity in honeybees, the quantification of fitness in the true sense is very difficult because of the complex socio-biology of reproduction in honeybees. In managed honeybee colonies, besides male mating success, swarming can be considered as a tangible proxy of fitness [92], which is in practice primarily linked to beekeeping management decisions though.

Here we experimentally assessed the effects of chronic dietary neonicotinoid exposure on honeybee colony performance and fitness on a temporal scale and in relation to the honeybees' genetic background. In a fully crossed experimental design 24 freely flying honeybee colonies, including two groups of sister-queens from different strains (14 and 10 colonies, respectively), were placed at a single apiary and were either exposed to control pollen or pollen that has been spiked with a combination of the two neonicotinoids thiamethoxam and clothianidin (on average 5.31 μg/kg and 2.05 μg/kg, respectively) via in-hive feeding over two brood cycles (see Figure S1). All colonies were then identically maintained and controlled against *V. destructor* throughout a one year monitoring period. During the study four detailed colony assessments, including estimates of numbers of adult bees and the amounts of brood and stores, were conducted to evaluate potential effects on colony performance and productivity in the short- (1.5 months), medium- (3.5 months) and long-term (1 year). We used this experimental design in order to contribute to better understand three currently poorly resolved aspects. First, while the majority of experiments at the colony level applied sublethal chronic neonicotinoid exposure through sucrose solution, we hypothesized that neonicotinoid-contaminated pollen provides stronger exposure of larval stages and nurse bees that may express sublethal effects when performing more complex tasks in later life cycle stages [53,93], thereby potentially resulting in delayed effects on colony performance. Second, contaminated pollen could result in sublethal exposure of honeybee queens that may affect their performance and subsequently cause failure. Therefore, we assessed the fate of queens one year subsequent to experimental feeding of neonicotinoid-spiked pollen, as well as the colonies' propensity to swarm as an indicator for colony fitness. Third, we addressed the question of whether neonicotinoid susceptibility at the honeybee colony level has a genetic basis.

Materials and Methods

Experimental setup and colony maintenance

Twenty-four honeybee colonies were established using artificial swarms (1.5 kg of bees) in summer 2010. Two groups of sister-queens originating from different, locally adapted breeding populations were introduced in order to control for the honeybees' genetic background and maternal effects: one group of 14 queens from a region in eastern Germany that is characterized by intense agriculture, and one group of 10 queens from an alpine region in central Switzerland. All queens were freely mated at apiaries in corresponding geographic regions during early summer 2010 and then individually tagged and clipped one forewing. The former group of colonies represented *A. m. carnica*, whereas the latter represented predominantly *A. m. mellifera*, and in the following they are referred to as strain A and B, respectively.

As permitted by the veterinary agency of the canton Zurich, we established an apiary on the land of the research station Agroscope Reckenholz-Tänniken in a rural area near the city of Zurich, Switzerland (47°25′38N 8°31′11E). Two groups of each 12 hives were placed in a single row, with all hive-entrances pointing in the same direction. To meet a fully-crossed experimental design, artificial swarms containing queens of the different strains were randomly allocated to the two experimental groups (N = 7 from strain A and N = 5 from strain B each). Hives containing queens of the two different strains A and B were ordered identically in each experimental group (see Figure S1 for details of the setup). Hives within groups were separated by 1 m, and both groups of hives were separated by approximately 20 m distance, including shrubs as landmarks to minimise forager drift between groups [94]. All colonies were equipped with brand new hive material, including polystyrene hive bodies, wooden frames (200×350 mm in size) and organically certified, pesticide-free wax foundations. Commercial pollen traps (Wienold, Lauterbach, Germany), painted in different colours, were installed at all hive entrances (identical colour sequence in each group), but only activated during the exposure phase (see below). All colonies were identically treated against *V. destructor* using oxalic acid (40 ml sucrose solution containing 3.5% w/w oxalic acid per colony) five days after establishment of artificial swarms (in the absence of capped brood), and fed with commercial sugar syrup (sugar beet based, 73% sugar content, containing equal proportions of glucose, fructose and sucrose; Hostettler's, Zurich, Switzerland) during summer 2010 to promote colony growth. Pollen was assumed to be available in sufficient quantities. All colonies overwintered on eleven combs, and oxalic acid treatment against *V. destructor* was repeated in December 2010.

During spring and summer 2011 colonies were not fed but left to freely collect nectar and pollen. All colonies were simultaneously provided with a second and third hive body containing 11 frames with wax-foundations for comb building in early April 2011 and in mid-May 2011, respectively. The upper hive body provided last was separated by a queen excluder to ensure honey storage only, and on the same day it was provided the experimental treatment was initiated and lasted until end of June 2011 (see below). In mid-July 2011 colonies were taken off their honey combs and subsequently maintained on 22 combs. They received 12.5 kg of sugar syrup during late July and late August 2011 (25 kg in total). After each feeding phase, colonies were simultaneously treated against *V. destructor* using 130 ml of formic acid (70% w/w) evaporating from commercial dispensers (Andermatt Biocontrol AG, Grossdietwil, Switzerland) for about one week each during early August and early September 2011. Colonies were then overwintered and treated with oxalic acid in December 2011 (see above). At no point during the study synthetic acaricides were used for varroa mite management. Subsequent to overwintering colonies were monitored until June 2012 without further intervention. No honey supers were provided in 2012 in order to increase the propensity for swarming, which served as a proxy of fitness one year after the treatment (see below).

Treatment procedures and residue analyses

In mid-May 2011 pollen traps were activated to vastly prevent pollen inflow, and in-hive pollen feeding was initiated. Pollen patties consisted of 55% honeybee pollen (common stock of commercial pollen with mixed floral content of at least 19 plants; Sonnentracht Imkerei, Bremen, Germany), 5% brewer's yeast and approximately 40% sucrose (two thirds 73% sugar syrup and one third powder sugar). Three times per week (each Monday, Wednesday and Friday) all colonies were provided with two 200 g pollen patties loosely packed in cellophane paper and placed between the two lower hive bodies (i.e. within the brood nest). Disturbance of the colonies was thus reduced to a minimum. The bees easily corroded the cellophane paper to access the content. Two pollen patties of 200 g were generally consumed completely within 48 hours by each colony. Prior to feeding, pollen was gamma ray irradiated (Leoni Studer Hard AG, Däniken, Switzerland) to prevent putative pathogen spill over (e.g., see [95]). One group of 12 colonies (see above) received plain pollen while the other received patties containing environmentally relevant residues of the two neonicotinoids thiamethoxam and clothianidin (see below). Chronic neonicotinoid exposure through in-hive pollen feeding was performed for 46 days (1.5 months) in order to cover two brood cycles, thereby resulting in total provisions of 8 kg of pollen patties per colony. Pollen traps were then deactivated to no longer prevent colonies from storing pollen collected outside.

For both neonicotinoids pure analytical standards (PESTANAL, Fluka; with purities of 99.7 and 99.9% for thiamethoxam and clothianidin, respectively) were purchased (Sigma-Aldrich, Seelze, Germany), dissolved in distilled water (1 mg/L) and then stored at room temperature and protected from light. Aliquots of a single stock solution for each parent compound were added to the sucrose solution, which was then thoroughly mixed into the pollen and yeast. A commercial kneader was used to produce a homogenous paste to be portioned in cellophane paper (200 g) and kept frozen until usage. In total, 20 mixtures of plain and neonicotinoid-spiked pollen were prepared and fed batch-wise over time. A subsample of each of these batches of pollen patty preparations was subjected to residue analyses performed by the United States Department of Agriculture, Agricultural Marketing Service, Science and Technology Laboratory Approval and Testing Division of the National Science Laboratories in Gastonia, North Carolina. All samples were extracted for analysis of agrochemicals using a refined methodology for the determination of pesticides using an approach of the official pesticide extraction method (AOAC OMA 2007.01) using an acetonitrile:water solution and analysed by liquid chromatography coupled with tandem mass spectrometry detection (LC/MS-MS) utilising the parent and confirmatory ions of thiamethoxam and clothianidin. Samples were analysed using certified standard reference materials for the presence of both compounds with a limit of detection of 4.0 ppb for thiamethoxam and 1.0 ppb for clothianidin. Our target concentrations were 5.0 and 2.0 ppb for thiamethoxam and clothianidin, respectively. Since clothianidin is the major metabolite of thiamethoxam [96,97], both bioactive compounds will co-occur in the pollen and nectar of thiamethoxam-treated crops and were therefore applied in combination. The concentrations used here match field-realistic levels of both compounds previously found in pollen of treated crops [41,42,46,80,82,98]. In order to confirm the absence of unexpected additional exposure, we also subjected six random samples of the sugar syrup used for late season feeding (2010 and 2011), six samples of the original pollen stock, as well as four pollen patty samples of the control group to residue analyses. Moreover, pollen trap contents collected during the experimental feeding were pooled across colonies of each experimental group and samples from five collection dates throughout the treatment were taken for residue analyses. Additional matrix endpoints at the end of the experimental pollen feeding phase for both treatment groups were forager bees (1 sample pooled across all colonies) and pupae close to adult emergence (3 samples pooled across 4 colonies each). Furthermore, in both treatments we sampled wax (2 samples pooled across 6 colonies each) and bee bread (4 samples pooled across 3 colonies each) 3 weeks after the pollen treatment when honey supers were removed, as well as one sample of honey from each colony of the neonicotinoid-exposed group (pooled from at least 3 different combs). All samples for residue analyses were stored frozen and shipped on dry ice.

Population estimates and data collection

Estimates of colony strength were performed using the 'Liebefelder Method' [99,100]. Specifically, we visually estimated the number of adult bees, the amount of capped brood (pupae) and un-capped brood (eggs and larvae), and the amount of honey and pollen stores in dm^2. Colony assessments were consistently performed by the same person and alternated between treatment groups during the day. During each colony assessment the presence of the original queen was checked. Successful queen replacement was counted as the presence of a non-tagged, egg-laying queen which possessed two intact forewings, either in the presence or absence of the originally tagged mother-queen. Based on 1 dm^2 comb containing 400 cells on average, the estimated proportion of comb area comprising of brood was converted into numbers of individuals in order to treat corresponding response variables as counts, whereas estimates of honey stores were converted into total weight (based on an average weight of 2 kg for fully filled honey combs of the used frame format).

In spring 2011 (mid-May) the first colony assessment was performed and three days later the experimental treatment was initiated. During the pollen feeding phase, contents of all pollen traps were collected and weighed each time when new pollen patties were provided, resulting in 20 pollen collection records per colony in total. In summer 2011 (beginning of July), two days after the last pollen patties were fed, the second colony assessment was conducted to evaluate short-term effects on colony performance. After the exposure phase the control and the neonicotinoid-treated colonies were maintained identically and the third colony assessment was performed 3.5 months after the exposure in autumn 2011 (mid-October), to evaluate medium-term effects colony performance before overwintering. Overwintering success was assessed end of March 2012 and thereafter surviving colonies were inspected on a weekly basis. Finally, the fourth colony assessment for all colonies that survived winter was performed one year after the treatment in spring 2012 (late April) to evaluate long-term effects on colony growth. Afterwards colonies were maintained until June 2012 and inspected for queen cells on a weekly basis and for swarming events at least every second day. Since original queens had one clipped forewing, swarms remained nearby the hive and could thus be easily recognized.

Statistical analyses

To investigate the effects of exposure to thiamethoxam and clothianidin on honeybee colony performance over time, we analyzed a set of sensitive endpoints within the framework of mixed models.

Model formulation and selection. The response variables (endpoints) were numbers of adult honeybees, pupae and eggs and larvae. These were modelled including the explanatory variables (factors) treatment (control and neonicotinoids), honeybee strain (A and B), and assessment date (spring 2011, summer 2011, autumn 2011 and spring 2012) as fixed effects, and colony as a random effect. Residual analysis of all response variables indicated the need for variance stabilization and variables were transformed accordingly. The data for the endpoints number of adult honeybees and pupae were square-root transformed. Residuals for eggs and larvae displayed a more complex pattern of a bow-shaped variance being largest for medium fitted values (~8000) and decreasing for larger and smaller fitted values. This pattern resembles that of a binomially distributed variable, which conforms well to the upper bounded egg-laying rate of a honeybee queen. In such cases effective counts of a given response variable can be divided by the expected maximum number to obtain binomially distributed variables. Based on Khoury *et al.* [101], we set the limit to a daily egg-laying rate of 2000 and, according to the honeybee life-cycle, 16000 eggs and larvae present at any time. Ratios of actually present and maximum possible numbers of eggs and larvae were arcsine square-root transformed to stabilize variances for further analyses, as commonly performed for binomially distributed variables.

Numbers of adult honeybees exhibited an increased variance at the fourth assessment date in spring 2012, which prompted us to use a weighted linear mixed model for this response variable. Weights were set as the inverse of the residual variances of the two groups (for the assessments between spring and autumn 2011 and the assessment in spring 2012, respectively).

For each endpoint, complete models were fitted based on the threefold interaction term of the explanatory variables (fixed effects) plus the random effect. Model simplification was evaluated by hierarchically removing interaction terms based on likelihood ratio tests. The goodness of corresponding Chi-squared approximations was confirmed by model based parametric bootstrapping. During all steps of the model selection, model assumptions and serial correlations of the residuals of colonies were inspected.

Hypotheses testing with contrasts. To test for effects of neonicotinoid exposure on colony performance and the influence of the honeybees' genetic background on responses to the neonicotinoid-treatment, one-sided contrasts and corresponding *P*-values (adjusted for multiple testing) were computed for the overall treatment effect at each individual assessment date and, when the threefold interaction significantly contributed to model a given response, also for treatment nested within honeybee strain. Since seasonal effects were expected, contrasts including assessment date were not performed.

Further statistical analyses. To investigate effects of chronic exposure to thiamethoxam and clothianidin on honey production, the difference of the log transformed total weights before and after the experimental pollen feeding was analysed using linear regression. The full model was fitted with neonicotinoid exposure and honeybee strain as fixed factors and the interaction between them. In the same way we compared comb areas in dm^2 comprising of pollen stores (bee bread) in the hives before and after the experimental pollen feeding in order to evaluate pollen consumptions during the treatment.

The time series of twenty pollen collections per colony sampled during the 1.5 months of experimental in-hive pollen feeding were converted into respective Areas Under the Curve (AUC) for further analysis. The AUC represents the overall colony-specific pollen foraging activity, with higher AUC values corresponding to higher collection performances. We analyzed AUC with a one-sided Mann-Whitney test for a difference between neonicotinoid-exposed and control colonies.

Supersedure of original queens (at any time) and swarming events in spring 2012 yield a yes/no value for each colony. The associations of these variables with neonicotinoid treatment were investigated using Fisher's exact tests for contingency tables of small sample sizes.

All statistical analysis were performed using R [102]. Mixed models were fitted using the lmer function of the *lme4* package [103], and contrasts were performed using the glht function of the *multcomp* package [104].

Results

Residue analyses

Original stocks of honeybee pollen and sugar syrup used to prepare pollen patties in our experiment did not contain traceable amounts of the two neonicotinoids thiamethoxam and clothianidin, even when the limit of detection was reduced to 0.1 ppb for both compounds. Thus, thiamethoxam and clothianidin are considered being absent in the pollen patties fed to the control colonies. In contrast, in all samples from the pollen patties that have been spiked with the two neonicotinoids both parent compounds were detected in the range of the target concentrations: The effective mean concentrations (± SD across different pollen patty batches) used during the neonicotinoid treatment were determined to be 5.31±0.75 ppb for thiamethoxam and 2.05±1.18 ppb for clothianidin. The residue analyses document constant chronic exposure to thiamethoxam and clothianidin at field-realistic levels in pollen over a period of two honeybee brood cycles. There was no unexpected additional exposure to thiamethoxam or clothianidin from the outside, as indicated by the lack of traceable residues of both compounds in the pollen collected from pollen traps of both treatment groups during the in-hive pollen feeding phase. In none of the forager bee and pupae samples collected directly after the treatment and in none of the hive samples collected 3 weeks after the treatment (i.e. bee bread, honey and wax) residues of either compound above respective limits of detection could be found in both the control and neonicotinoid treatment. The absence of residues in bees is not surprising given the low concentrations used here, yet the absence of in-hive residues 3 weeks after feeding contaminated pollen over two brood cycles indicates that low level residues may quickly disappear in the hive matrix (see also [80,82]) through consumption, dilution or degradation.

Colony growth

In the control group and in the group exposed to thiamethoxam and clothianidin each 1 colony of strain A lost their queen after the pollen feeding phase during the formic acid treatment against varroa mites in 2011. Moreover, in each experimental group 1 colony became queenless during winter (originating from strain B and A in the control and in the neonicotinoid-exposed group, respectively). Thus, mixed model analyses are based on 12 colonies per experimental group for the first and the second colony assessment (in both treatment groups 7 colonies originating from strain A and 5 from strain B), while 11 colonies per group were available for the third colony assessment (in both treatment groups 6 colonies originating from strain A and 5 from strain B), and 10 colonies were available for the fourth colony assessment (in the control 6 and 4 from strain A and B, respectively, and for the neonicotinoid treatment each 5 from strain A and B). Queenless colonies were removed immediately after queen loss was recognised.

The data for the three endpoints adult bees, pupae and eggs and larvae across assessment dates are summarized in Fig. 1A–C. Dynamics of colony strength and brood curves displayed the expected general pattern of seasonal variation. However, we detected strong effects of neonicotinoid exposure, as well as interactions of the honeybees' genetic background with neonicotinoid exposure. The number of adult bees and the number of eggs and larvae were each best explained by the threefold interaction term model, i.e. neonicotinoid exposure, honeybee strain and assessment date, while for the number of pupae the retained model included the twofold interactions of assessment date with honeybee strain and neonicotinoid exposure, respectively, but no threefold interaction. Model-based estimates of contrasts and corresponding significance levels are summarized in Table 1. After 1.5 months of experimental pollen feeding, there was a significantly negative influence of the exposure to thiamethoxam and clothianidin on the number of adult bees for both honeybee strains, whereas this effect was much stronger for honeybee strain B than for strain A (Fig. 1A). Overall, average worker populations were 28% smaller in the neonicotinoid treatment compared to the control. There was also a significant overall decrease of the number of eggs and larvae in the neonicotinoid treatment, yet, this effect was not significant when tested within either honeybee strain A or B (Fig. 1B). However, there was no significant effect of nenicotinoid treatment or honeybee strain on the amount of pupae after the experimental pollen feeding (Fig. 1C). Compared to the control, the average amount of total brood had declined by 13% in the colonies exposed to thiamethoxam and clothianidin. No effects of the previous neonicotinoid exposure on the amount of adult honeybees or honeybee brood were detected 3.5 months after the experimental pollen feeding (Fig. 1A–C). Interestingly though, one year after the experimental pollen feeding, the negative impact of the previous neonicotinoid treatment on the number of adult bees was even stronger than directly after exposure to thiamethoxam and clothianidin (Fig. 1A). These effects were significant within honeybee strains A and B, but again much more pronounced in strain B. Similarly, when the overall significant decrease of the amount of eggs and larvae one year after the neonicotinoid treatment was tested within strains, a significant effect was only detected for honeybee strain B (Fig. 1B). Moreover, contrasting to the finding directly after exposure to thiamethoxam and clothianidin, there was also a significantly detrimental effect of the neonicotinoid treatment in the previous year on the amount of pupae (independent of honeybee strain), see Fig. 1C and Table 1.

Honey production

At treatment initiation all colonies already harboured considerable honey stores due to comparatively early spring flowering in 2011. Strain A and B, respectively, had on average 24.8±2.9 and 27.0±2.9 kg in the control group, and 25.4±2.8 and 23.6±0.7 kg in the group subsequently exposed to thiamethoxam and clothianidin. During the experimental pollen feeding, honey stores in the control group increased by 7.7±4.4 kg per colony on average (10.3±3.6 and 4.1±2.2 kg for colonies of strain A and B, respectively). During the same period honey stores in the neonicotinoid-exposed group also slightly increased for colonies of strain A (1.8±2.1 kg on average), but decreased for neonicotinoid-exposed colonies of strain B (−4.9±1.0 kg on average), resulting in an overall decrease of −1.0±3.8 kg per colony on average. Honey production during the treatment was significantly influenced by both neonicotinoid exposure and honeybee strain: While strain B was significantly less productive than strain A independent of the treatment ($F_{1,21} = 40.40$, $P<0.001$), neonicotinoid exposure negatively affected honey production in both strains ($F_{1,21} = 68.18$, $P<0.001$). The interaction between both predictors was not significant ($F_{1,20} = 1.45$, $P = 0.24$) and was thus removed prior to testing the main effects. Overall, the mean honey production over the entire season (including honey production during the pre-treatment phase) remained 29% lower in the neonicotinoid-exposed colonies (23.7±2.5 kg) compared to the control (33.4±5.1 kg).

Pollen consumption

At treatment initiation, pollen stores (bee bread) in the control group comprised of 17.9±10.7 dm^2 and those in the group subsequently exposed to thiamethoam and clothianidin comprised

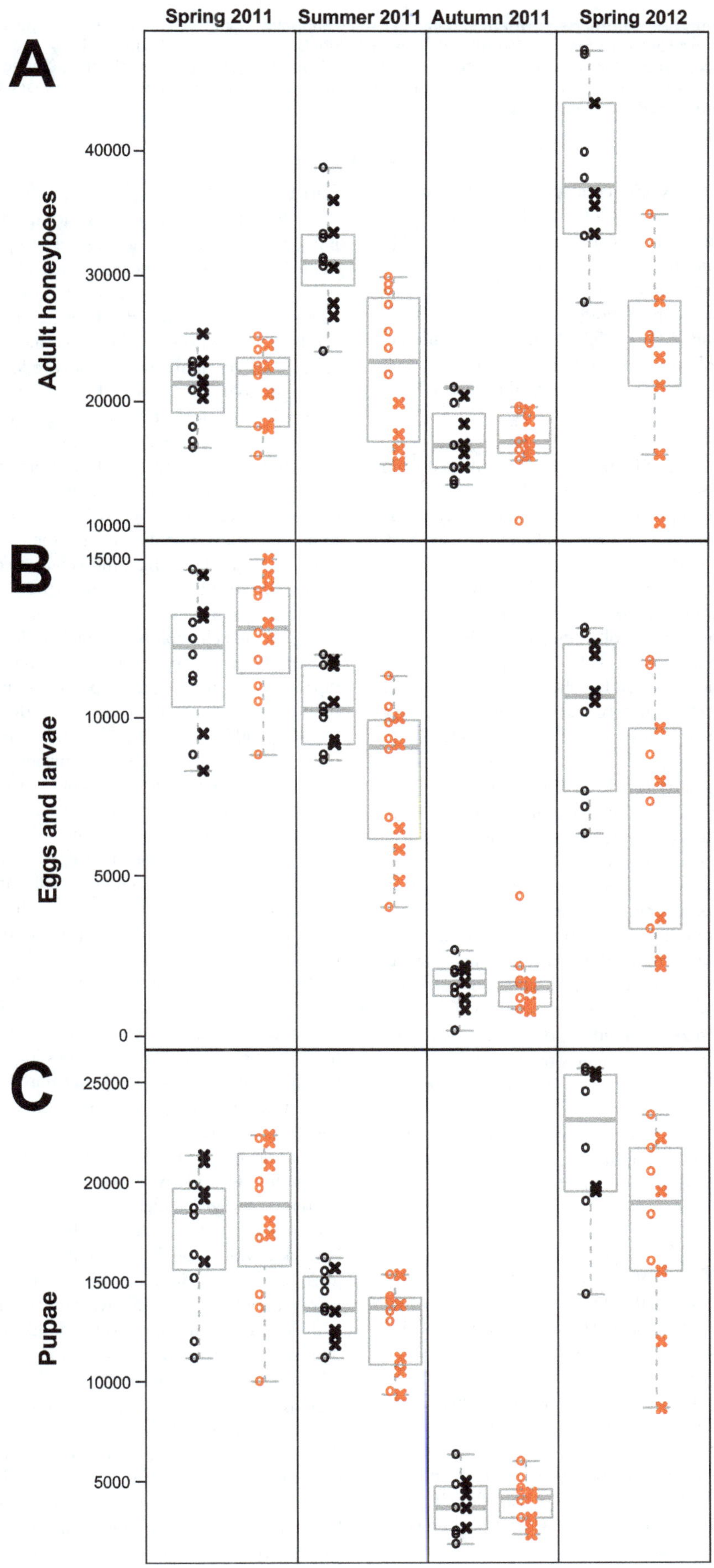
Spring 2011
Summer 2011
Autumn 2011
Spring 2012
A
Adult honeybees
B
Eggs and larvae
C
Pupae

Figure 1. Dynamics of honeybee colony performance. Data of all three endpoints number of adult bees (A), eggs and larvae (B) and pupae (C) for the different pollen feeding treatments (black = control; red = neonicotinoids) and honeybee strains (circles = strain A; crosses = strain B). The data were obtained at four successive colony assessment dates (X-axis subpanels within figures) performed before (Spring 2011) and directly after the 1.5 months of experimental pollen feeding (Summer 2011), 3.5 months after the treatment (Autumn 2011) and one year later (Spring 2012). Estimated numbers on the Y-axes are truncated for adult bees and pupae for better overview.

of 20.8±3.8 dm^2. After the experimental pollen feeding pollen stores within hives comprised of 29.8±8.9 dm^2 and 24.9±11.7 dm^2 in the control and neonicotinoid-exposed group, respectively. There was no indication that pollen storing and pollen consumption, respectively, during the experimental pollen feeding was influenced by neonicotinoid exposure ($F_{1,21} = 2.63$, $P = 0.12$) or honeybee strain ($F_{1,21} = 2.52$, $P = 0.13$). The interaction between the two predictors was not significant ($F_{1,21} = 0.74$, $P = 0.40$) and was thus removed prior to testing the main effects.

Pollen collections

Total mean pollen harvests (±SD) per colony, as inferred from pollen trap contents, were 4.4±0.47 kg and 3.58±0.43 kg for the control and neonicotinoid-exposed group, respectively. The colonies exposed to thiamethoxam and clothianidin had 19% lower total pollen collections on average. Pollen collections measured as AUCs were found to be significantly lower in neonicotinoid-exposed colonies ($P < 0.001$). While both treatment groups collected similar amounts of pollen during the first 3 weeks of the experimental pollen feeding, colonies exposed to thiamethoxam and clothianidin consistently collected less pollen later on, with mean pollen collections barely reaching more than 50% of the control group during the last week of exposure (Fig. 2).

Supersedure of queens and tendency to swarm

We found a significant association of neonicotinoid exposure and queen supersedure (in the absence of swarming) ($P = 0.01$): while all ten queens of the control group survived until the end of the experiment (~2 years or swarmed, see below), 6 out of 10 queens of the colonies experimentally exposed to thiamethoxam and clothianidin over 1.5 months were replaced within one year after treatment. The result remained significant when overall queen loss was assessed, i.e. also including the two colonies (one per treatment group) that lost their queen during winter ($P = 0.02$). A negative association of neonicotinoid exposure and swarming events during spring following experimental treatment was found ($P = 0.005$): in the control group 9 out of 10 colonies swarmed until end of May 2012 (5 out of 6 colonies of strain A and all 4 colonies of strain B), while only 2 colonies (one of strain A and B each) of the group that was exposed to thiamethoxam and clothianidin in the previous season swarmed.

Discussion

The major findings of this study using sublethal chronic exposure of honeybee colonies to thiamethoxam and clothianidin through feeding contaminated pollen were: (*i*) significant short-term (1.5 months) impacts at the colony level resulting in decreased colony performance and productivity; (*ii*) no negative influence in the medium-term (3.5 months) and on colony overwintering; (*iii*) significantly decelerated colony growth in the long-term (1 year) that was associated with higher queen supersedure rates and a reduced tendency to swarm; and (*iv*) significant interactions of the honeybee genetics with the observed effects of neonicotinoids on most parameters. In the following, these findings are discussed in context.

Short-term impact

At the colony level, honeybee foraging efficiency was negatively influenced during chronic exposure to pollen containing environmentally relevant concentrations of the two neonicotinoids thiamethoxam and clothianidin over two brood cycles (1.5 months). The detected decrease in pollen collection and honey production upon sublethal neonicotinoid exposure are in line with earlier findings of impaired honeybee foraging through impacts on neurophysiological traits and cognitive abilities, including sucrose responsiveness, foraging rates, waggle dancing and memory and learning [47,48,49,50,51,52,53,54,55,56,57,58,59]. In addition, increased forager losses resulting from decreased homing success [48] through compromised navigation memory [58] may have contributed to both reduced foraging efficiency and significantly smaller worker populations of the colonies exposed to thiamethoxam and clothianidin compared to controls (Fig. 1A, Table 1). Indeed, there were no significant effects on the numbers of pupae present at the end of the exposure phase (Fig. 1C, Table 1), which points at higher forager losses rather than decreased worker production of neonicotinoid-exposed colonies during the treatment. As opposed to known effects of neonicotinoid ingestion of foragers through nectar-substitutes [47,48,49,50,51,56,57,58], the overall reduced numbers of adult bees through pollen exposure is intriguing. Pollen is generally not stored extensively within hives but consumed quickly. There was no evidence for differences in pollen storing between treatment groups directly after the experimental feeding. Therefore, it can be assumed that control pollen and pollen spiked with thiamethoxam and clothianidin were similarly consumed within experimental colonies. Contaminated pollen may affect various life stages of honeybees [105], yet pollen is predominantly consumed by nurse bees and larvae, but not foragers. In this regard, the recent finding that sublethal neonicotinoid exposure of honeybee larvae impacts post-emergence olfactory associative behaviour of adults [53] is relevant, and might be one of the largely unresolved effects arising from altered larval gene expression profiles upon sublethal neonicotinoid exposure [93] that may help to explain the strong impediment of colony growth documented here. Delayed sublethal effects extending to later life-cycle stages could similarly apply to larvae and nurse bees consuming contaminated pollen [64] and, depending on colony exposure duration, be able to reinforce decreased foraging efficiency. Our observed pattern of increasing divergence of pollen collections between treatment groups after 2–3 weeks, which roughly corresponds to the adult in-hive phase after emergence [106], may be indicative of the recruitment of less efficient foragers, which have encountered pollen contaminated with thiamethoxam and clothianidin during their nursing phase. The successively greater decline of pollen collections of neonicotinoid-exposed colonies after 5 weeks, in turn coincides with the time frame during which foragers could be expected to be exposed to contaminated pollen from the young larva stage onwards and throughout their entire development. Further research is needed to evaluate the potential for delayed impact on implementing complex foraging tasks through altered metabolic networks caused by sublethal dietary neonicotinoid exposure to honeybee brood [53,93] and eventually also nurse bees [64], the developmental

Table 1. Model-based estimates of contrasts and corresponding significance levels of the treatment effect (neonicotinoid *versus* control) and honeybee genetics (strain A *vs.* strain B).

	Adult bees			Eggs and larvae			Pupae		
	Summer 2011	**Autumn 2011**	**Spring 2012**	**Summer 2011**	**Autumn 2011**	**Spring 2012**	**Summer 2011**	**Autumn 2011**	**Spring 2012**
Neonicotinoids *vs* Control	−60.56***	−0.73	−82.96***	−0.31*	−0.01	−0.49***	−4.36	1.84	−15.31**
Strain A *vs* strain B							5.31	2.65	7.91
Treatment within strain A	−14.07*	−1.33	−28.59*	−0.10	0.03	−0.06			
Treatment within strain B	−46.49***	0.59	−54.37***	−0.21·	−0.05	−0.42***			

Results are shown in the transformed scale for the three response variables adult bees, eggs and larvae and pupae assessed directly after the 1.5 months of treatment (Summer 2011), 3.5 months later (Autumn 2011) and 1 year later (Spring 2012). For adult bees and eggs and larvae (the models that included a significant threefold interaction between treatment, honeybee strain and assessment date) contrasts for treatment effects were also computed within individual honeybee strains at each assessment date. *P* values are adjusted for multiple testing. ***$P<0.001$; **$P<0.01$; *$P<0.05$; · $0.05<P<0.1$.

stages during which fundamental physiological processes required for adult olfaction and learning performance are settled [107].

The observation of strongly reduced pollen collection of the colonies exposed to thiamethoxam and clothianidin during the last week of the treatment could also be interpreted as a response to significantly reduced numbers of larvae (Fig. 1B, Table 1). However, a general decrease in foraging efficiency is also indicated by significantly reduced honey production. Because experimental pollen was provided constantly in sufficient amounts, significantly reduced investment in rearing larvae after 1.5 months of combined exposure to thiamethoxam and clothianidin is best explained by the declining numbers of workers: higher forager losses trigger premature forager recruitment, which results in fewer nurse bees available for brood rearing [101,108]. Although physiological changes in nurse bees may have played an additional role [54,55,93,109], reduced investment in brood rearing was probably reinforced by the reallocation of worker resources at the colony level towards the end of the exposure period rather than by adverse effects on the larvae themselves. Although there is some indication for negative effects of neonicotinoids and other pesticides on honeybee larvae [62,93,110], there is so far no evidence that field-realistic neonicotinoid exposure in the absence of additional stressors results in increased larval mortality [36,64]. The latter would also be difficult to reconcile with the observation that the numbers of pupae did not differ between treatments, even after 1.5 months of neonicotinoid exposure. Interestingly, short-term effects of the combined exposure to thiamethoxam and clothianidin on the number of adult bees were influenced by the honeybees' genetic background. While effects on colonies of strain A were only marginally significant, those on colonies of strain B were highly significant (Fig. 1, Table 1).

Medium-term impact

The colony assessment during autumn 2011, 3.5 months after the experimental pollen feeding, revealed that there were neither effects of the combined exposure to thiamethoxam and clothianidin nor of the honeybees' genetic background on colony strength and the amount of brood (Fig. 1A–C, Table 1). All colonies were strong and well-fed, and thus overwintered successfully, except one colony of each treatment which lost their queens during winter. This reiterates the general view that a sustainable varroa mite management is a major aspect of honeybee colony health, thereby limiting colony losses [25,26]. Our comprehensive varroa mite management, comprising of a combination of integrated actions using organic acids [27] but avoiding potentially detrimental synthetic acaricides [47,52,111,112], was apparently sufficient to limit *V. destructor*-associated damage during the sensitive overwintering period, and throughout the entire study. A thorough varroa mite control pre-supposed, the overcoming of the previously observed short-term effects of neonicotinoids on colony strength and brood rearing 4–5 brood cycles later shows that chronic sublethal neonicotinoid-exposure alone does not trigger elevated honeybee colony winter losses [17,20], although contrasting results have been found in other studies [113,114].

There were no obvious clinical symptoms of infections with widespread honeybee pathogens such as the ectoparasitic mite *V. destructor*, microsporidian gut parasites *Nosema* ssp., chalkbrood (the fungal pathogen *Ascophaera apis*) or European and American foulbrood (bacterial diseases caused by *Melissococcus plutonius* and *Paenibacillus larvae*, respectively) at any time during the study. Nevertheless, it cannot be excluded that some of the above described short-term effects on colony performance may have been influenced by detrimental neonicotinoid-pathogen interactions at the level of individual bees [36,68,69,70,71,72]. Higher

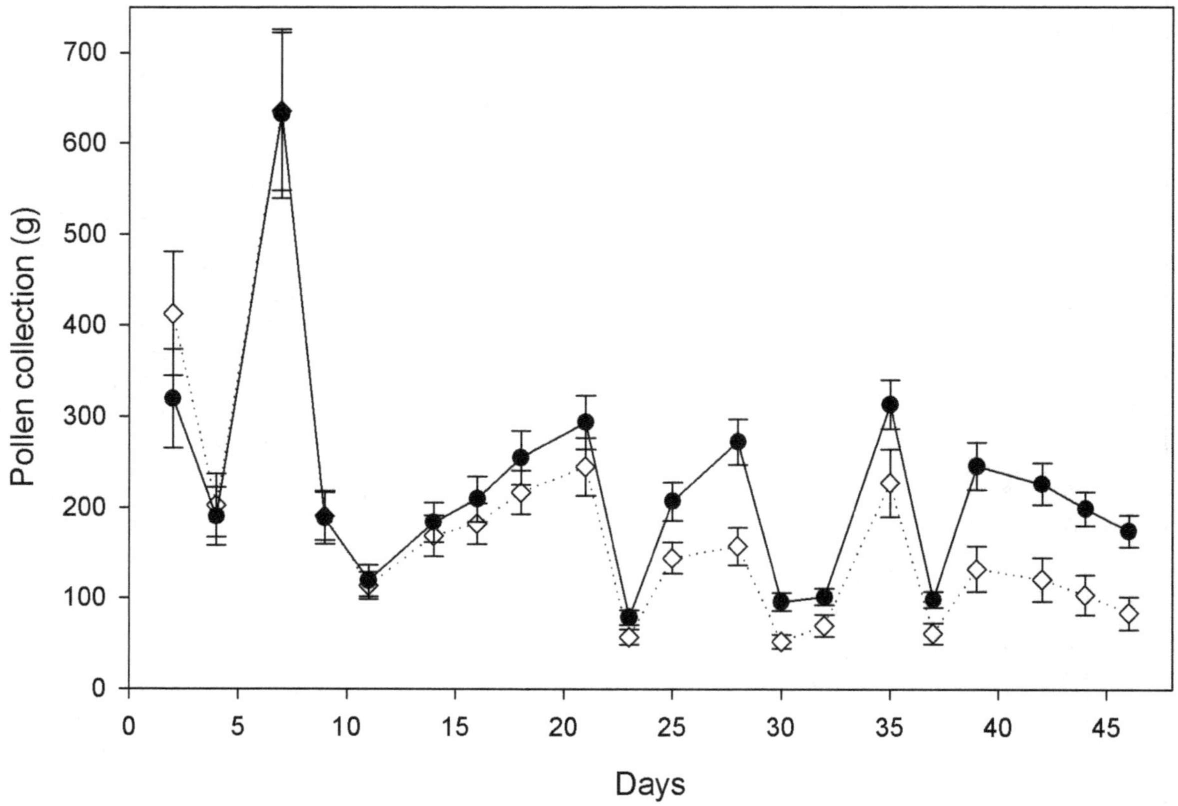

Figure 2. Pollen collections. Mean (±SD) fresh weights of pollen collections for control (black) and neonicotinoid-exposed (white) colonies over the course of the treatment period (pollen-trap contents were weighed in 2-2-3 days intervals throughout the study).

forager losses associated with overall shifts in forager age structure may also cause generally decreased immunological competence at the colony level [115]. However, these differentiations between individual drivers and their interactions are only of limited practical importance because free-flying honeybees will almost inevitably carry ubiquitous pathogens and thus encounter combined pressures. In fact, it is very likely that latent infections with the most common *V. destructor*-associated honeybee viruses and *Nosema* spp. have also been present in the experimental apiary. The common garden approach to maintain all colonies at the same isolated field site for almost one year prior to the experiments actually aimed at 'synchronizing' viral and microbial landscapes across colonies, thereby resulting in potential errors of systematic conservative nature. If multiple pressures were indeed present in our experiment, the observed recovery from decreased performance of previously neonicotinoid-exposed colonies after several brood cycles conforms to model predictions, showing that even detrimental interactions presumably can be tolerated to some extent and do not necessarily result in disrupting colony function [65].

Long-term impact

Given that significantly negative short-term impacts of combined exposure to thiamethoxam and clothianidin during summer 2011 had faded with respect to colony strength during autumn (medium-term) and overwintering success, the patterns observed during the subsequent spring were unexpected. Colonies that received pollen spiked with thiamethoxam and clothianidin during the previous spring exhibited significantly lower numbers of adult bees compared to controls one year later, whereas the effects were much stronger for strain B than for strain A (Fig. 1A, Table 1). In addition, there were significantly negative overall effects of last year's neonicotinoid exposure on the amount of pupae (Fig. 1C, Table 1) and eggs and larvae (Fig. 1B, Table 1). For the latter endpoint, however, significant effects were only found for strain B (Table 1). These patterns of decelerated colony growth are intriguing, because all hive samples collected 3 weeks after the experimental feeding of neonicotinoid-spiked pollen patties did not contain traceable residues of thiamethoxam and clothianidin. Although trace residues below corresponding limits of detection could have still been present within hives one year after the treatment, it is highly unlikely that this explains detrimental effects that far exceeded those observed directly after the treatment (Table 1). Instead, reduced performance of previously neonicotinoid-exposed queens appears to be a more plausible explanation for long-term effects. While all original, individually tagged and wing-clipped queens were recognized in autumn 2011, the assessment in spring 2012 revealed that there were non-tagged egg-laying queens with intact wings in some colonies previously exposed to thiamethoxam and clothianidin. This clearly shows queen supersedure during the previous autumn as a response to poor queen performance [86,87], which could pose a risk for successful overwintering. Yet, supersedure during autumn bears a considerable risk for colony failure as well, because virgin queens may not be sufficiently mated during their mating flights due to a comparatively lower number of available drones. Queen replacement in the neonicotinoid treatment group in the presence of original queens, and without swarming, was also observed during spring 2012. This indication of impaired performance of previously neonicotinoid-exposed queens, together with a likely reduced mating success of replacement queens from the previous autumn, is thus considered to be responsible for the overall decelerated colony growth of the neonicotinoid treatment group one year after exposure. The causal patterns of queen failure could be manifold, including compromised immunity that has been shown to result in increased pathogen loads in honeybee workers [36,68,69,72]. Taking into account that honeybee colony fate essentially depends on the queen, the long-term impact of neonicotinoids on queens we observed, resulting in 60% supersedure within one year, represents a novel finding of major importance that clearly deserves further research. Increased queen supersedure rates were shown upon sublethal pyrethroid exposure [116] and detrimental effects on queen development and performance have also been reported from exposure to commonly encountered in-hive acaricides [117,118,119,120], some of which are known to have similarly negative influence like neonicotinoids on worker bees [47,52,108,121]. General effects of neurotoxic insecticides on queens may thus not be fundamentally surprising. Queen failure has repeatedly been indicated to be an important aspect shaping the present enigma of widespread colony losses [22,25,122], which may also be influenced by neonicotinoids. While direct contact exposure to agrochemicals can be generally considered much more relaxed for queens compared to workers, this might be different regarding oral exposure to systemic compounds, such as neonicotinoids. Here, ingestion of contaminated food represents a principal risk for all developmental stages and different castes of honeybees. Moreover, the queen's life span as well as her level of trophallactic interactions far exceed that of workers [123], which may predestine her as a potential sink of sublethal exposure to systemic insecticides through pollen-based queen nutrition. Our results suggest that sublethal neonicotinoid effects on queens can jeopardize colony fate in the long-term, and should thus not be ignored.

Compared to the need for maintaining productive queens within colonies, swarming is less relevant for practical beekeeping, especially commercial operations. Nevertheless, apart from drone mating success, colony splitting through swarming represents a true fitness estimate in honeybees. According to overall reduced colony strength, colonies that were exposed to thiamethoxam and clothianidin in the previous season exhibited a significantly lower swarming success.

The role of honeybee genetics

The detection of significant interactions of the honeybees' genetic background with the effects of chronic neonicotinoid exposure on both colony performance in the short-term and queen performance in the long-term was a major insight of our study. Honeybee strain B, *A. m. mellifera* sister queens originating from a Swiss alpine region, was much more susceptible to the combination of thiamethoxam and clothianidin compared to strain A, *A. m. carnica* sister queens originating from a German region characterized by intense agriculture. For example, neonicotinoid-exposed colonies of strain B had the lowest numbers of adult bees directly after exposure (Fig. 1A), and none of their queens survived throughout the one year post-exposure period. This indicates that honeybee susceptibility to the here applied neonicotinoids may also include a genetic or epigenetic component, as has been previously suggested for neonicotinoids and other pesticides [17,93,111,124,125,126]. It remains unresolved to what extent the outcome of our study was influenced by the usage of different honeybee ecotypes and/or by their distinct breeding histories linked to different environments. It could be possible that *A. m. mellifera* tends to be more susceptible to oral neonicotinoid exposure than *A. m. carnica* bees, as similarly found in another recent study [126]. Yet, compared to strain B, the particular breeding regime of strain A prior to our study may have simply included an unintended selection for higher neonicotinoid tolerance as a non-lineage-specific trait. Further research is required to explore the potential genetic basis underlying variable responses to sublethal neonicotinoid exposure in honeybees. Causal patterns could include detoxification genes and corresponding expression profiles, e.g., cytochrome P450 monooxygenases [93], yet, compared to many other insects, honeybees are equipped with a limited set of detoxification genes [127] and specifically the pathways for nitroguanidine neonicotinoid metabolism in honeybees remain less resolved compared to other insecticidal compounds [61,111,128,129,130,131].

Conclusions

In line with a recent meta-analysis [44], our results clearly indicate that neonicotinoids negatively impact on honeybee colony performance after chronic sublethal exposure throughout two brood cycles. Virtually all tested contrasts (18 out of 21) produced negative estimates for the effects of exposure to thiamethoxam and clothianidin (Table 1). It is supposed that sublethal neonicotinoid exposure through pollen has a stronger impact at the honeybee colony level compared to nectar-substitute feeding (e.g., [132]). Therefore more studies focussing on effects of sublethal exposure of larvae or nurse bees extending to the performance of complex tasks of adult forager honeybees are needed. Similarly, sublethal effects of neonicotinoids on honeybee queens clearly deserve in depth investigation.

It remains uncertain whether the observed colony level responses were stronger influenced by either thiamethoxam or clothianidin, or by the possibility for interactive effects of the combination of these neonicotinoids, both being ranked as having high risk potential to honeybees [64]. Yet, since clothianidin is the major metabolite of thiamethoxam, both bioactive compounds will be present in pollen and nectar of crops treated with thiamethoxam [80,82,96,97,98]. Thus, the combined exposure as well as the residue levels administered in pollen patties in this study represent a biologically relevant exposure scenario.

Exposure to almost any sublethal dosage of these highly potent insecticides could trigger adverse chronic effects in a time-dependant context [133,134]. Our experimental exposure to contaminated pollen over 1.5 months can be considered as a worst-case scenario for agricultural settings, where honeybee colonies may encounter neonicotinoid-treated crops repeatedly throughout the season, but likely for shorter individual exposure periods. In bumblebees, it has recently been shown, that microcolonies can recover after short periods of sublethal exposure [135] to imidacloprid, which may well be similar, or even more pronounced in honeybee colonies. In a similar way, the supposedly exclusive exposure to pollen contaminated with neonicotinoids in our setup can be regarded as a worst case because in the field honeybee colonies generally exploit multiple available pollen resources at any time, some of which may only occasionally be contaminated with agricultural pesticides [38]. Nonetheless, it remains unclear whether repeated pulsed exposures over the entire season, either through consecutively available neonicotinoid-treated honeybee-attractive crops providing pollen and nectar (e.g., oilseed rape, sunflowers and maize that may each flower for 2–3 weeks) or through the general accumulation of neonicotinoid residues in the environment [38,41,42,82], could result in detrimental effects as found here after 1.5 months of continuous chronic exposure. Moreover, although distinguishing between continuous and shorter but repeated periods of neonicotinoid exposure could represent different risk potentials for the honeybee worker population succumbed to generally high turn-over rates [101], the suspected buffering capacities at the colony level may deplete in the long-term, if the queen was still affected through pulsed exposures. Thus, a worst case scenario that applies realistic exposure levels while settling at the upper possible range of overall exposure duration deserves consideration. Currently there is no evidence that field-realistic neonicotinoid exposure could be directly involved in colony losses [79,80,81,82,83]. However, available studies do not fully allow to address the question of whether neonicotinoids are really contributing to colony weakening, because several aspects in corresponding experimental designs remain unsettled, such as lacking sufficient statistical power [44], the putative influence of honeybee genetics (see above), too small distances between test fields and other factors that challenge the prerequisite of adequate control fields, such as no pesticide treatment at all [41,79,80,81,82], queen effects that remain elusive [25] or queen rotation practices that impede uncovering potential effects on queen performance [80]. Interestingly, this long-term impact detected in our study, notably supersedure of failing queens, compounds recent criticism that the presence of a given predictor may not necessarily correlate with impaired colony function [65] by showing that delayed effects can emerge also in the absence of causal stressors, in this case the lack of traceable amounts of the applied neonicotinoids within hives several weeks after exposure. There is an urgent need for more thoroughly designed studies to clarify the threats of neonicotinoids to honeybees, and pollinators in general [42]. The growing body of scientific awareness on sublethal side-effects of pesticides on non-target pollinators, ranging from gene expression profiles of individual developmental stages to entire life-time fitness performances of different species of bees, represents a unique opportunity to benefit the current framework of pesticide risk assessment [64,84,136,137].

Finally, the here detected interactions of honeybee genetics and impacts of chronic neonicotinoid exposure on colony performance suggest that there is genetic variability for neonicotinoid susceptibility, and thus potential to partly counteract negative effects through selective breeding of more tolerant honeybee strains.

Supporting Information

Figure S1 Colony set up at the experimental apiary. Two groups of honeybee colonies each comprising of 7 colonies originating from strain A (blue squares) and 5 colonies originating from strain B (yellow squares) were placed in a row in front of a small forest with entrances pointing in the same direction. All colonies were maintained approximately one year before and one year after the experimental feeding with either control or neonicotinoid-spiked pollen patties over two brood cycles.

Acknowledgments

We thank Jennifer Brandenburg, Rebecca Basile and Mario Waldburger for assistance and Nicolas Desneux, Werner Stahel and three anonymous reviewers for valuable comments. The infrastructure was courtesy provided by Agroscope Reckenholz-Tänniken ART, Switzerland.

Author Contributions

Conceived and designed the experiments: CS. Performed the experiments: CS AFM. Analyzed the data: MT LGT CS. Contributed reagents/materials/analysis tools: PN CS. Wrote the paper: CS PN SGP.

References

1. Bascompte J, Jordano P, Olesen JM (2006) Asymmetric coevolutionary networks facilitate biodiversity maintenance. Science 312: 431–433.
2. Fontaine C, Dajoz I, Meriguet J, Loreau M (2006) Functional diversity of plant-pollinator interaction webs enhances the persistence of plant communities. PLOS Biol 4: e1.
3. Garibaldi LA, Aizen MA, Klein AM, Cunningham SA, Harder LD (2011) Global growth and stability of agricultural yield decrease with pollinator dependence. Proc Natl Acad Sci USA 108: 5909–5914.
4. Klein AM, Vaissière BE, Cane JH, Steffan-Dewenter I, Cunningham SA, et al. (2007) Importance of pollinators in changing landscapes for world crops. Proc R Soc Lond B Biol Sci 274: 303–313.
5. Gallai N, Salles JM, Settele J, Vaissière BE (2009) Economic valuation of the vulnerability of world agriculture confronted with pollinator decline. Ecol Econ 68: 810–821.
6. Lautenbach S, Seppelt R, Liebscher J, Dormann CF (2012) Spatial and temporal trends of global pollination benefit. PLOS ONE 7: e35954.
7. Biesmeijer JC, Roberts SPM, Reemer M, Ohlemuller R, Edwards M, et al. (2006) Parallel declines in pollinators and insect-pollinated plants in Britain and the Netherlands. Science 313: 351–354.
8. Potts SG, Biesmeijer JC, Kremen C, Neumann P, Schweiger O, et al. (2010) Global pollinator declines: trends, impacts and drivers. Trends Ecol Evol 25: 345–353.
9. Cameron SA, Lozier JD, Strange JP, Koch JB, Cordes N, et al. (2011) Patterns of widespread decline in North American bumble bees. Proc Natl Acad Sci USA 108: 662–667.
10. Goulson D, Lye GC, Darvill B (2008) Decline and conservation of bumble bees. Annu Rev Entomol 53: 191–208.
11. Aizen MA, Garibaldi LA, Cunningham SA, Klein AM (2008) Long-term global trends in crop yield and production reveal no current pollination shortage but increasing pollinator dependency. Curr Biol 18: 1572–1575.
12. Aizen MA, Garibaldi LA, Cunningham SA, Klein AM (2009) How much does agriculture depend on pollinators? Lessons from long-term trends in crop production. Ann Bot 103: 1579–1588.
13. Potts SG, Roberts SPM, Dean R, Marris G, Brown MA, et al. (2010) Declines of managed honey bees and beekeepers in Europe. J Apic Res 49: 15–22.
14. Ellis JD, Evans JD, Pettis JS (2010) Colony losses, managed colony population decline and Colony Collapse Disorder in the United States. J Apic Res 49: 134–136.
15. Aizen MA, Harder LD (2009) The global stock of domesticated honey bees is growing slower than agricultural demand for pollination. Curr Biol 19: 915–918.
16. vanEngelsdorp D, Hayes J Jr., Underwood RM, Pettis J (2008) A survey of honey bee colony losses in the U.S., fall 2007 to spring 2008. PLOS ONE 3: e4071.
17. vanEngelsdorp D, Evans JD, Saegerman C, Mullin C, Haubruge E, et al. (2009) Colony collapse disorder: A descriptive study. PLOS ONE 4: e6481.
18. Cox-Foster DL, Conlan S, Holmes EC, Palacios G, Evans JD, et al. (2007) A metagenomic survey of microbes in honey bee colony collapse disorder. Science 318: 283–287.
19. Anderson D, East IJ (2008) The latest buzz about colony collapse disorder. Science 319: 724–725.
20. van der Zee R, Pisa L, Andronov S, Brodschneider R, Charrière J-D, et al. (2012) Managed honey bee colony losses in Canada, China, Europe, Israel and Turkey, for the winters of 2008–9 and 2009–10. J Apic Res 51: 100–114.
21. Neumann P, Carreck N (2010) Honey bee colony losses. J Apic Res 49: 1–6.
22. Brodschneider R, Moosbeckhofer R, Crailsheim K (2010) Surveys as a tool to record winter losses of honey bee colonies: a two-year case study in Austria and South Tyrol. J Apic Res 49: 23–30.
23. Johnson RM, Evans JD, Robinson GE, Berenbaum MR (2009) Changes in transcript abundance relating to colony collapse disorder in honey bees (*Apis mellifera*). Proc Natl Acad Sci USA 106: 14790–14795.
24. Vanbergen AJ, the Insect Pollinators Initiative (2013) Threats to an ecosystem service: pressures on pollinators. Front Ecol Environ 11: 251–259.
25. Genersch E, von der Ohe W, Kaatz H, Schroeder A, Otten C, et al. (2010) The German bee monitoring project: a long term study to understand periodically high winter losses of honey bee colonies. Apidologie 41: 332–352.
26. Le Conte Y, Ellis M, Ritter W (2010) *Varroa* mites and honey bee health: can Varroa explain part of the colony losses? Apidologie 41: 353–363.
27. Rosenkranz P, Aumeier P, Ziegelmann B (2010) Biology and control of *Varroa destructor*. J Invertebr Pathol 103 Suppl 1: S96–119.
28. Nazzi F, Brown SP, Annoscia D, Del Piccolo F, Di Prisco G, et al. (2012) Synergistic parasite-pathogen interactions mediated by host immunity can drive the collapse of honeybee colonies. PLOS Pathog 8: e1002735.
29. Martin SJ, Highfield AC, Brettell L, Villalobos EM, Budge GE, et al. (2012) Global honey bee viral landscape altered by a parasitic mite. Science 336: 1304–1306.

30. Higes M, Martin-Hernandez R, Garrido-Bailon E, Gonzalez-Porto AV, Garcia-Palencia P, et al. (2009) Honeybee colony collapse due to *Nosema ceranae* in professional apiaries. Environ Microbiol Rep 1: 110–113.
31. Antunez K, Martin-Hernandez R, Prieto L, Meana A, Zunino P, et al. (2009) Immune suppression in the honey bee (*Apis mellifera*) following infection by *Nosema ceranae* (Microsporidia). Environ Microbiol 11: 2284–2290.
32. Higes M, Meana A, Bartolome C, Botias C, Martin-Hernandez R (2013) *Nosema ceranae* (Microsporidia), a controversial 21st century honey bee pathogen. Environ Microbiol Rep 5: 17–29.
33. Evans JD, Schwarz RS (2011) Bees brought to their knees: microbes affecting honey bee health. Trends Microbiol 19: 614–620.
34. Bromenshenk JJ, Henderson CB, Wick CH, Stanford MF, Zulich AW, et al. (2010) Iridovirus and microsporidian linked to honey bee colony decline. PLOS ONE 5: e13181.
35. Cornman RS, Tarpy DR, Chen Y, Jeffreys L, Lopez D, et al. (2012) Pathogen webs in collapsing honey bee colonies. PLOS ONE 7: e43562.
36. Doublet V, Labarussias M, De Miranda JR, Moritz RFA, Paxton JR (2014) Bees under stress: sublethal doses of a neonicotinoid pesticide and pathogens interact to elevate honey bee mortality across the life cycle. Environ Microbiol. (in press): DOI:10.1111/1462-2920.12426.
37. Mullin CA, Frazier M, Frazier JL, Ashcraft S, Simonds R, et al. (2010) High levels of miticides and agrochemicals in North American apiaries: implications for honey bee health. PLOS ONE 5: e9754.
38. Krupke CH, Hunt GJ, Eitzer BD, Andino G, Given K (2012) Multiple routes of pesticide exposure for honey bees living near agricultural fields. PLOS ONE 7: e29268.
39. Elbert A, Haas M, Springer B, Thielert W, Nauen R (2008) Applied aspects of neonicotinoid uses in crop protection. Pest Manag Sci 64: 1099–1105.
40. Jeschke P, Nauen R, Schindler M, Elbert A (2011) Overview of the status and global strategy for neonicotinoids. J Agric Food Chem 59: 2897–2908.
41. van der Slujs JP, Simon-Delso N, Goulson D, Maxim L, Bonmatin JM, et al. (2013) Neonicotinoids, bee disorders and the sustainability of pollinator services. Curr Opin Environ Sustain 5: 293–305.
42. Goulson D (2013) An overview of the environmental risks posed by neonicotinoid insecticides. J Appl Ecol 50: 977–987.
43. Matsuda K, Buckingham SD, Kleier D, Rauh JJ, Grauso M, et al. (2001) Neonicotinoids: insecticides acting on insect nicotinic acetylcholine receptors. Trends Pharmacol Sci 22: 573–580.
44. Cresswell JE (2011) A meta-analysis of experiments testing the effects of a neonicotinoid insecticide (imidacloprid) on honey bees. Ecotoxicology 20: 149–157.
45. Desneux N, Decourtye A, Delpuech JM (2007) The sublethal effects of pesticides on beneficial arthropods. Annu Rev Entomol 52: 81–106.
46. Blacquière T, Smagghe G, van Gestel CA, Mommaerts V (2012) Neonicotinoids in bees: a review on concentrations, side-effects and risk assessment. Ecotoxicology 21: 973–992.
47. Williamson SM, Wright GA (2013) Exposure to multiple cholinergic pesticides impairs olfactory learning and memory in honeybees. J Exp Biol 216: 1799–1807.
48. Henry M, Beguin M, Requier F, Rollin O, Odoux JF, et al. (2012) A common pesticide decreases foraging success and survival in honey bees. Science 336: 348–350.
49. Belzunces LP, Tchamitchan S, Brunet J (2012) Neural effects of insecticides in the honey bee. Apidologie 43: 348–370.
50. Decourtye A, Devillers J (2010) Ecotoxicity of neonicotinoid insecticides to bees. In: Thany SH, editor. Insect nicotinic acetylcholine receptors. New York: Springer. 85–95.
51. Schneider CW, Tautz J, Grünewald B, Fuchs S (2012) RFID tracking of sublethal effects of two neonicotinoid insecticides on the foraging behavior of *Apis mellifera*. PLOS ONE 7: e30023.
52. Palmer MJ, Moffat C, Saranzewa N, Harvey J, Wright GA, et al. (2013) Cholinergic pesticides cause mushroom body neuronal inactivation in honeybees. Nat Commun 4: 1634.
53. Yang EC, Chang HC, Wu WY, Chen YW (2012) Impaired olfactory associative behavior of honeybee workers due to contamination of imidacloprid in the larval stage. PLOS ONE 7: e49472.
54. Hatjina F, Papaefthimiou C, Charistos L, Dogaroglu T, Bouga M, et al. (2013) Sublethal doses of imidacloprid decreased size of hypopharyngeal glands and respiratory rhythm of honeybees in vivo. Apidologie 44: 467–480.
55. Oliveira RA, Roat TC, Carvalho SM, Malaspina O (2013) Side-effects of thiamethoxam on the brain and midgut of the africanized honeybee *Apis mellifera* (Hymenoptera: Apidae). Environ Toxicol. (in press): DOI:10.1002/tox.21842.
56. Eiri DM, Nieh JC (2012) A nicotinic acetylcholine receptor agonist affects honey bee sucrose responsiveness and decreases waggle dancing. J Exp Biol 215: 2022–2029.
57. Ramirez-Romero R, Chaufaux J, Pham-Delègue MH (2005) Effects of Cry1Ab protoxin, deltamethrin and imidacloprid on the foraging activity and the learning performances of the honeybee *Apis mellifera*, a comparative approach. Apidologie 36: 601–611.
58. Fischer J, Müller T, Spatz AK, Greggers U, Grünewald B, et al. (2014) Neonicotinoids interfere with specific components of navigation in honeybees. PLOS ONE 9: e91364.
59. Han P, Niu CY, Lei CL, Cui JJ, Desneux N (2010) Use of an innovative T-tube maze assay and the proboscis extension response assay to assess sublethal effects of GM products and pesticides on learning capacity of the honey bee *Apis mellifera* L. Ecotoxicology 19: 1612–1619.
60. Gill RJ, Ramos-Rodriguez O, Raine NE (2012) Combined pesticide exposure severely affects individual- and colony-level traits in bees. Nature 491: 105–108.
61. Iwasa T, Motoyama N, Ambrose JT, Roe RM (2004) Mechanism for the differential toxicity of neonicotinoid insecticides in the honey bee, *Apis mellifera*. Crop Prot 23: 371–378.
62. Zhu W, Schmehl DR, Mullin CA, Frazier JL (2014) Four common pesticides, their mixtures and a formulation solvent in the hive environment have high oral toxicity to honey bee larvae. PLOS ONE 9: e77547.
63. Thompson HM, Fryday SL, Harkin S, Milner S (2014) Potential impacts of synergism in honeybees (*Apis mellifera*) of exposure to neonicotinoids and sprayed fungicides in crops. Apidologie (in press): DOI:10.1007/s13592-014-0273-6.
64. Sànchez-Bayo F, Goka K (2014) Pesticide residues and bees - a risk assessment. PLOS ONE 9: e94482.
65. Bryden J, Gill RJ, Mitton RA, Raine NE, Jansen VA (2013) Chronic sublethal stress causes bee colony failure. Ecol Lett. 16: 1463–1469.
66. James RR, Xu J (2012) Mechanisms by which pesticides affect insect immunity. J Invertebr Pathol 109: 175–182.
67. Mason R, Tennekes H, Sànchez-Bayo F, Jepsen PU (2013) Immune suppression by neonicotinoid insecticides at the root of global wildlife declines. J Environ Immunol Toxicol 1: 3–12.
68. Vidau C, Diogon M, Aufauvre J, Fontbonne R, Vigues B, et al. (2011) Exposure to sublethal doses of fipronil and thiacloprid highly increases mortality of honeybees previously infected by *Nosema ceranae*. PLOS ONE 6: e21550.
69. Pettis JS, vanEngelsdorp D, Johnson J, Dively G (2012) Pesticide exposure in honey bees results in increased levels of the gut pathogen *Nosema*. Naturwissenschaften 99: 153–158.
70. Alaux C, Brunet JL, Dussaubat C, Mondet F, Tchamitchan S, et al. (2010) Interactions between *Nosema* microspores and a neonicotinoid weaken honeybees (*Apis mellifera*). Environ Microbiol 12: 774–782.
71. Aufauvre J, Misme-Aucouturier B, Viguès B, Texier C, Delbac F, et al. (2014) Transcriptome analyses of the honeybee response to *Nosema ceranae* and insecticides. PLOS ONE 9: e91686.
72. Di Prisco G, Cavaliere V, Annoscia D, Varricchio P, Caprio E, et al. (2013) Neonicotinoid clothianidin adversely affects insect immunity and promotes replication of a viral pathogen in honey bees. Proc Natl Acad Sci USA 110: 18466–18471.
73. Naug D (2009) Nutritional stress due to habitat loss may explain recent honeybee colony collapses. Biol Conserv 142: 2369–2372.
74. Alaux C, Dantec C, Parrinello H, Le Conte Y (2011) Nutrigenomics in honey bees: digital gene expression analysis of pollen's nutritive effects on healthy and varroa-parasitized bees. BMC Genomics 12: 496.
75. Alaux C, Ducloz F, Crauser D, Le Conte Y (2010) Diet effects on honeybee immunocompetence. Biol Lett 6: 562–565.
76. Mao W, Schuler MA, Berenbaum MR (2013) Honey constituents up-regulate detoxification and immunity genes in the western honey bee *Apis mellifera*. Proc Natl Acad Sci USA 110: 8842–8846.
77. Chauzat MP, Martel AC, Blanchard P, Clément MC, Schurr F, et al. (2010) A case report of a honey bee colony poisoning incident in France. J Apic Res 49: 113–115.
78. Tremolada P, Mazzoleni M, Saliu F, Colombo M, Vighi M (2010) Field trial for evaluating the effects on honeybees of corn sown using Cruiser and Celest xl treated seeds. Bull Environ Contam Toxicol 85: 229–234.
79. Cutler GC, Scott-Dupree CD (2007) Exposure to clothianidin seed-treated canola has no long-term impact on honey bees. J Econ Entomol 100: 765–772.
80. Pilling E, Campbell P, Coulson M, Ruddle N, Tornier I (2013) A four-year field program investigating long-term effects of repeated exposure of honey bee colonies to flowering crops treated with thiamethoxam. PLOS ONE 8: e77193.
81. Nguyen BK, Saegerman C, Pirard C, Mignon J, Widart J, et al. (2009) Does imidacloprid seed-treated maize have an impact on honey bee mortality? J Econ Entomol 102: 616–623.
82. Pohorecka K, Skubida P, Miszczak A, Semkiw P, Sikorski P, et al. (2012) Residues of neonicotinoid insecticides in bee collected plant materials from oilseed rape crops and their effect on bee colonies. Journal of Apicultural Science 56: 115–134.
83. Cresswell JE, Desneux N, vanEngelsdorp D (2012) Dietary traces of neonicotinoid pesticides as a cause of population declines in honey bees: an evaluation by Hill's epidemiological criteria. Pest Manag Sci 68: 819–827.
84. Cressey D (2013) Europe debates risk to bees. Nature 496: 408.
85. Stokstad E (2013) Pesticides under fire for risks to pollinators. Science 340: 674–676.
86. Butler CG (1957) The process of queen supersedure in colonies of honeybees (*Apis mellifera* Linn.). Insectes Soc 4: 211–223.
87. Pettis JS, Higo H, Winston ML, Pankiw T (1997) Queen rearing suppression in the honey bee - evidence for a fecundity signal. Insectes Soc 44: 311–322.
88. Whitehorn PR, O'Connor S, Wackers FL, Goulson D (2012) Neonicotinoid pesticide reduces bumble bee colony growth and queen production. Science 336: 351–352.

89. Larson JL, Redmond CT, Potter DA (2013) Assessing insecticide hazard to bumble bees foraging on flowering weeds in treated lawns. PLOS ONE 8: e66375.
90. Fauser-Misslin A, Sadd BM, Neumann P, Sandrock C (2014) Influence of combined pesticide and parasite exposure on bumblebee colony traits in the laboratory. J Appl Ecol 51: 450–459.
91. Sandrock C, Tanadini LG, Pettis J, Biesmeijer JC, Potts SG, et al. (2014) Sublethal neonicotinoid insecticide exposure reduces solitary bee reproductive success. Agric For Entomol 16: 119–128.
92. Moritz RFA, Southwick EE (1992) Bees as superorganisms: an evolutionary reality. Berlin: Springer-Verlag. 395p.
93. Derecka K, Blythe MJ, Malla S, Genereux DP, Guffanti A, et al. (2013) Transient exposure to low levels of insecticide affects metabolic networks of honeybee larvae. PLOS ONE 8: e68191.
94. Neumann P, Moritz RFA, Mautz D (2000) Colony evaluation is not affected by drifting of drone and worker honeybees (*Apis mellifera* L.) at a performance testing apiary. Apidologie 31: 67–79.
95. Higes M, Martin-Hernandez R, Garrido-Bailon E, Garcia-Palencia P, Meana A (2008) Detection of infective *Nosema ceranae* (Microsporidia) spores in corbicular pollen of forager honeybees. J Invertebr Pathol 97: 76–78.
96. Maienfisch P, Angst M, Brandl F, Fischer W, Hofer D, et al. (2001) Chemistry and biology of thiamethoxam: a second generation neonicotinoid. Pest Manag Sci 57: 906–913.
97. Nauen R, Ebbinghaus-Kintscher U, Salgado VL, Kaussmann M (2003) Thiamethoxam is a neonicotinoid precursor converted to clothianidin in insects and plants. Pestic Biochem Phys 76: 55–69.
98. Dively GP, Kamel A (2012) Insecticide residues in pollen and nectar of a cucurbit crop and their potential exposure to pollinators. J Agric Food Chem 60: 4449–4456.
99. Imdorf A, Buehlmann G, Gerig L, Kilchenmann V, Wille H (1987) A test of the method of estimation of brood areas and number of worker bees in free-flying colonies. Apidologie 18: 137–146.
100. Delaplane KS, van der Steen J, Guzman E (2013) Standard methods for estimating strength parameters of *Apis mellifera* colonies. In: Dietemann V, Ellis JD, Neumann P, editors. The COLOSS BEEBOOK, Volume 1: standard methods for *Apis mellifera* research.
101. Khoury DS, Myerscough MR, Barron AB (2011) A quantitative model of honey bee colony population dynamics. PLOS ONE 6: e18491.
102. R Core Development_Team (2012) R: A language and environment for statistical computing. R Foundation for Statistical computing, Vienna, Austria. Available: http://cran.r-project.org. Accessed 27 April 2014.
103. Bates D, Maechler M, Bolker B, Walker S (2013) lme4: Linear mixed-effects models using Eigen and S4 classes. R package version 10-4. Available: http:// CRANR-projectorg/package = lme4.
104. Hothorn T, Bretz F, Westfall P (2008) Simultaneous inference in general parametric models. Biometrical Journal 50: 346–363.
105. Rortais A, Arnold G, Halm MP, Touffet-Briens F (2005) Modes of honeybees exposure to systemic insecticides: estimated amounts of contaminated pollen and nectar consumed by different categories of bees. Apidologie 36: 71–83.
106. Seeley TD (1982) Adaptive significance of the age polyethism schedule in honeybee colonies. Behav Ecol Sociobiol 11: 287–293.
107. Masson C, Pham-Delègue MH, Fonta C, Gascuel J, Arnold G, et al. (1993) Recent advances in the concept of adaptation to natural odour signals in the honeybee, *Apis mellifera* L. Apidologie 24: 169–194.
108. Wu JY, Anelli CM, Sheppard WS (2011) Sub-lethal effects of pesticide residues in brood comb on worker honey bee (*Apis mellifera*) development and longevity. PLOS ONE 6: e14720.
109. Smodis Skerl MI, Gregorc A (2010) Heat shock proteins and cell death in situ localisation in hypopharyngeal glands of honeybee (*Apis mellifera carnica*) workers after imidacloprid or coumaphos treatment. Apidologie 41: 73–86.
110. Gregorc A, Ellis JD (2011) Cell death localization *in situ* in laboratory reared honey bee (*Apis mellifera* L.) larvae treated with pesticides. Pesticide Biochemistry and Physiology 99: 200–207.
111. Johnson RM, Dahlgren L, Siegfried BD, Ellis MD (2013) Acaricide, fungicide and drug interactions in honey bees (*Apis mellifera*). PLOS ONE 8: e54092.
112. Hawthorne DJ, Dively GP (2011) Killing them with kindness? In-hive medications may inhibit xenobiotic efflux transporters and endanger honey bees. PLOS ONE 6: e26796.
113. Lu C, Warchol KM, Callahan RA (2012) *In situ* replication of honey bee colony collapse disorder. Bull Insectology 65: 99–106.
114. Lu C, Warchol KM, Callahan RA (2014) Sub-lethal exposure to neonicotinoids impaired honey bees winterization before proceeding to colony collapse disorder. Bull Insectology 67: 125–130.
115. Wilson-Rich N, Dres ST, Starks PT (2008) The ontogeny of immunity: development of innate immune strength in the honey bee (*Apis mellifera*). J Insect Physiol 54: 1392–1399.
116. Bendahou N, Fleche C, Bounias M (1999) Biological and biochemical effects of chronic exposure to very low levels of dietary cypermethrin (Cymbush) on honeybee colonies (Hymenoptera: Apidae). Ecotoxicol Environ Saf 44: 147–153.
117. Pettis JS, Collins AM, Wilbanks R, Feldlaufer M (2004) Effects of coumaphos on queen rearing in the honey bee, *Apis mellifera*. Apidologie 35: 605–610.
118. Haarmann T, Spivak M, Weaver D, Weaver B, Glenn T (2002) Effects of fluvalinate and coumaphos on queen honey bees (Hymenoptera: Apidae) in two commercial queen rearing operations. J Econ Entomol 95: 28–35.
119. DeGrandi-Hoffman G, Chen Y, Simonds R (2013) The effects of pesticides on queen rearing and virus titers in honey bees (*Apis mellifera* L.). Insects 4: 71–89.
120. Collins AM, Pettis JS, Wilbanks R, Feldlaufer M (2004) Performance of honey bee (*Apis mellifera*) queens reared in beeswax cells impregnated with coumaphos. J Apic Res 43: 128–134.
121. Garrido PM, Antunez K, Martin M, Porrini MP, Zunino P, et al. (2013) Immune-related gene expression in nurse honey bees (*Apis mellifera*) exposed to synthetic acaricides. J Insect Physiol 59: 113–119.
122. vanEngelsdorp D, Tarpy DR, Lengerich EJ, Pettis JS (2013) Idiopathic brood disease syndrome and queen events as precursors of colony mortality in migratory beekeeping operations in the eastern United States. Prev Vet Med 108: 225–233.
123. Crailsheim K (1998) Trophallactic interactions in the adult honeybee (*Apis mellifera* L.). Apidologie 29: 97–112.
124. Elzen PJ, Elzen GW, Rubink W (2003) Comparative susceptibility of European and Africanized honey bee (Hymenoptera: Apidae) ecotypes to several insecticide classes. Southwest Entomol 28: 255–260.
125. Suchail S, Guez D, Belzunces LP (2000) Characteristics of imidacloprid toxicity in two *Apis mellifera* subspecies. Environ Toxicol Chem 19: 1901–1905.
126. Laurino D, Manino A, Patetta A, Porporato M (2013) Toxicity of neonicotinoid insecticides on different honey bee genotypes. Bull Insectology 66: 119–126.
127. Claudianos C, Ranson H, Johnson RM, Biswas S, Schuler MA, et al. (2006) A deficit of detoxification enzymes: pesticide sensitivity and environmental response in the honeybee. Insect Mol Biol 15: 615–636.
128. Johnson RM, Mao W, Pollock HS, Niu G, Schuler MA, et al. (2012) Ecologically appropriate xenobiotics induce cytochrome P450s in *Apis mellifera*. PLOS ONE 7: e31051.
129. Mao W, Schuler MA, Berenbaum MR (2011) CYP9Q-mediated detoxification of acaricides in the honey bee (*Apis mellifera*). Proc Natl Acad Sci USA 108: 12657–12662.
130. Suchail S, Debrauwer L, Belzunces LP (2004) Metabolism of imidacloprid in *Apis mellifera*. Pest Manag Sci 60: 291–296.
131. Johnson RM, Pollock HS, Berenbaum MR (2009) Synergistic interactions between in-hive miticides in *Apis mellifera*. J Econ Entomol 102: 474–479.
132. Faucon JP, Aurieres C, Drajnudel P, Mathieu L, Ribière M, et al. (2005) Experimental study on the toxicity of imidacloprid given in syrup to honey bee (*Apis mellifera*) colonies. Pest Manag Sci 61: 111–125.
133. Tennekes H, Sànchez-Bayo F (2012) Time-dependent toxicity of neonicotinoids and other toxicants: implications for a new approach to risk assessment. J Environ Anal Toxicol S4: S4-001.
134. Tennekes HA, Sànchez-Bayo F (2013) The molecular basis of simple relationships between exposure concentration and toxic effects with time. Toxicology 309: 39–51.
135. Laycock I, Cresswell JE (2013) Repression and recuperation of brood production in *Bombus terrestris* bumble bees exposed to a pulse of the neonicotinoid pesticide imidacloprid. PLOS ONE 8: e79872.
136. Decourtye A, Henry M, Desneux N (2013) Environment: Overhaul pesticide testing on bees. Nature 497: 188.
137. Osborne JL (2012) Ecology: Bumblebees and pesticides. Nature 491: 43–45.

3

Associations between Rice, Noodle, and Bread Intake and Sleep Quality in Japanese Men and Women

Satoko Yoneyama[1]*, Masaru Sakurai[1], Koshi Nakamura[1], Yuko Morikawa[1], Katsuyuki Miura[2], Motoko Nakashima[3], Katsushi Yoshita[4], Masao Ishizaki[5], Teruhiko Kido[6], Yuchi Naruse[7], Kazuhiro Nogawa[8], Yasushi Suwazono[8], Satoshi Sasaki[9], Hideaki Nakagawa[1]

1 Department of Epidemiology and Public Health, Kanazawa Medical University, Ishikawa, Japan, **2** Department of Health Science, Shiga University of Medical Science, Otsu, Japan, **3** Department of Community Health Nursing, School of Nursing, Kanazawa Medical University, Ishikawa, Japan, **4** Department of Food and Human Health Science Osaka City University, Graduate School of Human Life Science, Osaka, Japan, **5** Department of Social and Environmental Medicine, Kanazawa Medical University, Ishikawa, Japan, **6** School of Health Science, College of Medical, Pharmaceutical and Health Science, Kanazawa University, Kanazawa, Japan, **7** Department of Human Science and Fundamental Nursing, Toyama University School of Nursing, Toyama, Japan, **8** Department of Occupational and Environmental Medicine, Graduate School of Medicine, Chiba University, Chiba, Japan, **9** Department of Social and Preventive Epidemiology, the University of Tokyo, Tokyo, Japan

Abstract

Background: Previous studies have shown that a diet with a high-glycemic index is associated with good sleep quality. Therefore, we investigated the association of sleep quality with the intake of 3 common starchy foods with different glycemic indexes–rice, bread, and noodles–as well as the dietary glycemic index in a Japanese population.

Methods: The participants were 1,848 men and women between 20 and 60 years of age. Rice, bread, and noodle consumption was evaluated using a self-administered diet history questionnaire. Sleep quality was evaluated by using the Japanese version of the Pittsburgh Sleep Quality Index, and a global score >5.5 was considered to indicate poor sleep.

Results: Multivariate-adjusted odds ratios (95% confidence intervals) for poor sleep across the quintiles of rice consumption were 1.00 (reference), 0.68 (0.49–0.93), 0.61 (0.43–0.85), 0.59 (0.42–0.85), and 0.54 (0.37–0.81) (p for trend = 0.015); those for the quintiles of noodle consumption were 1.00 (reference), 1.25 (0.90–1.74), 1.05 (0.75–1.47), 1.31 (0.94–1.82), and 1.82 (1.31–2.51) (p for trend = 0.002). Bread intake was not associated with sleep quality. A higher dietary glycemic index was significantly associated with a lower risk of poor sleep (p for trend = 0.020).

Conclusion: A high dietary glycemic index and high rice consumption are significantly associated with good sleep in Japanese men and women, whereas bread intake is not associated with sleep quality and noodle consumption is associated with poor sleep. The different associations of these starchy foods with sleep quality might be attributable to the different glycemic index of each food.

Editor: Guy Brock, University of Louisville, United States of America

Funding: This research was supported by a Grant-in-Aid from the Ministry of Health, Labour, and Welfare, Health and Labor Sciences research grants, Japan (H18-Junkankitou[Seishuu]- Ippan-012, H19-Junkankitou [Seishuu]-Ippan-012, H19-Junkankitou [Seishuu]-Ippan- 021, H20-Junkankitou [Seishuu]-Ippan-013, H22-Junkankitou [Seishuu]-Ippan-005, H23-Junkankitou [Seishuu]-Ippan-005) and the Japan Arteriosclerosis Prevention Fund. The funders had no role in study design, data collection and analysis.

Competing Interests: The authers have declared that no competing interests exist.

* Email: yoneyama@kanazawa-med.ac.jp

Introduction

Sleep quality is known to be a function of sleep duration and latency [1]. Epidemiological studies have shown that short sleep duration is associated with increased mortality [2,3], poor mood [2,4], chronic health conditions (e.g., obesity and metabolic syndrome) [2,5], cardiovascular disease and diabetes [2,6], hypertension [2,7], and poor self-related health and quality of life [2,8]. Moreover, previous studies have shown that dietary factors affect sleep quality. A cross-sectional study of children younger than 2 years of age showed that the consumption of a meal with a high-glycemic index (GI) in the evening was associated with longer sleep duration [9]. In addition a clinical trial showed that sleep onset latency is reduced by approximately 10 minutes after the consumption of a carbohydrate-rich evening meal with a high-GI compared with an evening meal with a low-GI [10]. These data suggest that sleep quality is influenced by the carbohydrate-based GI of the meals.

The dietary GI of the general Japanese population is approximately 70 [11–13], this is considerably higher than the dietary GI in predominantly Western populations (i.e., European, Australian, and North American), which ranges from 48 to 60 [14–16]. This difference may be due to disparities in the average intakes of different foods that contribute to the GI. Rice is a common starchy food in the Japanese diet, as approximately 70% of the cereals consumed are rice [17], and rice accounts for 59% of the dietary GI [11–13]. However, no studies have evaluated the associations of rice or other common staple foods such as bread and noodles with sleep quality in a Japanese population.

This study investigated the associations between sleep quality and intake of carbohydrate-based staple foods (i.e., rice, bread, and noodles) as well as the dietary GI and glycemic load (GL) in a Japanese population.

Methods

Participants

The study population comprised 7,306 employees of a factory that produces zippers and aluminum sashes in Toyama Prefecture, Japan. The Industrial Health and Safety Law in Japan requires that employers offer annual health examinations to all of their employees. The present study included data on 2,255 white-collar daytime workers between 20 and 60 years of age. White-collar workers were studied because many blue-collar workers are involved in shift work, making it difficult to evaluate sleep quality.

A questionnaire about diet was completed by 1,977 (88%) of the white-collar daytime workers in 2003, and a questionnaire about sleep was completed by 2003 (94%) of the worker in 2004. In total, 1,858 (82%) of the workers provided complete data on both questionnaires. Ten participants with extremely low or high energy intake (i.e., <500 or >4,000 kcal/day) were excluded from the study. Thus, data on 1,848 white-collar daytime workers (1,164 men and 684 women) were included in the analysis.

Data collection

The annual health examination included a medical history, physical examination, and anthropometric measurements. Body mass index was calculated as weight divided by height squared (kg/m^2). A questionnaire was used to identify health-related behaviors including smoking status (i.e., current, previous, or never), and habitual exercise; habitual exercise was assessed as hours per week spent on leisure time physical activities and was expressed as metabolic equivalent hours per week (MET-h/week).

Dietary assessment and calculation of the dietary GI and GL

A self-administered diet history questionnaire (DHQ) was used to assess dietary habits during the preceding month. [18,19]. The DHQ was developed to estimate the respondents' dietary intake of macronutrients and micronutrients for use in epidemiological studies in Japan. Detailed descriptions of the methods used to calculate dietary intakes and the validity of the DHQ have been reported previously [18,19]. Estimates of dietary intake for 147 food and beverage items, energy, protein, fat, total carbohydrate, and alcohol in 2003 were calculated using an ad hoc computer algorithm developed for the DHQ that was based on the Standard Tables of Food Composition in Japan [20]. The DHQ evaluates the consumption of 19 staple foods (i.e., rice, noodles, and other wheat foods). The intake frequency of each staple food for breakfast, lunch, dinner, and snack/midnight snack in 1 week was evaluated. For rice, the type of rice (i.e., white rice, white rice mixed with barley, white rice with germ, 50% polished rice, 70% polished rice, or brown rice) and serving size (i.e., number and size; cups for children, women, and men, and small and large bowls were defined as 110, 140, 170, 220, and 250 g, respectively) were evaluated. Similarly, the types of bread and noodles were evaluated. Bread was classified as white bread, buttered bread, cake bread, bread containing cream and sweet bean paste, pizza, *okonomiyaki* (Japanese "pizza," which contains shredded cabbage and dough cooked in a frying pan), or Japanese-style pancakes (small pancakes containing flour, sugar, and egg, cooked in a frying pan). Noodles were classified as Japanese noodles (i.e., buckwheat and Japanese white noodles), instant noodles, Chinese noodles, or pasta [12]. The DHQ also includes the frequencies of skipping breakfast, lunch, dinner per week. Of the 147 food and beverage items included in the DHQ, 6 (4.1%) are alcoholic beverages, 8 (5.4%) contain no available carbohydrates, and 63 (42.9%) contain less than 3.5 g available carbohydrate per serving. Therefore, the dietary GI and GL were calculated on the basis of the remaining 70 items [11,21]. The GI databases used were an international table of GI [22], a report on the GI values of Japanese foods [23], a report on GI values published after the publication of the international GI tables [24], and an online database provided by the Sydney University Glycemic Index Research Service [25]. The GIs of all foods in the DHQ have been published elsewhere [11]. Although there are concerns regarding the utility of the GI for mixed meals (i.e., overall diet) [26,27], many studies have shown that the GI of mixed meals can be predicted on the basis of the GI value of each of the component foods [28]. We calculated the dietary GI as the sum of the percentage contribution of each food multiplied by their respective GI values. Dietary GL was calculated by multiplying the dietary GI by the total daily carbohydrate intake and dividing by 100. We used energy-adjusted values calculated using the density method (per 1,000 kcal) for GL [21]. The reproducibility and relative validity of the dietary GI and GL assessed using the DHQ have been reported elsewhere [21].

Sleep assessment

Sleep quality in the previous month was assessed by using the Japanese version of the Pittsburgh Sleep Quality Index questionnaire (PSQI-J) [29], which was developed from the original questionnaire, the PSQI [1]. In brief, the PSQI-J is a standardized self-administered questionnaire for assessing sleep quality that includes the following 7 components: subjective sleep quality, sleep latency, sleep duration, habitual sleep efficiency, sleep disturbances, use of sleep medication, and daytime dysfunction. Each component is weighted equally on a scale of 0 to 3, and the scores for each component are then summed to yield a PSQI-J global score ranging from 0 to 21, higher scores indicate poorer sleep quality. Participants completed the PSQI-J at home in 5–10 minutes, and the responses were then reviewed by a well-trained nurse.

Statistical analysis

When the PSQI-J component scores of the male and female participants were compared, sleep duration was significantly shorter in men than in women ($p = 0.011$); however, there were no significant differences in the other component scores including the PSQI-J global score between sexes. Therefore, all analyses were performed in the whole population, (i.e., not stratified by sex). In this study, we used energy density values for macronutrients and alcohol (% of energy [% energy]) and for food intakes (weight per 1000 kcal [g/1000 kcal]).

"Poor sleep," was defined as a PSQI-J global score >5.5 [29]. In a previous study, using a cut-off of 5.5 for the PSQI-J global score provided estimates with a sensitivity and specificity of 85.7% and 86.6% for primary insomnia, 80.0% and 86.6% for major depression, and 83.3% and 86.6% for schizophrenia, respectively [29]. Rice, bread, and noodle intake as well as the GI and GL were categorized into quintiles. Analysis of covariance was used to evaluate the means of each PSQI-J component score adjusted for age, sex and total energy intake. The prevalence of poor sleep in each quintile was compared using the χ^2 test. Odds ratios (ORs) with 95% confidence intervals (95% CIs) for poor sleep were

Table 1. Characteristics of study participants by quintiles of dietary rice, bread, and noodle intake as well as dietary glycemic index and glycemic load ($N = 1,848$).

	Q1 (lowest)	Q2	Q3 (middle)	Q4	Q5 (highest)	p value[a]
Rice (range, g/1,000 kcal)	<132.7	132.7–168.4	168.5–202.2	202.3–249.1	≥249.2	
Male (%)	48.0	54.5	61.7	74.1	76.7	<0.001
Age (years)	37.6 ± 10.1	39.2 ± 9.5	39.9 ± 9.8	39.9 ± 9.9	41.7 ± 10.2	0.001
Body mass index (kg/m^2)	22.4 ± 3.1	22.5 ± 3.0	23.1 ± 3.2	22.9 ± 3.2	23.0 ± 3.0	0.060
Habitual exercise level (METs/week)	1.0 ± 12.1	1.1 ± 8.7	0.6 ± 4.0	0.8 ± 9.5	1.2 ± 8.5	0.823
Current smokers (%)	28.0	26.6	30.4	32.8	37.5	0.026
Skip breakfast (%)	64.5	42.1	35.9	18.3	11.7	<0.001
Total energy intake (kcal/day)	2012 ± 582	2034 ± 491	1942 ± 452	1870 ± 410	1731 ± 414	<0.001
Protein intake (%kcal)	17.9 ± 2.9	17.8 ± 2.6	17.2 ± 2.5	16.5 ± 2.4	15.5 ± 2.4	<0.001
Fat intake (%kcal)	31.8 ± 6.4	29.7 ± 5.4	26.9 ± 5.4	23.8 ± 5.0	19.8 ± 4.9	<0.001
Carbohydrate intake (%kcal)	52.0 ± 7.1	54.5 ± 5.6	57.3 ± 5.4	60.3 ± 5.6	65.3 ± 5.9	<0.001
Alcohol consumption (%kcal)	5.0 ± 7.5	4.4 ± 6.4	4.5 ± 6.6	4.7 ± 5.8	4.1 ± 6.1	0.603
Bread intake (g/1,000 kcal)	44.9 ± 32.2	35.4 ± 24.5	30.2 ± 24.0	20.9 ± 21.8	12.9 ± 18.9	<0.001
Noodle intake (g/1,000 kcal)	47.9 ± 38.1	37.7 ± 30.4	34.4 ± 29.6	37.3 ± 35.7	27.0 ± 29.0	<0.001
Dietary GI	63.8 ± 4.1	66.6 ± 2.7	68.1 ± 2.9	69.7 ± 2.5	71.6 ± 3.0	<0.001
Dietary GL (/1,000 kcal)	141 ± 46	157 ± 40	163 ± 42	171 ± 39	179 ± 44	<0.001
Bread (range, g/1,000 kcal)	0	0.1–14.8	14.9–30.1	30.2–47.2	≥47.3	
Male (%)	73.9	66.1	58.0	58.0	58.5	<0.001
Age (years)	41.1 ± 10.0	39.9 ± 9.8	39.7 ± 9.9	39.5 ± 10.2	38.9 ± 9.8	0.045
Body mass index (kg/m^2)	23.1 ± 3.0	23.0 ± 3.3	22.8 ± 3.2	22.6 ± 3.2	22.5 ± 2.9	0.082
Habitual exercise level (METs/week)	1.3 ± 10.7	0.5 ± 2.4	1.3 ± 10.5	0.7 ± 5.1	0.9 ± 10.3	0.610
Current smokers (%)	40.7	29.5	29.2	26.0	29.2	0.284
Skip breakfast (%)	17.3	10.7	20.6	50.9	72.4	<0.001
Total energy intake (kcal/day)	1811 ± 445	2031 ± 508	1995 ± 508	1927 ± 405	1803 ± 472	<0.001
Protein intake (%kcal)	16.3 ± 3.0	17.0 ± 2.7	17.2 ± 2.7	17.3 ± 2.4	16.8 ± 2.3	<0.001
Fat intake (%kcal)	22.5 ± 7.1	25.7 ± 6.5	27.3 ± 6.5	27.8 ± 6.2	26.6 ± 6.2	<0.001
Carbohydrate intake (%kcal)	59.0 ± 8.6	57.8 ± 7.5	58.2 ± 7.0	57.4 ± 6.5	59.2 ± 6.9	0.003
Alcohol consumption (%kcal)	7.43 ± 8.36	5.15 ± 6.80	3.12 ± 4.61	3.40 ± 4.86	3.28 ± 5.38	<0.001
Rice intake (g/1,000 kcal)	239.1 ± 71.4	206.3 ± 62.9	185.6 ± 61.3	165.1 ± 52.7	154.8 ± 59.5	<0.001
Noodle intake (g/1,000 kcal)	35.3 ± 39.6	35.6 ± 27.5	37.9 ± 29.8	36.1 ± 32.1	34.7 ± 33.0	0.733
Dietary GI	70.1 ± 4.2	68.9 ± 3.6	67.9 ± 3.6	67.3 ± 3.6	67.2 ± 3.6	<0.001
Dietary GL (/1,000 kcal)	160 ± 44	172 ± 45	170 ± 46	161 ± 39	157 ± 42	<0.001
Noodles (range, g/1,000 kcal)	<7.4	7.4–23.3	23.4–36.5	36.6–57.4	≥57.5	
Male (%)	66.0	56.5	62.8	63.3	66.4	0.330
Age (years)	40.9 ± 10.2	39.9 ± 10.0	40.2 ± 9.5	38.6 ± 10.0	39.7 ± 9.9	0.037

Table 1. Cont.

	Q1 (lowest)	Q2	Q3 (middle)	Q4	Q5 (highest)	p value[a]
Body mass index (kg/m^2)	22.9 ± 3.1	22.9 ± 3.1	22.6 ± 2.9	22.7 ± 3.1	23.0 ± 3.4	0.498
Habitual exercise level (METs/week)	0.6 ± 7.2	1.2 ± 10.9	0.8 ± 5.4	1.2 ± 8.7	0.8 ± 9.8	0.864
Current smokers (%)	26.2	27.3	32.2	33.0	27.9	0.801
Skip breakfast (%)	39.5	37.8	28.8	33.4	32.8	0.584
Total energy intake (kcal/day)	1833 ± 455	1945 ± 470	1997 ± 421	1917 ± 509	1861 ± 509	<0.001
Protein intake (%kcal)	16.6 ± 2.9	17.3 ± 2.6	17.0 ± 2.6	16.9 ± 2.8	16.8 ± 2.4	0.006
Fat intake (%kcal)	25.5 ± 6.9	27.4 ± 6.5	26.9 ± 6.6	26.0 ± 6.7	23.9 ± 6.5	<0.001
Carbohydrate intake (%kcal)	58.8 ± 7.6	57.8 ± 6.9	57.1 ± 6.8	58.3 ± 7.3	59.8 ± 7.9	<0.001
Alcohol consumption (%kcal)	4.72 ± 6.90	3.48 ± 5.39	4.86 ± 6.77	4.52 ± 6.38	4.95 ± 6.40	0.012
Rice intake (g/1,000 kcal)	220.1 ± 72.8	188.8 ± 66.3	185.1 ± 64.0	184.3 ± 64.5	174.7 ± 69.0	<0.001
Bread intake (g/1,000 kcal)	25.9 ± 28.2	31.9 ± 27.9	25.6 ± 22.1	27.0 ± 25.0	27.4 ± 26.7	0.008
Dietary GI	70.5 ± 4.0	68.9 ± 3.5	68.5 ± 3.4	67.6 ± 3.4	66.0 ± 3.7	<0.001
Dietary GL (/1,000 kcal)	163 ± 41	166 ± 43	168 ± 41	163 ± 44	159 ± 50	0.094
Dietary GI (range)	<65.3	65.3–67.7	67.8–69.5	69.6–71.6	≥71.7	
Male (%)	52.4	53.5	62.3	69.2	77.5	0.011
Age (years)	38.7 ± 10.3	40.2 ± 9.6	39.1 ± 9.6	39.6 ± 10.0	41.6 ± 9.9	<0.001
Body mass index (kg/m^2)	22.6 ± 3.3	22.7 ± 3.2	22.7 ± 2.9	23.0 ± 3.3	23.1 ± 2.8	0.172
Habitual exercise level (METs/week)	1.3 ± 12.7	0.4 ± 1.9	1.1 ± 10.6	0.6 ± 3.8	1.2 ± 8.9	0.466
Current smokers (%)	27.5	24.9	33.7	31.5	38.3	0.605
Skip breakfast (%)	50.8	39.2	35.5	28.4	18.4	<0.001
Total energy intake (kcal/day)	2017 ± 560	1977 ± 469	1896 ± 449	1858 ± 426	1804 ± 439	<0.001
Protein intake (%kcal)	17.7 ± 2.7	17.9 ± 2.5	16.8 ± 2.3	16.5 ± 2.5	15.7 ± 2.6	<0.001
Fat intake (%kcal)	28.7 ± 6.6	27.9 ± 6.2	26.4 ± 6.4	24.5 ± 6.2	22.3 ± 6.4	<0.001
Carbohydrate intake (%kcal)	56.0 ± 7.4	56.9 ± 6.9	58.8 ± 7.1	59.0 ± 6.9	61.1 ± 7.4	<0.001
Alcohol consumption (%kcal)	4.1 ± 6.3	3.6 ± 5.3	3.6 ± 5.2	5.5 ± 7.5	5.7 ± 7.1	<0.001
Rice intake (g/1,000 kcal)	128.9 ± 55.5	160.4 ± 44.0	187.3 ± 50.2	214.9 ± 46.8	261.7 ± 61.5	<0.001
Bread intake (g/1,000 kcal)	35.5 ± 29.2	32.6 ± 24.8	30.6 ± 26.0	24.5 ± 24.1	14.6 ± 20.6	<0.001
Noodle intake (g/1,000 kcal)	53.9 ± 40.2	46.5 ± 34.0	34.5 ± 28.8	27.3 ± 23.7	17.4 ± 19.3	<0.001
Dietary GL (range,/1,000 kcal)	<128	128–149	150–169	170–194	≥195	
Male (%)	47.8	48.1	64.8	70.3	84.0	<0.001
Age (years)	37.7 ± 9.7	39.4 ± 9.7	40.4 ± 9.6	41.3 ± 10.1	40.4 ± 10.2	<0.001
Body mass index (kg/m^2)	22.0 ± 3.1	22.5 ± 3.1	23.1 ± 3.3	23.1 ± 3.0	23.4 ± 2.9	<0.001
Habitual exercise level (METs/week)	0.4 ± 2.6	0.8 ± 7.7	0.3 ± 1.1	1.3 ± 12.4	2.0 ± 12.3	<0.001
Current smokers (%)	33.7	27.4	27.7	33.9	33.2	0.301
Skip breakfast (%)	58.9	36.8	31.7	24.1	20.9	<0.001

Table 1. Cont.

	Q1 (lowest)	Q2	Q3 (middle)	Q4	Q5 (highest)	p value[a]
Total energy intake (kcal/day)	1472 ± 305	1695 ± 272	1870 ± 302.9	2052 ± 331	2465 ± 450	<0.001
Protein intake (%kcal)	17.5 ± 3.0	17.2 ± 2.6	17.1 ± 2.6	16.8 ± 2.5	15.9 ± 2.4	<0.001
Fat intake (%kcal)	28.2 ± 7.1	26.6 ± 6.4	25.9 ± 6.6	25.1 ± 6.6	24.0 ± 6.4	<0.001
Carbohydrate intake (%kcal)	53.8 ± 7.4	57.6 ± 6.5	58.5 ± 6.8	59.8 ± 6.8	62.1 ± 6.7	<0.001
Alcohol consumption (%kcal)	6.5 ± 8.8	4.3 ± 5.7	4.2 ± 6.1	4.0 ± 5.2	3.5 ± 5.0	<0.001
Rice intake (g/1,000 kcal)	154.3 ± 64.4	189.4 ± 64.3	197.1 ± 66.5	203.4 ± 65.0	208.9 ± 71.6	<0.001
Bread intake (g/1,000 kcal)	30.7 ± 28.5	27.1 ± 24.7	29.8 ± 28.1	24.4 ± 23.5	25.9 ± 25.2	0.004
Noodle intake (g/1,000 kcal)	41.8 ± 35.7	36.3 ± 30.9	31.1 ± 30.9	34.3 ± 31.1	36.1 ± 34.4	<0.001

GI: glycemic index, GL: glycemic load, METs/week: metabolic equivalent hours per week; Q: quintile.
[a]The χ^2 test was used to analyze categorical variables, and linear regression analysis was used to calculate *p*-values for trends for continuous variables.

calculated using multiple logistic regression analyses. ORs were first adjusted for age (years; continuous) and sex (age- and sex-adjusted model) and then for body mass index (kg/m^2; continuous), smoking status (i.e., current, previous, or never; dummy variable), habitual exercise (MET-h/week; continuous), alcohol consumption (percentage of energy; continuous), frequency of breakfast consumption per week (i.e., 0–3, 4–6, or 7 days/week; dummy variable), rice intake (for the multivariate analyses of bread and noodle intake; continuous), bread intake (for the multivariate analyses of rice and noodle intake; continuous), and noodle intake (for the multivariate analyses of rice and bread intake; continuous). The *p*-values for linear trends were calculated by using the median value of each quintile. Furthermore, each food, dietary GI, and dietary GL was included in the logistic regression analyses as continuous variables, and the ORs for an increment of 1 standard deviation in these variables were calculated. Statistical analyses were performed with Statistical Analysis System version 9.3 (SAS Institute Inc., Cary, NC, USA). The level of significance was set at $p<0.05$.

Ethical considerations

Written informed consent was not obtained from the participants. The design of the present study was approved by the occupational safety and health committee of the subject company, which consisted of employee representatives. Employees were informed of the study design and of the right to refuse to participate in the study in the study documents. Participants who answered the questionnaire were regarded as having consented to the survey. Linkable anonymized data were provided by the company to ensure that individuals would not be identifiable by the researchers. This study was approved by the Institutional Review Committee of Kanazawa Medical University for Ethical Issues.

Results

Table 1 shows the characteristics of the 1,848 study participants stratified by rice, bread, and noodle consumption quintiles as well as dietary GI and GL quintiles. Higher rice intake was significantly associated with older age ($p = 0.001$), higher carbohydrate intake ($p<0.001$), higher dietary GI ($p<0.001$), higher GL ($p<0.001$), lower bread intake ($p<0.001$), lower noodle intake ($p<0.001$), lower frequency of breakfast consumption ($p<0.001$), and a lower probability of being a current smoker ($p = 0.026$). Body mass index, alcohol consumption, and habitual exercise were not significantly associated with rice intake. Higher bread intake was significantly associated with a higher frequency of breakfast consumption ($p<0.001$), female sex ($p<0.001$), younger age ($p = 0.045$), lower alcohol consumption ($p<0.001$), lower rice intake ($p<0.001$), lower dietary GI ($p<0.001$), and lower dietary GL ($p<0.001$). Habitual exercise and smoking status were not significantly associated with bread intake. Higher noodle intake was significantly associated with higher carbohydrate intake ($p<0.001$), higher bread intake ($p = 0.008$), higher alcohol consumption ($p = 0.012$), lower rice intake ($p<0.001$), and lower dietary GI ($p<0.001$). Sex, smoking status, and frequency of breakfast consumption were not significantly associated with noodle intake. Increasing GI quintiles were significantly associated with older age ($p<0.001$), alcohol consumption ($p<0.001$), higher carbohydrate intake ($p<0.001$), higher rice intake ($p<0.001$), lower bread intake ($p<0.001$), lower noodle intake ($p<0.001$), and lower frequency of breakfast consumption ($p<0.001$). Habitual exercise and smoking status were not significantly associated with the dietary GI.

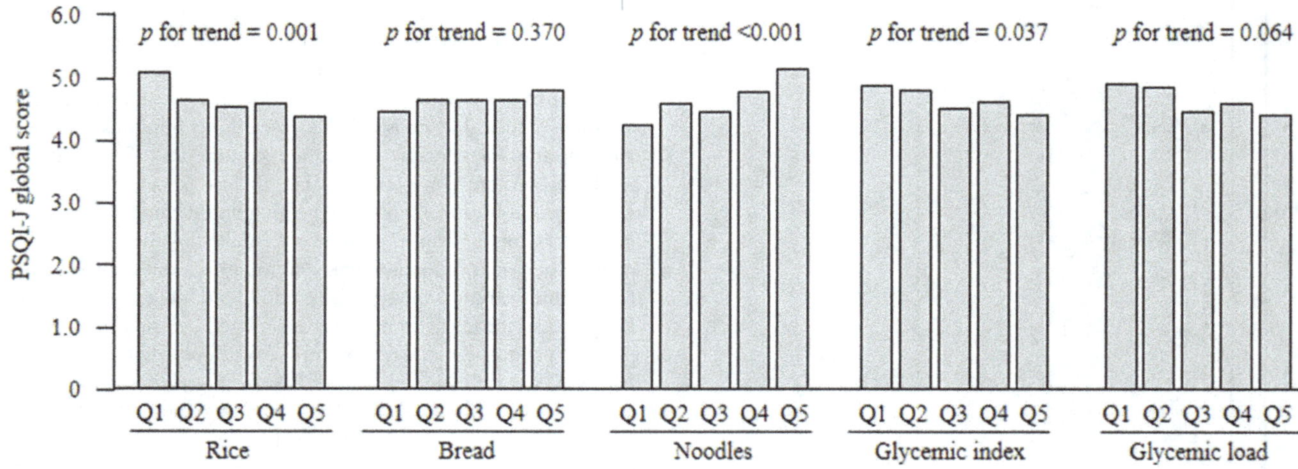

Figure 1. PSQI-J global scores for quintiles of starchy food intake, dietary glycemic index, and glycemic load. Mean PSQI-J global scores were adjusted for age, sex, and total energy intake (kcal/day, continuous), by using the analysis of covariance model. PSQI-J: Japanese version of the Pittsburgh Quality Index; Q: quintile.

Figure 1 shows the mean PSQI-J global score according to rice, bread, and noodle consumption quintile as well as dietary GI and GL quintiles adjusted for age, sex and total energy intake. Higher rice intake and higher GI were significantly associated with a lower PSQI-J global score ($p = 0.001$ and $p = 0.037$, respectively), and higher noodle intake was significantly associated with a higher PSQI-J global score ($p<0.001$). Table 2 shows sleep duration and PSQI-J component scores according to rice, bread, and noodle consumption quintile as well as dietary GI and GL quintile. Higher rice intake was significantly associated with lower scores for poor sleep duration ($p = 0.003$) but was not associated with any other component of sleep quality. Higher noodle intake was significantly associated with a higher frequency of sleep disturbance ($p<0.001$), higher levels of daytime dysfunction ($p = 0.005$), increased use of sleep medication ($p = 0.008$), poorer subjective sleep quality ($p = 0.021$), and longer sleep latency ($p = 0.049$). A higher dietary GI was significantly associated with lower scores for poor sleep duration ($p = 0.013$) but not with other PSQI-J components. These associations remained even after adjusting for age, sex, and total energy intake (data not tabulated).

The multivariate-adjusted ORs (quintile, 95%CI) for the prevalence of poor sleep across the quintiles of rice intake were 1.00 (reference), 0.68 (0.49–0.93), 0.61 (0.43–0.85), 0.59 (0.42–0.85), and 0.54 (0.37–0.81), respectively, indicating that rice intake had a significant positive association with better sleep (p for linear trend = 0.015) (Table 3). In contrast, the multivariate-adjusted ORs across the quintiles of noodle intake were 1.00 (reference), 1.25 (0.90–1.74), 1.05 (0.75–1.47), 1.31 (0.94–1.82), and 1.82 (1.31–2.51), respectively, indicating that noodle consumption was significantly associated with poor sleep (p for linear trend = 0.002) (Table 3). These associations did not change even after further adjusting for vegetable, meat, and fish intake (data not shown). Dietary GI was also associated with good sleep (p for trend = 0.020), whereas dietary GL was not (p for trend = 0.092).

Discussion

This study evaluated the association between sleep quality and the intake of common starchy foods (i.e., rice, bread, and noodles) as well as the dietary GI and GL in a Japanese population. Rice consumption was positively associated with sleep quality. In contrast, noodle consumption had a significant inverse association with sleep quality. Furthermore, a significant positive relationship between dietary GI and sleep quality was observed. Because rice is a major contributor to the dietary GI among Japanese people, differences between the GI values of rice, bread, and noodles may influence their sleep quality.

The present results show that higher consumption of rice, which is the main contributor to the dietary GI in Japanese foods, and the dietary GI itself are closely associated with a lower PSQI-J global score, i.e., good sleep. In a previous cross-sectional study of children younger than 2 years of age, the consumption of an evening meal with a high-GI was associated with longer sleep duration compared with the consumption of an evening meal with a low-GI [9]. The present results are consistent with these previous findings, because rice intake and the dietary GI were associated with sleep duration but not sleep latency in the present study. In contrast, in a clinical trial of 12 healthy young men, a carbohydrate-based meal with a high-GI was significantly associated with a shortening of sleep onset latency compared with a meal with a low-GI and was most effective when consumed 4 hours before going to sleep [10]. We assessed daily rice consumption and the dietary GI, but not rice consumption or the GI of evening meals, which may have affected the present results.

A high dietary GI may affect sleep quality via the effects of tryptophan (TRP) and melatonin [30–36]. A previous study showed that both carbohydrate intake and a meal with a high-GI increase the ratio of TRP to other large neutral amino acids (TRP/LNAA) after the meal, compared with a meal with a low-GI [37]. LNAA and TRP are competitively transported across the blood–brain barrier, and a higher TRP/LNAA ratio would result in more TRP being transported into the brain. In the brain, TRP is converted into serotonin and then to melatonin, which induces sleep [30–36].

Similar to the dietary GI, rice consumption was significantly associated with a low PSQI-J global score in the present study. Rice, especially white rice, is a common starchy food eaten by Japanese people; it accounts for approximately 28% of the daily energy intake and 70% of cereal intake [17]. Furthermore, white rice accounts for 59% of the dietary GI for in the Japanese diet [11–13]. Therefore, rice intake would affect sleep quality via the effect of the GI. In addition, rice contains high levels of melatonin [38], which may also favor good sleep.

Table 2. PSQI-J component scores by quintiles of rice, bread, and noodle intake as well as dietary glycemic index and glycemic load.

	Q1 (lowest)	Q2	Q3 (middle)	Q4	Q5 (highest)	P value[a]
Rice						
Sleep duration (hours)	6.2 ± 0.9	6.3 ± 0.8	6.4 ± 0.8	6.4 ± 0.9	6.4 ± 0.8	0.008
PSQI-J						
Subjective sleep quality	1.26 ± 0.69	1.16 ± 0.64	1.18 ± 0.68	1.15 ± 0.64	1.08 ± 0.63	0.063
Sleep latency	0.72 ± 0.77	0.70 ± 0.74	0.70 ± 0.77	0.67 ± 0.74	0.67 ± 0.75	0.630
Sleep duration	1.04 ± 0.84	0.91 ± 0.74	0.81 ± 0.70	0.84 ± 0.75	0.79 ± 0.73	0.003
Habitual sleep efficiency	0.13 ± 0.50	0.06 ± 0.25	0.07 ± 0.31	0.08 ± 0.34	0.09 ± 0.40	0.787
Sleep disturbances	0.93 ± 0.51	0.94 ± 0.51	0.90 ± 0.50	0.89 ± 0.49	0.86 ± 0.51	0.290
Use of sleep medication	0.08 ± 0.40	0.04 ± 0.26	0.05 ± 0.33	0.06 ± 0.36	0.03 ± 0.29	0.773
Daytime dysfunction	0.99 ± 0.73	0.91 ± 0.67	0.87 ± 0.74	0.96 ± 0.72	0.86 ± 0.71	0.211
Bread						
Sleep duration (hours)	6.4 ± 0.8	6.4 ± 0.8	6.3 ± 0.8	6.3 ± 0.8	6.2 ± 0.8	0.007
PSQI-J						
Subjective sleep quality	1.13 ± 0.69	1.17 ± 0.60	1.14 ± 0.64	1.17 ± 0.65	1.22 ± 0.69	0.407
Sleep latency	0.71 ± 0.76	0.71 ± 0.75	0.64 ± 0.73	0.69 ± 0.73	0.72 ± 0.78	0.570
Sleep duration	0.77 ± 0.75	0.83 ± 0.74	0.90 ± 0.74	0.92 ± 0.78	0.97 ± 0.78	0.003
Habitual sleep efficiency	0.07 ± 0.30	0.10 ± 0.39	0.10 ± 0.37	0.09 ± 0.41	0.08 ± 0.37	0.706
Sleep disturbances	0.88 ± 0.50	0.94 ± 0.52	0.93 ± 0.50	0.89 ± 0.50	0.90 ± 0.51	0.383
Use of sleep medication	0.05 ± 0.33	0.05 ± 0.32	0.05 ± 0.33	0.04 ± 0.29	0.06 ± 0.38	0.905
Daytime dysfunction	0.89 ± 0.72	0.94 ± 0.71	0.97 ± 0.73	0.91 ± 0.71	0.89 ± 0.69	0.491
Noodles						
Sleep duration (hours)	6.38 ± 0.83	6.32 ± 0.81	6.37 ± 0.80	6.30 ± 0.86	6.27 ± 0.82	0.275
PSQI-J						
Subjective sleep quality	1.11 ± 0.66	1.14 ± 0.66	1.13 ± 0.63	1.22 ± 0.68	1.23 ± 0.65	0.021
Sleep latency	0.64 ± 0.72	0.65 ± 0.70	0.67 ± 0.75	0.72 ± 0.79	0.79 ± 0.78	0.049
Sleep duration	0.82 ± 0.75	0.91 ± 0.76	0.82 ± 0.73	0.90 ± 0.77	0.94 ± 0.78	0.114
Habitual sleep efficiency	0.05 ± 0.28	0.07 ± 0.37	0.10 ± 0.39	0.09 ± 0.39	0.12 ± 0.40	0.069
Sleep disturbances	0.81 ± 0.52	0.94 ± 0.51	0.87 ± 0.50	0.95 ± 0.49	0.96 ± 0.50	<0.001
Use of sleep medication	0.02 ± 0.23	0.03 ± 0.27	0.03 ± 0.28	0.06 ± 0.36	0.10 ± 0.46	0.008
Daytime dysfunction	0.83 ± 0.72	0.91 ± 0.70	0.92 ± 0.72	0.90 ± 0.71	1.03 ± 0.70	0.005
Dietary GI						
Sleep duration (hours)	6.3 ± 0.8	6.3 ± 0.8	6.3 ± 0.8	6.4 ± 0.8	6.4 ± 0.8	0.025
PSQI-J						
Subjective sleep quality	1.21 ± 0.68	1.17 ± 0.62	1.16 ± 0.65	1.17 ± 0.70	1.11 ± 0.63	0.279
Sleep latency	0.73 ± 0.76	0.74 ± 0.76	0.64 ± 0.76	0.66 ± 0.74	0.69 ± 0.72	0.382

Table 2. Cont.

	Q1 (lowest)	Q2	Q3 (middle)	Q4	Q5 (highest)	P value[a]
Sleep duration	0.98 ± 0.78	0.91 ± 0.78	0.88 ± 0.74	0.84 ± 0.76	0.79 ± 0.73	0.013
Habitual sleep efficiency	0.09 ± 0.38	0.10 ± 0.42	0.09 ± 0.36	0.08 ± 0.34	0.07 ± 0.36	0.923
Sleep disturbances	0.93 ± 0.51	0.94 ± 0.50	0.88 ± 0.51	0.91 ± 0.50	0.87 ± 0.50	0.204
Use of sleep medication	0.06 ± 0.32	0.09 ± 0.45	0.03 ± 0.29	0.05 ± 0.35	0.02 ± 0.21	0.065
Daytime dysfunction	0.96 ± 0.71	0.91 ± 0.71	0.88 ± 0.71	0.94 ± 0.72	0.89 ± 0.71	0.561
Dietary GL						
Sleep duration (hours)	6.3 ± 0.8	6.3 ± 0.8	6.3 ± 0.8	6.4 ± 0.8	6.4 ± 0.8	0.067
PSQI-J						
Subjective sleep quality	1.15 ± 0.66	1.19 ± 0.66	1.13 ± 0.62	1.15 ± 0.64	1.20 ± 0.71	0.515
Sleep latency	0.71 ± 0.75	0.76 ± 0.77	0.62 ± 0.74	0.67 ± 0.73	0.71 ± 0.77	0.159
Sleep duration	0.94 ± 0.81	0.91 ± 0.74	0.87 ± 0.72	0.82 ± 0.76	0.85 ± 0.77	0.241
Habitual sleep efficiency	0.12 ± 0.46	0.09 ± 0.39	0.07 ± 0.34	0.09 ± 0.35	0.07 ± 0.30	0.370
Sleep disturbances	0.87 ± 0.50	0.92 ± 0.48	0.86 ± 0.52	0.96 ± 0.48	0.91 ± 0.53	0.041
Use of sleep medication	0.04 ± 0.33	0.07 ± 0.37	0.05 ± 0.32	0.06 ± 0.40	0.02 ± 0.20	0.388
Daytime dysfunction	0.94 ± 0.72	0.88 ± 0.70	0.89 ± 0.71	0.92 ± 0.71	0.96 ± 0.73	0.537

PSQI-J, the Japanese version of the Pittsburgh Sleep Quality Index; GI, glycemic index; GL, glycemic load; Q: quintile.
[a]Linear regression analyses were used to assess the linear trends between sleep duration and each PSQI-J component score across the quintiles of starchy food intake, dietary GI, and dietary GL by using the median value of each quintile.

Table 3. ORs for the prevalence of poor sleep[a] in each quintile of dietary rice, bread, and noodle intake as well as dietary glycemic index and glycemic load.

	Q1	Q2	Q3	Q4	Q5	p^b value	Continuous[c]	P value
	(lowest)		(middle)		(highest)		(1 SD increment)	
Rice								
Prevalence of poor sleep (%)	39.0	30.7	28.0	28.0	26.0	<0.001		
Age-, sex-adjusted OR	1	0.69	0.60	0.59	0.54	0.001	0.85	0.010
(95%CI)	(reference)	(0.51, 0.94)	(0.44, 0.82)	(0.43, 0.81)	(0.39, 0.74)		(0.76, 0.96)	
Multivariate-adjusted OR[d]	1	0.68	0.61	0.59	0.54	0.015	0.87	0.045
(95%CI)	(reference)	(0.49, 0.93)	(0.43, 0.85)	(0.42, 0.85)	(0.37, 0.81)		(0.76, 1.00)	
Bread								
Prevalence of poor sleep (%)	27.7	30.1	29.5	31.3	33.3	0.284		
Age-, sex-adjusted OR	1	1.13	1.10	1.19	1.31	0.545	1.06	0.312
(95%CI)	(reference)	(0.82, 1.55)	(0.80, 1.51)	(0.87, 1.63)	(0.96, 1.78)		(0.95, 1.19)	
Multivariate-adjusted OR[d]	1	1.14	1.04	1.05	1.14	0.921	1.01	0.885
(95%CI)	(reference)	(0.81, 1.60)	(0.74, 1.47)	(0.74, 1.50)	(0.79, 1.63)		(0.89, 1.14)	
Noodle								
Prevalence of poor sleep (%)	24.6	30.5	26.4	31.3	39.0	<0.001		
Age-, sex-adjusted OR	1	1.35	1.10	1.38	1.95	<0.001	1.21	0.001
(95%CI)	(reference)	(0.97, 1.87)	(0.79, 1.53)	(1.00, 1.91)	(1.42, 2.67)		(1.09, 1.35)	
Multivariate-adjusted OR[d]	1	1.25	1.05	1.31	1.82	0.002	1.21	<0.001
95%CI)	(reference)	(0.90, 1.74)	(0.75, 1.47)	(0.94, 1.82)	(1.31, 2.51)		(1.09, 1.35)	
Dietary GI								
Prevalence of poor sleep (%)	35.4	34.3	24.7	28.9	28.5	0.016		
Age-, sex-adjusted OR	1	0.96	0.59	0.73	0.72	0.006	0.82	<0.001
(95%CI)	(reference)	(0.71, 1.30)	(0.43, 0.81)	(0.54, 1.00)	(0.52, 0.99)		(0.74, 0.91)	
Multivariate-adjusted OR[d]	1	0.96	0.60	0.77	0.77	0.020	0.85	0.006
(95%CI)	(reference)	(0.71, 1.31)	(0.44, 0.84)	(0.56, 1.07)	(0.55, 1.07)		(0.76, 0.95)	
Dietary GL								
Prevalence of poor sleep (%)	31.1	30.0	25.8	31.1	33.9	0.379		
Age-, sex-adjusted OR	1	0.96	0.78	1.02	1.14	0.215	1.02	0.721
(95%CI)	(reference)	(0.70, 1.32)	(0.56, 1.08)	(0.74, 1.40)	(0.83, 1.57)		(0.91, 1.14)	
Multivariate-adjusted OR[d]	1	0.98	0.79	1.09	1.27	0.092	1.07	0.284
(95%CI)	(reference)	(0.71, 1.35)	(0.56, 1.11)	(0.77, 1.54)	(0.88, 1.82)		(0.95, 1.21)	

GI, glycemic index; GL, glycemic load, CI, confidence interval; SD, standard deviation; OR: odds ratio; PSQI-J: Japanese version of the Pittsburgh Sleep Quality Index; Q: quintile;

[a]A PSQI-J global score >5.5 indicate poor sleep.

[b]The χ^2 test was used to analyze the prevalence of poor sleep, and logistic regression analysis was used to assess the linear trends of ORs by using the median value of each quintile.

[c]Differences of SD for rice, bread, noodles, dietary GI, and dietary GL were 69.1 g/1,000 kcal, 26.2 g/1,000 kcal, 32.8 g/1,000 kcal, 3.9, and 43.8/1,000 kcal, respectively.

[d]Multivariate models included age (continuous), sex (continuous), Body mass index (kg/m^2; continuous), smoking status (i.e., current, previous, or never; dummy variable), habitual exercise (MET-h/week; continuous), alcohol consumption (percentage of energy; continuous), frequency of breakfast consumption (i.e., 0–3, 4–6, or 7 days/week; dummy variable), rice intake (for the multivariate analyses of bread and noodles; continuous), bread intake (for the multivariate analyses of rice and noodles; continuous), and noodle intake (for the multivariate analyses of rice and bread; continuous).

In contrast, bread intake was not significantly associated with sleep quality, whereas noodle intake was significantly associated with poor sleep. The GIs of the breads and noodles used in the analyses ranged from 51 to 74 and 46 to 47, respectively; these values are lower than 77, which is the GI of Japanese white rice [11]. In a previous study, the TRP/LNAA ratio increased by 17% after a mixed-macronutrient meal with a high-GI (GI = 70) and was higher than that after a mixed-macronutrient meal with a low-GI (GI of 50; 8% increase), even though the amount of carbohydrates was the same in both meals (66.5% energy) [37]. Although noodles are major starchy foods, the GI of noodles is too low to increase the postprandial TRP/LNAA ratio. Furthermore, noodle intake was inversely associated with rice intake. In the present study, higher noodle intake was associated with poor sleep even after adjusting for rice intake. However, it is possible that the adjustment using statistical models is insufficient; thus, the low sleep quality of subjects with higher noodle intake may be due to a lower rice intake. An interventional study is required to investigate the differences in the associations of starchy foods with sleep quality.

Shorter sleep duration is associated with a relative increase and decrease in calories derived from fat and carbohydrates, respectively [39]. In Japan, breakfast often consists of foods low in fat but high in carbohydrates and fiber. Japanese people who eat breakfast generally consume more rice [40]. People with good sleep quality tend to eat breakfast, which may affect the association between rice intake and sleep quality. However, in the present study, lower rice intake was significantly associated with poor sleep even after adjusting for the frequency of breakfast consumption.

In this study, diets with high rice intake and a high GI were significantly associated with good sleep; however, such diets are also reported to be associated with several health problems including obesity, diabetes mellitus, cardiovascular disease, and some cancers [11–16,41–43]. Furthermore, obesity induced by the long-term consumption of a diet with a high-GI may cause sleep apnea syndrome, which may also affect sleep quality. Accordingly, the association between the long-term consumption of meals with a high-GI and sleep quality should be analyzed in greater detail.

One of the strengths of the present study is that we examined rice consumption in a large Japanese population. Japanese people consume approximately 10 times more rice than European and North American people [44]. Thus, it is important to evaluate the association between rice and sleep in people with high rice consumption. Further, this is the first study to investigate the association between rice, bread, and noodle consumption and sleep quality. In addition, the GI and GL were calculated by using responses to a validated questionnaire [21]. Nevertheless, the present study also has several limitations. First, we restricted the final study population to white-collar workers; white-collar work is reported to be strongly correlated with poor sleep quality [45]. Compared with the general Japanese population, the study participants had a similar mean PSQI-J global score but shorter mean sleep duration [46]. Therefore, the results of this study cannot necessarily be generalized to the overall Japanese population. Second, sleep quality is reported to be related to physiological actions and eating behaviors such as skipping meals, eating speed, and watching television during meals [47]; we did not have data on these variables. Third, the DHQ and PSQI-J were evaluated approximately 1 year apart. However, lifestyle factors such as dietary habits and sleep quality are unlikely to change much in 1 year among steadily employed middle-aged people. Fourth, women are reported to have difficulty sleeping at the beginning and end of their menstrual cycle [48,49]; in the present study, we did not obtain data on the menstrual cycles of the female participants. However, when we compared the PSQI-J component and global scores of men and women, nearly identical trends were observed (data not shown). Fifth, the dietary GI and rice consumption data used in this study were daily values, not evening values. As mentioned in the preceding text, the consumption of a meal with a high-GI within 4 hours of going to bed may be an effective way of facilitating sleep [10]. In the present study, the dietary GI and rice intake were significantly associated with sleep duration but not sleep latency. However, dietary intake at dinner may be more closely associated with sleep quality.

In conclusion, the present study indicate that high consumption of rice and a high dietary GI are associated with good sleep, especially good sleep duration. Meanwhile, higher noodle consumption is associated with poor sleep quality. The effects of starchy foods on sleep may differ according to their GI values. Diets with a high-GI, especially those with high rice intake, may contribute to good sleep. Nevertheless, further interventional studies are required to determine appropriate carbohydrate intake during the evening meal to facilitate good sleep.

Author Contributions

Conceived and designed the experiments: SY MS K. Nakamura YM KM MN HN. Performed the experiments: MS K. Nakamura YM KM MN KY MI TK YN HN. Analyzed the data: SY. Contributed reagents/materials/analysis tools: SY MS K. Nakamura YM KM MN KY MI TK YN K. Nogawa YS SS HN. Wrote the paper: SY MS.

References

1. Buysse DJ, Reynolds CF III, Monk TH, Berman SR, Kupfer DJ (1989) The Pittsburgh Sleep Quality Index: a new instrument for psychiatric practice and research. Psychiatry Res 28: 193–213.
2. Bixler E (2009) Sleep and society: an epidemiological perspective. Sleep Med 10: S3–S6.
3. Hublin C, Parlinen M, Koskenvuo M, Kaprio J (2007) Sleep and mortality: a population-based 22-year follow-up study. Sleep 30: 1245–1253.
4. Banks S, Dinges DF (2007) Behavioral and physiological consequences of sleep restriction. J Clin Sleep Med 3: 519–528.
5. Hall MH, Muldoon MF, Jennings JR, Buysse DJ, Flory JD, et al. (2008) Self-reported sleep duration is associated with the metabolic syndrome in midlife adults. Sleep 31: 635–643.
6. Gangwisch JE, Heymsfield SB, Boden-Albala B, Bujs RM, Kreier F, et al. (2007) Sleep duration as a risk factor for diabetes incidence in a large US sample. Sleep 30: 1667–1673.
7. Gangwisch JE, Heymsfield SB, Boden-Albala B, Buijs RM, Kreier F, et al. (2006) Short sleep duration as a risk factor for hypertension. Analyses of the first national health and nutrition examination survey. Hypertension 47: 833–839.
8. Magee CA, Caputi P, Iverson DC (2011) Relationships between self-rated health, quality of life and sleep duration in middle aged and elderly Australians. Sleep Med 12: 346–350.
9. Diethelm K, Remer T, Jilani H, Kunz C, Buyken AE (2011) Associations between the macronutrient composition of the evening meal and average daily sleep duration in early childhood. Clin Nutr 30: 640–646.
10. Afaghi A, O'Connor H, Chow CM (2007) High-glycemic-index carbohydrate meals shorten sleep onset. Am J Clin Nutr 85: 426–430.
11. Murakami K, Sasaki S, Takahashi Y, Okubo H, Hosoi Y, et al. (2006) Dietary glycemic index and load in relation to metabolic risk factors in Japanese female farmers with traditional dietary habits. Am J Clin Nutr 83: 1161–1169.
12. Nakashima M, Sakurai M, Nakamura K, Miura K, Yoshita K, et al. (2010) Dietary glycemic index, glycemic load and blood lipid levels in middle-aged Japanese men and women. J Atheroscler Thromb 17: 1082–1095.
13. Sakurai M, Nakamura K, Miura K, Takamura T, Yoshita K, et al. (2012) Dietary glycemic index and risk of type 2 diabetes mellitus in middle-aged Japanese men. Metabolism 61: 47–55.
14. Willett W, Manson J, Liu S (2002) Glycemic index, glycemic load, and risk of type 2 diabetes. Am J Clin Nutr 76: 274S–280S.

15. Barclay AW, Petocz P, McMillan-Price J, Flood VM, Prvan T, et al. (2008) Glycemic index, glycemic load, and chronic disease risk–a meta-analysis of observational studies. Am J Clin Nutr 87: 627–637.
16. Krishnan S, Rosenberg L, Singer M, Hu FB, Djousse L, et al. (2007) Glycemic index, glycemic load, and cereal fiber intake and risk of type 2 diabetes in US black women. Arch Intern Med 167: 2304–2309.
17. Office for Life-style Related Diseases Control, General Affairs Division, Health Service Bureau, Ministry of Health, Labour and Welfare (2013) The National Health and Nutrition Survey in Japan, 2011. (in Japanese). Ministry of Health, Labour and Welfare.
18. Sasaki S, Yanagibori R, Amano K (1988) Self-administered diet history questionnaire developed for health education: a relative validation of the test-version by comparison with 3-day diet record in women. J Epidemiol 8: 203–215.
19. Sasaki S, Ushio F, Amano K, Morihara M, Todoroki O, et al. (2000) Serum biomarker-based validation of a self-administered diet history questionnaire for Japanese subjects. J Nutr Sci Vitaminol (Tokyo) 46: 285–296.
20. Science and Technology Agency, Japan (2000) Standard Tables of Food Composition in Japan, 5th ed. Tokyo: Printing Bureau of the Ministry of Finance. [In Japanese.].
21. Murakami K, Sasaki S, Takahashi Y, Okubo H, Hirota N, et al. (2008) Reproducibility and relative validity of dietary glycemic index and load assessed with a self-administered diet-history questionnaire in Japanese adults. Br J Nutr 99: 639–648.
22. Foster-Powell K, Holt SH, Brand-Miller JC (2002) International table of glycemic index and glycemic load values. Am J Clin Nutr 76: 5–56.
23. Sugiyama M, Tang AC, Wakaki Y, Koyama W (2003) Glycemic index of single and mixed meal foods among common Japanese foods with white rice as a reference food. Eur J Clin Nutr 57: 743–752.
24. Fernandes G, Velangi A, Wolever TM (2005) Glycemic index of potatoes commonly consumed in North America. J Am Diet Assoc 105: 557–562.
25. Sydney University Glycemic Index Research Service (2007) The official website of glycemic index and GI database. Available: http://www.glycemicindex.com. Accessed February 1, 2007.
26. Henry CJ, Lightowler HJ, Strik CM, Renton H, Hails S (2005) Glycaemic index and glycaemic load values of commercially available products in the UK. Br J Nutr 94: 922–930.
27. Coulston AM, Hollenbeck CB, Swislocki AL, Reaven GM (1987) Effect of source of dietary carbohydrate on plasma glucose and insulin responses to mixed meals in subjects with NIDDM. Diabetes Care 10: 395–400.
28. Wolever TM, Jenkins DJ, Jenkins AL, Josse RG (1991) The glycemic index: methodology and clinical implications. Am J Clin Nutr 54: 846–854.
29. Doi Y, Minowa M, Uchiyama M, Okawa M, Kim K, et al. (2000) Psychometric assessment of subjective sleep quality using the Japanese version of the Pittsburgh Sleep Quality Index (PSQI-J) in psychiatric disordered and control subjects. Psychiatry Res 97: 165–172.
30. Fernstrom JD, Wurtman RJ (1971) Brain serotonin content: physiological dependence on plasma tryptophan levels. Science 173: 149–152.
31. Fernstrom JD, Wurtman RJ (1972) Brain serotonin content: physiological regulation by plasma neutral amino acids. Science 178: 414–416.
32. Madras BK, Cohen EL, Fernstrom JD, Larin F, Munro HN, et al. (1973) Letter: Dietary carbohydrate increases brain tryptophan and decreases free plasma tryptophan. Nature 244(5410): 34–35.
33. Hartmann E, Spinweber CL (1979) Sleep induced by L-tryptophan. Effect of dosages within the normal dietary intake. J Nerv Ment Dis 167: 497–499.
34. Wurtman RJ, Wurtman JJ, Regan MM, McDermott JM, Tsay RH, et al. (2003) Effects of normal meals rich in carbohydrates or proteins on plasma tryptophan and tyrosine ratios. Am J Clin Nutr 77: 128–132.
35. Berry EM, Growdon JH, Wurtman JJ, Caballero B, Wurtman RJ (1991) A balanced carbohydrate: protein diet in the management of Parkinson's disease. Neurology 41: 1295–1297.
36. Lyons PM, Truswell AS (1988) Serotonin precursor influenced by type of carbohydrate meal in healthy adults. Am J Clin Nutr 47: 433–439.
37. Herrera CP, Smith K, Atkinson F, Ruell P, Chow CM, et al. (2011) High-glycemic index and -glycaemic load meals increase the availability of tryptophan in healthy volunteers. Brit J Nutr 105: 1601–1606.
38. Badria FA (2002) Melatonin, serotonin, and tryptamine in some Egyptian food and medicinal plants. J Med Food 5: 153–157.
39. Weiss A, Xu F, Storfer-Isser A, Thomas A, Ievers-Landis CE, et al. (2010) The association of sleep duration with adolescents' fat and carbohydrate consumption. Sleep 33: 1201–1209.
40. Taniguchi A, Yamanaka-Okumura H, Nishida Y, Yamamoto H, Kaketani Y, et al. (2008) Natto and viscous vegetables in a Japanese style meal suppress postprandial glucose and insulin response. Asia Pac J Clin Nutr 17: 663–668.
41. Esfahani A, Wong JM, Mirrahimi A, Srichaikul K, Jenkins DJ, et al. (2009) The glycemic index: physiological significance. J Am Coll Nutr Suppl 28: 439S–445S.
42. Nanri A, Mizoue T, Noda M, Takahashi Y, Kato M, et al. (2010) Rice intake and type 2 diabetes in Japanese men and women: the Japan Public Health Center-based Prospective Study. Am J Clin Nutr 92: 1468–1477.
43. Eshak ES, Iso H, Date C, Yamagishi K, Kikuchi S, et al. (2011) Rice intake is associated with reduced risk of mortality from cardiovascular disease in Japanese men but not women. J Nutr 141: 595–602.
44. Food and Agriculture Organization of the United Nations (FAOSTAT) (2014) Available: http://faostat.fao.org/#. Accessed March 20, 2014.
45. Doi Y, Minowa M, Tango T (2003) Impact and correlates of poor sleep quality in Japanese white-collar employees. Sleep 26: 467–471.
46. Doi Y, Minowa M, Uchiyama M, Okawa M (2001) Subjective sleep quality and sleep problems in the general Japanese adult population. Pshychiatry Clin Neurosci 3: 213–215.
47. Sato-Mito N, Sasaki S, Murakami K, Okubo H, Takahashi Y, et al. (2011) The midpoint of sleep is associated with dietary intake and dietary behavior among young Japanese women. Sleep Med 12: 289–294.
48. Kravitz HM, Janssen I, Santoro N, Bromberger JT, Schocken M, et al. (2005) Relationship of day-to-day reproductive hormone levels to sleep in midlife women. Arch Intern Med 165: 2370–2376.
49. Baker FC, Driver HS (2004) Self-reported sleep across the menstrual cycle in young, healthy women. J Psychosom Res 56: 239–243.

4

Honeybee Colony Disorder in Crop Areas: The Role of Pesticides and Viruses

Noa Simon-Delso[1,2]*, Gilles San Martin[3], Etienne Bruneau[1], Laure-Anne Minsart[1], Coralie Mouret[1], Louis Hautier[3]

1 Beekeeping Research and Information Centre, Louvain la Neuve, Belgium, **2** Environmental Sciences, Copernicus Institute, Utrecht University, Utrecht, The Netherlands, **3** Plant Protection and Ecotoxicology Unit, Life Sciences Department, Walloon Agricultural Research Centre, Gembloux, Belgium

Abstract

As in many other locations in the world, honeybee colony losses and disorders have increased in Belgium. Some of the symptoms observed rest unspecific and their causes remain unknown. The present study aims to determine the role of both pesticide exposure and virus load on the appraisal of unexplained honeybee colony disorders in field conditions. From July 2011 to May 2012, 330 colonies were monitored. Honeybees, wax, beebread and honey samples were collected. Morbidity and mortality information provided by beekeepers, colony clinical visits and availability of analytical matrix were used to form 2 groups: healthy colonies and colonies with disorders (n = 29, n = 25, respectively). Disorders included: (1) dead colonies or colonies in which part of the colony appeared dead, or had disappeared; (2) weak colonies; (3) queen loss; (4) problems linked to brood and not related to any known disease. Five common viruses and 99 pesticides (41 fungicides, 39 insecticides and synergist, 14 herbicides, 5 acaricides and metabolites) were quantified in the samples.The main symptoms observed in the group with disorders are linked to brood and queens. The viruses most frequently found are Black Queen Cell Virus, Sac Brood Virus, Deformed Wing Virus. No significant difference in virus load was observed between the two groups. Three acaricides, 5 insecticides and 13 fungicides were detected in the analysed samples. A significant correlation was found between the presence of fungicide residues and honeybee colony disorders. A significant positive link could also be established between the observation of disorder and the abundance of crop surface around the beehive. According to our results, the role of fungicides as a potential stressor for honeybee colonies should be further studied, either by their direct and/or indirect impacts on bees and bee colonies.

Editor: Fabio S. Nascimento, Universidade de São Paulo, Faculdade de Filosofia Ciências e Letras de Ribeirão Preto, Brazil

Funding: The Walloon Region was the only funder of this study. The funders had no role in study design, data collection and analysis, or preparation of the manuscript.

Competing Interests: The authors have declared that no competing interests exist.

* Email: simon@cari.be

Introduction

The evolution of pollinator populations has been the subject of an increasing number of studies, most of them showing worrying negative trends [1–4]. Furthermore, beekeepers have long been notifying enhanced bee winter losses and disorders [5–8]. Bees contribute to ecosystem services and their decline thus threatens pollination of both wild and cultured plants, endangering biodiversity, food and fibre production [9,10]. This decline may also have an impact on the production of other goods with pharmacological uses (e.g. honey, propolis) [11,12], and scientific and technological inspiration (e.g. development of visual guided flight robotics) [13]. Bees are also part of our culture (e.g. culinary, hobby occupation, etc.), contributing to the dynamism of rural and urban areas [14] and providing a source of inspiration and well-being for many [15].

Belgium shares the trends observed worldwide both in terms of wild and reared pollinators [8,16], with enhanced winter mortality observed from 1999 [8,17,18]. However, apart from colony mortality, Walloon beekeepers have reported a number of imprecise symptoms: colony weakness, mainly in spring; fast renewal of young queens; rapid loss of individuals in the colony, mainly foragers, or slow loss of individuals in the colony. In many cases brood and food remains in the colony. Sometime a small cluster of bees with the queen survives [17]. Some beekeepers described unspecific brood abnormalities not characteristic to any known disease (Baudoin and Lequeux, pers. com.). Other studies describe similar mortality trends [8,19,20] as well as unspecific symptoms: increased colony mortality and/or weakening [21–23], queen failure [21,23–25] or honey yield reduction [21].

Multifarious factors have been proposed to provide a cause to such a phenomenon. Climate change is proposed as one of them, together with a decrease of genetic variability of the bee colonies, electromagnetic radiation, pathogens and parasites or the impact of intensive agricultural systems (nutritional lack, GM plants or pesticides) [26]. Previous studies developed in the region discard some of these factors as causes of bee losses, specifically *Nosema* spp and American Foulbrood [27]. However, pesticide residues and certain viruses were detected in bee colonies [28,27]. These elements were the most relevant to us.

Countless studies have shown lethal and sub-lethal effects of pesticides on bees [29–31]. Insecticides are often the most studied for obvious reasons. However other substances (fungicides, herbicides) deserve analysis for their specific toxicity, individually or in synergy with other substances [32,33] or pathogens [34–36], or their extensive exposure given their large scale and/or repeated use. Indeed, residue analyses show that these types of substance are found in the hives, even though the crops in which they were applied would suggest no bee exposure [37–40].

Beside pesticides, bee viruses are often mentioned as a putative cause of decline of the colonies, or at least to reside among the presumed multi-factorial causes [41]. In Europe, at least 12 viruses infecting bees have been compiled [21]. Many honeybee viruses commonly occur in seemingly healthy populations that continue to run well. Viruses may remain latent and confined within certain cells or tissues with no active replication and no disruption of cellular function. Likewise, they may be replicating at low level in permissive cells but in non-vital sites or in honeybee life stages that do not exhibit any symptoms or obvious pathology [21,42,43]. Nevertheless, two viruses, ABPV and DWV, are able of inducing serious disorders to honeybees and have been shown to cause -in association with *V. destructor* - winter losses in Germany [23].

In this paper, we first studied the relationship of in-hive viral prevalence as well as the presence of pesticide residues on honeybee colonies' health. As a next step, we focused on the relationship between the environment surrounding the monitored apiaries and the health condition of their colonies.

Materials and Methods

Field work – colony follow up

A group of voluntary beekeepers were requested to participate in the study. All of them shared the following criteria: (1) have a minimum of 5 production colonies per apiary in June 2011; (2) regularly follow up the health status and development of their colonies; and (3) monitor the varroa infestation level and carry out officially recommended varroa treatments (treatment in July-August with veterinary medicaments based on thymol and winter treatment with veterinary medicaments based on oxalic acid). A total of 330 colonies distributed among 66 apiaries (5 colonies/ apiary) in Walloon and Brussels regions (Belgium) were followed. In those apiaries composed of 5 or more colonies, the 5 well-developed colonies at the beginning of the study were selected.

Colonies received three visits along the study, the first one from mid-July to mid-August 2011, the second one from mid-September to mid-October 2011 and the third one from March to April 2012. State official beekeeping technicians specialised in bee health were trained in the framework of the project in order to minimise as far as possible the variability of the results due to handling and observations. For each of the visits, beekeepers were requested to fulfil a form asking information about the health history of the apiary and of the followed-up colonies, as well as about their beekeeping practices. Honeybee colony disorder symptoms were reported in the questionnaire. These include the following symptoms for which no causal agent could obviously be identified:

(1) dead and disappeared colonies : (1a) death of part or the whole colony, where dead bees can be found close to the hive or inside it. Beekeepers also describe the (1b) disappearance of part or the whole colony, leaving behind food reserves and brood, a phenomenon similar to the one described in North-American apiaries (Colony Collapse Disorder (CCD) [24];

(2) weak colonies : weakening of the colony, showing in occasions a slow development in spring under optimal conditions (e.g. optimal weather, low varroa pressure, etc) with as consequence the loss of the spring production, but in occasions showing abnormally small colonies or colonies with low activity;

(3) queen loss : replacement of young queens sometimes leading to queen-less colonies or interruption of the egg-laying activity of the queen [17];

(4) problems linked to brood and not related to any known disease.

The form also included requests about other symptoms typically linked to known diseases (e.g. diarrhoea, mummified larvae, varroa presence, presence of deformed wing bees, etc). Each of the questions requested further characterisation of the symptoms (e.g. population size, population dynamics, bees behaviour, etc.).

In addition, a thorough clinical inspection was carried out for each colony in the mentioned period. Special attention was given to the strength of the colony in terms of bee numbers, brood surface and reserves content, the presence of the queen and the varroa infestation level. Finally, two different samples were collected before and after the winter: (1) in-hive bees (minimum of 100 bees); (2) a section of the frame containing beebread and honey (about 100 cm^2). Samples were collected in hermetic plastic bags, cooled after collection and stored at $-20°C$.

Case choice – hierarchical sample clustering

Information available from bee colonies comprised field observations, beekeeper answers to the questionnaire and results from the analyses of the samples of beekeeping matrices (honey, beebread, wax and bees). Colonies for which this information was available were considered for our analyses. Colonies with well identified problems (heavy varroa infestation, lack of food or drone-laying queens) were discarded. After that, two groups were made: a group with disorders and another with healthy colonies. In order to constitute these groups and to limit variations due to potential different bee management, a hierarchical classification was made. The criteria used were the amount of food stores before the winter, the year of colony creation, the subspecies and the age of the queen. This classification was made by using Ward aggregation method. This method allows to build group with the lower variation within the group and the higher variation between groups [44].

Virus analyses

The viruses under investigation were the Black Queen Cell Virus (BQCV), the Chronic Bee Paralysis Virus (CBPV), the Acute Bee Paralysis Virus (ABPV), the Deformed Wings Virus (DWV), and the Sac Brood Virus (SBV). Viral analyses were conducted on the honeybee workers collected before the winter, during the first and second periods (July–August and September–October). The samples were analysed with a quantitative RT-PCR by the National Bee Unit laboratory, Food and Environment Research Agency (Sand Hutton, York, United-Kingdom).

Total Nucleic acid (TNA) was extracted from 60 bees homogenised for 12 minutes with 20 ml GITC Lysis Buffer (5 M Guandine Thiocynate, 0.05 M Tris base, 0.02 M EDTA, pH 8.0) in a 30 ml bottle containing 3, 7/16″ ball bearings. GITC Lysis buffer also contained 17.3 mM SDS buffer (173 mM Sodium dodecyl sulphate (SDS) in 100 ml MGW). The SDS buffer is added prior to use in warmed GITC Lysis Buffer. The homogenate was then incubated at 65°C for 40 minutes and then spun at 6189 g for 5 minutes. Polypropylene 96 -deep well plates (DT850301 Elkay Laboratory Products Ltd) were prepared as follows (1 well/extract); plate A: 800 µl extract, and 100 µl MagneSil^{TM} beads (MD1441, Promega); plate B: 1 ml of GITC wash buffer (5 M Guandine Thiocynate, 0.05 M Tris base); plates C, D, E: 1 ml 70%v/v ethanol (E/00665DF/17, Fisher Scientific); plate F: 1 ml 5 M Betaine (B2629, Sigma), plate G, 300 ul 1×TE

Buffer (stock 100X TE (EC-862 National Diagnostics). Plates were loaded onto the Kingfisher Flex and processed as follows: Plate A – Bind 5 mins (fast dual mix), Plate B – Wash 3 mins (fast dual mix), Plate C, D, E – Wash 2 mins (fast dual mix), collect beads at 1 min intervals, Plate F – Wash 20 secs (medium), without releasing beads, Plate G – Mix 1 min then incubate at 65°C for 5 mins with mixing. All steps of the process are looped through twice. TNA was collected from plate G of each reaction and stored at −80°C prior to use in real-time PCR.

Reactions were set up in 96 well reaction plates using Absolute Blue QPCR ROX mix (AB-4139, Thermo Scientific) following the protocols supplied. 0.1 mM of 0.1 M Dithiothreitol (165680250, Arcos Organics) and 0.33 unit of MMLV (EPO441: Fermentas) were added to each reaction. The primers (Table 1) were all used at 400 nM and probes at 200 nM final concentration. Total nucleic acid (5 μl) was added to each reaction, giving a final reaction volume of 20 μl. Plates were cycled for 48°C/30 min, 95°C/10 min and 40 cycles of 60°C/1 min, 95°C/15 sec within the 7900 HT Sequence Detection System (Applied Biosystems), using real time data collection. The results were recorded as the cycle threshold (Ct) or cycle number after which a significant accumulation of florescence over the baseline was observed; an average (of duplicate wells) Ct value below 40 was regarded as a positive result with a threshold ΔRn setting of 0.2. Given the absence of internal standard, we assumed that the extraction method had the same efficiency towards bee DNA/RNA and viral RNA.

Virus primers and probes used for all pathogens tested have been previously described in Chantawannakul et al., 2006 [45]. Additional APBV primers are described in Martin et al., 2012. [46].

Pesticide analyses

Samples collected before the winter were sent to Eurofins Chemiphar NV, Brugge, Belgium and analysed by SOFIA GmbH Chemisches Labor für Softwareentwicklung und Intelligente Analytik, Berlin, Germany. Two multi-residues methods (SF146 and SF150) were used searching for 99, 93 and 96 pesticides residues in wax (54 samples), beebread (108 samples) and honey (107 samples – one sample did not contain enough matrix) respectively (LOQ in Table 2).

For SF146 method, 10 ml of water was added to 10 g of samples. Methanol was added and the preparation was mixed. The mixture was filtered and centrifuged. Next, for analysis by gas chromatography coupled with mass spectrometry (GC-MS), the filtrate was mixed with sodium chloride and ethyl acetate solution 1:1 (v/v). All was dried with sodium sulfate and filtrated. This filtrate was then concentrated and analysed by GC-MS. For analysis with liquid chromatography coupled with tandem mass spectrometry (LC-MS/MS), 5 ml of sample were transferred in ChemElut column and eluted with dichloromethane. After concentration, 1 ml of water-methanol 1:1 (v/v) was added and this solution was analysed by LC-MS/MS. For the wax, some modifications were made. For GC-MS, sodium chloride was replaced by hexane to dissolve wax and the mixture was frozen until a precipitate appears. For LC-MS/MS, 0.2 g of sample were extracted with 30 ml of mixture of naphtha:acetonitrile 1:2 (v/v). 10 ml of acetonitrile phase was isolated and concentrated before the analysis by LC-MS/MS.

For SF150 method, 10 ml of water was added to 10 g of samples as well as methanol and hydrochloric acid. All was mixed, filtrated and centrifuged. A solution of sodium chloride (20%) was added and 5 ml of sample were transferred in ChemElut column and eluted with dichloromethane. After concentration, 1 ml of water-methanol 1:1 (v/v) was added and this solution was analysed by LC-MS/MS.

Descriptive analyses

A descriptive analysis of virus prevalence and pesticide residues was first carried out. The relationship between disorder and these stressing factors was then assessed. For each virus type, a linear model (two way ANOVA) was used, with the cycle threshold value as dependent variable and the visit (first or second), group (with disorder or healthy) and their interaction as explanatory variables. For the pesticides residues, we used a similar model with the total number of residues as dependent variable and type (fungicide or insecticide/acaricide), group (with disorder or healthy) and their interaction as explanatory variable. Based on these models, we constructed a contrast matrix to test explicit post-hoc hypotheses (e.g. compare virus load between groups within each visit…). As several dependent variables had a strongly asymmetric distribution (i.e. non-normal), we computed all p-values by permutation ($n = 1000$). We applied a Bonferoni correction on the post-hoc tests p-values to take into account the multiplicity of the tests.

Relationship between bee colony disorders and potential stressors or surrounding environment of the apiary

We used two separate generalized linear mixed models with a binomial distribution and logit link function. In both models, the "group" (with disorder or healthy) was used as dependent binary variable and the apiary was used as random effect (grouping

Table 1. List of primers used for virus analyses.

Target	Primer Name	Sequence (5′-3′)
BQCV	BQCV 9195F	GGT GCG GGA GAT GAT ATG GA
	BQCV 8265R	GCC GTC TGA GAT GCA TGA ATA C
	BQCV 8217T	TTT CCA TCT TTA TCG GTA CGC CGC C
SBV	SBV 311F	AAG TTG GAG GCG CGy AAT TG
	SBV 380R	CAA ATG TCT TCT TAC dAG AGG yAA GGA TTG
	SBV 331T (MGB)	CGG AGT GGA AAG AT
CPV	CPV 304F	TCT GGC TCT GTC TTC GCA AA
	CPV 371R	GAT ACC GTC GTC ACC CTC ATG
	CPV 325T	TGC CCA CCA ATA GTT GGC AGT CTG C

Table 2. Active ingredients or metabolite included in the multi-residue analyses by beekeeping matrix (A = Acaricide; F = Fungicide; H = Herbicide; I = Insecticide; S = Synergist).

Active ingredient or metabolite*	Class	LOQ (mg/kg)		
		Wax	Beebread	Honey
2,4-D	H	0.1	–	0.01
Abamectin	I	0.1	0.1	0.005
Acetamiprid	I	0.1	0.1	0.005
Aldicarb	I	0.1	0.1	0.005
Alpha-cypermethrin	I	0.1	0.1	0.005
Amitraz	A	0.1	0.1	0.01
Azoxystrobin	F	0.1	0.1	0.005
Bentazone	H	0.2	–	0.02
Benthiavalicarb	F	0.1	0.1	0.005
Beta-cyfluthrin	I	0.1	0.1	0.01
Bifenthrin	I	0.1	0.1	0.005
Boscalid	F	0.1	0.1	0.005
Captan	F	0.1	0.1	0.01
Carbaryl	I	0.1	0.1	0.005
Chlorpyriphos	I	0.1	0.1	0.005
Chlorpyriphos-methyl	I	0.1	0.1	0.005
Chlorothalonil	F	0.1	0.1	0.005
Clothianidin	I	0.1	0.1	0.01
Coumaphos	A	0.1	0.1	0.05
Coumaphos oxon *	A	0.1	0.1	–
Coumaphos phenolic*	A	0.1	0.1	–
Cyazofamid	F	0.2	0.2	0.02
Cyfluthrin	I	0.1	0.1	0.01
Cymoxanil	F	0.1	0.1	0.01
Cypermethrin	I	0.1	0.1	0.005
Cyproconazole	F	0.1	0.1	0.005
Cyprodinil	F	0.1	0.1	0.01
DDT	I	0.1	0.1	0.005
Deltamethrine	I	0.1	0.1	0.005
Dichlorprop-P	H	0.1	–	0.01
Difenoconazole	F	0.1	0.1	0.005
Diflubenzuron	I	0.2	0.2	0.02
Dimethenamid-P	H	0.1	0.1	0.005
Dimethoate	I	0.1	0.1	0.005
Dimethomorph	F	0.1	0.1	0.01
Dimoxystrobin	F	0.1	0.1	0.005
Epoxiconazole	F	0.1	0.1	0.005
Esfenvalerate	I	0.1	0.1	0.005
Ethofumesate	H	0.5	0.5	0.05
Famoxadone	F	0.1	0.1	0.01
Fenhexamid	F	0.1	0.1	0.005
Fenoxycarb	F	0.1	0.1	0.005
Fenpropidin	F	0.1	0.1	0.01
Fenpropimorph	F	0.1	0.1	0.005
Fipronil	I	0.1	0.1	0.01
Flonicamid	I	2	2	0.2
Fluazinam	F	0.1	0.1	0.01
Flufenacet	H	0.1	0.1	0.01

Table 2. Cont.

Active ingredient or metabolite*	Class	LOQ (mg/kg)		
		Wax	Beebread	Honey
Fluopicolide	F	0.1	0.1	0.01
Flusilazole	F	0.1	0.1	0.005
Heptenophos	I	0.1	0.1	0.01
Imidacloprid	I	0.1	0.1	0.005
Indoxacarb	I	0.1	0.1	0.005
Iprodione	F	0.1	0.1	0.005
Kresoxim-methyl	I	0.1	0.1	0.005
Lambda-cyhalothrin	I	0.1	0.1	0.005
Lindane	I	0.1	0.1	0.005
Linuron	H	0.1	0.1	0.005
MCPA	H	0.1	–	0.01
Mecoprop-P	H	0.1	–	0.01
Metalaxyl-M	F	0.1	0.1	0.005
Metamitron	H	0.1	0.1	0.005
Metconazole	F	0.2	0.2	0.02
Methiocarb	I	0.1	0.1	0.005
Methoxyfenozide	F	0.1	0.1	0.005
Metribuzin	H	0.1	0.1	0.005
Penconazole	F	0.1	0.1	0.005
Pendimethalin	H	0.1	0.1	0.005
Permethrin	I	0.2	0.2	0.02
Picoxystrobin	F	0.1	0.1	0.005
Piperonyl butoxide	S	0.1	0.1	0.01
Pirimicarb	I	0.1	0.1	0.005
Prochloraz	F	0.1	0.1	0.005
Propamocarb	F	0.1	0.1	0.005
Propiconazole	F	0.1	0.1	0.01
Propyzamide	F	0.1	0.1	0.01
Pymetrozine	I	0.1	0.1	0.005
Pyraclostrobin	F	0.1	0.1	0.005
Pyrethrin	I	0.2	0.2	0.02
Pyrimethanil	F	0.1	0.1	0.005
Rotenone	I	0.1	0.1	0.01
Spinosad	I	0.1	0.1	–
Spirodiclofen	I	0.1	0.1	0.01
Spirotetramat	F	0.1	0.1	0.01
Spiroxamine	F	0.1	0.1	0.005
Sulcotrione	H	0.1	–	0.01
Tau-fluvalinate	IA	0.1	0.1	0.01
Tebuconazole	F	0.1	0.1	0.005
Tebufenozide	I	0.1	0.1	0.005
Tefluthrine	I	0.1	0.1	0.005
Terbuthylazine	H	0.1	0.1	0.01
Tetraconazole	F	0.1	0.1	0.01
Thiabendazole	F	0.1	0.1	0.005
Thiacloprid	I	0.1	0.1	0.005
Thiamethoxam	I	0.1	0.1	0.005
Thiophanate-methyl	F	0.1	0.1	0.005
Trifloxystrobin	F	0.1	0.1	0.01

Table 2. Cont.

Active ingredient or metabolite*	Class	LOQ (mg/kg)		
		Wax	Beebread	Honey
Zeta-cypermethrin	I	0.1	0.1	0.005
Zoxamide	F	0.1	0.1	0.01

factor) to take into account the non-independence between colonies from the same apiary and allow the intercept to vary between apiaries [47].

With the first model, we explored the relationship between the probability of disorder in a colony and potential stress factors, i.e. pesticides or viruses total load into the colonies. We used as explanatory variables the total number of fungicides residues, the total number of insecticides or acaricides (pooled together) residues, the total number of viruses detected for both visits and all first level interactions between these three explanatory variables. The insecticides and acaricides were pooled together because the most frequently found active ingredient, namely tau-fluvalinate, is authorized in Belgium for both purposes.

With the second model, we investigated the relationship between the probability of disorder in a colony and the structure of the agricultural landscape around the beehive. The surfaces of all different kinds of agricultural soil occupancy in a circle with a radius of 1500 m around each apiary were calculated according to the information provided by the farmers to the Walloon administration (Land Parcel Identification System). The different soil occupancy categories were pooled into two categories defined according to the potential frequency of plant protection product use: (1) grasslands (low pesticides use), (2) crops *sensu lato* (potentially higher pesticides use), including major crops (mainly: cereals, potatoes, beet, oilseed rape, maize, flax, …) but also surfaces dedicated to fruit or vegetables production, fodder production (mainly legumes) and to horticulture. The surfaces of these two land use options, grasslands and crops (*sensu lato*), were used as explanatory variables in the model. The 1500 m radius was chosen accordingly to the mean pollen and nectar collecting distance for the honeybee [48,49]. As the agricultural soil occupancy data was available only for Wallonia, we eliminated from the analysis the apiaries whose buffer had less than 70% of their surface within the administrative boundaries of Wallonia (n = 2).

We used Likelihood Ratio (LR) Tests to evaluate the significance of the explanatory variables [47,50]. We respected the marginality rules, i.e. all main effects were tested after removing from the model the interactions in which they are involved [51].

All analyses were performed with R (R Core Team 2013) and the mixed models were fitted with the package lme4 [52].

Results

Description of honeybee colony disorders

We gathered all sources of information, i.e. questionnaires, analytical matrices and information from clinical visits, for 173 colonies. After the clustering, 54 colonies coming from 21 apiaries (Figure 1) were considered for the study: 25 presenting bee disorders and 29 not presenting them, defined as healthy group. Their data and samples were collected by 8 beekeeping technicians.

In the group presenting disorders, 6 colonies were dead or unviable -with only a handful of bees remaining with the queen- at the spring visit (Table 3). Pre-wintering weakness, winter worker losses, late-season re-queening were reported in these cases. One colony was dead due to queen failure without re-queening in spring. Furthermore, a number of colonies were weak in spring. They were characterised by a low number of individuals and a slow development. In total, nine colonies lost their queens during the study, five of them leading to queenless colonies. These were considered as "disorder colonies" in the framework of the study. Finally, brood abnormalities not linked to known disease were observed in 10 colonies, most of them both before and after the winter.

Symptoms of other diseases or bee parasite observation remained low within the selected colonies. Wax moths were observed in two cases, one in each group. *Varroa destructor* was present in all colonies of the study. All of them were treated according to official veterinary advice. Diarrhoea was observed in one of the colonies showing brood abnormalities. Anatomical modifications (i.e. deformed or undeveloped wings, small abdomens) were observed in 6 colonies, half of them being healthy and half of them showing disorders. No symptoms of any of the foulbroods were observed.

Virus content

One bees sample from the "disorder" group could not be analysed due to a lack of sufficient matrix. The three most abundantly found viruses were the Deformed Wings Virus (DWV), the Black Queen Cell Virus (BQCV) and the Sac Brood Virus (SBV) (Figure 2). The Acute Bee Paralysis Virus (ABPV) and the Chronic Bee Paralysis Virus (CBPV) were found only in a very

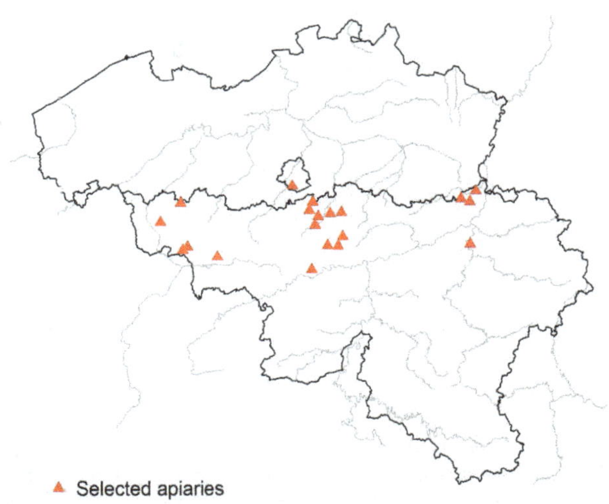

Figure 1. Spatial distribution of selected apiaries.

Table 3. Symptoms observed in the group with disorders.

Symptoms of disorder	Frequency
Mortality	2*
Weakening	3
Queen failure	5
Brood problems	9
Mortality+Weakening	2
Mortality+Weakening+Queen failure	2
Mortality+Queen failure	1
Queen failure+Brood problems	1
Total	25

* One of these colonies not considered in the model due to a lack of viral results.

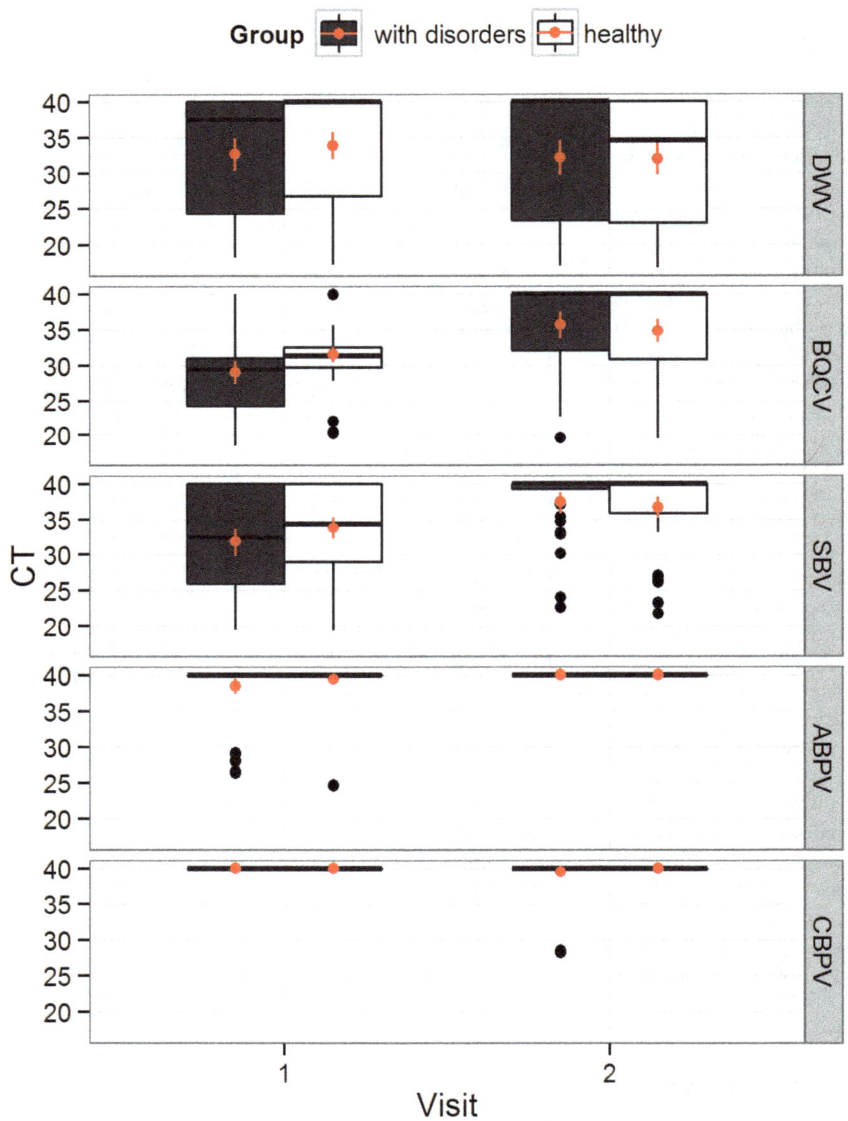

Figure 2. Virus content according to the Cycle Threshold (CT) for the groups "with disorder" and "healthy". Boxplot of Cycle Threshold for the first and second visits (visit 1 - mid-July to mid-august and visit 2 - mid-September to mid-October) and the group with disorders (grey, n = 24 colonies) and the healthy one (white, n = 29 colonies). Deformed Wings Virus (DWV), Black Queen Cell Virus (BQCV), SacBrood Virus (SBV), Acute Bee Paralysis Virus (ABPV), Chronic Bee Paralysis Virus (CBPV). In red, mean with confidence interval estimated by boostrap method. Note: CT values below 40 were regarded as positive results and the lowest CT values correspond to the higher virus contents.

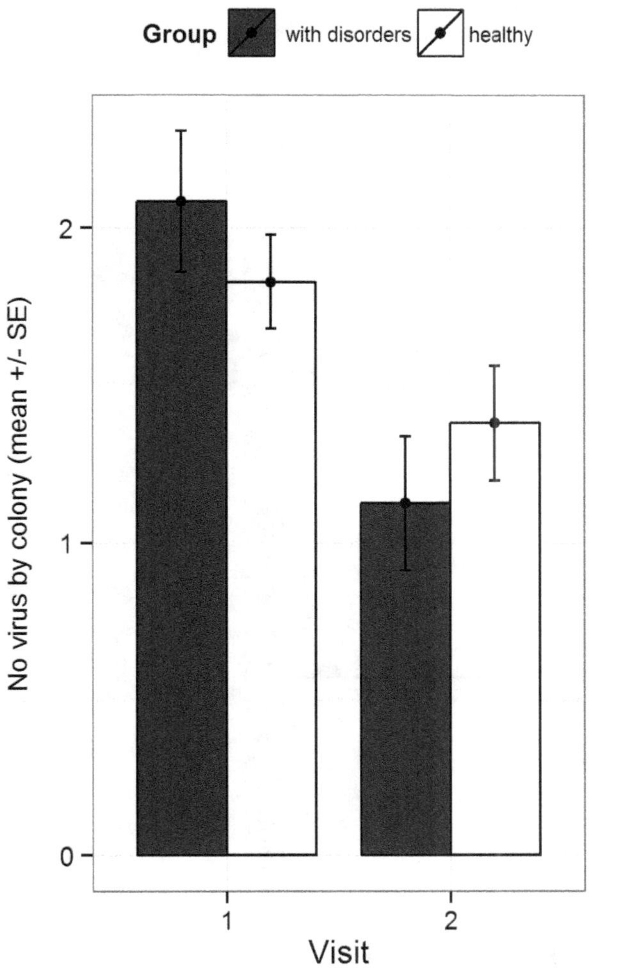

Figure 3. Average number of different viruses per colony. Data shown for the first and second visits (visit 1 - mid-July to mid-august and visit 2 - mid-September to mid-October) and the group with disorders (grey, n = 24 colonies) and the healthy one (white, n = 29 colonies). Whiskers show the standard error (SE).

limited number of samples and did not allowed particular statistical analyses on these two viruses.

There was no significant difference in viral content between the group with disorders or the healthy one, and independently of the visit for any of the three most abundant viruses (2-way ANOVA tested by permutations, DWV: $p = 0.731$, BQCV: $p = 0.373$, SBV: $p = 0.54$). We observed a decrease of virus content from summer to fall 2011, independently of the group, for BQCV ($p<0.001$) and SBV ($p<0.001$) but not for DWV ($p = 0.271$). For BQCV only, we observed a significant ($p = 0.036$) group×visit interaction indicating that the decrease of the virus abundance from visit 1 to visit 2 was higher in the group "with disorder" than in the group "healthy". Overall, the number of virus changed between visit 1 and visit 2 and a significant decrease was observed in the group with disorders ($p<0.001$) (Figure 3).

Pesticide analysis

172 agrochemical residues of 23 different active ingredients were detected in 94 out of 269 samples. Wax was the most contaminated matrix: 109 residues of 15 different active ingredients; while 39 and 24 residues of 10 and 8 substances were detected in beebread and honey, respectively (Figures 4 & 5).

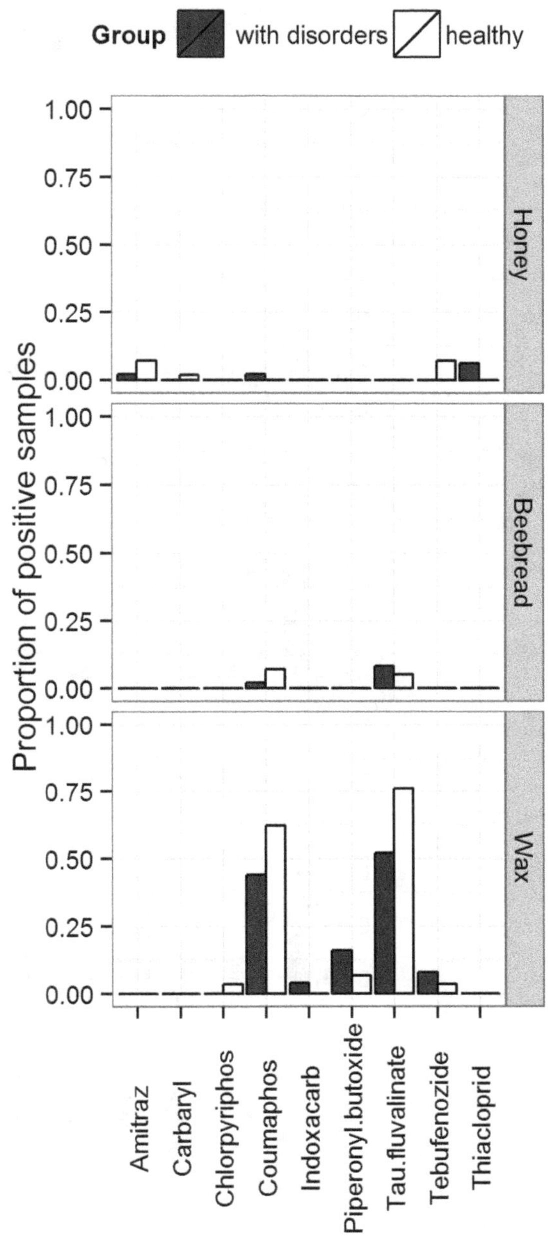

Figure 4. Proportion of samples containing residues of acaricides/insecticides in the different beekeeping matrices (honey, beebread and wax). Data shown for the group with disorders (grey, n = 25 colonies) and the healthy one (white, n = 29 colonies).

Residue levels contained in wax and beebread were higher (0.21–3.1 mg/kg) than those in honey (0.001–0.058 mg/kg).

For the subsequent statistical analysis, the results obtained for insecticide and acaricides residues were pooled together because the most frequently found active ingredient, tau-fluvalinate (n = 46), can be used in Belgium as an acaricide against varroa mite and as an insecticide to control *Meligethes aeneus* in rape. The second most frequently found residue was the coumaphos (n = 35), followed by two fungicides, boscalid (n = 33), iprodione (n = 13) (Table 4). Some residues of neonicotinoid insecticides, synergist and herbicide were also detected: thiacloprid (n = 3), piperonyl butoxide (n = 6), terbuthylazine (n = 1). The highest

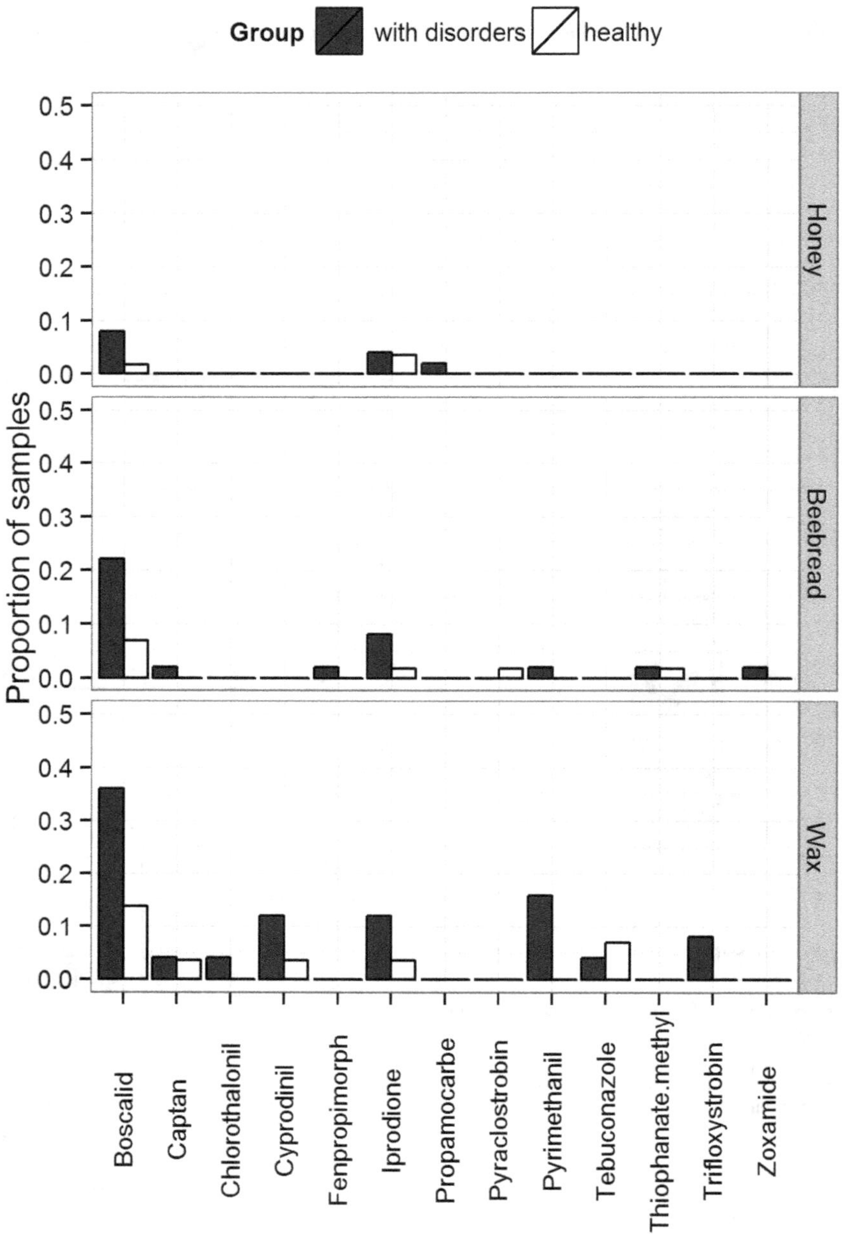

Figure 5. Proportion of samples containing residues of fungicides in the different beekeeping matrices (honey, beebread and wax). Data shown for the group with disorders (grey, n = 25 colonies) and the healthy one (white, n = 29 colonies).

residue level concerned captan with 3.1 and 1.9 mg/kg in the wax and bee bread of the same colony, respectively. Despite of being the most frequently found in matrices, tau-fluvalinate and coumaphos residues never exceeded 0.71 and 0.58 mg/kg, respectively. Boscalid, the most commonly found fungicide, ranged from 0.005 to 1.3 mg/kg.

There was a significant difference ($p = 0.01$) in terms of number of fungicide substances found between the "disorder" group (mean = 2.0) and the "healthy" one (mean = 0.7) as presented in Figure 6. The total number of insecticides/acaricides residues was slightly higher in the disorder group (mean = 2.1) than in the healthy group (mean = 1.64) but this difference is not statistically significant ($p = 0.79$). The most frequent fungicides in the group with disorders were boscalid and iprodione, detected in the three investigated matrices (Figure 5). However, for single active substances, no significant difference of number of residues was observed between the groups "with disorder" and "healthy".

Probability of disorders in relation to potential stressors

There is clearly a significant positive relationship between the probability of a colony showing disorders and the total number of fungicides (Figure 7, LR = 7.128, df = 1, $p = 0.008$). The estimated probability for a colony to be in the "with disorder" group is 0.26 without fungicides residues, 0.60 with 2 fungicides residues and 0.88 with 4 fungicides residues when the insecticides-acaricides residues number and virus load are fixed to their observed mean value (Figure 7). None of the other variables (total number of viruses, total number of insecticides-acaricides) and none of the first level interactions seem to have any explanatory power on the probability of disorders in a colony (Table 5). No direct link could

Table 4. Residues of active ingredients found in wax, beebread and honey samples from colonies with disorders (Group D, n = 25 colonies) and healthy ones (Group H, n = 29 colonies).

Active ingredient	Group	Wax							Bee bread							Honey						
		LOQ (mg/kg)	Number of samples (n = 54)			Residues amount (mg/kg)			LOQ (mg/kg)	Number of samples (n = 108)			Residues amount (mg/kg)			LOQ (mg/kg)	Number of samples (n = 107)			Residues amount (mg/kg)		
			<LOD	Detected	Quantified	Range	Mean	s.d.		<LOD	Detected	Quantified	Range	Mean	s.d.		<LOD	Detected	Quantified	Range	Mean	s.d.
Amitraz	D	0.1	–	–	–				0.1	–	–	–				0.01	49	–	1	0.022	0.02	
	H		–	–	–					–	–	–					53	–	4	0.01–0.028	0.02	0.01
Boscalid	D	0.1	16	8	1	0.29	0.29	–	0.1	39	7	4	0.4–1.3	0.68	0.42	0.005	46	–	4	0.005–0.026	0.01	0.01
	H		25	4	–	–	–	–		54	4	–	–	–	–		56	–	1	0.058	0.06	–
Captan	D	0.1	24	–	1	3.1	3.1	–	0.1	48	–	1	1.9	1.90	–	0.01	–	–	–			
	H		28	1	–	–	–	–		58	–	–	–	–	–		–	–	–			
Carbaryl	D	0.1	–	–	–				0.1	–	–	–				0.005	50	–				
	H		–	–	–					–	–	–					56	–	1	0.02	0.02	–
Chlorpyriphos	D	0.1	25	–	–				0.1	–	–	–				0.005	–	–	–			
	H		28	1	–					–	–	–										
Chlorothalonil	D	0.1	24	1	–				0.1	–	–	–				0.005	–	–	–			
	H		29	–	–					–	–	–					–	–	–			
Coumaphos	D	0.1	14	9	2	0.32–0.34	0.33	0.01	0.1	48	1	–				0.05	49	–	1	0.012	0.01	–
	H		11	10	8	0.23–0.58	0.37	0.01		54	4	–					57	–	–			
Cyprodinil	D	0.1	22	3	–				0.1	–	–	–				0.01	–	–	–			
	H		28	1	–					–	–	–					–	–	–			
Fenpropimorph	D	0.1	–	–	–				0.1	49	1	–				0.005	–	–	–			
	H		–	–	–					58	–	–					–	–	–			
Indoxacarb	D	0.1	24	1	–				0.1	–	–	–				0.005	–	–	–			
	H		29	–	–					–	–	–					–	–	–			
Iprodione	D	0.1	22	1	2	0.24–1.5	0.87	0.89	0.1	45	–	4	0.34–1.5	0.90	0.48	0.005	48	–	2	0.017–0.022	0.02	0.00
	H		28	1	–	–	–	–		57	1	–	–	–	–		55	–	2	0.022–0.04	0.03	0.01
Piperonyl butoxide	D	0.1	21	4	–				0.1	–	–	–				0.01	–	–	–			
	H		27	2	–					–	–	–					–	–	–			
Propamocarbe	D	0.1	–	–	–				0.1	–	–	–				0.005	49	–	1	0.008	0.01	0.00

Table 4. Cont.

Active ingredient	Group	Wax							Bee bread							Honey						
		LOQ (mg/kg)	Number of samples (n = 54)			Residues amount (mg/kg)			LOQ (mg/kg)	Number of samples (n = 108)			Residues amount (mg/kg)			LOQ (mg/kg)	Number of samples (n = 107)			Residues amount (mg/kg)		
			<LOD	Detected	Quantified	Range	Mean	s.d.		<LOD	Detected	Quantified	Range	Mean	s.d.		<LOD	Detected	Quantified	Range	Mean	s.d.
	H		–	–	–					–	–	–					57	–	–	–	–	–
Pyraclostrobin	D	0.1	–	–	–				0.1	50	–	–				0.005	–	–	–			
	H		–	–	–					57	1	–					–	–	–			
Pyrimethanil	D	0.1	21	4	–				0.1	49	1	–				0.005	–	–	–			
	H		29	–	–					58	–	–					–	–	–			
Tau-fluvalinate	D	0.1	12	9	4	0.29–0.46	0.4	0.08	0.1	45	4	–				0.01	50	–	–	–	–	–
	H		7	13	9	0.21–0.71	0.5	0.08		55	3	–					53	–	4	0.011–0.02	0.02	0.00
Tebuconazole	D	0.1	24	1	–				0.1	–	–	–				0.005	–	–	–			
	H		27	2	–					–	–	–					–	–	–			
Tebufenozide	D	0.1	23	2	–				0.1	–	–	–				0.005	–	–	–			
	H		28	1	–					–	–	–					–	–	–			
Terbuthylazine	D	0.1	24	1	–				0.1	–	–	–				0.01	–	–	–			
	H		29	–	–					–	–	–					–	–	–			
Thiacloprid	D	0.1	–	–	–				0.1	–	–	–				0.005	47	–	3	0.009–0.013	0.01	0.00
	H		–	–	–					–	–	–					57	–	–	–	–	–
Thiophanate-methyl	D	0.1	–	–	–				0.1	49	1	–				0.005	–	–	–			
	H		–	–	–					57	–	1	0.38	0.38	–		–	–	–			
Trifloxystrobin	D	0.1	23	2	–				0.1	–	–	–	–	–	–	0.01	–	–	–			
	H		29	–	–					–	–	–					–	–	–			
Zoxamide	D	0.1	–	–	–				0.1	49	1	–				0.01	–	–	–			
	H		–	–	–					58	–	–					–	–	–			

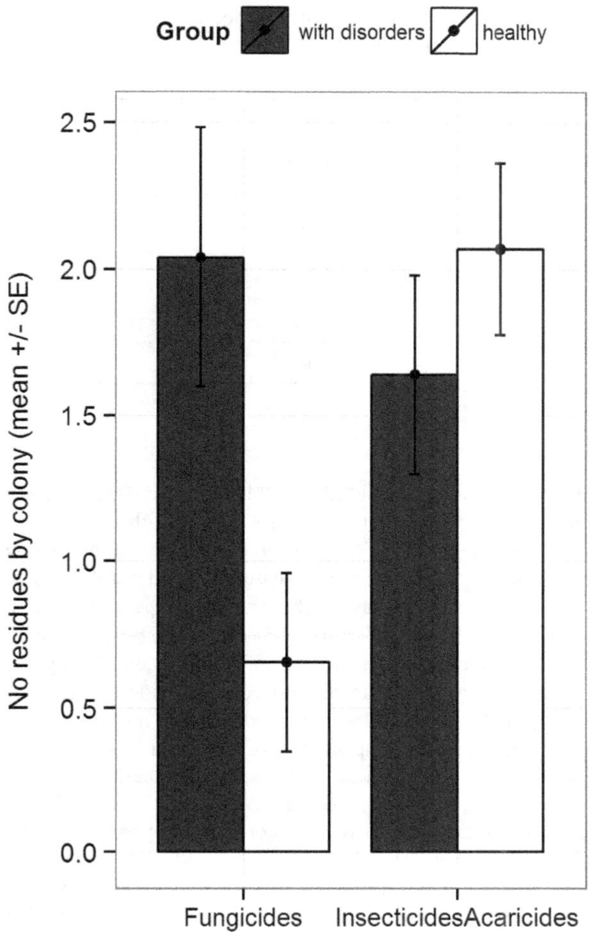

Figure 6. Average number of residues per colony. Data shown for the group with disorders (grey, n = 25 colonies) and the healthy ones (white, n = 29 colonies). Whiskers show the standard error (SE).

be established between bee colony disorders and the amount (in µg/kg) of residues found in the matrices.

Probability of disorders and crop/grassland surface

Our data clearly show a significant increase in disorder probability with the increase of crop surfaces (*sensu lato*, i.e. including fruit, vegetables, fodder production and horticulture) in the surrounding of the apiary (Figure 8, LR = 8.052, df = 1, p = 0.0045). The predicted probability of disorders is close to 0.1 for a crop surface of 0 ha in the radius of 1500 m and increases up to 0.8 for a surface of 500 ha of crops when fixing the grasslands surface to its observed mean.

On the contrary, the probability of disorders strongly decreases when the grassland surfaces increases (Figure 8, LR = 14.527, df = 1, p = 0.0001) after controlling for the crop surface. The predicted probability of disorders is close to 1 for a grassland surface of 0 ha in a radius of 1500 m and drops to ~0.1 for a surface of 150 ha of grasslands when fixing the crops surface to its observed mean.

Very similar results were found with a 3000 m buffer around the apiary (results not shown).

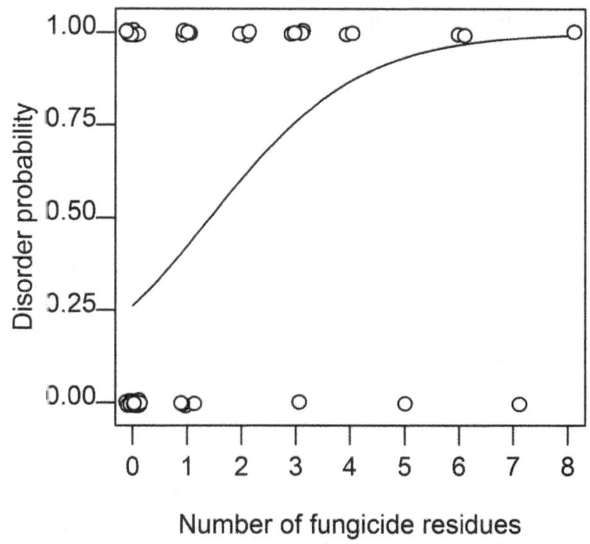

Figure 7. Probability of honeybee colony disorders depending on the number of fungicide residues detected. Model based on averaged coefficients and median value both for the number of insecticides-acaricides residues and total number of virus detected for both visits (n = 53 colonies).

Discussion

The bee disorders observed after the winter in the Walloon region happened despite of normal climatic conditions. The autumn of 2011 was dry (140.4 mm rainfall water from October to December, average being 219.9 mm), sunny and warm for Belgian conditions (12.4°C on average, which is normally 10.9°C for this period), followed by average winter and spring 2012 in terms of temperature, rainfall, with the exception of a cold wave lasting twelve days in February [53]. These conditions would not induce, *a priori*, a risk for honeybee colonies. Furthermore, based on studies carried out on the palynological diversity of the pollens collected by these colonies before the winter (Table S1), the hypothesis of nutritional lack is unlikely. All samples analysed contained at least 8 different botanic sources of pollen, including rich protein content as oilseed rape, ivy and *Phacelia*.

Viruses infections has often been mentioned as a source of stress for honeybee colonies [7]. However no significant difference in quantity or occurrence was observed between the healthy and the "with disorder" groups. DWV is one of the most commonly detected virus in *A. mellifera*. The prevalence of this virus is even more important at colonies infested by *Varroa destructor*, a well-established vector of this virus [7]. In accordance with the present study, further studies run on Belgian apiaries show DWV, BQCV and SBV as the most frequently found viruses [54]. Unlike DWV, we observed that the amount of SBV and BQCV has dropped significantly between the first and second visits for each group. In the case of BQCV, this is of no surprise as the cycle of incidence of this virus has been shown to increase in late winter, with a peak in May or June followed by a rapid decline [55]. The observed decrease of SBV has also been reported in other studies [42] in which the authors suggested that bees could develop a molecular defensive mechanism to reduce virus multiplication, or that the change in bee susceptibility to the virus could result from environmental conditions such as the quality of pollen.

We cannot prove any causal relationship between any of these viruses analysed and bee disorders, nor does the interaction

Table 5. Analysis of deviance table for generalized linear binomial models describing the relationships between the colony disorder probability and three variables: the total number of (1) fungicide residues (totfungicides), (2) insecticide-acaricide residues (totinsaca) and (3) virus detected for both visits (totvirus).

	LR	df	p(>Chisq)
totfungicides	7.13	1	0.008
totinsaca	0.005	1	0.943
totvirus	0.136	1	0.712
totfungicides:totvirus	2.222	1	0.136
totinsaca:totvirus	0.975	1	0.323
totfungicides:totinsaca	0.901	1	0.342

LR = likelihood ratio.

between these two factors. Cox-Foster et al., 2007 [41] found no clear correlation between a variety of pathogens, including *Nosema* spp., DWV, CBPV, ABPV, BQCV, *Mellisococcus pluton* and *Paenibacillus larvae* ssp and CCD. No specific spore counts were carried out in our study. However, no signs of nosemosis or foulbrood could be linked to colonies presenting bee disorders. It is noteworthy that a monitoring run at Belgian level found *Nosema* spp spores in one out of four colonies [56]. Nevertheless, Cox-Foster et al., 2007 [41], show a positive correlation between IAPV and CCD, which *a priori* would not be relevant in our conditions given the low prevalence of IAPV in this country [27,54]. A recent publication [36] shows a positive correlation between the presence of fungicides in pollen loads and the presence of spores of *Nosema ceranae*. We do not exclude the potential involvement of *Nosema* spp. in the case of bee disorders. However, in the framework of our study, *N. ceranae* seems either to play a role in the development of this weakening, while remaining asymptomatic, or not to play a decisive role in it.

When considering pesticide residues, no direct link could be established between bee colony disorders and the amount (in μg/kg) of residues found in the matrices. Neither could we identify any specific molecule as cause of bee disorders. Nevertheless, the study of the residue load of pesticides, specifically fungicides, opens new avenues for a better understanding of honeybee colony disorders.

Even if insecticides/acaricides were the most numerous residues detected in hives mainly in wax, no significant difference in the number of accumulated residues was observed between colonies with disorders and the healthy ones. Indeed the two most abundant active ingredients, tau-fluvalinate and coumaphos, came most probably from varroa control measures even if tau-fluvalinate is used as an insecticide (Mavrik 2F) against *Meligethes aeneus* in oilseed rape. These active ingredients seem to be a frequent outcome of residue analyses studies [57,58,39,38,40,59]. Synergistic effects have been shown between acaricides and other molecules [33,60]. Nevertheless, our modelling did not suggest any synergistic effects in the appearance of bee disorders occurring between residues of fungicides and insecticides-acaricides. Residues of synergist, piperonyl butoxide, were also detected that indicates a prior exposure to synthetic or natural pyrethroids even though residues were not found in the analysed matrix, probably due to a fast degradation of these active ingredients [61]. A non-authorised active ingredient was also detected: carbaryl, forbidden in Belgium since 2007, indicating an illegal agricultural or gardening use.

The only neonicotinoid found, thiacloprid, was detected in honey during the sampling period of July-August in two colonies. However, the limits of detection achieved in our study do not allow to determine the presence of neonicotinoids -with the exception of acetamiprid- or fipronil at levels in the range of the acute toxicity of these substances (30–40 μg/Kg). Residues of these substances could be present at lower levels and thus an exposure to these substances cannot be excluded.

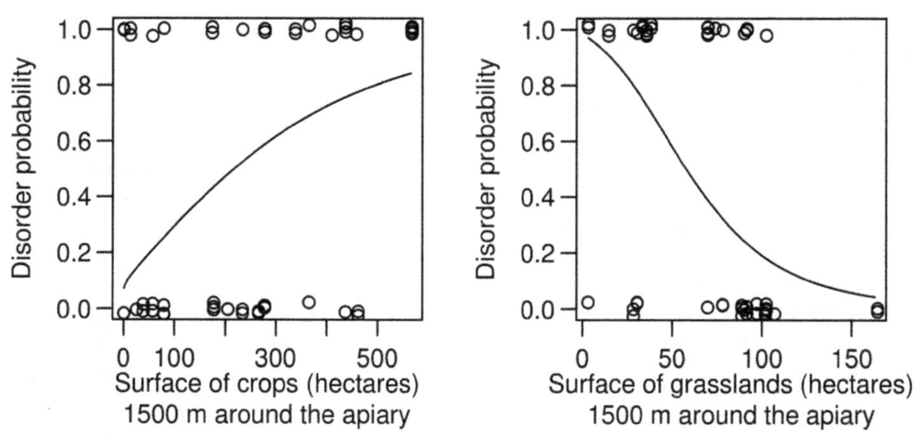

Figure 8. Probability of honeybee colony disorders depending on the apiary's environment. Consideration of crop surface *vs.* grassland surface in a radius of 1500 m around the apiary. Crops include fruit, vegetables, fodder production and horticulture. For each graph, the value of the variable not displayed is fixed to its observed mean (n = 53 colonies).

According to our results, the number of fungicide residues seems to plays a role in the appearance of honeybee colony disorder.

Significantly, more fungicides residues were detected in colonies with disorders than in the healthy ones. Mainly four active ingredients, frequently used in plant protection, were detected: boscalid, iprodione, pyrimethanil and cyprodinil. Fungicides are often considered safe for honeybees based on their acute toxicity. However some direct toxic effects on bees either by the mother compounds or their metabolites have been reported in the past [62]. For example, boscalid shows low acute toxicity to bees [63], despite the fact that beekeepers in the USA have already reported losses and adverse effects on bee brood development related to the foliar application of this systemic active ingredient [64]. Incidents were often linked to the use of a co-formulation boscalid – pyraclostrobin. However, both molecules appeared above detection levels in only two colonies of our study and could not explain the general trend. Interestingly, one metabolite of boscalid, the 2-chloronicotinic acid, is similar to the 6-chloronicotinic acid, a metabolite of imidacloprid. The latter has proved to be lethal to bees at low concentrations (0.1 µg/L) following chronic exposure [65]. Further research should be carried out in order to clarify the mechanism of bee toxicity of boscalid. Indeed, boscalid has proved toxic to other aquatic invertebrates, reducing daphnid fecundity and *Chironomid* emergence [64]. In addition, synergism with other active ingredients like insecticides are possible and increase the toxicity for honeybee [66,32,67]. Two other fungicides were also detected at very high levels in wax and beebread: iprodione and captan. The former is known for its synergistic effects in collaboration with insecticidal compounds [33]. The latter has been shown to induce effects on growth and development of larval honeybees [68,69]. Chronic and larval toxicity studies would be interesting at this stage in order to evaluate possible direct toxic effects on bee individuals and their behaviour. Indeed, a recent study showed increased larval mortality following chronic exposure to tau-fluvalinate, coumaphos, chlorpyriphos and chlorotalonyl or some of their combinations [70]. All these substances were found in our study. Increased mortality rates in the fall may compromise the size and age structure of the wintering cluster, which could lead to winter losses.

The indirect effects of fungicides on bees or on bee colonies are relatively little-known to date.

Fungicides may have an impact on the colony by modifying the existing microflora present in the food stores or in the bee intestinal tract [71]. Studies have already shown the possible modification of microbial composition both at beebread level [62,72] and at intestinal level [73]. This modification in the composition of microbiota may lead to dysbiosis [74]. The impact that such an unbalance in the bee gut microflora may have on bee health has already been considered. The link between the unspecific symptoms observed in our study and a possible microbial alteration could be subject of further research.

In parallel, the potential impact of microbial modification on digestibility and availability of nutrients should be a target for further research. Indeed, the content of essential amino acids might be altered when beebread is contaminated with fungicides (DeGrandi-Hoffman, 2013, pers com.). Given the importance of nutrition, especially pollen, in the good development of the colony [75] alterations in composition or lack of essential nutrients would put the homeostasis of the colony at stake. Some studies have already shown the impact of nutritional lack on bee development and health [76]. Provided that pollen is the unique source of amino acids for honeybees, royal jelly production could also be affected [77,78] with unexpected potential consequences for its main consumers, larvae and the queen. A poor nutrition of the queen, could have as a result an impact in its activity. Likewise, a poor nutrition of the larvae has been shown to impact their development [76]. As a result, the presence of fungicides on beebread and honey may have both a direct effect on their health, but also an indirect one on the colony development.

Fungicides are widely used in agriculture and are broadly present in bee matrices, sometimes at high concentrations at levels of mg/kg [79,80,38,59]. Boscalid, cyprodinil, iprodione are used to control a broad range of fungal pathogens including *Botrytis* spp., *Alternaria* spp. and *Sclerotinia* spp. on a wide range of crops including fruits, vegetables and ornamentals. Pyrimethanil is more specifically used to control grey mould on fruits, vegetables and ornamentals, and leaf scab on apple trees [81]. These active ingredients were already reported in bee matrices in Europe and in the USA [23,39,62]. Their frequent presence in bee matrices might be an indication of chemical plant protection intensity in all agricultural landscapes. Fungicides could also be markers of exposure to other active ingredients with higher toxicity to bees. Mixes of products like fungicides – insecticides are often applied to reduce the number of spray applications. As a result, other pesticides often used in combination with the fungicides found or applied in the same crops could have been at the origin of the effects observed in this study. However, the sensibility of the residue analyses used in our study might explain the lack of detection of such components. Further intensive monitoring and a thorough record of the agricultural practices on pesticide application in tank mixes would help clarifying this alternative explanation.

Factors different from fungicides are most likely involved in the development of bee disorders. According to our model, the disorder probability was not absent when fungicides residues were not detected in presence of insecticide residues and virus. Non identified pathogens, chemicals or factors of different nature could be operating as silent stressors. Ravoet and colleagues (2013) [82] reported the presence of new pathogens in Belgium that were not taken into consideration in our analyses (i.e. *Crithidia mellificae* or the Lake Sinai Virus (LSV)). Other stressing factors could be also linked to the intensive agriculture. In fact, we observed an increase of colony disorders in the area with high density of crops in comparison with areas with grassland. Some studies and beekeeper claims go in line with our outcome regarding the concentration of bee problems in areas with intensive agriculture [83–86]. Furthermore, the same negative trends on pollinators and biodiversity in areas with intensive agriculture have already been described as the result of as increased pesticide use, decreased landscape heterogeneity, loss and fragmentation of natural habitat [87,88].

In conclusion, the five virus studied (ABPV, CBPV, QBCV, SBV DWV) do not seem determinant in the appearance of bee disorders in our study. These disorders seem clearly linked to the environment of the apiaries and were observed mainly in agricultural crop areas. We observed also that the number of fungicide residues appears as the main potential stress factor linked to bee disorder. However other stressing factors could be acting or interacting at the same time: insecticides exposure, a lack of amino acids and oligo-elements, etc. Our results open new avenues for future research in order to better understand the side effects of fungicides on the bee colony and questions the sustainability of intensive agriculture model and its impact on bees. Specific toxicological studies on both adult bees and larvae would be recommendable in order to better characterise the toxicity of fungicides.

Acknowledgments

We would like to salute and to thank the beekeepers and beekeeping technicians for their dedication and active contribution to our study. Likewise, we thank Gloria DiGrandi-Hoffman, Gerard Arnold, Szaniszlo Szöke and Martin Dermine for their critical and constructive review of the article. We would like also to thank the Direction Générale Opérationnelle Agriculture, Ressources Naturelles et Environnement (DGO3), Département des Aides (D4), Direction des Surfaces (D42), Service 42/3 - LPIS (Land Parcel Identification System) - Service Public de Wallonie for the spatial data. We would also like to thank the Molecular Technology Unit at The Food and Environment Research Agency, Sand Hutton, York, YO41 1LZ for Bee Pathogen Screening Services. Finally, we would like to thank the reviewers for their helpful comments.

Author Contributions

Conceived and designed the experiments: NS LH EB. Performed the experiments: NS LH CM. Analyzed the data: GSM LH. Wrote the paper: LH NS LAM GSM.

References

1. Biesmeijer JC, Roberts SPM, Reemer M, Ohlemüller R, Edwards M, et al. (2006) Parallel declines in pollinators and insect-pollinated plants in Britain and the Netherlands. Science 313: 351–354.
2. Potts SG, Biesmeijer JC, Kremen C, Neumann P, Schweiger O, et al. (2010) Global pollinator declines: trends, impacts and drivers. Trends Ecol Evol 25: 345–353.
3. Goulson D, Lye GC, Darvill B (2008) Decline and conservation of bumble bees. Annu Rev Entomol 53: 191–208.
4. Carvalheiro LG, Kunin WE, Keil P, Aguirre-Gutiérrez J, Ellis WN, et al. (2013) Species richness declines and biotic homogenisation have slowed down for NW-European pollinators and plants. Ecol Lett 16: 870–878. doi:10.1111/ele.12121.
5. Kluser S, Peduzzi P (2007) Global pollinator decline: a literature review. UNEP/GRID- Europe. © UNEP 2007. Switzerland.
6. Maxim L, van der Sluijs JP (2010) Expert explanations of honeybee losses in areas of extensive agriculture in France: Gaucho ® compared with other supposed causal factors. Environ Res Lett 5: 014006. doi:10.1088/1748-9326/5/1/014006.
7. vanEngelsdorp D, Meixner MD (2010) A historical review of managed honey bee populations in Europe and the United States and the factors that may affect them. J Invertebr Pathol 103: S80–S95.
8. Van der Zee R, Pisa L, Andonov S, Brodschneider R, Charriere J-D, et al. (2012) Managed honey bee colony losses in Canada, China, Europe, Israel and Turkey, for the winters of 2008–9 and 1009–10. J Apic Res Bee World 51: 100–114.
9. Klein A-M, Müller C, Hoehn P, Kremen C (2009) Understanding the role of species richness for crop pollination services. Biodiversity, ecosystem function and human wellbeing. New York. 195–208.
10. Lautenbach S, Seppelt R, Liebscher J, Dormann CF (2012) Spatial and temporal trends of global pollination benefit. PloS One 7: e35954.
11. Banskota AH, Tezuka Y, Kadota S (2001) Recent progress in pharmacological research of propolis. Phytother Res 15: 561–571. doi:10.1002/ptr.1029.
12. Jull AB, Rodgers A, Walker N (2008) Honey as a topical treatment for wounds. Cochrane Database of Systematic Reviews. Chichester, UK: John Wiley & Sons, Ltd. 1–43.
13. Srinivasan MV (2011) Honeybees as a Model for the Study of Visually Guided Flight, Navigation, and Biologically Inspired Robotics. Physiol Rev 91: 413–460. doi:10.1152/physrev.00005.2010.
14. Bradber N (1990) Beekeeping in rural development. International Bee Research Association. 15 pp.
15. UNEP (2005) Ecosystems and Human Well-Being: Our Human Planet: Summary for Decision Makers. Island Press. Washington: Island Press.
16. Rasmont P, Pauly A, Terzo M, Patiny S, Michez D, et al. (2005) The survey of wild bees (Hymenoptera, Apoidea) in Belgium and France. Food Agric Organ Rome: 18.
17. Lefevbre M, Bruneau E (2004) État des lieux du phénomène de dépérissement des ruchers en Région wallonne. Louvain la Neuve.
18. Nguyen BK, Mignon J, Laget D, de Graaf D, Jacobs F, et al. (2010) Honey bee colony losses in Belgium during the 2008–9 winter. J Apic Res 49: 337–339. doi:10.3896/IBRA.1.49.4.07.
19. Neumann P, Carreck NL (2010) Honey bee colony losses. J Apic Res 49: 1–6.
20. Vanengelsdorp D, Hayes J, Underwood RM, Caron D, Pettis J (2011) A survey of managed honey bee colony losses in the USA, fall 2009 to winter 2010. J Apic Res 50: 1–10.
21. Aubert M, Faucon J-P, Chauzat M-P (2008) Enquête prospective multi-factorielle: influence des agents microbiens et parasitaires, et des résidus de pesticides sur le devenir de colonies d'abeilles domestiques en conditions naturelles. AFSSA.
22. Higes M, Martín-Hernández R, Garrido-Bailón E, González-Porto AV, García-Palencia P, et al. (2009) Honeybee colony collapse due to *Nosema ceranae* in professional apiaries. Environ Microbiol Rep 1: 110–113. doi:10.1111/j.1758-2229.2009.00014.x.
23. Genersch E, von der Ohe W, Kaatz H, Schroeder A, Otten C, et al. (2010) The German bee monitoring project: a long term study to understand periodically high winter losses of honey bee colonies. Apidologie 41: 332–352.
24. vanEngelsdorp D, Speybroeck N, Evans JD, Nguyen BK, Mullin C, et al. (2010) Weighing Risk Factors Associated With Bee Colony Collapse Disorder by Classification and Regression Tree Analysis. J Econ Entomol 103: 1517–1523. doi:10.1603/EC09429.
25. Pettis JS (2013) The Role Of Pesticides In Queen Health & Sperm Viability. Apimondia 2014, Kiev.
26. Farooqui T (2013) A potential link among biogenic amines-based pesticides, learning and memory, and colony collapse disorder: A unique hypothesis. Neurochem Int 62: 122–136. doi:10.1016/j.neuint.2012.09.020.
27. Nguyen BK, Ribiere M, Vanengelsdorp D, Snoeck C, Saegerman C, et al. (2011) Effects of honey bee virus prevalence, Varroa destructor load and queen condition on honey bee colony survival over the winter in Belgium. J Apic Res 50: 195–202.
28. Nguyen BK, Saegerman C, Pirard C, Mignon J, Widart J, et al. (2009) Does imidacloprid seed-treated maize have an impact on honey bee mortality? J Econ Entomol 102: 616–623.
29. Desneux N, Decourtye A, Delpuech J-M (2007) The Sublethal Effects of Pesticides on Beneficial Arthropods. Annu Rev Entomol 52: 81–106. doi:10.1146/annurev.ento.52.110405.091440.
30. Belzunces LP, Tchamitchian S, Brunet J-L (2012) Neural effects of insecticides in the honey bee. Apidologie 43: 348–370. doi:10.1007/s13592-012-0134-0.
31. Van der Sluijs JP, Simon-Delso N, Goulson D, Maxim L, Bonmatin J-M, et al. (2013) Neonicotinoids, bee disorders and the sustainability of pollinator services. Curr Opin Environ Sustain 5: 293–305. doi:10.1016/j.cosust.2013.05.007.
32. Pilling ED, Jepson PC (1993) Synergism between EBI fungicides and a pyrethroid insecticide in the honeybee (Apis mellifera). Pestic Sci 39: 293–297.
33. Fischer R, Wachendorff-Neumann U (2003) Active ingredient combinations with insecticidal, fungicidal and acaricidal properties.
34. Alaux C, Brunet J-L, Dussaubat C, Mondet F, Tchamitchan S, et al. (2010) Interactions between *Nosema* microspores and a neonicotinoid weaken honeybees (*Apis mellifera*). Environ Microbiol 12: 774–782. doi:10.1111/j.1462-2920.2009.02123.x.
35. Vidau C, González-Polo RA, Niso-Santano M, Gómez-Sánchez R, Bravo-San Pedro JM, et al. (2011) Fipronil is a powerful uncoupler of oxidative phosphorylation that triggers apoptosis in human neuronal cell line SHSY5Y. NeuroToxicology 32: 935–943. doi:10.1016/j.neuro.2011.04.006.
36. Pettis JS, Lichtenberg EM, Andree M, Stitzinger J, Rose R (2013) Crop pollination exposes honey bees to pesticides which alters their susceptibility to the gut pathogen Nosema ceranae. PloS One 8: e70182.
37. Bogdanov S (2005) Contaminants of bee products. Apidologie 37: 1–18. doi:10.1051/apido:2005043.
38. Johnson RM, Ellis MD, Mullin CA, Frazier M (2010) Pesticides and honey bee toxicity – USA. Apidologie 41: 312–331. doi:10.1051/apido/2010018.
39. Mullin CA, Frazier M, Frazier JL, Ashcraft S, Simonds R, et al. (2010) High Levels of Miticides and Agrochemicals in North American Apiaries: Implications for Honey Bee Health. PLoS ONE 5: e9754. doi:10.1371/journal.pone.0009754.
40. Chauzat M-P, Martel A-C, Cougoule N, Porta P, Lachaize J, et al. (2011) An assessment of honeybee colony matrices, Apis mellifera (Hymenoptera: Apidae) to monitor pesticide presence in continental France. Environ Toxicol Chem 30: 103–111. doi:10.1002/etc.361.
41. Cox-Foster DL, Conlan S, Holmes EC, Palacios G, Evans JD, et al. (2007) A metagenomic survey of microbes in honey bee colony collapse disorder. Science 318: 283–287.
42. Tentcheva D, Gauthier L, Zappulla N, Dainat B, Cousserans F, et al. (2004) Prevalence and seasonal variations of six bee viruses in Apis mellifera L. and Varroa destructor mite populations in France. Appl Environ Microbiol 70: 7185–7191.
43. Gauthier L, Tentcheva D, Tournaire M, Dainat B, Cousserans F, et al. (2007) Viral load estimation in asymptomatic honey bee colonies using the quantitative RT-PCR technique. Apidologie 38: 426–435.
44. Zuur AF, Ieno EN, Smith GM (2007) The Analysis of Ecological Data. Springer-Verlag.
45. Chantawannakul P, Ward L, Boonham N, Brown M (2006) A Scientific Note on the Detection of Honeybee Viruses Using real-time PCR (TaqMan®) in Varroa

Mites Collected from a Thai Honeybee (Apis mellifera) Apiary. Journal of Invertebrate Pathology: 91: 69–73.
46. Martin SJ, Highfield AC, Brettell L, Villalobos EM, Budge GE, et al. (2012) Global honey bee viral landscape altered by a parasitic mite. Science 336: 1304–1306.
47. Zuur AF, Ieno EN, Elphick CS (2010) A protocol for data exploration to avoid common statistical problems. Methods Ecol Evol 1: 3–14.
48. Beekman M, Ratnieks FLW (2000) Long-range foraging by the honey-bee, Apis mellifera L. Funct Ecol 14: 490–496.
49. Steffan-dewenter I, Kuhn A (2003) Honeybee foraging in differentially structured landscapes. Proc R Soc Lond B Biol Sci 270: 569–575.
50. Pinheiro JC, Bates DM (2000) Mixed-Effects Models in S and S-PLUS. Springer. 560 p.
51. Fox J (2002) An R and S-Plus companion to applied regression. Sage Publications, Inc. Available: http://books.google.be/books?hl = en&lr = &id = xWS8kgRjGcAC &oi = fnd&pg = PR9&dq = Fox+2002+An+R+and+S+Plus+&ots = o5qCjIMtOb &sig = lvi2jQFv4iDIBrv0QtaWiRIlRBM. Accessed 2012 Sep 18.
52. Bates D (2013) Linear mixed model implementation in lme4. Ms Univ Wis. Available: http://debianmirror.wwi.dk/cran/web/packages/lme4/vignettes/Implementation.pdf. Accessed 2014 Feb 3.
53. IRM IR de M (2013) Bilan climatologique annuel. Available: http://www.meteo.be/meteo/view/fr/1317239-Bilan+climatologique+annuel.html. Accessed 2013 Dec 15.
54. De Smet L, Ravoet J, de Miranda JR, Wenseleers T, Mueller MY, et al. (2012) BeeDoctor, a versatile MLPA-based diagnostic tool for screening bee viruses. PloS One 7: e47953.
55. Bailey L, Ball BV, Perry JN (1981) The prevalence of viruses of honey bees in Britain. Ann Appl Biol 97: 109–118.
56. Verhoeven B (2014) Projet pilote de surveillance de la mortalité des abeilles 2012–2013 Premiers résultats. AFSCA. Journé apicole 26 janvier 2014, Namur.
57. Chauzat M-P, Faucon J-P, Martel A-C, Lachaize J, Cougoule N, et al. (2006) A survey of pesticide residues in pollen loads collected by honey bees in France. J Econ Entomol 99: 253–262.
58. Chauzat M-P, Faucon J-P (2007) Pesticide residues in beeswax samples collected from honey bee colonies (Apis mellifera L.) in France. Pest Manag Sci 63: 1100–1106. doi:10.1002/ps.1451.
59. Wiest L, Buleté A, Giroud B, Fratta C, Amic S, et al. (2011) Multi-residue analysis of 80 environmental contaminants in honeys, honeybees and pollens by one extraction procedure followed by liquid and gas chromatography coupled with mass spectrometric detection. J Chromatogr A 1218: 5743–5756. doi:10.1016/j.chroma.2011.06.079.
60. Johnson RM, Pollock HS, Berenbaum MR (2009) Synergistic interactions between in-hive miticides in Apis mellifera. J Econ Entomol 102: 474–479.
61. Yu SJ (2008) The toxicology and biochemistry of insecticides. CRC N Y NY USA. Available: http://www.lavoisier.fr/livre/notice.asp?ouvrage = 1795057. Accessed 2014 Jan 31.
62. DeGrandi-Hoffman G, Chen Y, Simonds R (2013) The Effects of Pesticides on Queen Rearing and Virus Titers in Honey Bees (Apis mellifera L.). Insects 4: 71–89. doi:10.3390/insects4010071.
63. Pesticide Properties Database (PPDB) (2014) Boscalid (Ref: BAS 510F). Available: http://sitem.herts.ac.uk/aeru/ppdb/en/86.htm. Accessed 2014 Jan 3.
64. Aubee C, Lieu D (2010) Environmental Fate and Ecological Risk Assessment for Boscalid New Use on Rapeseed, Including Canola (Seed Treatment). U.S. EPA - Washington.
65. Suchail S, Guez D, Belzunces LP (2001) Discrepancy between acute and chronic toxicity induced by imidacloprid and its metabolites in Apis mellifera. Environ Toxicol Chem SETAC 20: 2482–2486.
66. Belzunces LP, Colin ME (1992) Les phenoménes d'affaiblissement de ruchers.
67. Meled M, Thrasyvoulou A, Belzunces LP (1998) Seasonal variations in susceptibility of Apis mellifera to the synergistic action of prochloraz and deltamethrin. Environ Toxicol Chem 17: 2517–2520.
68. Thompson HM (2003) Behavioural effects of pesticides in bees–their potential for use in risk assessment. Ecotoxicology 12: 317–330.
69. Mussen EC, Lopez JE, Peng CY (2004) Effects of selected fungicides on growth and development of larval honey bees, Apis mellifera L.(Hymenoptera: Apidae). Environ Entomol 33: 1151–1154.
70. Zhu W, Schmehl DR, Mullin CA, Frazier JL (2014) Four Common Pesticides, Their Mixtures and a Formulation Solvent in the Hive Environment Have High Oral Toxicity to Honey Bee Larvae. PloS One 9: e77547.
71. Batra LR, Batra SWT, Bohart GE (1973) The mycoflora of domesticated and wild bees (Apoidea). Mycopathol Mycol Appl 49: 13–44.
72. Yoder JA, Jajack AJ, Rosselot AE, Smith TJ, Yerke MC, et al. (2013) Fungicide Contamination Reduces Beneficial Fungi in Bee Bread Based on an Area-Wide Field Study in Honey Bee, *Apis mellifera*, Colonies. J Toxicol Environ Health A 76: 587–600. doi:10.1080/15287394.2013.798846.
73. Anderson KE, Sheehan TH, Eckholm BJ, Mott BM, DeGrandi-Hoffman G (2011) An emerging paradigm of colony health: microbial balance of the honey bee and hive (Apis mellifera). Insectes Sociaux 58: 431–444. doi:10.1007/s00040-011-0194-6.
74. Sartor RB (2008) Therapeutic correction of bacterial dysbiosis discovered by molecular techniques. Proc Natl Acad Sci 105: 16413–16414.
75. Di Pasquale G, Salignon M, Le Conte Y, Belzunces LP, Decourtye A, et al. (2013) Influence of Pollen Nutrition on Honey Bee Health: Do Pollen Quality and Diversity Matter? PLoS ONE 8: e72016. doi:10.1371/journal.pone.0072016.
76. Brodschneider R, Crailsheim K (2010) Nutrition and health in honey bees. Apidologie 41: 278–294.
77. Standifer LN (1967) A comparison of the protein quality of pollens for growth-stimulation of the hypopharyngeal glands and longevity of honey bees, Apis mellifera L. (Hymenoptera: Apidae). Insectes Sociaux 14: 415–425. doi:10.1007/BF02223687.
78. Liming W, Jinhui Z, Xiaofeng X, Yi L, Jing Z (2009) Fast determination of 26 amino acids and their content changes in royal jelly during storage using ultra-performance liquid chromatography. J Food Compos Anal 22: 242–249.
79. Kubik M, Nowacki J, Pidek A, Warakomska Z, Michalczuk L, et al. (1999) Pesticide residues in bee products collected from cherry trees protected during blooming period with contact and systemic fungicides. Apidologie 30: 12. doi:10.1051/apido:19990607.
80. Kubik M, Nowacki J, Pidek A, Warakomska Z, Michalczuk L, et al. (2000) Residues of captan (contact) and difenoconazole (systemic) fungicides in bee products from an apple orchard. Apidologie 31: 531–542.
81. Pesticide Properties Database (PPDB) (2014) Pyrimethanil (Ref: SN 100309). Available: http://sitem.herts.ac.uk/aeru/ppdb/en/573.htm. Accessed 2014 Jan 3
82. Ravoet J, Maharramov J, Meeus I, De Smet L, Wenseleers T, et al. (2013) Comprehensive bee pathogen screening in Belgium reveals Crithidia mellificae as a new contributory factor to winter mortality. PloS One 8: e72443.
83. Comen PA, Belzunces L, Pélissier C, Lewis G (2001) Honey bee poisoning incidents over the last ten years, as reported by bee keepers in The Netherlands. Les Colloques 98: 129–136.
84. Brittain CA, Vighi M, Bommarco R, Settele J, Potts SG (2010) Impacts of a pesticide on pollinator species richness at different spatial scales. Basic Appl Ecol 11: 106–115.
85. CRA-API (2011) Effects of coated maize seed on honey bees. Report based on results obtained from the first year of activity of the APENET project. Italy.
86. Maxim L, van der Sluijs J (2013) Seed-dressing systemic insecticides and honeybees. Late Lessons from Early Warnings: Science, Precaution, Innovation. Copenhagen. 401–438. Available: http://www.beekeeping.com/articles/us/late_lessons_from_early_warnings_2.pdf. Accessed 2014 Feb 10.
87. Holzschuh A, Steffan-Dewenter I, Tscharntke T (2008) Agricultural landscapes with organic crops support higher pollinator diversity. Oikos 117: 354–361.
88. Kleijn D, Kohler F, Báldi A, Batáry P, Concepcion ED, et al. (2009) On the relationship between farmland biodiversity and land-use intensity in Europe. Proc R Soc B Biol Sci 276: 903–909.

5

Dietary Sources of Methylated Arsenic Species in Urine of the United States Population, NHANES 2003–2010

B. Rey deCastro*, Kathleen L. Caldwell, Robert L. Jones, Benjamin C. Blount, Yi Pan, Cynthia Ward, Mary E. Mortensen

Centers for Disease Control and Prevention, National Center for Environmental Health, Division of Laboratory Sciences, Atlanta, Georgia, United States of America

Abstract

Background: Arsenic is an ubiquitous element linked to carcinogenicity, neurotoxicity, as well as adverse respiratory, gastrointestinal, hepatic, and dermal health effects.

Objective: Identify dietary sources of speciated arsenic: monomethylarsonic acid (MMA), and dimethylarsinic acid (DMA).

Methods: Age-stratified, sample-weighted regression of NHANES (National Health and Nutrition Examination Survey) 2003–2010 data (~8,300 participants ≥6 years old) characterized the association between urinary arsenic species and the additional mass consumed of USDA-standardized food groups (24-hour dietary recall data), controlling for potential confounders.

Results: For all arsenic species, the rank-order of age strata for median urinary molar concentration was children 6–11 years > adults 20–84 years > adolescents 12–19 years, and for all age strata, the rank-order was DMA > MMA. Median urinary molar concentrations of methylated arsenic species ranged from 0.56 to 3.52 µmol/mol creatinine. Statistically significant increases in urinary arsenic species were associated with increased consumption of: fish (DMA); fruits (DMA, MMA); grain products (DMA, MMA); legumes, nuts, seeds (DMA); meat, poultry (DMA); rice (DMA, MMA); rice cakes/crackers (DMA, MMA); and sugars, sweets, beverages (MMA). And, for adults, rice beverage/milk (DMA, MMA). In addition, based on US (United States) median and 90th percentile consumption rates of each food group, exposure from the following food groups was highlighted: fish; fruits; grain products; legumes, nuts, seeds; meat, poultry; and sugars, sweets, beverages.

Conclusions: In a nationally representative sample of the US civilian, noninstitutionalized population, fish (adults), rice (children), and rice cakes/crackers (adolescents) had the largest associations with urinary DMA. For MMA, rice beverage/milk (adults) and rice cakes/crackers (children, adolescents) had the largest associations.

Editor: David O. Carpenter, Institute for Health & the Environment, United States of America

Funding: The authors have no funding or support to report.

Competing Interests: The authors have declared that no competing interests exist.

* Email: rdecastro@cdc.gov

Introduction

Arsenic is an ubiquitous metalloid element present in the environment as inorganic species with different oxidation states, or as part of organic compounds. Inorganic arsenic species of greatest environmental health concern have oxidation states of +3 (As(III) or arsenite) or +5 (As(V) or arsenate), and are classified as human carcinogens [1,2]. People with chronic exposure to high levels of inorganic arsenic species in drinking water have manifested neurotoxicity, skin lesions, gastrointestinal and liver dysfunction, and cardiovascular disease [3–6]. In the United States, regulations limit arsenic in public water systems and in bottled water to 10 µg/L [7,8]. The methylated arsenic species dimethylarsinic acid (DMA) and monomethylarsonic acid (MMA) have both been detected in soils, fresh and marine waters, and fish and shellfish.

Human metabolic biotransformation of inorganic arsenic involves reduction from As(V) to As(III), followed by oxidative methylation to monomethyarsinic acid (MMA) and dimethylarsinic acid (DMA) [5,9]. Since most arsenic species absorbed from the gastrointestinal tract is excreted in urine within 1–3 days [10–15], urinary arsenic is well-suited as an exposure biomarker to correlate with NHANES 24-hour dietary recall data. Although inorganic species have been a focus of concern because of their carcinogenicity [16], certain methylated arsenic species may be carcinogenic [17,18]. Indeed, there is greater awareness that methylation of inorganic arsenic species may also affect susceptibility to arsenic-induced disease and may vary among individuals depending on genetic polymorphism, dose, age, selenium intake, as well as folate and homocysteine status [5,17,19–27]. Exposure to DMA [28] and MMA [29–35] have produced tumors in animal studies, resulting in concerns about human carcinogenicity.

Several studies have examined selected US (United States) foods for total and inorganic arsenic species content [36–40], or have examined the relationship between consumption of selected foods and total urinary arsenic [36,39] and speciated arsenic [41–43]. Using US FDA's (Food and Drug Administration) Total Diet Study 1991–1996, Tao and Bolger [44] reported that total arsenic concentration in food was highest in seafood, followed by rice/rice cereal, mushrooms, and poultry. We analyzed NHANES (National Health and Nutrition Examination Survey) data from 2003–2010 for associations between increased consumption of a comprehensive set of food groups and urinary concentrations of arsenic species that share human metabolic biotransformation pathways [9]. This approach was successfully utilized for a similar assessment of dietary exposure to perchlorate in NHANES 2001–2008 data [45].

Materials and Methods

Study Design

NHANES, conducted by the National Center for Health Statistics (NCHS) of the Centers for Disease Control and Prevention (CDC), collects serial cross-sectional data from a complex, multistage probability sample representative of the civilian, non-institutionalized population of the United States. The data used in this study are publicly available for download at http://www.cdc.gov/nchs/nhanes.htm. This website also provides details on the study design and recommended statistical techniques for analyzing NHANES data. Food consumption information was collected from participants using structured questionnaires administered by trained interviewers. Urinary arsenic species were measured in a single spot urine sample obtained from a one-third subsample of participants 6 years and older who provided spot urine specimens during physical examinations in the NHANES 2003–2010 cycles. Urine was collected and stored in arsenic-free containers and shipped on dry ice to CDC's National Center for Environmental Health laboratory, where samples were stored at or below −20°C until analyzed and typically analyzed within three weeks of collection (total urinary arsenic concentrations are stable at approximately −70°C for up to three years [46]). Arsenic species in urine were separated by high performance liquid chromatography, then directed to an ELAN DRC II ICP-MS (PerkinElmer SCIEX, Concord, Ontario, Canada) [47]. The limits of detection (LOD) were: As (III) 1.2 μg/L; As (V) 1.0 μg/L; DMA 1.7 μg/L; and MMA 0.9 μg/L [47,48]. Measurements below the LOD were substituted with the quotient of the LOD divided by the square-root of two. Urine creatinine measurements in NHANES 2003–2006 were made using a CX3 Analyzer that employed the Jaffe reaction [49]; in NHANES 2007–2010 these measurements were made using a Roche/Hitachi Modular P Chemistry analyzer that employed an enzymatic method using creatinase [50]. Serum folate measurements in NHANES 2003–2006 were made using the BioRad Quantaphase II Radioassay [51]; in NHANES 2007–2010 these measurements were made using a microbiologic assay [52,53]. Reported measurements met the accuracy and precision specifications of the quality-control/quality-assurance program of the CDC National Center for Environmental Health, Division of Laboratory Sciences [54].

Statistical Analysis

NHANES is a complex survey where participants are recruited through a multistage sampling design that involves stratification, clustering, and oversampling of specific population subgroups. It is therefore necessary to account for this complex design in order to properly estimate variances of regression coefficients and to produce unbiased, nationally representative statistics [55]. Robust estimation may be accomplished through Taylor series linearization and applying survey sample weights to each survey participant. We used this estimation approach as it was implemented in the DESCRIPT and REGRESS subroutines of SUDAAN version 11.0.0 [56] called from the SAS version 9.3 statistical software application [57]. We fit a set of sample-weighted, age-stratified linear regression models to publicly available NHANES data from the 2003–2010 survey cycles [58] where the dependent variable was the urinary molar concentration of one of four arsenic species [nmol/L]: As(III) (arsenous acid), As(V) (arsenic acid), DMA (dimethylarsinic acid), and MMA (monomethylarsonic acid). Using molar units enables concentrations to be directly compared between arsenic species. We refer to As(III) and As(V) as "inorganic" arsenic species, and DMA and MMA as "methylated" arsenic species. Since urinary concentrations can be influenced by urine dilution, which can vary markedly throughout the day within each individual [59], we accounted for urinary dilution by normalizing urinary arsenic molar concentrations to urinary molar creatinine (Cre) for the summary statistics in Tables 1–3 [μmol/mol Cre]. For the same reason, we accounted for urinary dilution by including urinary creatinine [g/L] as a model predictor in the regression models. In addition, because the distribution of urinary arsenic measurements were highly right-skewed, these data were transformed with the natural log for evaluating the statistical significance of regression slopes and we report the p-values from the ln-transformed regression models. To facilitate interpretability, however, we report slopes and their 95% confidence intervals estimated from identical un-transformed regression models. Statistical significance was set to $p \leq 0.05$, and marginal significance was set to $0.05 < p \leq 0.15$.

Dietary Consumption by Food Group. Primary interest was in the mass NHANES participants consumed within each USDA (US Department of Agriculture) food group for the 24-hour period (midnight to midnight) preceding the dietary recall interview conducted in-person as part of the physical examination. Data for the 24-hour recall period are contained in the publicly available NHANES Individual Foods – First Day file, which provides a record describing each food, water, or beverage consumed by the participant, including the mass reported consumed and eight-digit USDA food code. Standardized hierarchical food groups can be identified from the USDA code, where the first digit represents one of nine major food groups, and each subsequent digit represents subgroups of increasing specificity [60]. The mass consumed in each food group was summed so that each participant was represented by a single record describing their dietary intake for the previous 24 hours. Each participant's dietary intake was first apportioned over nine food groups: milk products; meat, poultry; eggs; legumes, nuts, seeds; grain products; fruits; vegetables; fats, oils, salad dressings; and sugars, sweets, beverages. In addition, we distinguished several food subgroups known or suspected of concentrating arsenic from the environment: fish (comprising both shellfish and finfish); rice (equivalent to the rice food subgroup defined by the USDA Food Surveys Research Group); rice cakes and crackers; rice beverage and milk; fruit juice and drink; and water (not bottled) consumed at home (i.e., residential tap water). To avoid double counting, the mass consumed in each subgroup was subtracted from the mass consumed in their respective food group. The USDA food codes and logic for apportioning dietary intake are detailed in Table S1.

Linear Regression Models. Additional predictors representing potential confounders were included in the regression models: sex, race/ethnicity, serum folate [mg/L], body mass index (BMI), poverty income ratio (PIR; ratio of self-reported family income to the US Census poverty threshold), education, fasting

Table 1. Sample-weighted statistics for creatinine-adjusted urinary arsenic species [μmol/mol Cre] in NHANES 2003–2010 data used in the regression models displayed in Tables 3 and 4.

	Median (25 percentile, 75 percentile)		
Arsenic Species	**Adults**	**Adolescents**	**Children**
DMA	2.97 (1.97, 4.81)	2.18 (1.55, 3.18)	3.52 (2.54, 5.36)
MMA	0.66 (0.42, 1.07)	0.56 (0.37, 0.85)	0.78 (0.50, 1.23)

Cre: creatinine.

time (time elapsed since participant last ate or drank anything other than water and the time of specimen collection), tobacco/ nicotine use in the five days prior to the physical examination, and NHANES study cycle. Information for potential confounders was self-reported, except for BMI (measured during the physical examination), urinary creatinine, and serum folate. Serum selenium and plasma homocysteine were not included because data were available for limited age groups and NHANES study cycles. Educational attainment for 20–84 year-olds was based on self-report, but for 6–19 year-olds educational attainment was based on the highest degree attained among the household reference person and their spouse. The models were stratified by age: children (6–11 years), adolescents (12–19 years), and adults (20–84 years). There were no age predictors in the children and adolescent models, but because the adult models encompassed a relatively broad age range, an age predictor was included with the categories 20–39 years, 40–59 years, and 60–84 years. No predictor for tobacco/nicotine use was included in the 6–11 years models because NHANES does not collect this information for this age group.

Regression models require complete information on all dependent and predictor data for each subject, which were available for about 8,268 of 10,868 participants in NHANES 2003–2010 depending on arsenic species. Missing data may introduce bias to model estimates depending on the degree of non-randomness in the pattern of missingness. To ameliorate this, the original NHANES survey sample weights were adjusted using the WTADJUST subroutine of SUDAAN version 11.0.0, which treats those participants with complete information as a random subsample of the entire sample. The probability of a sampled participant being in this subsample was assumed to be a logistic function of covariates, which was estimated implicitly by WTADJUST in computing the adjusted analysis weights. Because all models reported here used analysis weights adjusted in this manner, results may be considered statistically representative of the NHANES study population [61].

Table 2. Sample-weighted 25th, 50th, and 75th percentiles for creatinine-adjusted urinary DMA [μmol/mol Cre] for NHANES 2003–2010 data used in the regression models displayed in Tables 3 and 4.

	DMA					
	Adults		**Adolescents**		**Children**	
Percent ≥ LOD Used in Analysis		**84.2**		**87.4**		**86.0**
	Sample Size	**Median (25%ile, 75%ile)**	**Sample Size**	**Median (25%ile, 75%ile)**	**Sample Size**	**Median (25%ile, 75%ile)**
Age at Screening [years]						
6–11					1,044	3.52 (2.54, 5.36)
12–19			1,709	2.18 (1.55, 3.18)		
20–39	1,906	2.65 (1.76, 4.32)				
40–59	1,758	3.07 (2.05, 5.07)				
60–84	1,851	3.30 (2.24, 5.20)				
Race/Ethnicity						
Mexican American	1,016	3.35 (2.23, 4.99)	498	2.57 (1.86, 3.67)	326	4.28 (3.08, 5.73)
Non-Hispanic Black	1,091	2.35 (1.58, 3.92)	536	1.87 (1.28, 2.80)	288	3.08 (2.24, 4.51)
Non-Hispanic White	2,819	2.84 (1.94, 4.61)	499	2.05 (1.53, 2.95)	280	3.36 (2.46, 5.03)
Other Hispanic	381	4.39 (2.89, 6.90)	101	3.08 (1.86, 4.49)	81	3.85 (2.80, 5.82)
Other/Multiracial	208	5.18 (3.27, 9.50)	75	3.20 (1.85, 6.67)	69	4.72 (3.15, 8.39)
Sex						
Female	2,798	3.28 (2.17, 5.26)	822	2.29 (1.59, 3.25)	524	3.51 (2.49, 5.34)
Male	2,717	2.65 (1.77, 4.28)	887	2.08 (1.52, 3.07)	520	3.53 (2.62, 5.37)

Cre: creatinine.

Table 3. Sample-weighted 25th, 50th, and 75th percentiles for creatinine-adjusted urinary MMA [μmol/mol Cre] for NHANES 2003–2010 data used in the regression models displayed in Tables 3 and 4.

	MMA					
	Adults		Adolescents		Children	
Percent ≥ LOD Used in Analysis		32.9		42.4		29.2
	Sample Size	Median (25%ile, 75%ile)	Sample Size	Median (25%ile, 75%ile)	Sample Size	Median (25%ile, 75%ile)
Age at Screening [years]						
6–11					1,044	0.78 (0.50, 1.23)
12–19			1,709	0.56 (0.37, 0.85)		
20–39	1,906	0.60 (0.39, 0.96)				
40–59	1,757	0.66 (0.42, 1.14)				
60–84	1,851	0.74 (0.49, 1.20)				
Race/Ethnicity						
Mexican American	1,016	0.66 (0.40, 1.03)	498	0.58 (0.38, 0.85)	326	0.78 (0.54, 1.36)
Non-Hispanic Black	1,091	0.44 (0.32, 0.66)	536	0.45 (0.29, 0.62)	288	0.64 (0.41, 1.03)
Non-Hispanic White	2,818	0.69 (0.45, 1.11)	499	0.58 (0.37, 0.87)	280	0.80 (0.50, 1.28)
Other Hispanic	381	0.73 (0.47, 1.14)	101	0.58 (0.43, 0.86)	81	0.92 (0.58, 1.32)
Other/Multiracial	208	0.89 (0.53, 1.35)	75	0.73 (0.49, 1.24)	69	0.83 (0.54, 1.18)
Sex						
Female	2,798	0.75 (0.47, 1.29)	822	0.58 (0.36, 0.91)	524	0.78 (0.49, 1.32)
Male	2,716	0.59 (0.38, 0.90)	887	0.55 (0.37, 0.80)	520	0.78 (0.51, 1.18)

Cre: creatinine.

Median & 90th Percentile Diets. The sample-weighted percentile mass consumed in each food group adjusted for body weight [kg consumed/kg body weight] was computed by age stratum from NHANES 2003–2010 data to create a nationally representative percentile dietary consumption profile. Then, for each food group, multiplying the percentile mass by the slope for urinary arsenic species estimated from the regression models [nmol/L per kg consumed] produced arsenic species exposure via the percentile diet for the United States [nmol/L per kg body weight]. For this analysis, food group consumption was estimated for the 50th and 90th percentile diets.

Ethics Statement

The NCHS Research Ethics Review Board (ERB) protected the rights and welfare of NHANES participants. In accordance with Federal regulations, the NCHS ERB reviewed and approved NHANES protocols and any changes made to them: Protocols #98-12, #2005-06, #2011-17, and their respective continuations. Signed informed consent was obtained from each participant or their parent/guardian prior to collecting any data.

Results

Summary Statistics and Demographic Differences

There were 10,868 participants ages 6 years and older in NHANES 2003–2010. The proportion of participants with measurements greater than the LOD differed by age stratum and arsenic species: As(III) (2.8–5.3 percent depending on age stratum); As(V) (3.0–4.9 percent); DMA (84.2–87.4 percent); and MMA (29.2–42.4 percent). Since the inorganic species data had such low detection frequency, substantial bias could be introduced to statistical analysis [62,63]. Therefore, no further results on inorganic species are reported here, although results from statistical analyses analogous to those reported for methylated species are available from the corresponding author upon request.

Table 1 displays the sample-weighted 25th, 50th, and 75th percentiles for creatinine-adjusted urinary molar concentration [μmol/mol Cre] for each arsenic species by age stratum. Across all age strata, the rank-order for urinary molar concentration was DMA > MMA, and across all arsenic species concentrations, the rank-order for age was children > adults > adolescents. The median molar concentration was highest for DMA in children at 3.52 μmol/mol Cre and lowest for MMA in adolescents at 0.56 μmol/mol Cre. For each methylated arsenic species, the difference in the geometric mean creatinine-adjusted molar concentration was statistically significant between adults *vs.* adolescents and adults *vs.* children.

Tables 2–3 display the sample-weighted 25th, 50th, and 75th percentiles for creatinine-adjusted molar concentrations of urinary arsenic species by age stratum, race/ethnicity, and sex for the same data used in the regression models reported in Tables 4–5. The statistical significance of differences in urinary arsenic species between levels of each demographic characteristic were evaluated in regression models and controlled for all other variables in the models. For p-values, refer to Tables S2–S3. Urinary DMA was significantly higher in Mexican Americans and Other/Multiracial participants in all age strata compared to non-Hispanic Whites, and significantly elevated among adult and adolescent Other Hispanics. Among adults, males had significantly lower urinary DMA than females. Adults 40–59 years and 60–84 years had significantly elevated urinary DMA compared to 20–39 years participants. Urinary MMA among adults, adolescents, and children was significantly lower in non-Hispanic Blacks compared

Table 4. Summary of food groups with DMA regression slope p-values ≤0.15 (results identical to those in Table S2).

		DMA					
Regression Slope		**Adults**		**Adolescents**		**Children**	
Sign	**p-Value**	**Food Group**	**Slope**	**Food Group**	**Slope**	**Food Group**	**Slope**
Positive	**Significant**	Fish	181.16	Rice cakes/crackers	872.55	Rice	115.38
		Rice	105.58	Rice	101.05	Rice cakes/crackers	82.20
		Rice beverage/milk*	84.15	Fish	85.14	Fish	46.99
		Fruits	13.55	Legumes, Nuts, Seeds	24.96	Fruits	33.13
		Legumes, Nuts, Seeds	4.15	Meat, Poultry	7.82	—	—
		Meat, Poultry	2.23	—	—	—	—
		Grain Products	1.88	—	—	—	—
	Marginally Significant	—	—	Grain Products	2.37	Meat, Poultry	8.08
Negative	**Marginally Significant**	Vegetables	−1.36	Sugars, Sweets, Beverages	−0.72	Sugars, Sweets, Beverages	−3.23
		Milk Products	−2.34	—	—	—	—
	Significant	—	—	—	—	—	—

Complete tabulation of model slopes is in Table S2–S3.
Significant: p-Value ≤0.05.
Marginally Significant: 0.05 < p-Value ≤0.15.
*: Data on rice beverage/milk consumption available for adults only during NHANES 2003–2010.

Table 5. Summary of food groups with MMA regression slope p-values ≤0.15 (results identical to those in Table S3).

Regression Slope		MMA					
		Adults		Adolescents		Children	
Sign	p-Value	Food Group	Slope	Food Group	Slope	Food Group	Slope
Positive	Significant	Rice beverage/milk*	6.45	Rice cakes/crackers	103.04	Rice cakes/crackers	65.59
		Rice	5.75	Rice	11.71	Grain Products	2.22
		Fruits	1.24	—	—	—	—
		Sugars, Sweets, Beverages	0.14	—	—	—	—
	Marginally Significant	—	—	Milk Products	0.47	Rice	11.10
		—	—	Fruit juice/drink	0.31	Eggs	3.14
Negative	Marginally Significant	—	—	—	—	Sugars, Sweets, Beverages	−0.40
	Significant	Milk Products	−0.69	—	—	—	—

Complete tabulation of model slopes is in Table S2–S3.
Significant: p-Value ≤0.05.
Marginally Significant: 0.05 < p-Value ≤0.15.
*: Data on rice beverage/milk consumption available for adults only during NHANES 2003–2010.

to non-Hispanic Whites, and significantly elevated among Other Hispanic and Other/Multiracial adults.

Food Groups Associated with Urinary Methylated Arsenic

The creatinine-adjusted associations between food group consumed and urinary arsenic species were estimated with sample-weighted regression model slopes, which are displayed in Tables 4–5 (complete tabulation of slopes are in Tables S2–S3), controlling for potential confounders. To facilitate interpretation, Tables 4–5 display only the food groups for slopes with p-values ≤ 0.15, ordered by magnitude. The creatinine-adjusted food group slopes represent the change in urinary molar arsenic concentration attributable to one additional kilogram consumed of a food group [nmol/L per kg consumed]. The displayed p-values are from identical models except that the dependent variable was ln-transformed. No parameter estimates are available for adolescents and children consuming rice beverage/milk because no NHANES 2003–2010 participants in these age strata reported consuming this food group.

Several continuous potential confounders were influential predictors in the regression models (Tables S2–S3; categorical potential confounders were discussed in the summary statistics section). Urinary creatinine was a positive and statistically significant predictor across all age strata and arsenic species. Serum folate was a significant positive predictor for DMA and MMA among adolescents. BMI was a statistically significant negative predictor for DMA among adults and for MMA among all age strata. Fasting time was a statistically significant negative predictor for DMA among adolescents and a positive predictor for DMA and MMA among adults.

The largest significant increase in urinary molar concentration of methylated arsenic species was for DMA (872.55 nmol/L per kg) attributable to rice cakes/crackers consumed by adolescents (Table 4). The next largest molar increase among methylated species was associated with fish consumption among adults: 181.16 nmol DMA/L per kg. The third largest molar increase was for rice consumption among children at 115.38 nmol DMA/L per kg, followed by 105.58 nmol DMA/L per kg rice consumed by adults. At the fifth rank, MMA appears for the first time with 103.04 nmol MMA/L per kg rice cake/crackers consumed by adolescents (Table 5). The magnitude of association for the remaining food groups associated with significant increases in methylated arsenic ranged from 0.14 nmol MMA/L to 101.05 nmol DMA/L per kg for fish; fruits; grain products; legumes, nuts, seeds; meat, poultry; rice; rice cakes/crackers; rice beverage/milk (adults only); and sugars, sweets, beverages.

Only one food group was associated with a significant decrease in methylated arsenic: −0.69 nmol MMA/L per kg milk products consumed by adults.

Arsenic Exposure for the Median & 90th Percentile Diets

Arsenic species exposure [nmol/L per kg body weight (bw)] are tabulated for the median (Table 6) and 90th percentile (Table 7) United States diets, where asterisks indicate food groups significantly associated with creatinine-adjusted changes in urinary arsenic species, as shown by the regression model slopes (Tables 4–5). The net total dietary urinary arsenic species for each age stratum is also shown.

Median Diet. The net effect of all food groups on urinary arsenic can be appreciated by combining the regression slopes quantifying the contribution of each food group to urinary arsenic with information on the amount of each food group consumed. For the methylated arsenic species, children (1.28E-2 nmol MMA/L per kg bw), adolescents (9.32E-3 nmol DMA/L and

Table 6. Sample-weighted change in urinary methylated arsenic species [nmol/L per kg body weight] attributable to consuming each food group at the median amount estimated from NHANES 2003–2010 data.

	DMA			MMA		
Food Group	**20–84**	**12–19**	**6–11**	**20–84**	**12–19**	**6–11**
Milk Products	−3.70E-3	−8.21E-3	−7.77E-2	−1.09E-3*	1.37E-3	−4.30E-3
Meat, Poultry	4.17E-3*	1.58E-2*	2.34E-2	−9.46E-4	−4.64E-5	1.16E-3
Eggs	—	—	—	—	—	—
Legumes, Nuts, Seeds	—*	—*	—	—	—	—
Grain Products	5.30E-3*	1.06E-2	7.27E-2	−1.28E-3	2.69E-4	1.73E-2*
Fruits	—*	—	—*	—*	—	—
Vegetables	−2.05E-3	−2.24E-5	−2.20E-2	4.54E-4	−9.62E-4	1.63E-4
Fats, Oils, Salad Dressings	—	—	—	—	—	—
Sugars, Sweets, Beverages	5.07E-3	−8.85E-3	−3.66E-2	2.45E-3*	−2.94E-4	−4.49E-3
Fish	—*	—*	—*	—	—	—
Rice	—*	—*	—*	—*	—*	—
Rice cakes/crackers	—	—*	—*	—	—*	—*
Rice beverage/milk	—*	NA	NA	—*	NA	NA
Fruit juice/drink	—	—	4.84E-3	—	—	2.93E-3
Water (Not Bottled) At Home	—	—	—	—	—	—
NET TOTAL	**8.78E-3**	**9.32E-3**	**−3.54E-2**	**−4.14E-4**	**3.35E-4**	**1.28E-2**

*: food group significantly associated with urinary arsenic species in regression models reported in Tables 3a and 3b.
—: food group data insufficient to estimate sample-weighted percentile consumption.
NA: rice beverage/milk was only evaluated in adults 20–84 years because no NHANES participants <20 years reported consuming this food group.

Table 7. Sample-weighted change in urinary methylated arsenic species [nmol/L per kg body weight] attributable to consuming each food group at the 90th percentile amount estimated from NHANES 2003–2010 data.

	DMA			MMA		
Food Group	**20–84**	**12–19**	**6–11**	**20–84**	**12–19**	**6–11**
Milk Products	−1.74E-2	−3.45E-2	−2.17E-1	−5.13E-3*	5.75E-3	−1.20E-2
Meat, Poultry	1.32E-2*	5.38E-2*	7.57E-2	−2.99E-3	−1.58E-4	3.74E-3
Eggs	−7.47E-4	2.57E-3	−3.31E-2	−1.69E-3	−3.17E-3	6.61E-3
Legumes, Nuts, Seeds	6.27E-3*	1.95E-2*	2.98E-2	−1.50E-3	1.84E-3	−1.43E-3
Grain Products	1.52E-2*	2.92E-2	1.79E-1	−3.68E-3	7.39E-4	4.26E-2*
Fruits	4.71E-2*	1.31E-3	2.41E-1*	4.29E-3*	−2.67E-4	5.83E-3
Vegetables	−7.39E-3	−1.01E-4	−1.02E-1	1.64E-3	−4.33E-3	7.59E-4
Fats, Oils, Salad Dressings	−1.11E-2	−1.90E-3	3.52E-2	−2.12E-3	−1.81E-3	1.31E-2
Sugars, Sweets, Beverages	1.26E-2	−2.53E-2	−1.00E-1	6.10E-3*	−8.42E-4	−1.23E-2
Fish	7.26E-2*	—*	—*	3.72E-4	—	—
Rice	—*	—*	—*	—*	—*	—
Rice cakes/crackers	—	—*	—*	—	—*	—*
Rice beverage/milk	—*	NA	NA	—*	NA	NA
Fruit juice/drink	−9.83E-4	2.85E-2	1.72E-2	3.13E-3	4.30E-3	1.04E-2
Water (Not Bottled) At Home	−4.59E-3	6.79E-3	−2.29E-2	1.07E-3	−2.10E-3	9.65E-3
NET TOTAL	**1.25E-1**	**7.99E-2**	**1.02E-1**	**−5.09E-4**	**−5.92E-5**	**6.69E-2**

*: food group significantly associated with urinary arsenic species in regression models reported in Tables 3a and 3b.
—: food group data insufficient to estimate sample-weighted percentile consumption.
NA: rice beverage/milk was only evaluated in adults 20–84 years because no NHANES participants <20 years reported consuming this food group.

3.35E-4 nmol MMA/L per kg bw), and adults (8.78E-3 nmol DMA/L per kg bw) had a net increase in urinary arsenic from the median diet (Table 6).

Molar contributions from the median diet to net urinary methylated arsenic species was greatest among children eating grain products (7.27E-2 nmol DMA/L per kg bw, followed by 1.73E-2 nmol MMA/L per kg bw), followed by DMA in adolescents eating meat, poultry (1.58E-2 nmol DMA/L per kg bw). The regression slopes, however, were significant only for children who ate grain products (DMA slope p-value = 0.0333) and adolescents who ate meat, poultry (DMA slope p-value = 0.0024).

90th Percentile Diet. Several food groups with positive and statistically significant regression slopes — fish; fruits; legumes, nuts, seeds; rice; rice beverage/milk; rice cakes/crackers; and sugar, sweets, beverages — were not represented or were not estimable in the median dietary consumption profile, most likely due to sparse numbers of NHANES participants who reported consuming these foods. In order to evaluate the influence of high dietary consumption, we examined the 90th percentile dietary consumption profile for the United States (Table 7). Fish; fruits; legumes, nuts, seeds; and sugar, sweets, beverages now appear in the profile, but rice; rice beverage/milk; and rice cakes/crackers were still absent across all arsenic species and age strata.

Reviewing the net changes in urinary arsenic species for the 90th percentile United States diet, methylated arsenic species (Table 7) increased for adults (1.25E-1 nmol DMA/L per kg bw), adolescents (7.99E-2 nmol DMA/L per kg bw), and children (1.02E-1 nmol DMA/L per kg bw and 6.69E-2 nmol MMA/L per kg bw).

Increases in urinary methylated arsenic species for the 90th percentile diet comprised several food groups with positive and statistically significant regression slopes. The greatest molar increase among methylated species was associated with increased fruit consumption among children (2.41E-1 nmol DMA/L per kg bw), followed by fish eaten by adults (7.26E-2 nmol DMA/L per kg bw), meat, poultry eaten by adolescents (5.38E-2 nmol DMA/L per kg bw), fruits eaten by adults (4.71E-2 nmol DMA/L per kg bw), grain products eaten by children (4.26E-2 nmol MMA/L per kg bw), and legumes, nuts, seeds eaten by adolescents (1.95E-2 nmol DMA/L per kg bw). The next largest increase was associated with grain products consumed by adults (1.52E-2 nmol DMA/L per kg bw), followed by meat, poultry (1.32E-2 nmol DMA/L per kg bw), legumes, nuts, seeds (6.27E-3 nmol DMA/L per kg bw), sugars, sweets, beverages (6.10E-3 nmol MMA/L per kg bw), and fruits (4.29E-3 nmol MMA/L per kg bw).

Discussion

This analysis provides the most comprehensive model of NHANES data characterizing the association of food consumption with methylated urinary arsenic, while accounting for numerous potential confounders (urinary creatinine, serum folate, sex, race, BMI, poverty income ratio, education, fasting time, recent tobacco/nicotine use, and NHANES study cycle). Our analysis details which food groups contribute to each urinary arsenic species and how these dietary contributions vary among age groups in the US population. Similar to previous studies examining populations without high arsenic exposure from drinking water, we found that increased rice and fish consumption were associated with increased urinary methylated arsenic [36,41–44,64]. We also found that consuming either home tap water or fruit juice/drink was not significantly associated with any of the two urinary arsenic species (Tables S2–S3). The absence of a significant association with home tap water consumption reflects the comparatively low concentration of arsenic in United States drinking water, which averages 2 μg/L [9]. In addition, we assessed urinary arsenic excretion attributable to dietary sources based on 50th and 90th percentile rates of food consumption for the US population in combination with the rates of dietary arsenic exposure estimated in the regression models.

The methylated arsenic species selected for analysis are associated with public health concerns for potential carcinogenicity and other adverse health effects [1,2,65]. Of the two methylated species, DMA was observed at the highest concentrations and detected among the most participants. Rice, rice cakes/crackers, and fish were the most prominent sources of urinary DMA (Table 4). Other food groups that contributed significantly to urinary DMA, but to a lesser degree, were fruits (adults, children); meat, poultry (adults, adolescents); and legumes, nuts, seeds (adults, adolescents). For urinary MMA, the most prominent contributions came from rice cakes/crackers eaten by adolescents and children, followed by adults consuming rice beverage/milk and rice (Table 5). Other food groups that contributed significantly to urinary MMA were fruits (adults) and sugars, sweets, beverages (adults).

The food groups and the magnitudes of their contributions to urinary arsenic species vary markedly with age. For example, increased fish consumption was associated with the greatest change in urinary DMA among adults (181.16 nmol DMA/L per kg), but diminished to 85.14 nmol DMA/L per kg among adolescents, then to 46.99 nmol DMA/L per kg among children. The greatest increase in urinary DMA associated with increased consumption of rice cakes/crackers was among adolescents (872.55 nmol DMA/L per kg), but diminished sharply to 82.20 nmol DMA/L per kg among children.

Age-dependent variations like these may be due to variation in the types and amounts of food consumed, and although the USDA food classification scheme standardizes references to the diverse cornucopia of food consumed throughout the United States, the composition of food in each category, which in some cases is broad, could vary considerably in arsenic content. Consider, for example, that arsenic in soil varies spatially in relation to underlying geology, or through anthropogenic deposition associated with such activities as pesticide application, mining, discharge of metal processing waste, and fossil fuel combustion [66,67]. The same type of food harvested in one area may therefore have a different arsenic species concentration profile than another area. Rice, for example, varies markedly in arsenic species content depending on where it is obtained [68], or whether it is brown or white (polished) rice [69,70]. In the south central United States, arsenic is present in soil where arsenical pesticides were applied to cotton crops for decades since the 1930s [71–73]. This acreage has been given over to rice varieties that provide favorable yields in arsenical-pesticide-treated soils [74,75], and the relatively high arsenic content of rice grown in this region may be attributable to historical arsenical pesticide use [40,76]. Such compositional variations in dietary exposure may vary sufficiently with age to affect the statistical association of aggregate food groups with urinary arsenic species.

Indeed, the potential for exploring exposure to arsenic species from the numerous USDA food groups represented in NHANES data has not been exhausted by this analysis. Yet, while examining narrower food group designations would yield greater specificity, this would be counterbalanced by diminishing mass attributable to the food group.

The geographic and age-dependent variation just discussed also introduces a degree of exposure misclassification that reduces the overall statistical power of the study, and this reduction may be accentuated for food groups that comprise a relatively small proportion of the diet or a small population subgroup. Similarly, recall data is less precise than objectively measuring, say, the amount of arsenic species consumed via each food group [77].

The proportion of analyzed data with urinary concentrations exceeding the LOD ranged from 29.2 percent for MMA in children to 87.4 percent for DMA in adolescents (Tables 2–3). Diminished detection frequency potentially admits statistical bias, especially since measurements below the LOD were substituted with a fixed value (the quotient of the LOD divided by the square-root of 2) [62,63]. In a similar vein, the data are limited to the extent that NHANES participants consumed sufficient quantities of each food group to detect a significant change in urinary arsenic species. Since food groups are consumed disproportionately, it is possible that underrepresented food groups that were found in the regression models to not have significant influence on urinary arsenic species may nevertheless be important dietary sources of arsenic exposure. The clearest example of this was for rice beverage/milk, which was not reported consumed by adolescents and children in the NHANES 2003–2010 cycles and so its contribution to arsenic exposure could not be evaluated.

Another consideration is that food groups found to have significant influence on urinary arsenic species may not be consumed in quantities sufficient to appreciably affect population exposure. Conversely, food groups with relatively low rates of association with urinary arsenic may be consumed in great enough quantities to affect population exposure. We also found that increased consumption of some food groups was associated with reductions in urinary arsenic species, so the net effect on urinary arsenic would be expected to depend on the mix of food groups in a population's diet. Alternatively, it is possible the reductions apparent in the regression model results could have arisen from bias associated with substituting measurements below LOD with the quotient of the LOD divided by the square-root of two.

To evaluate the influence of population food consumption patterns on arsenic exposure, we combined urinary arsenic regression slopes for food consumption with statistical estimates of US population consumption of each food group. This approach highlighted a different set of food groups. For people who eat food groups at typical rates, as represented by the median diet (Table 6), increases in urinary arsenic species among adults were significantly attributable to meat, poultry (DMA); grain products (DMA); and sugars, sweets, beverages (MMA). Among adolescents, increases in urinary arsenic species were significantly attributable to meat, poultry (DMA). Among children, increases in urinary arsenic species were significantly attributable to grain products (MMA). For people who eat certain food groups at high rates, as represented by the 90th percentile diet (Table 7), increases in urinary arsenic species among adults were significantly attributable to fish (DMA); fruits (DMA, MMA); grain products (DMA); legumes, nuts, seeds (DMA); meat, poultry (DMA); and sugars, sweets, beverages (MMA). Among adolescents, increases in urinary arsenic species were significantly attributable to legumes, nuts, seeds (DMA) and meat, poultry (DMA), and among children to fruits (DMA) and grain products (MMA).

Figure 1 displays inorganic and methylated arsenic species on a diagram depicting two biotransformation pathways adapted from Figures 3–7 and 3–8 of ATSDR's Toxicological Profile for Arsenic [9], which in turn were adapted from Aposhian et al. [78] (Pathway I), as well as Hayakawa et al. [79] and Thomas et al. [80] (Pathway II). Although determination of the exact metabolic pathway(s) for the methylation of inorganic arsenic is still the subject of study [81], simple attribution of speciated arsenic exposure to particular food groups is clouded by the metabolic interrelationship depicted in Figure 1. The concentration of each species may increase either directly by exposure to exogenous dietary or non-dietary sources, or — for As(III), DMA, and MMA — indirectly by endogenous biotransformation from precursors. Alternatively, arsenic species may decrease by endogenous biotransformation to subsequent metabolites. It is therefore impossible to identify with NHANES data whether the source of measured arsenic species is exogenous or endogenous. For example, since methylated arsenic species are end products of the biotransformation pathways, it would have been desirable if their concentration — expressed perhaps as DMA or DMA + MMA — could be interpreted as a measure of cumulative exposure to inorganic arsenic species, which have usually been of greatest human health concern. Yet, because methylated species may arise either from endogenous biotransformation of inorganic species or from environmental exposure, it cannot be said that methylated species concentration is a simple proportional measure of risk from inorganic species. Conversely, the low detection frequency of inorganic arsenic species among NHANES 2003–2010 participants does not necessarily indicate an absence of exposure to these species from diet. While this difficulty in discriminating endogenous from exogenous sources may admittedly be irrelevant to the ultimate risk posed by all arsenic exposure, it nevertheless complicates attribution of arsenic species to specific dietary sources.

Rice is prominent in certain ethnic cuisines, most notably in Spanish and Asian cooking, while fish is a staple of Asian cooking. Racial/ethnic patterns in molar concentrations of urinary arsenic species were compared to non-Hispanic Whites in the linear regression models, controlling for all other predictors in the models (Tables S2–S3). Mexican Americans across all age strata had significantly elevated urinary DMA molar concentrations compared to non-Hispanic Whites. Other Hispanic adults and adolescents had significantly elevated urinary DMA molar concentrations, while Other Hispanic adults had significantly elevated urinary MMA. Also, although comprising a relatively small number of participants, Other/Multi-Racial participants (which include those of Asian ethnicity) across all age strata had significantly elevated urinary DMA, while Other/Multi-Racial adults had significantly elevated urinary MMA molar concentrations. These racial/ethnic elevations may be attributable to ethnic dietary patterns favoring arsenic-rich food groups like rice and fish (although diet would have been accounted for to a fair degree by the food group predictors included in the regression models), racial/ethnic differences in biotransformation of arsenic species, or a combination. Further research is needed to elucidate the causes for these racial/ethnic differences.

We evaluated the relative impact of different demographic and dietary factors on urinary arsenic species. Including urinary creatinine concentration as a predictor variable in all regression models accounted for varying rates of fluid consumption and excretion, as well as varying duration of when the urine specimen accumulated before micturition [62,82]. Additionally, fasting time and serum folate were included in the regression models and found to be statistically significant predictors in several models. Serum folate's statistical significance was consistent with its demonstrated role in metabolic methylation of arsenic [21]. Other contemporary analyses of NHANES data examining dietary exposure to arsenic have omitted fasting time and serum folate [42,43,83,84]. In addition, although availability of NHANES data on selenium and serum homocysteine was too restrictive for the scope of our analysis, future research should consider including these measurements because of their role in arsenic metabolism [17,19,21,22].

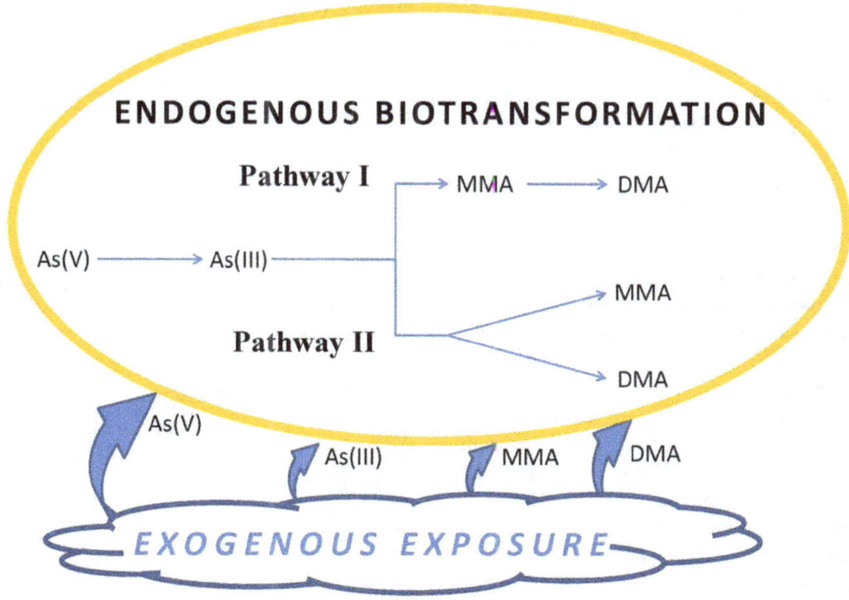

Figure 1. Biotransformation pathways for arsenic species As(III), As(V), DMA, and MMA.

The large size of the NHANES sample used for this study — approximately 8,300 participants— not only permitted control for several potential confounders in the statistical analysis, but also allowed age-stratified analyses, which revealed different excretion patterns among age strata. The data used in this report also comprise the largest number of NHANES cycles used for examining dietary exposure to arsenic compared to other contemporary analyses [42,43,83,84].

Conclusions

In a comprehensive evaluation of dietary sources of arsenic exposure in a representative sample of the United States civilian, non-institutionalized population observed 2003–2010, certain food groups were found to have been significantly associated with increases in urinary methylated arsenic species concentration: fish (DMA); fruits (DMA, MMA); grain products (DMA, MMA); legumes, nuts, seeds (DMA); meat, poultry (DMA); rice (DMA, MMA); rice cakes/crackers (As(III), DMA, MMA); sugars, sweets, beverages (MMA). Rice beverage/milk (DMA, MMA) contributed significantly among adults, but this food group could not be evaluated for the other age strata because child and adolescent NHANES participants during the 2003–2010 study cycles did not report consuming this food group. Different food groups in each age stratum contributed to each arsenic species with differing magnitudes. Fruit juice/drinks and home tap water were not significantly associated with changes in urinary arsenic.

This study also examined how dietary exposure to arsenic species depends on the amount consumed of each food group, as represented by typical (median) and high (90th percentile) dietary intake patterns in the United States. This perspective focused attention on a subset of food groups. At typical (median) dietary intakes, statistically significant sources of arsenic species were: grain products; meat, poultry; and sugars, sweets, beverages. At high (90th percentile) dietary intakes, statistically significant sources of arsenic species were: fish; fruits; grain products; legumes, nuts, seeds; meat, poultry; and sugars, sweets, beverages. Dietary intakes of these food groups were also found to vary between age strata.

Supporting Information

Table S1 USDA Food Codes and Logic for Apportioning Dietary Intake. To prepare the data for analysis, we summed the mass consumed in each food group so that each participant was represented by a single record describing their dietary intake for the previous 24 hours. Each participant's dietary intake was first apportioned over nine food groups: milk products; meat, poultry; eggs; legumes, nuts, seeds; grain products; fruits; vegetables; fats, oils, salad dressings; and sugars, sweets, beverages. In addition, we distinguished several food subgroups known or suspected of concentrating arsenic from the environment: fish (USDA food codes 261, 262, and 263, comprising both shellfish and finfish); rice (comprising multiple food codes equivalent to the rice food subgroup defined by the USDA Food Surveys Research Group); rice cakes and crackers (comprising multiple food codes); rice beverage and milk (USDA food code 92205000); and fruit juice and drink (comprising multiple food codes). Each of these subgroups is a constituent of a broader food group in the USDA food code hierarchy, so to avoid double counting the mass consumed in these subgroups was subtracted from the mass consumed in their respective food group. The food codes and logic for apportioning dietary intake are detailed in Table S1. We distinguished one more food subgroup of special interest as a route of arsenic exposure: water (not bottled) consumed at home (i.e., residential tap water) as an additional food subgroup. This subgroup was identified when the food code equaled 940 and the subject answered "yes" to whether water (not bottled) was consumed at home. Water (not bottled) is a constituent of the sugars, sweets, and beverages group (USDA food code 9), so for each participant, the mass consumed at home of water (not bottled) was subtracted from the mass consumed of the sugars, sweets, and beverages group to avoid double counting.

Table S2 Change in urinary DMA [nmol/L per kg] attributable to mass consumed estimated from sample-weighted, multiple regression models of NHANES 2003–2010 data. Estimates adjusted for urine volume by including urinary creatinine as a predictor in the models. Slopes are in units of nmol arsenic species/L per kg food consumed. CI: confidence interval HS: high school. NA: rice beverage/milk was only evaluated in adults 20–84 years old because no NHANES participants <20 years old reported consuming this food group. YO: years-old. a: p-Values estimated from identical models where the dependent variable was ln-transformed urinary arsenic species. Hypothesis tests represent comparisons with a slope equal to zero.

Table S3 Change in urinary MMA [nmol/L per kg] attributable to mass consumed estimated from sample-weighted, multiple regression models of NHANES 2003–2010 data. Estimates adjusted for urine volume by including urinary creatinine as a predictor in the models. Slopes are in units of nmol arsenic species/L per kg food consumed. CI: confidence interval. HS: high school. NA: rice beverage/milk was only evaluated in adults 20–84 years old because no NHANES participants <20 years old reported consuming this food group. YO: years-old. a: p-Values estimated from identical models where the dependent variable was ln-transformed urinary arsenic species. Hypothesis tests represent comparisons with a slope equal to zero.

Acknowledgments

Disclaimer: The findings and conclusions in this article are those of the authors and do not necessarily represent the views of the Centers for Disease Control and Prevention. The authors also wish to thank the staff of the Inorganic Analytical Toxicology Laboratory at CDC for their dedication and commitment to high quality measurements, as well as CDC's Sam Caudill and Yutaka Aoki for their statistical review. We are grateful to the NHANES staff who work tirelessly to maintain high participation in NHANES and who produce extensive amounts of data from each of the thousands of Survey participants. The authors would also like to convey thanks to staff of the Agency for Toxic Substances and Disease Registry for their guidance and expertise: Selene Chou, Carolyn Harper, and Kenneth Orloff.

Author Contributions

Conceived and designed the experiments: BRdC BCB MEM. Analyzed the data: BRdC YP. Wrote the paper: BRdC MEM. Conception and design: BRdC BCB MEM. Interpretation of results: BRdC KLC RLJ BCB MEM. Critical revising: BRdC KLC RLJ BCB YP CW MEM. Final approval: BRdC KLC RLJ BCB YP CW MEM. Conducted the experiments: KLC RLJ CW.

References

1. IARC Working Group on the Evaluation of Carcinogenic Risks to Humans (2012) Arsenic, metals, fibres, and dusts. Volume 100 C. A review of human carcinogens. Lyon, France. Available: http://monographs.iarc.fr/ENG/Monographs/vol100C/mono100C.pdf. Accessed 7 November 2011.
2. National Toxicology Program (2011) Arsenic and inorganic arsenic compounds. Report on Carcinogens 12th ed. Research Triangle Park, NC. Available: http://ntp.niehs.nih.gov/ntp/roc/twelfth/profiles/Arsenic.pdf. Accessed 2012 November 7.
3. Chen CJ, Hsueh YM, Lai MS, Shyu MP, Chen SY, et al. (1995) Increased prevalence of hypertension and long-term arsenic exposure. Hypertension 25: 53–60.
4. Jensen GE, Hansen ML (1998) Occupational arsenic exposure and glycosylated haemoglobin. Analyst 123: 77–80.
5. National Research Council Subcommittee on Arsenic in Drinking Water (1999) Arsenic in Drinking Water. Washington DC. Available: http://www.nap.edu/openbook.php?record_id=6444. Accessed 2012 November 7.
6. Vahidnia A, van der Voet GB, de Wolff FA (2007) Arsenic neurotoxicity–a review. Hum Exp Toxicol 26: 823–832.
7. US Environmental Protection Agency (2001) NPDES Final arsenic rule. Washington, DC. Available: http://www.epa.gov/fedrgstr/EPA-WATER/2001/January/Day-22/w1668.htm. Accessed 2012 November 7.
8. US Food and Drug Administration (2005) Bottled water quality standards: Arsenic monitoring. Washington, DC. Available: http://www.gpo.gov/fdsys/pkg/FR-2005-06-09/pdf/05-11406.pdf. Accessed 2012 November 7.
9. Agency for Toxic Substances and Disease Registry (2007) Toxicological profile for arsenic. Atlanta, GA. Available: http://www.atsdr.cdc.gov/ToxProfiles/tp2.pdf. Accessed 11 June 2013.
10. Apostoli P, Alessio L, Romeo L, Buchet JP, Leone R (1997) Metabolism of arsenic after acute occupational arsine intoxication. J Toxicol Environ Health 52: 331–342.
11. Bettley FR, O'Shea JA (1975) The absorption of arsenic and its relation to carcinoma. Br J Dermatol 92: 563–568.
12. Buchet JP, Lauwerys R, Roels H (1981) Comparison of the urinary excretion of arsenic metabolites after a single oral dose of sodium arsenite, monomethylarsonate, or dimethylarsinate in man. Int Arch Occup Environ Health 48: 71–79.
13. Crecelius EA (1977) Changes in the chemical speciation of arsenic following ingestion by man. Environ Health Perspect 19: 147–150.
14. Mappes R (1977) [Experiments on excretion of arsenic in urine (author's transl)]. Int Arch Occup Environ Health 40: 267–272.
15. Tam GK, Charbonneau SM, Bryce F, Pomroy C, Sandi E (1979) Metabolism of inorganic arsenic (^{74}As) in humans following oral ingestion. Toxicol Appl Pharmacol 50: 319–322.
16. Cohen SM, Arnold LL, Beck BD, Lewis AS, Eldan M (2013) Evaluation of the carcinogenicity of inorganic arsenic. Crit Rev Toxicol 43: 711–752.
17. Coppin JF, Qu W, Waalkes MP (2008) Interplay between cellular methyl metabolism and adaptive efflux during oncogenic transformation from chronic arsenic exposure in human cells. J Biol Chem 283: 19342–19350.
18. Del Razo LM, Styblo M, Cullen WR, Thomas DJ (2001) Determination of trivalent methylated arsenicals in biological matrices. Toxicol Appl Pharmacol 174: 282–293.
19. Basu A, Mitra S, Chung J, Guha Mazumder DN, Ghosh N, et al. (2011) Creatinine, diet, micronutrients, and arsenic methylation in West Bengal, India. Environ Health Perspect 119: 1308–1313.
20. Chen CJ, Wang SL, Chiou JM, Tseng CH, Chiou HY, et al. (2007) Arsenic and diabetes and hypertension in human populations: a review. Toxicol Appl Pharmacol 222: 298–304.
21. Gamble MV, Liu X, Ahsan H, Pilsner JR, Ilievski V, et al. (2006) Folate and arsenic metabolism: a double-blind, placebo-controlled folic acid-supplementation trial in Bangladesh. Am J Clin Nutr 84: 1093–1101.
22. Gamble MV, Liu X, Ahsan H, Pilsner R, Ilievski V, et al. (2005) Folate, homocysteine, and arsenic metabolism in arsenic-exposed individuals in Bangladesh. Environ Health Perspect 113: 1683–1688.
23. Steinmaus C, Yuan Y, Liaw J, Smith AH (2009) Low-level population exposure to inorganic arsenic in the United States and diabetes mellitus: a reanalysis. Epidemiology 20: 807–815.
24. Tseng CH (2008) Arsenic exposure and diabetes mellitus in the United States. JAMA 300: 2728; author reply 2728–2729.
25. Ghose N, Majumdar KK, Ghose AK, Saha CK, Nandy AK, et al. (2014) Role of folic Acid on symptoms of chronic arsenic toxicity. Int J Prev Med 5: 89–98.
26. Howe CG, Niedzwiecki MM, Hall MN, Liu X, Ilievski V, et al. (2014) Folate and cobalamin modify associations between S-adenosylmethionine and methylated arsenic metabolites in arsenic-exposed Bangladeshi adults. J Nutr 144: 690–697.
27. Niedzwiecki MM, Hall MN, Liu X, Slavkovich V, Ilievski V, et al. (2014) Interaction of plasma glutathione redox and folate deficiency on arsenic methylation capacity in Bangladeshi adults. Free Radic Biol Med 73: 67–74.
28. Chen GQ, Zhou L, Styblo M, Walton F, Jing Y, et al. (2003) Methylated metabolites of arsenic trioxide are more potent than arsenic trioxide as apoptotic but not differentiation inducers in leukemia and lymphoma cells. Cancer Res 63: 1853–1859.
29. Kligerman AD, Doerr CL, Tennant AH, Harrington-Brock K, Allen JW, et al. (2003) Methylated trivalent arsenicals as candidate ultimate genotoxic forms of arsenic: induction of chromosomal mutations but not gene mutations. Environ Mol Mutagen 42: 192–205.
30. Le XC, Ma M, Cullen WR, Aposhian HV, Lu X, et al. (2000) Determination of monomethylarsonous acid, a key arsenic methylation intermediate, in human urine. Environ Health Perspect 108: 1015–1018.
31. Mass MJ, Tennant A, Roop BC, Cullen WR, Styblo M, et al. (2001) Methylated trivalent arsenic species are genotoxic. Chem Res Toxicol 14: 355–361.
32. Nesnow S, Roop BC, Lambert G, Kadiiska M, Mason RP, et al. (2002) DNA damage induced by methylated trivalent arsenicals is mediated by reactive oxygen species. Chem Res Toxicol 15: 1627–1634.
33. Styblo M, Del Razo LM, Vega L, Germolec DR, LeCluyse EL, et al. (2000) Comparative toxicity of trivalent and pentavalent inorganic and methylated arsenicals in rat and human cells. Arch Toxicol 74: 289–299.
34. Tokar EJ, Diwan BA, Thomas DJ, Waalkes MP (2012) Tumors and proliferative lesions in adult offspring after maternal exposure to methylarsonous acid during gestation in CD1 mice. Arch Toxicol 86: 975–982.
35. Valenzuela OL, Borja-Aburto VH, Garcia-Vargas GG, Cruz-Gonzalez MB, Garcia-Montalvo EA, et al. (2005) Urinary trivalent methylated arsenic species

in a population chronically exposed to inorganic arsenic. Environ Health Perspect 113: 250–254.
36. Gilbert-Diamond D, Cottingham KL, Gruber JF, Punshon T, Sayarath V, et al. (2011) Rice consumption contributes to arsenic exposure in US women. Proc Natl Acad Sci U S A 108: 20656–20660.
37. Jackson BP, Taylor VF, Karagas MR, Punshon T, Cottingham KL (2012) Arsenic, organic foods, and brown rice syrup. Environ Health Perspect 120: 623–626.
38. Meacher DM, Menzel DB, Dillencourt MD, Bic LF, Schoof RA, et al. (2002) Estimation of multimedia inorganic arsenic intake in the US population. Human and Ecological Risk Assessment 8: 1697–1721.
39. Schoof RA, Yost LJ, Eickhoff J, Crecelius EA, Cragin DW, et al. (1999) A market basket survey of inorganic arsenic in food. Food Chem Toxicol 37: 839–846.
40. Williams PN, Raab A, Feldmann J, Meharg AA (2007) Market basket survey shows elevated levels of As in South Central U.S. processed rice compared to California: consequences for human dietary exposure. Environ Sci Technol 41: 2178–2183.
41. Cleland B, Tsuchiya A, Kalman DA, Dills R, Burbacher TM, et al. (2009) Arsenic exposure within the Korean community (United States) based on dietary behavior and arsenic levels in hair, urine, air, and water. Environ Health Perspect 117: 632–638.
42. Davis MA, Mackenzie TA, Cottingham KL, Gilbert-Diamond D, Punshon T, et al. (2012) Rice consumption and urinary arsenic concentrations in US children. Environ Health Perspect 120: 1418–1424.
43. Navas-Acien A, Francesconi KA, Silbergeld EK, Guallar E (2011) Seafood intake and urine concentrations of total arsenic, dimethylarsinate and arsenobetaine in the US population. Environ Res 111: 110–118.
44. Tao SS, Bolger PM (1999) Dietary arsenic intakes in the United States: FDA Total Diet Study, September 1991-December 1996. Food Addit Contam 16: 465–472.
45. Lau FK, deCastro BR, Mills-Herring L, Tao L, Valentin-Blasini L, et al. (2013) Urinary perchlorate as a measure of dietary and drinking water exposure in a representative sample of the United States population 2001–2008. J Expo Sci Environ Epidemiol 23: 207–214.
46. Yu LL, Verdon CP, Davis WC, Turk GC, Caldwell KL, et al. (2011) A human urine standard reference material for accurate assessment of arsenic exposure. Analytical Methods 3: 1107–1115.
47. Verdon CP, Caldwell KL, Fresquez MR, Jones RL (2009) Determination of seven arsenic compounds in urine by HPLC-ICP-DRC-MS: a CDC population biomonitoring method. Anal Bioanal Chem 393: 939–947.
48. Caldwell KL, Jones RL, Verdon CP, Jarrett JM, Caudill SP, et al. (2009) Levels of urinary total and speciated arsenic in the US population: National Health and Nutrition Examination Survey 2003–2004. J Expo Sci Environ Epidemiol 19: 59–68.
49. Beckman Instruments Beckman Synchron CX3 Clinical System Operating and Service Instruction. Brea, CA: Beckman Instruments.
50. Roche/Hitachi Diagnostics (2006) Modular Analytics Operator's Manual. Indianapolis, IN: Roche/Hitachi Diagnostics.
51. Bio-Rad Laboratories (1993) Bio-Rad Quantaphase II Folate Radioassay Manual. Hercules, CA: Bio-Rad Laboratories.
52. Molloy AM, Scott JM (1997) Microbiological assay for serum, plasma, and red cell folate using cryopreserved, microtiter plate method. Methods Enzymol 281: 43–53.
53. O'Broin S, B K (1992) Microbiological assay on microtitre plates of folate in serum and red cells. J Clin Pathol 45: 344–347.
54. Caudill SP, Schleicher RL, Pirkle JL (2008) Multi-rule quality control for the age-related eye disease study. Stat Med 27: 4094–4106.
55. CDC National Center for Health Statistics (2006) The National Health and Nutrition Examination Survey (NHANES) Analytic and Reporting Guidelines. Atlanta, GA. Available: http://www.cdc.gov/nchs/data/nhanes/nhanes_03_04/nhanes_analytic_guidelines_dec_2005.pdf. Accessed 7 November 2012.
56. Research Triangle Institute (2012) SAS-Callable SUDAAN. Research Triangle Park, NC.
57. SAS Institute (2010) SAS. Cary, NC.
58. CDC National Center for Health Statistics (2003–2010) National Health and Nutrition Examination Survey Data. Hyattsville, MD. Available: http://www.cdc.gov/nchs/nhanes.htm. Accessed 11 June 2013.
59. Barr DB, Wilder LC, Caudill SP, Gonzalez AJ, Needham LL, et al. (2005) Urinary creatinine concentrations in the U.S. population: implications for urinary biologic monitoring measurements. Environ Health Perspect 113: 192–200.
60. Ahuja JKA, Montville JB, Omolewa-Tomobi G, Heendeniya KY, Martin CL, et al. (2012) USDA Food and Nutrient Database for Dietary Studies, 5.0. Beltsville, MD. Available: http://www.ars.usda.gov/Services/docs.htm?docid=22370. Accessed 2013 June 11.
61. Folsom RE, Singh AC The generalized exponential model for sampling weight calibration for extreme values, nonresponse, and poststratification. In: Proceedings of the Joint Statistical Meetings 2000, Section on Survey Research Methods, 2000, American Statistical Association, 598–603.
62. Boeniger MF, Lowry LK, Rosenberg J (1993) Interpretation of Urine Results Used to Assess Chemical-Exposure with Emphasis on Creatinine Adjustments - a Review. American Industrial Hygiene Association Journal 54: 615–627.
63. Helsel DR (2006) Fabricating data: how substituting values for nondetects can ruin results, and what can be done about it. Chemosphere 65: 2434–2439.
64. Cascio C, Raab A, Jenkins RO, Feldmann J, Meharg AA, et al. (2011) The impact of a rice based diet on urinary arsenic. J Environ Monit 13: 257–265.
65. Moon KA, Guallar E, Umans JG, Devereux RB, Best LG, et al. (2013) Association between exposure to low to moderate arsenic levels and incident cardiovascular disease: A prospective cohort study. Ann Intern Med.
66. Cappuyns V, Van Herreweghe S, Swennen R, Ottenburgs R, Deckers J (2002) Arsenic pollution at the industrial site of Reppel-Bocholt (north Belgium). Science of the Total Environment 295: 217–240.
67. Fergusson JE (1990) The heavy elements: chemistry, environmental impact, and health effects. Oxford; New York: Pergamon Press. vii, 614 p. p.
68. US Food and Drug Administration (2012) Arsenic in Rice: Full Analytical Results from Rice/Rice Product Sampling - September 2012. Available: http://www.fda.gov/Food/FoodSafety/FoodContaminantsAdulteration/Metals/ucm319916.htm. Accessed 2013 June 11.
69. Carey AM, Norton GJ, Deacon C, Scheckel KG, Lombi E, et al. (2011) Phloem transport of arsenic species from flag leaf to grain during grain filling. New Phytol 192: 87–98.
70. Sun GX, Williams PN, Carey AM, Zhu YG, Deacon C, et al. (2008) Inorganic arsenic in rice bran and its products are an order of magnitude higher than in bulk grain. Environ Sci Technol 42: 7542–7546.
71. Epps EA, Sturgis MB (1939) Arsenic compounds toxic to rice. Soil Sci Soc Am Pro 4: 215–218.
72. Loebenstein JR (1994) The Materials Flow of Arsenic in the United States. Washington, DC. Available: http://books.google.com/books?id=1RbHGwAACAAJ. Accessed 11 June 2013.
73. Marcus-Wyner L, Rains DW (1982) Uptake, accumulation, and translocation of arsenical compounds by cotton. J Environ Qual 11: 715–719.
74. Wells BR, Gilmour JT (1977) Sterility, in rice cultivars as influenced byMSMA rate and water management. Agron J 69: 451–454.
75. Yan WG, Dilday RH, Tai TH, Gibbons JW, McNew RW, et al. (2005) Differential response of rice germplasm to straighthead induced by arsenic. Crop Science 45: 1223–1228.
76. Williams PN, Price AH, Raab A, Hossain SA, Feldmann J, et al. (2005) Variation in arsenic speciation and concentration in paddy rice related to dietary exposure. Environ Sci Technol 39: 5531–5540.
77. Lovreglio P, D'Errico MN, Gilberti ME, Drago I, Basso A, et al. (2012) The influence of diet on intra and inter-individual variability of urinary excretion of arsenic species in Italian healthy individuals. Chemosphere 86: 898–905.
78. Aposhian HV, Zheng B, Aposhian MM, Le XC, Cebrian ME, et al. (2000) DMPS-arsenic challenge test. II. Modulation of arsenic species, including monomethylarsonous acid (MMA(III)), excreted in human urine. Toxicol Appl Pharmacol 165: 74–83.
79. Hayakawa T, Kobayashi Y, Cui X, Hirano S (2005) A new metabolic pathway of arsenite: arsenic-glutathione complexes are substrates for human arsenic methyltransferase Cyt19. Arch Toxicol 79: 183–191.
80. Thomas DJ, Li J, Waters SB, Xing W, Adair BM, et al. (2007) Arsenic (+3 oxidation state) methyltransferase and the methylation of arsenicals. Exp Biol Med (Maywood) 232: 3–13.
81. Cullen WR (2014) Chemical mechanism of arsenic biomethylation. Chem Res Toxicol 27: 457–461.
82. Mage DT, Allen RH, Gondy G, Smith W, Barr DB, et al. (2004) Estimating pesticide dose from urinary pesticide concentration data by creatinine correction in the Third National Health and Nutrition Examination Survey (NHANES-III). J Expo Anal Environ Epidemiol 14: 457–465.
83. Navas-Acien A, Silbergeld EK, Pastor-Barriuso R, Guallar E (2008) Arsenic exposure and prevalence of type 2 diabetes in US adults. JAMA 300: 814–822.
84. Navas-Acien A, Silbergeld EK, Pastor-Barriuso R, Guallar E (2009) Rejoinder: Arsenic exposure and prevalence of type 2 diabetes: updated findings from the National Health Nutrition and Examination Survey, 2003–2006. Epidemiology 20: 816–820; discussion e811–812.

6

Cross-Sectional Study of Malnutrition and Associated Factors among School Aged Children in Rural and Urban Settings of Fogera and Libo Kemkem Districts, Ethiopia

Zaida Herrador[1,2], Luis Sordo[3,4,5], Endalamaw Gadisa[6], Javier Moreno[7], Javier Nieto[7], Agustín Benito[1,2], Abraham Aseffa[6], Carmen Cañavate[7], Estefania Custodio[1,2]*

1 National Centre of Tropical Medicine, Instituto de Salud Carlos III (ISCIII), Madrid, Spain, **2** Tropical Diseases Research Network (RICET in Spanish), Madrid, Spain, **3** National Centre of Epidemiology, ISCIII, Madrid, Spain, **4** Department of Preventive Medicine and Public Health, Faculty of Medicine, Complutense University, Madrid, Spain, **5** Network Biomedical Research Centers, Epidemiology and Public Health (CIBERESP in Spanish), Madrid, Spain, **6** Armauer Hansen Research Institute, Addis Ababa, Ethiopia, **7** National Centre of Microbiology, ISCIII, Madrid, Spain

Abstract

Introduction: Little information is available on malnutrition-related factors among school-aged children ≥5 years in Ethiopia. This study describes the prevalence of stunting and thinness and their related factors in Libo Kemkem and Fogera, Amhara Regional State and assesses differences between urban and rural areas.

Methods: In this cross-sectional study, anthropometrics and individual and household characteristics data were collected from 886 children. Height-for-age z-score for stunting and body-mass-index-for-age z-score for thinness were computed. Dietary data were collected through a 24-hour recall. Bivariate and backward stepwise multivariable statistical methods were employed to assess malnutrition-associated factors in rural and urban communities.

Results: The prevalence of stunting among school-aged children was 42.7% in rural areas and 29.2% in urban areas, while the corresponding figures for thinness were 21.6% and 20.8%. Age differences were significant in both strata. In the rural setting, fever in the previous 2 weeks (OR: 1.62; 95% CI: 1.23–2.32), consumption of food from animal sources (OR: 0.51; 95% CI: 0.29–0.91) and consumption of the family's own cattle products (OR: 0.50; 95% CI: 0.27–0.93), among others factors were significantly associated with stunting, while in the urban setting, only age (OR: 4.62; 95% CI: 2.09–10.21) and years of schooling of the person in charge of food preparation were significant (OR: 0.88; 95% CI: 0.79–0.97). Thinness was statistically associated with number of children living in the house (OR: 1.28; 95% CI: 1.03–1.60) and family rice cultivation (OR: 0.64; 95% CI: 0.41–0.99) in the rural setting, and with consumption of food from animal sources (OR: 0.26; 95% CI: 0.10–0.67) and literacy of head of household (OR: 0.24; 95% CI: 0.09–0.65) in the urban setting.

Conclusion: The prevalence of stunting was significantly higher in rural areas, whereas no significant differences were observed for thinness. Various factors were associated with one or both types of malnutrition, and varied by type of setting. To effectively tackle malnutrition, nutritional programs should be oriented to local needs.

Editor: Heather B. Jaspan, University of Cape Town, South Africa

Funding: The authors gratefully acknowledge the financial support of the UBS-Optimus Foundation in Switzerland, (www.ubs.com/global/en/wealth_management/optimusfoundation.html), via the Visceral Leishmaniasis and Malnutrition in Amhara State, Ethiopia project, and the Tropical Diseases Research Network in Spain (www.ricet.es/es/) via the VI PN de I+D+I 2008–2011, ISCIII -Subdirección General de Redes y Centros de Investigación Cooperativa RD12/0018/0001 and RD12/0018/0003. The funders had no role in study design, data collection and analysis, decision to publish, or preparation of the manuscript.

Competing Interests: The authors have declared that no competing interests exist.

* Email: ecustodio2014@gmail.com

Introduction

Adequate nutrition is essential during childhood to ensure healthy growth, proper organ formation and function, a strong immune system, and neurological and cognitive development [1]. Nutritional status has a major impact on children's survival mainly due to the synergistic relationships between malnutrition and diseases [2,3]. In Eastern and Southern Africa, malnutrition is a major underlying cause of the persistently high child mortality, contributing to more than a third of all deaths among children under age 5 [4].

The two main anthropometric indicators used to define malnutrition– stunting, and wasting or thinness– represent different histories of nutritional insult to the child. Linear growth retardation (chronic malnutrition or stunting) is frequently associated with repeated exposure to adverse economic conditions, poor sanitation, and the interactive effects of poor nutrient intakes and infection. Low weight-for-height or low body mass index (BMI) for age (acute malnutrition, wasting or thinness) is generally associated with recent illness and/or food deprivation [5].

The causes of childhood malnutrition are diverse, multidimensional, and interrelated. An analytical framework suggested by the

United Nations Children's Fund (UNICEF) categorizes the causes into (a) immediate causes: inadequate dietary intake and illness, (b) underlying causes: insufficient access to food in a household; inadequate health services and unhealthy environment; and inadequate care for children and women at the household level, and (c) basic causes: insufficient current and potential resources at societal level [6]. In Sub-Saharan Africa, various indicators of social economic status have been associated with children's nutritional status, such as maternal and paternal educational level, parental income, and family assets [7–9]. In addition, child nutrition outcomes in developing countries have been characterized by large rural-urban disparities over the last few decades [10].

In Ethiopia, child malnutrition continues to be a major public health problem. According to the Ethiopian National Demographic Health Survey (2011), the prevalence of both wasting and stunting in children under 5 years is very high (10% and 44% respectively) [11], while the situation in older children is not so well known [12,13]. Furthermore, rural-urban disparities in child nutrition, as well as growing urbanization that results in increasing inequalities in urban areas, underlines the need to improve our knowledge of the main drivers of urban-rural differences [14].

The Amhara Region is one of the four primary agricultural regions in Ethiopia [15], and most households rely upon livestock and crop sales to generate cash income. This region, and especially the Tana Zuria Zone, has a moderate population density, fertile soils and good rainfall. For this reason, it is amongst the most food self-sufficient regions in the country [16]. Despite this good regional profile, other factors may be determining the high prevalence of infant malnutrition in this area [17]. According to the Food and Agriculture Organization of the United Nations (FAO), the four pillars of food security are food availability, stability of the food supply, food access and the utilization of food by the body [18]. In our context, availability is strongly affected by seasonality; many households are only able to produce sufficient food to meet their food requirements for less than six months of the year [19]. Food access may be affected by market conditions, but also by cultural and religious practices. For example, the high number of fasting days commemorated by the Ethiopian Orthodox Church, the main religion in the country, may have repercussions on the nutritional status of the community, particularly in rural Ethiopia [20].

Even if people get enough to eat, good nutrition requires access to a sufficient, supply of varied, safe and nutritious food to meet daily nutritional requirements [21]. Although diet diversity questionnaires are extensively used in Ethiopia to investigate relationships between food intake and nutritional status, there is limited knowledge of nutrition outcomes, dietary practices and socioeconomic factors among school-aged children in this specific context [17].

The present study aimed to [22] describe the prevalence of stunting and thinness, and their related factors, including dietary habits, and [23] document the differences in nutritional status across urban and rural areas accounting for household and individual characteristics in school-aged children in Libo Kemkem and Fogera, Amhara regional State, Ethiopia.

Material and Methods

Study area and population

The study was carried out during May–June 2009 in the districts (*woredas*) of Libo Kemkem and Fogera (Amhara regional state, Ethiopia). Libo Kemkem and Fogera woredas are located in the Tana Zuria Livelihood Zone, within the Amhara Regional State, northwestern Ethiopia at an altitude of 2,000 m above sea level. According to the 2009 census, the population was 198,374 and 226,595 for Libo Kemkem and Fogera, respectively.

These two districts are located in a black cotton clay soil flat plain. Temperatures are relatively high, but rainfall is unusually abundant, with a mean of 1173 mm per annum. Agricultural activities are dependent on a single rainy season (from June to September). Maize, barley and millet are the main food crops, while rice, vetch and chickpea are the main cash crops. Livestock holdings in sheep and cattle are relatively modest, but livestock and butter sales make a substantial complement to the predominant crop sales. The major hazards to crop production and livestock are pests, occasional flooding, and zoonosis such as anthrax, trypanosomiasis, pasteurellosis and black leg [16].

Study design

This cross-sectional survey was part of a UBS Optimus Foundation funded project called Visceral Leishmaniasis (VL) and Malnutrition in Amhara State, Ethiopia. Among its specific objectives, the project aimed to characterize nutritional, immunological, and parasitological factors in school-aged children in the districts of Fogera and Libo Kemkem. Other methodological aspects have previously been published [24–26].

Sampling was carried out by multistage cluster survey. A total of 886 children aged 4 to 15 years were recruited. Primary sampling units were sub-districts (*kebeles*) with a high incidence of VL according to the 2008 register of the Addis Zemen VL Treatment Centre: one urban (Addis Zemen) and the rest rural: Bura, Yifag Akababi and Agita from Libo Kemkem, and Sifatra and Rib Gebriel from Fogera. Secondary sampling units were randomly selected villages (*gotts*) in each of the selected sub-districts. Third-stage sampling units were randomly selected households in each of the villages. All children with reported age between 4 and 15 years living in the household at the time of the survey were recruited. Sample size was calculated according to previous estimates of malnutrition for children under age 5 in the area and taking into account a design effect of 2, corresponding to the complex design.

Data collection

All children were measured and weighed according to standard WHO procedures [27]. Weight was measured to the nearest 0.1 kg on a battery-powered digital scale (SECA 881©). Standing height was measured to the nearest 0.1 cm using a portable adult/infant measuring unit (PE-AIM-101©).

A pre-tested questionnaire translated into Amharic, the local language, was administered to the caretaker/head of household (HH) of each child in the study by trained medical personnel (nurses and health officers).

We asked about individual demographic characteristics, health status and behavior determinants. The following household variables were also recorded: household socio-demographic characteristics, person in charge of food preparation (PCFP), house construction material and assets (land and cultivation, domestic animal assets) and community variables. Dietary data was collected through a 24-hour diet recall.

Statistical analysis

Stunting and thinness were the main outcomes of interest, defined as height-for-age z-score (HAZ) <-2 and BMI-for-age z-score (BAZ) <-2 respectively. The z-scores were calculated using the WHO 2007 reference (for children $\geq$5 years) and the WHO Growth Standards (for children $<$5 years old), both computed by WHO Anthro Plus software.

The dietary data collected through the 24-hour diet recall were computed into 9 food groups (1. Basic staples, 2. Vitamin A rich fruits and vegetables, 3. Other fruits, 4. Other vegetables, 5. Legumes and pulses, 6. Meat or Fish, 7. Oil, 8. Dairy and 9. Eggs) based on the FAO/FANTA Household Dietary Diversity Questionnaire and Guidelines [21].

Frequencies and percentages were used to summarize data and to explore the differences between rural and urban communities. These differences were assessed by Student's t-test and χ^2 tests for continuous and categorical variables, respectively.

Bivariate analyses for thinness and stunting and their related factors were performed, with stratification by setting. Age and sex, considered biologically relevant, and all variables associated with each of the outcomes at the p<0.10 level were included in the multivariable analysis. Logistic regression models stratified by setting for stunting and thinness were obtained by using a manual backward stepwise procedure. P-values less than or equal to 0.05 were considered statistically significant.

Data analysis was performed using Anthro Plus v1.02 (WHO, Geneva, Switzerland) and SPSS version 18.0 (SPSS Inc., Chicago, Illinois, USA).

Ethical considerations

The study was approved by the ethical review boards of the *Instituto de Salud Carlos III* (ISCIII), the Armauer Hansen Research Institute, and the Ethiopian National Ethical Review Committee. Support letters were obtained from the Amhara Regional State and the *woreda* health bureaus. Parents/guardians gave written informed consent before enrollment of their children in the study.

Results

Description of the sample

The study included a total of 886 children aged 4 to 15 years, of which 462 (52.0%) were males. Around 80% lived in the rural setting and 50.6% presented malnutrition. The prevalence of malnutrition was significantly higher in rural than in urban communities (53% and 42.1% respectively; p = 0.006).

The mean HAZ and BAZ for the overall study population were below the WHO references [28], −1.62 (SD = 1.34, range −6.12–5.74, p≤0.05) and −1.28 (SD = 1.00, range −4.95–3.82, p≤0.05), respectively.

Individual characteristics, including demographic data, nutritional status and diet habits are summarized in Table 1, disaggregated by rural and urban strata.

There were several differences between children living in rural and urban settings regarding child health status, behavior and dietary habits. Children living in rural areas slept under a bed net less frequently than urban children (41.1% vs. 67.4% respectively, p<0.001). On the day before the survey, 18.1% of children in the rural setting had consumed food from animal sources vs. 64% of those in the urban setting.. The proportion of children who had consumed food from four or more food groups was 16.3% vs. 39.9%, respectively (p<0.001 for each comparison).

Household characteristics are summarized in Table 2. The proportion of rural households that owned land was 97.6% vs. 10.1% in urban households, while the corresponding figures for ownership of domestic animals or chickens were 96.3% vs. 36.5%, respectively (p<0.001 for each). The distribution of the rest of the socio-demographic and household variables but one (years of education of the HH) also differed significantly between urban and rural areas.

Chronic malnutrition

The prevalence of stunting was 42.7% in the rural setting and 29.2% in the urban setting (p = 0.001).

Chronic malnutrition in rural communities. In the bivariate analysis (Table S1), the prevalence of chronic malnutrition was similar in males and females, however it was significantly higher inchildren age 10 and over than in those under 10 years of age (OR: 2.28; 95% CI: 1.66–3.11) in the rural group. Stunting was significantly more frequent in children with a previous history of splenomegaly (OR: 2.26; 95% CI: 1.11–4.59) or fever (OR: 1.59; 95% CI: 1.15–2.18), and less common in those who slept under a bed net (OR: 0.68; 95% CI: 0.50–0.92) or herded the cattle (OR: 0.70; 95% CI: 0.52–0.95). Regarding dietary habits in rural communities, the consumption of vitamin A rich fruits and vegetables and the consumption of any meat or fish the day before the survey were associated with a lower prevalence of chronic malnutrition (OR: 0.34 (95% CI: 0.13–0.93) and OR: 0.59 (95% CI: 0.36–0.97), respectively).

Results from the multivariable logistic analysis are presented in Table 3. The difference between the two age groups remained significant in the final model (OR: 3.12; 95% CI: 2.15–4.51), showing that the prevalence of chronic malnutrition was higher in children age 10 and over. Children with fever in the two weeks prior to the survey were 1.62 times more likely to be stunted (95% CI: 1.23–2.32). Herding cattle (OR: 0.43; 95% CI: 0.30–0.63) and the consumption of any food from animal sources (OR: 0.51; 95% CI: 0.29–0.91) showed a significant negative association with stunting. With regard to household socio demographic characteristics, children from rural areas were 2.97 times more likely to have chronic malnutrition if the HH was female (95%CI: 1.47–5.98). The number of people living in the house was positively associated with the prevalence of stunting (p = 0.042), while millet production (OR: 0.50; 95% CI: 0.27–0.93) and consumption of products from the family's own cattle (OR: 0.67; 95% CI: 0.46–0.96) were negatively associated.

Chronic malnutrition in urban communities. In the urban setting, the significant age differences (OR: 3.73; 95% CI: 1.89–7.39) found in the bivariate analysis occurred in the same direction as in the rural area (Table S1). Furthermore, the prevalence of stunting was significantly higher among children living in a house where the HH (OR: 1.58; 95% CI: 1.00–2.53) or the PCFP (OR: 1.60; 95% CI: 0.99–2.66) had not attended school.

Table 3 summarizes the results adjusted by logistic regression. Older children were more prone to stunting than younger children (OR: 4.62; 95% CI: 2.09–10.21). Years of school attendance of the PCFP was negatively associated with chronic malnutrition among children living in urban communities (OR: 0.88; 95% CI: 0.79–0.97).

Acute malnutrition

The prevalence of thinness was 21.6% in the rural setting and 20.8% in the urban setting (p>0.05).

Acute malnutrition in rural communities. In the bivariate analysis (Table S2), the prevalence of acute malnutrition was higher in children age 10 and over (OR: 4.74; 95% CI: 3.24–6.94) and among boys (OR: 1.58; 95% CI: 1.18–2.12). Children from rural communities who herded the cattle were 2.43 times more likely to be thin (95%CI: 1.63–3.61) than those who did not. The number of children living in the house (p = 0.007) and teff cultivation (OR: 1.53; 95% CI: 1.02–2.30) were positively associated with higher prevalence of thinness, while living with a HH under 40 years old and rice farming showed an inverse association with thinness (OR: 0.75; 95% CI: 0.56–0.99 and 0.63; 95% CI: 0.42–0.95, respectively).

Table 1. Individual characteristics, behavioral determinants and dietary habits of school-aged children in rural and urban areas of at Libokemkem and Fogera districts, Ethiopia, May–June 2009.

CHARACTERISTICS	RURAL (n = 711)		URBAN (n = 178)		p value
	No.	(%)	No.	(%)	
Sex (female)	339	47,68	88	49,44	0,676
Age group (≥10 years)	259	36,43	58	32,58	0,193
Stunting	302	42,66	52	29,21	0,001
Wasting	153	21,61	37	20,79	0,450
Splenomegaly	34	4,79	1	0,56	0,004
Fever in the last 15 days	223	31,41	37	20,79	0,003
Sleeps under a bed net	292	41,13	120	67,42	<0.001
Herds the cattle	413	58,17	7	3,93	<0.001
Consumption on day before survey of:					
Food of animal source	129	18,14	114	64,04	<0.001
Basic staples	708	99,58	178	100	0,511
VitA rich fruits and vegetables	24	3,38	11	6,18	0,071
Other fruits	0	0	3	1,69	0,008
Other vegetables	53	7,45	22	12,36	0,029
Legumes and pulses	643	90,44	106	59,55	<0.001
Meat/fish	79	11,11	103	57,87	<0.001
Oil	644	90,58	166	93,26	0,164
Dairy	53	7,45	15	8,43	0,381
Eggs	5	0,7	5	2,81	0,032
5 or more food groups	28	3,94	16	8,99	0,007
4 or more food groups	116	16,32	71	39,89	<0.001
	Mean	**s.d.**	**Mean**	**s.d.**	**p value**
Sum of food groups	3,12	0,60	3,42	0,77	<0.001

After adjusting for socio demographic and household characteristics in the model, sex differences lost significance, and the relationship between thinness and age was slightly weakened (OR: 4.11; 95% CI: 2.74–6.16) (Table 4). Children from rural communities were significantly less likely to be thin if the HH was female (OR: 0.40; 95% CI: 0.16–0.70). The number of children living in the house showed a positive relationship with thinness in this setting ($p = 0.027$), while children from households that cultivate rice were less likely to be thin (OR: 0.64; 95% CI: 0.41–0.99).

Acute malnutrition in urban communities. In the bivariate analysis (Table S2), no significant associations with thinness were found apart from age group (OR: 2.76; 95% CI: 1.13–5.80).

After adjusting the analysis, age group remained significantly related to thinness (OR: 3.67; 95% CI: 1.63–8.30). Food consumption from animal sources on the day before the survey was inversely associated with acute malnutrition (OR: 0.26; 95% CI: 0.10–0.67) and thinness prevalence was lower among in households headed by literate persons (OR: 0.24; 95% CI: 0.09–0.65) (Table 4).

Discussion

Our study shows that there is a high prevalence of stunting (39.8%) and thinness (21.4%) among school-aged children in Libo Kemkem and Fogera regions of Ethiopia. The prevalence of stunting was significantly higher in rural areas (42.7% vs. 29.2%), but no significant differences were observed for thinness. These results are similar to those observed in other developing countries [29]. Various intermediate and distal factors like age, consumption of food from animal sources and family size were associated with both types of malnutrition in one or both settings. Other determinants such as years of school attendance of the PCFP and consumption of the family's own cattle products were related to only one kind of malnutrition. Although malnutrition among pre-school children has been well documented in Ethiopia [5,30,31], to our knowledge this is the first research to assess factors related to acute and chronic malnutrition stratified by setting in school aged children. These results may assist stakeholders in planning and undertaking contextual and evidence-based policy initiatives.

We found that the probability of a child being malnourished increases with age. Age-group differences were significant in both strata for stunting and thinness. No sex differences were found in either strata. As children mature, household socioeconomic characteristics may emerge in conjunction with behavioral and biological variables as important risk factors [32].

Chronic malnutrition

The prevalence of stunting in rural areas in our study was higher (42.7%) than that found in a study conducted in the same age group in rural settings of Fogera in 2012 (30.7%) [33]. Our study was carried out in 2009, which may partially explain this difference due to possible improvements in local conditions;

Table 2. Parental and household characteristics of school-aged children in rural and urban areas of Libo Kemkem and Fogera districts, Ethiopia, May–June 2009.

CHARACTERISTICS	RURAL (n = 711)		URBAN (n = 178)		p value
	No.	(%)	No.	(%)	
Sex head of household (HH)					
Female	52	7.31	75	42.13	<0.001
Age HH					
≥40 years	351	49.72	65	36.93	0.008
HH literacy (read and write)					
Yes	282	39.83	97	54.49	<0.001
Person in charge of food preparation (PCFP)					
Wife or HH(she)	690	97.05	144	80.9	<0.001
Other	21	2.95	34	19.1	
Years of HH education	**Mean**	**s.d.**	**Mean**	**s.d.**	**p value**
	2.70	12.6	4.27	4.92	0.106
Years of education of the PCFP					
	0.22	1	3.30	4.53	<0.001
Number of people living in the house					
	6.41	1.71	5.24	1.58	<0.001
Number children in the house					
	2.85	1.13	2.17	0.89	<0.001
Does the household own land?	**No.**	**(%)**	**No.**	**(%)**	**p value**
Yes	694	97.61	18	10.11	<0.001
Have domestic animals or chickens?					
Yes	685	96.34	65	36.52	<0.001
Does the household....					
cultivate teff?					
Yes	481	67.65	4	2.25	<0.001
cultivate rice?					
Yes	231	32.49	2	1.12	<0.001
cultivate millet?					
Yes	70	9.85	5	2.81	<0.001
cultivate beans?					
Yes	22	3.09	1	0.56	0.038
consume products from their own cattle?					
Do not consume own cattle products	224	31.68	0		
Consume own cattle products	419	59.26	11	6.29	<0.001
Do not have cattle	64	9.05	164	93.71	
consume products from their own goats?					
Do not consume own goat products	35	4.96	0		
Consume own goat products	34	4.82	7	3.93	0.008
Do not have goats	637	90.23	171	96.07	
consume products from their own sheep?					
Do not consume own sheep products	62	8.81	2	1.12	
Consume own sheep products	90	12.78	6	3.37	<0.001
Do not have sheep	552	78.41	170	95.51	
consume products from their own chickens?					
Do not consume own chicken products	80	11.28	2	1.12	
Consume own chicken products	343	48.38	47	26.40	<0.001
Do not have chickens	286	40.34	129	72.47	

Table 3. Multivariable logistic regression analysis of stunting in school-aged children stratified by setting in Libo Kemkem and Fogera districts, Ethiopia, May–July 2009.

VARIABLES		RURAL (N=711)				URBAN (N=178)			
		n (%)	AOR	95% CI	p value	n (%)	AOR	95% CI	p value
CHILD CHARACTERISTICS									
Sex	**male**	166 (44.86)	1			27 (30.00)	1		
	female	136 (40.24)	0.78	(0.55–1.10)	0.160	25 (28.41)	1.29	(0.56–2.96)	0.554
Age group	**<10 years**	159 (35.24)	1			24 (20.01)	1		
	≥10 years	143 (55.26)	3.12	(2.15–4.51)	0.000	28 (48.39)	4.62	(2.09–10.21)	0.000
Fever in the last 15 days?	**No**	112 (50.45)	1			13 (35.14)	1		
	Yes	190 (39.09)	1.62	(1.23–2.32)	0.009	39 (27.66)	1.80	(0.73–4.47)	0.204
Does the child herd the cattle?	**No**	141 (47.64)	1			39 (29.24)	1		
	Yes	160 (38.93)	0.43	(0.30–0.63)	0.000	13 (28.57)	0.75	(0.07–7.71)	0.811
DOES THE CHILD CONSUME...									
Any food from animal sources*	**No**	254 (43.87)	1			20 (31.25)	1		
	Yes	48 (37.21)	0.51	(0.29–0.91)	0.022	32 (28.07)	0.72	(0.31–1.71)	0.463
vit A rich fruits and vegetables*	**No**	297 (43.42)	1			48 (28.74)	1		
	Yes	5 (20.83)	0.29	(0.83–1.04)	0.057	4 (36.36)	1.32	(0.29–5.99)	0.717
Other vegetables*	**No**	284 (43.36)	1			42 (26.92)	1		
	Yes	18 (33.96)	1.08	(0.49–2.38)	0.855	10 (45.45)	3.00	(0.97–9.38)	0.058
HOUSEHOLD AND LAND PRODUCTION									
Sex of head of household	**Male**	267 (40.70)	1			29 (28.16)	1		
	Female	35 (67.31)	2.97	(1.47–5.98)	0.002	23 (30.67)	0.66	(0.27–1.64)	0.370
Age of head of household	**<40 years**	151 (42.66)	1			37 (28.16)	1		
	≥40 years	147 (42.14)	0.73	(0.50–1.06)	0.097	23 (30.67)	0.43	(0.17–1.06)	0.069
Years of school-person in charge of food preparation		**Mean (sd)**	**AOR**	**95% CI**	**p value**	**Mean (sd)**	**AOR**	**95% CI**	**p value**
		0.16 (0.86)	0.84	(0.70–1.01)	0.065	2.19 (4.0)	0.88	(0.79–0.97)	0.014
Number of people living in the house									
		6.43 (1.85)	1.12	(1.01–1.25)	0.042	5.08 (1.41)	0.84	(0.63–1.13)	0.260
		n (%)	**AOR**	**95% CI**	**p value**	**n (%)**	**AOR**	**95% CI**	**p value**
Does the family cultivate millet?	**No**	280 (43.82)	1			50 (28.90)	1		
	Yes	22 (31.88)	0.50	(0.27–0.93)	0.029	2 (40.00)	2.35	(0.27–20.19)	0.435
Does the family consume products from their own cattle?	**Do not consume own products**	39 (60.94)	1			47 (28.66)	1		
	Consume own products	107 (48.20)	0.67	(0.46–0.96)	0.030	0	-	-	N.A.
	Do not have cattle	154 (36.84)	1.36	(0.72–2.56)	0.348	3 (27.27)	1.07	(0.11–9.23)	0.989

Table 3. Cont.

VARIABLES		RURAL (N = 711)				URBAN (N = 178)			
		n (%)	AOR	95% CI	p value	n (%)	AOR	95% CI	p value
Does the family consume products from their own goats?	Do not consume own products	277 (43.69)	1			52 (30.41)	1		
	Consume own products	16 (45.71)	0.37	(0.12–1.16)	0.090	0	-	-	N.A.
	Do not have goats	8 (23.53)	0.92	(0.43–1.96)	0.833	0	-	-	N.A.

*day before the survey.

another reason may be that children in the Fogera study had to be enrolled in school in order to participate, which could result in selection bias. In addition, our sampling was done in sub-districts with a high incidence of VL, a characteristic that may be associated with fewer resources and worse health status in children. The prevalence of chronic malnutrition in the urban area (29.2%) could not be compared to previous data due to the lack of research targeting this particular age group in this setting.

In rural communities, the setting with the highest stunting prevalence, we found several factors associated with chronic malnutrition: age group, fever in the previous 15 days, herding the cattle, consumption of any food from animal sources, sex of the HH, family size, cultivation of millet and consumption of the family's own cattle products. These factors should be considered when targeting chronic malnutrition in this region.

Children who had fever in the previous 15 days were 62% more likely to be stunted than those who did not. Infection and malnutrition are intricately linked through extensive, synergistic, antagonistic, and cyclical interactions [34,35]. Although our study area is known to be a low endemic area for malaria and leishmaniasis [25,36], other specific infections associated with malnutrition (such as chronic parasitic infestations) are highly prevalent [37,38]. Infectious diseases manifested in the form of fever affect both dietary intake and utilization, which may affect child growth. Not having empirical data on specific infections is a limitation, but we considered fever in the previous 15 days could act as a proxy for non-specific infection. On the other hand, stunted growth and related immunosuppression may lead to intermittent fever [39].

In our research, children who herd the cattle were less likely to be stunted. This could be explained by better activity levels in non-stunted children, given that stunted children show behavioral differences in early childhood including apathy and reduced activity, play and exploration [40].

Finally, children from households with millet farming and from families who consume their own cattle products were less likely to be stunted in rural communities. Although most rural families own land and animals (97.6% and 96.3% respectively), we observed that they do not consume their own products as often. Only 11.1% of the children had eaten any meat or fish over the last 24 hours, while 99.6% and 90.4%, respectively, had consumed basic staples and legumes and/or pulses respectively. In Ethiopia, child diet is based mainly based on plant foods like the traditional Ethiopian staple food called "*injera*", a yeast-risen flatbread made of a blend of cereals, usually served with legumes or pulses. This may not provide all the nutritional requirements of children [41]. We are aware that market access in this livelihood zone is poor; moreover what little trade interaction exists is restricted to cash crops that are attractive for their high price (i.e. rice and teff), while other essential crops cultivated mainly for personal consumption face disincentives [16,42].

In urban communities, age group and years of school of the PCFP were significantly associated with chronic malnutrition in children. This educational factor may operate indirectly to affect children's nutritional status by determining the quality of the child's diet, care and physical environment [30]. The level of education of the PCFP may have a positive impact on his/her knowledge on food facilities, controlling contamination, time and temperature parameters for controlling pathogens, and advice on good dietary habits [43].

Acute malnutrition

The prevalence of acute malnutrition in the rural settings of Fogera and Libo Kemkem was 21.6%. The prevalence of

Table 4. Multivariable logistic regression analysis of thinness in school-aged children, stratified by setting in Libo Kemkem and Fogera districts, Ethiopia, May–July 2009.

VARIABLES		RURAL (N=711)				URBAN (N=178)			
		n (%)	Adjusted OR	95% CI	p value	n (%)	Adjusted OR	95% CI	p value
CHILD CHARACTERISTICS									
Sex	**male**	97 (26.22)	1			21 (23.33)	1		
	female	56 (16.57)	0.69	(0.46–1.03)	0.073	16 (18.18)	0.86	(0.39–1.92)	0.717
Age group	**<10 years**	53 (11.83)	1			18 (15.02)	1		
	≥10 years	100 (38.84)	4.11	(2.74–6.16)	0.000	19 (32.81)	3.67	(1.63–8.30)	0.002
Does the child herd the cattle?	**No**	40 (13.51)	1			36 (21.05)	1		
	Yes	113 (27.49)	1.50	(0.96–2.36)	0.076	1 (14.29)	0.55	(0.06–5.03)	0.598
DOES THE CHILD CONSUME...									
Any food from animal sources	**No**	129 (22.28)	1			18 (28.13)	1		
	Yes	24 (18.60)	0.83	(0.49–1.41)	0.493	19 (16.67)	0.26	(0.10–0.67)	0.005
HOUSEHOLD AND LAND PRODUCTION									
Sex of head of household	**Male**	146 (22.26)	1			23 (22.33)	1		
	Female	7 (13.46)	0.40	(0.16–0.70)	0.043	14 (18.67)	0.67	(0.26–1.72)	0.407
Literacy of head of household (can read and write)	**No**	93 (21.83)	1			25 (25.77)	1		
	Yes	60 (21.51)	1.39	(0.91–2.11)	0.127	12 (14.81)	0.24	(0.09–0.65)	0.005
Number of people living in the house		**Mean (sd)**	**AOR**	**95% CI**	**p value**	**Mean (sd)**	**AOR**	**95% CI**	**p value**
		6.45 (1.68)	0.87	(0.75–1.00)	0.054	5.14 (1.72)	0.87	(0.64–1.20)	0.403
Number of children in the house									
		3.06 (1.14)	1.28	(1.03–1.60)	0.027	2.19 (0.94)	1.02	(0.61–1.70)	0.955
		n (%)	**AOR**	**95% CI**	**p value**	**n (%)**	**AOR**	**95% CI**	**p value**
Does the family cultivate rice?	**No**	115 (24.01)	1			36 (20.45)	1		
	Yes	38 (16.59)	0.64	(0.41–0.99)	0.045	1 (50.00)	3.26	(0.15–72.94)	0.456

underweight found in the study conducted in Fogera was 37.2% [33]. These results cannot be directly compared as different anthropometric indices were used. And again, we did not find any data on thinness to compare with our results in the urban population.

In rural settings, age group, sex of the HH, number of children in the house and rice cultivation were factors associated with thinness. The number of children in a household and the prevalence of thinness were positively associated. Larger family size may put children at higher risk for acute malnutrition, which could be due to the imbalance between family size and resources [44].

Those whose families cultivate rice were less likely to be thin in rural communities. In this zone, rice production might be acting as a proxy for better socioeconomic status, as rice consumption is relatively recent but is one of the main cash crops in the area [16]. The low consumption of animal source foods and its association with acute malnutrition has been previously identified as a major contributing factor to delayed growth in children [45] and suboptimal dietary practices among adolescents in Ethiopia [17].

In urban areas, children with a literate HH were 4 times less likely to be thin than those living in houses headed by illiterate adults. Some studies have shown that parental education is associated with more efficient management of limited household resources, improved utilization of available health care services, and better health-promoting behaviors, all of which are associated with better child nutrition [46,47]. This result is similar to what we previously observed for stunting and PCFP years of education in the urban setting. A possible explanation could be the existence of an educational gap in urban but not in rural areas.

Stunting versus thinness: associated factors

Clear differences among risk factors for stunting (Table 3) and thinness (Table 4) emerged from this study. The literature on the causes of stunting is vast, and conventional thinking is summarized in the *Lancet* series on maternal and child under-nutrition [48]. Recognized causal factors include prenatal and postnatal periods. Stunting is seen as closely tied to poverty and access to services. Less knowledge is available on risk factors for thinness [1]. In our research, risk factors for chronic malnutrition encompass a wide range of variables.. The relatively consistent pattern of related factors for stunting suggests that continued exposure to adverse conditions retards children's linear growth. Conversely, the greater diversity observed in the factors associated with thinness is consistent with the fact that a relatively short period of risk exposure can precipitate its onset in children [32].

In rural communities, children from male-headed households were more likely to be thin than children from female-headed households ($p = 0.043$), while stunting was significantly more frequent in female-headed households ($p = 0.002$). The disparate sample size in rural and urban areas may have influenced these results. However, the result in the rural area is consistent with the study conducted in North Ethiopia by Haidar et al. [49]. This study found a significantly higher proportion of stunted and underweight pre-school children in female headed-households, whereas the prevalence of thinness was similar [48–50]. Women who are single HH may be removed from their support structures and may face constraints in accessing services, including food, as a result of insecurity, cultural discrimination and limited mobility [48,50]. This situation may have a long-term impact in child nutrition.

Rural versus urban: associated factors

Ethiopia remains one of the least urbanized countries in the world [42]. Globally, malnutrition is less common in urban areas [2,31]. We found that malnutrition in rural communities was associated with food habits and the lack of material resources whereas in the urban area, it was better predicted by socio demographic factors. Inequalities in child health outcomes are known to vary between rural and urban areas, and are often due to unequal allocation of resources [51].

Significant urban-rural differences remained in the multivariable model. This shows that even in the presence of important individual factors and socioeconomic variables, area of residence is still a predictor of children's nutritional status. Our results highlight the need to stratify data when rural and urban communities are targeted in nutritional research in this kind of context.

Limitations

The present study was conducted in two single districts in Ethiopia, thus, the findings may not be generalizable to a larger population. Additionally, the cross-sectional nature of this data does not allow us to examine causality in the relationship between malnutrition and diverse risk factors. Seasonality should be given special attention; the season of the year has a significant effect not only on food security and nutritional status, but also on patterns and trends of infectious disease incidence. Therefore, consecutive measurements are desirable..

This research is part of a project which aimed to characterize nutritional, immunological, and parasitological aspects in school-aged children from urban and rural villages with a high incidence of VL in 2005–07. However, the VL prevalence found in the study was very low [25], and no association was found between nutritional status and asymptomatic infection [24]. Therefore, we are confident that this limitation does not alter our general conclusions.

Conclusions

Our findings suggest that improving food availability is a necessary but not sufficient condition to improve the nutritional status of school-aged children in this region. Especially in rural areas, the challenge will be for health and development extension workers to build on this knowledge through educational campaigns when advising households about balanced diet, food production and consumption, and hygienic behavior. It is also important to emphasize that nutritional programs should not be biased towards rural areas at the cost of excluding the urban poor.

To effectively tackle malnutrition, nutritional programs should be oriented to the local needs. Our findings can be used to help policy makers plan and undertake regional initiatives to streamline recommendations.

Supporting Information

Table S1 Factors related to stunting in school-aged children by setting in Libokemkem and Fogera districts, Ethiopia, May–June 2009. Bivariate analysis.

Table S2 Factors related to thinness in school-aged children by setting in Libokemkem and Fogera districts, Ethiopia, May–June 2009. Bivariate analysis.

Acknowledgments

We thank the study participants for volunteering to participate in the study; the data collectors for performing field work; the Armauer Hansen Research Institute/All Africa Leprosy Rehabilitation and Training Center and the Fundación Española para la Cooperación Internacional, Salud y Política Social for providing logistic and technical support; the Amhara Regional State Laboratory for allowing us to use their laboratory facility and for creating a conducive environment during the field work.

Author Contributions

Conceived and designed the experiments: LS EG JM JN AA CC EC. Performed the experiments: ZH AB LS EG EC. Analyzed the data: ZH AB LS EC. Contributed reagents/materials/analysis tools: AB JM AA JN CC. Wrote the paper: ZH EC LS. Critically reviewed the manuscript: EG JM JN AB AA CC.

References

1. United Nations Children's Fund, World Health Organization, The World Bank (2012) UNICEF-WHO-World Bank Joint Child Malnutrition Estimates. UNICEF, New York; WHO, Geneva; The World Bank, Washington, DC; 2012. Available: http://www.who.int/nutgrowthdb/jme_unicef_who_wb.pdf. Accessed: 2013 Aug 19.
2. de Onis M, Blossner M, Borghi E (2012) Prevalence and trends of stunting among pre-school children, 1990–2020. Public Health Nutr 15: 142–148.
3. de Onis M, Onyango A, Borghi E, Siyam A, Blossner M, et al. (2012) Worldwide implementation of the WHO Child Growth Standards. Public Health Nutr 15: 1603–1610.
4. Ezzati M, Hoorn SV, Lopez AD, Danaei G, Rodgers A, et al. (2006) Comparative Quantification of Mortality and Burden of Disease Attributable to Selected Risk Factors. In: Lopez AD, Mathers CD, Ezzati M, et al., editors. Global Burden of Disease and Risk Factors. Washington (DC): World Bank; 2006. Chapter 4. Available: http://www.ncbi.nlm.nih.gov/books/NBK11813/. Accessed: 2013 Sep 1.
5. United Nations System Standing Committee on Nutrition (2010) Progress in Nutrition: 6th Report on the World Nutrition Situation (Geneva, Switzerland: UNSCN Secretariat, 2010), Available: www.unscn.org/files/Publications/RWNS6/report/SCN_report.pdf. Accessed: 2013 Aug 19.
6. United Nations Children's Fund (UNICEF) (1991) Strategy for improved nutrition of children and women in developing countries: a UNICEF policy review. New York, USA: 1991. Available: http://repository.forcedmigration.org/show_metadata.jsp?pid=fmo:3066. Accessed: 2013 Aug 19.
7. Owusu WB, Lartey A, de Onis M, Onyango AW, Frongillo EA (2004) Factors associated with unconstrained growth among affluent Ghanaian children. Acta Paediatr 93: 1115–1119.
8. Abubakar A, Uriyo J, Msuya SE, Swai M, Stray-Pedersen B (2012) Prevalence and risk factors for poor nutritional status among children in the Kilimanjaro region of Tanzania. Int J Environ Res Public Health 9: 3506–3518.
9. Engebretsen IM, Tylleskar T, Wamani H, Karamagi C, Tumwine JK (2008) Determinants of infant growth in Eastern Uganda: a community-based cross-sectional study. BMC Public Health 8: 418.
10. Van de Poel E, O'Donnell O, Van DE (2007) Are urban children really healthier? Evidence from 47 developing countries. Soc Sci Med 65: 1986–2003.
11. Central Statistical Agency [Ethiopia] and ICF International (2012) Ethiopia Demographic and Health Survey 2011. Addis Ababa, Ethiopia and Calverton, Maryland, USA: Central Statistical Agency and ICF International. Available: http://www.usaid.gov/sites/default/files/documents/1860/Demographic%20Health%20Survey%202011%20Ethiopia%20Final%20Report.pdf. Accessed: 2013 Aug 20.
12. Demissie T, Ali A, Mekonnen Y, Haider J, Umeta M (2009) Demographic and health-related risk factors of subclinical vitamin A deficiency in Ethiopia. J Health Popul Nutr 27: 666–673.
13. Woldehanna T, Mekonnen A, Alemu T (2008) Young Lives: Ethiopia Round 2 Survey Report. University of Oxford, UK; 2008. Available: http://www.younglives.org.uk/files/country-reports/country-report-ethiopia-2008. Accessed: 2013 Aug 23.
14. Fotso JC (2006) Child health inequities in developing countries: differences across urban and rural areas. Int J Equity Health 5: 9.
15. Frank E (1999) Gender, Agricultural Development and Food Security in Amhara, Ethiopia: The Contested Identity of Women Farmers in Ethiopia. Agency for International Development, Washington, DC. Available: http://pdf.usaid.gov/pdf_docs/pnacg552.pdf. Accessed: 2013 Aug 23.
16. Tools for Food Security and Nutrition Analysis, Household Economy Approach and Cost of the Diet (2007) Livelihood Profile Amhara Region, Ethiopia. Tana Zuria Livelihood Zone (TZA). Available: http://www.heawebsite.org/countries/ethiopia/reports/hea-lz-profile-tana-zuria-livelihood-zone-tza-amhara-region-ethiopia-2007. Accessed: 2013 Aug 23.
17. Belachew T, Lindstrom D, Gebremariam A, Hogan D, Lachat C, et al. (2013) Food insecurity, food based coping strategies and suboptimal dietary practices of adolescents in Jimma zone Southwest Ethiopia. PLoS One 8 [2]: e57643.
18. Food and Agriculture Organization of the United Nations (FAO) (2009) Declaration of the World Summit on Food Security. Rome, Italy; 16–18 November 2009. Available: http://www.fao.org/fileadmin/templates/wsfs/Summit/Docs/Final_Declaration/WSFS09_Declaration.pdf. Accessed: 2013 Aug 20.
19. USAID Collaborative Research Support Programs Team (2000) Amhara National Regional State Food Security- Research Assessment Report. Available: http://www.ctahr.hawaii.edu/sm-crsp/phase1/pdf/amhara.pdf. Accessed 2013 Sep 1.
20. International Food Policy Research Institute (2005) An assessment of the causes of malnutrition in Ethiopia. A contribution to the formulation of a National Nutrition Strategy for Ethiopia. Washington, DC, USA Available: http://www.ifpri.org/sites/default/files/publications/ethionutrition.pdf. Accessed: 2013 Sep 1.
21. Food and Agriculture Organization of the United Nations and Food and Nutrition Technical Assistance Project (2008) Guidelines for Measuring Household and Individual Dietary Diversity. FAO, Rome, Italy; Reprinted 2013..Available: http://www.fao.org/docrep/014/i1983e/i1983e00.pdf. Accessed 2013 Sep 2.
22. Lyons S, Veeken H, Long J (2003) Visceral leishmaniasis and HIV in Tigray, Ethiopia. Trop Med Int Health 8: 733–739.
23. Amati L, Cirimele D, Pugliese V, Covelli V, Resta F, et al. (2003) Nutrition and immunity: laboratory and clinical aspects. Curr Pharm Des 9: 1924–1931.
24. Custodio E, Gadisa E, Sordo L, Cruz I, Moreno J, et al. (2012) Factors associated with Leishmania asymptomatic infection: results from a cross-sectional survey in highland northern Ethiopia. PLoS Negl Trop Dis 6: e1813.
25. Sordo L, Gadisa E, Custodio E, Cruz I, Simon F, et al. (2012) Low prevalence of Leishmania infection in post-epidemic areas of Libo Kemkem, Ethiopia. Am J Trop Med Hyg 86: 955–958.
26. Gadisa E, Custodio E, Canavate C, Sordo L, Abebe Z, et al. (2012) Usefulness of the rK39-immunochromatographic test, direct agglutination test, and leishmanin skin test for detecting asymptomatic Leishmania infection in children in a new visceral leishmaniasis focus in Amhara State, Ethiopia. Am J Trop Med Hyg 86: 792–798.
27. World Health Organization Working Group (1986) Use and interpretation of anthropometric indicators of nutritional status. Bull World Health Organ 64: 929–941.
28. de Onis M, Garza C, Victora CG, Onyango AW, Frongillo EA, et al. (2004) The WHO Multicentre Growth Reference Study: planning, study design, and methodology. Food Nutr Bull 25: S15–S26.
29. Food and Agriculture Organization of the United Nations (FAO) (2010) Assessment of Nutritional Status in Urban Areas. Available: http://www.fao.org/ag/agn/nutrition/urban_assessment_en.stm. Accessed: 2013 Sep 2.
30. Girma W, Genebo T (2002) Determinants of Nutritional Status of Women and Children in Ethiopia. ORC Macro, Calverton, Maryland, USA. Available: http://dhsprogram.com/pubs/pdf/FA39/02-nutrition.pdf. Accessed: 2013 Sep 2.
31. World Health Organization (WHO) (2006) The African Regional Health Report. WHO, Geneva, Switzerland; 2007. Available: http://www.who.int/mediacentre/news/releases/2006/pr68/en/. Accessed: 2013 Sep 2.
32. Ricci JA, Becker S (1996) Risk factors for wasting and stunting among children in Metro Cebu, Philippines. Am J Clin Nutr 63: 966–975.
33. Mekonnen H, Tadesse T, Kisi T (2013) Malnutrition and its Correlates among Rural Primary School Children of Fogera District, Northwest Ethiopia. J NutrDisorders Ther S12: 002.
34. Custodio E, Descalzo MA, Villamor E, Molina L, Sanchez I, et al. (2009) Nutritional and socio-economic factors associated with Plasmodium falciparum infection in children from Equatorial Guinea: results from a nationally representative survey. Malar J 8: 225.
35. Katona P, Katona-Apte J (2008) The interaction between nutrition and infection. Clin Infect Dis 46: 1582–1588.
36. Ayele DG, Zewotir TT, Mwambi HG (2012) Prevalence and risk factors of malaria in Ethiopia. Malar J 11: 195.
37. Amare B, Ali J, Moges B, Yismaw G, Belyhun Y, et al. (2013) Nutritional status, intestinal parasite infection and allergy among school children in Northwest Ethiopia. BMC Pediatr 13: 7.
38. Mahmud MA, Spigt M, Mulugeta BA, Lopez P, Dinant GJ, et al. (2013) Risk factors for intestinal parasitosis, anaemia, and malnutrition among school children in Ethiopia. Pathog Glob Health 107: 58–65.
39. Ehrhardt S, Burchard GD, Mantel C, Cramer JP, Kaiser S, et al. (2006) Malaria, anemia, and malnutrition in african children–defining intervention priorities. J Infect Dis 194: 108–114.
40. Black RE, Victora CG, Walker SP, Bhutta ZA, Christian P, et al. (2013) Maternal and child undernutrition and overweight in low-income and middle-income countries. Lancet 382: 427–451.
41. Mekonnen A, Jones N, Tefera B (2005) Tackling child malnutrition in Ethiopia: do the Sustainable development poverty reduction programme's underlying policy assumptions reflect local realities? Young Lives-Save the Children Working Paper 19, London, UK. Available: http://www.younglives.org.uk/

files/working-papers/wp19-tackling-child-malnutrition-in-ethiopia-do-the-sustainable-development-poverty-reduction-programme2019s-underlying-policy-assumptions-reflect-local-realities. Accessed: 2013 Sept 7.
42. Dorosh P, Schmidt E (2010) The Rural-Urban Transformation in Ethiopia. Development Strategy and Governance Division, International Food Policy Research Institute.. Working Paper 13. Addis Ababa, Ethiopia; Washington, DC, USA; 2010. Available: http://www.ifpri.org/sites/default/files/publications/esspwp013.pdf. Accessed 2013 Sep 7.
43. Coates J, Swindale A, Bilinsky P (2007) Household Food Insecurity Access Scale (HFIAS) for Measurement of Food Access: Indicator Guide. Food and Nutrition Technical Assistance Project (FANTA). USAID, Washington, DC, USA; August 2007. Available: http://www.fao.org/fileadmin/user_upload/eufao-fsi4dm/doc-training/hfias.pdf. Accessed: 2013 Sep 7.
44. Filmer D, Friedman J, Schady N (2009) Development, Modernization, and Childbearing: The Role of Family Sex Composition. World Bank Econ Rev 23: 371–398.
45. Ayele Z, Peacock C (2003) Improving access to and consumption of animal source foods in rural households: the experiences of a women-focused goat development program in the highlands of Ethiopia. J Nutr 133: 3981S–3986S.
46. Glewwe P (2005) The impact of child health and nutrition on education in developing countries: theory, econometric issues, and recent empirical evidence. Food Nutr Bull 26: S235–S250.
47. Abuya BA, Onsomu EO, Kimani JK, Moore D (2011) Influence of maternal education on child immunization and stunting in Kenya. Matern Child Health J 15: 1389–1399.
48. Inter-agency Standing Committee (IASC) (2006) Women, Girls, Boys and Men. Different Needs. Equal Opportunities. Gender Handbook in Humanitarian Action. IASC, December 2006. Available: http://www.humanitarianinfo.org/iasc/gender. Accessed: 2013 Sep 8.
49. Haidar J, Kogi-Makau W (2009) Gender differences in the household-headship and nutritional status of pre-school children. East Afr Med J 86: 69–73.
50. Woldehann T, Tefera B, Jones N, Bayrau A (2005) Child labour, gender inequality and rural/urban disparities: how can Ethiopia national development strategies best address negative spill-over impacts on child education and well-being?. Young Lives-Save the Children Working Paper No 20; Addis Ababa, Ethiopia; London, UK. Available: http://r4d.dfid.gov.uk/PDF/Outputs/YoungLives/wp20-execsummary.pdf. Accessed: 2013 Oct 8.
51. Siddiqi A, Irwin LG, Hertzman C (2007) Early child development: a powerful equalizer. Final Report for the World Health Organization's Commission on the Social Determinants of Health. WHO, Geneva, Switzerland, June 2007. Available: http://www.who.int/social_determinants/resources/ecd_kn_report_07_2007.pdf. Accessed: 2013 OCt 8.

7

Light Scattering Sensor for Direct Identification of Colonies of *Escherichia coli* Serogroups O26, O45, O103, O111, O121, O145 and O157

Yanjie Tang[1¤a], Huisung Kim[2], Atul K. Singh[1], Amornrat Aroonnual[1¤b], Euiwon Bae[2], Bartek Rajwa[3], Pina M. Fratamico[4], Arun K. Bhunia[1,5*]

1 Molecular Food Microbiology Laboratory, Department of Food Science, Purdue University, West Lafayette, Indiana, United States of America, **2** School of Mechanical Engineering, Purdue University, West Lafayette, Indiana, United States of America, **3** Bindley Bioscience Center, Purdue University, West Lafayette, Indiana, United States of America, **4** USDA-ARS, Eastern Regional Research Center, Wyndmoor, Pennsylvania, United States of America, **5** Department of Comparative Pathobiology, Purdue University, West Lafayette, Indiana, United States of America

Abstract

Background: Shiga-toxin producing *Escherichia coli* (STEC) have emerged as important foodborne pathogens, among which seven serogroups (O26, O45, O103, O111, O121, O145, O157) are most frequently implicated in human infection. The aim was to determine if a light scattering sensor can be used to rapidly identify the colonies of STEC serogroups on selective agar plates.

Methodology/Principal Findings: Initially, a total of 37 STEC strains representing seven serovars were grown on four different selective agar media, including sorbitol MacConkey (SMAC), Rainbow Agar O157, BBL CHROMagarO157, and R&F *E. coli* O157:H7, as well as nonselective Brain Heart Infusion agar. The colonies were scanned by an automated light scattering sensor, known as BARDOT (BActerial Rapid Detection using Optical scattering Technology), to acquire scatter patterns of STEC serogroups, and the scatter patterns were analyzed using an image classifier. Among all of the selective media tested, both SMAC and Rainbow provided the best differentiation results allowing multi-class classification of all serovars with an average accuracy of more than 90% after 10–12 h of growth, even though the colony appearance was indistinguishable at that early stage of growth. SMAC was chosen for exhaustive scatter image library development, and 36 additional strains of O157:H7 and 11 non-O157 serovars were examined, with each serogroup producing unique differential scatter patterns. Colony scatter images were also tested with samples derived from pure and mixed cultures, as well as experimentally inoculated food samples. BARDOT accurately detected O157 and O26 serovars from a mixed culture and also from inoculated lettuce and ground beef (10-h broth enrichment +12-h on-plate incubation) in the presence of natural background microbiota in less than 24 h.

Conclusions: BARDOT could potentially be used as a screening tool during isolation of the most important STEC serovars on selective agar plates from food samples in less than 24 h.

Editor: Dongsheng Zhou, State Key Laboratory of Pathogen and Biosecurity, Beijing Institute of Microbiology and Epidemiology, China

Funding: The project was supported by funds from the Agriculture Research Service of the United States Department of Agriculture project number 1935-42000-072-02G, and the Center for Food Safety Engineering (CFSE) at Purdue University. The funders had no role in study design, data collection and analysis, decision to publish, or preparation of the manuscript.

Competing Interests: Prof. Bhunia has recently gained partial ownership of Advanced Bioimaging Systems, West Lafayette, Indiana, United States of America on March 14, 2014. His contribution to the study design and execution of the research was done prior to his ownership of this company.

* Email: bhunia@purdue.edu

¤a Current address: Microbiological & Molecular Analytics, Nestlé Research Centre, Nestec Ltd, Vers-chez-les-Blanc, Lausanne, Switzerland
¤b Current address: Department of Tropical Nutrition & Food Science, Mahidol University, Bangkok, Thailand

Introduction

Shiga-toxin producing *Escherichia coli* (STEC) strains are recognized as serious foodborne pathogens and comprise of a diverse group of organisms, related to their O-group designations and virulence gene profiles. Although STEC O157 is the most widely recognized, other serogroups have been increasingly implicated in cases of foodborne human diseases [1–4]. The proportion of illnesses linked to non-O157 STEC (% = number of non-O157/total STEC infections) is estimated to be 10–80%, but the percentages differ greatly based on geographical areas, which range from 30–80% in European countries [5–8] and 50–63% in North America [9,10]. The most common non-O157 STEC serogroups identified as causes of human infections include O26,

O45, O103, O111, O121 and O145 [11,12]. Foods from which non-O157 STEC have been isolated include sausage, ice cream, milk, lettuce, and cucumber [13–17]. In 2011, the US Department of Agriculture Food Safety and Inspection Service (USDA-FSIS) declared the presence of these serogroups in beef trimmings to be adulterants, and testing for these serogroups became effective in June 2012 [18,19]. These ongoing events serve as a constant reminder for the need of reliable, user-friendly, and low cost screening tools for major STEC strains to prevent outbreaks.

Use of traditional cultural methods utilizing selective and chromogenic differential media is still considered a "gold standard" for isolation and detection of STEC, regardless of whether or not other immunological or/and molecular typing methods are employed in the testing protocol. Sorbitol MacConkey (SMAC) agar supplemented with or without cefixime-tellurite (CT) was formulated to exploit the fermentative features of *E. coli* serotypes that result in chromogenic differentiation of most O157 from non-O157 serovars [20,21]. While most O157 colonies are sorbitol negative and appear colorless, non-O157 serotypes appear as bright pink to mauve, making it difficult to distinguish non-O157 STEC from non-pathogenic *E. coli* based on color alone. Furthermore, sorbitol fermenting O157 variants also exist [22], and thus this property cannot be used as a firm diagnostic trait. A similar differential medium, R&F *E. coli* O157:H7 (R&F Laboratories, West Chicago, IL, USA), was designed to increase the specific isolation of both sorbitol-positive and negative O157 by introducing more fermentable carbohydrate sources [23]. However, differentiation of non-O157 STEC still remains a challenge. Other chromogenic media have been introduced, allowing color-based differentiation of non-O157 STEC serogroups, such as CHROMagar O157, Rainbow Agar and many other media developed by various academic laboratories [24–27]. Although these chromogenic media provide optimum recovery, improved selectivity, sensitivity, and overall accuracy for presumptive identification of most serogroups, some remain undistinguishable, for example, O157 and O111 both appear gray on Rainbow agar. Moreover, bacteria may need to be grown for 18–24 h or longer before the colony pigments are fully developed for differentiation.

Various analytical methods have been combined with selective and differential plating media for accurate detection and identification of the major serovars of STEC. Multiplex polymerase chain reaction (mPCR) methods have been widely used that target the *wzx* and other genes that are involved in encoding for O-antigen gene cluster-related proteins [28]. Recently, a DNA microarray [29] and Luminex microbead–based suspension array [30] were used to detect O-antigen gene clusters of *E. coli* serogroups (O26, O45, O91, O103, O104, O111, O113, O121, O128, O145, and O157) or an antibody microarray [31] was used to detect the organisms. These methods are laborious and costly when large amounts of samples are to be tested thus may have limitations for rapid high throughput screening applications. More recently, research suggested that microscopic variations in surface antigens can result in macroscopic differences in comprehensive colony morphology [32–34]. Therefore, it would be highly valued if colony morphology could be captured as a differentiator for various *E. coli* O-antigenic groups. Recently, a hyperspectral imaging method has been described for differentiation of STEC on agar plates that requires pure cultures of each test organism in separate plates. This method captures the spectral reflectance using visible-near infrared of all the collective colonies in the entire plate containing pure cultures and is used for differentiation of non-O157 STEC serovars [35]. This method is not suitable for detecting individual colonies present in a mixture on the same plate as is performed by classical microbiological testing.

Our group has designed and built a novel laser-based light scattering device (**Fig 1**) that detects/identifies a single target colony in the presence of a mixture of colonies formed by other bacterial species and can be easily integrated with traditional culture-based methods [36]. By shining a laser (635 nm) on the center of a colony, this instrument generates scatter patterns in a 2-dimensional plane, which is mathematically expressed as Fourier transform of the input aperture field that is dependent on the macromolecular composition/structure such as shape, chromogen, and colony composition (O-antigen, peptidoglycan or metabolic by-products) to produce species or serovar-specific scatter signatures [37–39]. This method is label-free and does not require any specialized reagents or antibodies, but requires a scatter image library for detection or identification of an unknown organism. Thus, this system has the potential for high throughput screening of multiple microorganisms if grown on the same plate. Furthermore, since laser scatter patterns are used as an identification fingerprint, minute structural changes in the single cell is amplified in the colony morphotype, allowing for automated classification of serovars differentiated by metabolic activities and surface carbohydrate profiles.

Our previous research demonstrated that the light-scattering system is able to differentiate colonies of *E. coli* O157:H7 from bacteria belonging to other genera such as *Listeria*, *Salmonella*, *Vibrio*, *Staphylococcus*, etc. [38]. In addition, BARDOT was able to detect and identify different species within a genus or different serovars within a species. For example, BARDOT was used for detection of different species of *Listeria* [37,38], *Vibrio* [40], and the top 20 *Salmonella* serovars [41]. The objective of this study was to evaluate the application of the BARDOT for real-time detection and differentiation of colonies of the top seven STEC serogroups (O26, O45, O103, O111, O121, O145 and O157) on selective and differential chromogenic media based on optical scatter patterns.

Results

Selection of appropriate media for differentiation of STEC serovars using the light scattering sensor, BARDOT

BARDOT (**Fig 1**) uses a laser to generate scatter patterns of bacterial colonies of about 1 mm diameter on agar plates for detection and identification of bacteria at the genus, species, and even at the serovar levels [38]. In this study, our initial goal was to identify a solid agar medium that would yield suitable colony scatter patterns to differentiate seven serovars of STEC (O26, O45, O103, O111, O121, O145 and O157) with high accuracy (**Table 1**). We examined commercial chromogenic differential agar media including CHROMagar O157, R&F *E. coli* O157:H7, Rainbow Agar O157 and sorbitol MacConkey (SMAC), as well as BHI agar that is nonselective. The colony morphology and scatter patterns of a representative strain from each serovar were compared on different media and each serovar produced scatter patterns that were visually distinct (**Fig 2**). With further image analysis using the accompanied software, the accuracy of discrimination among the seven serovars was represented by positive precision values (PPV) ranging from 0.91–1.0 for SMAC and 0.89–0.98 for BHI (**Table 2**). The colony scatter patterns on Rainbow and R&F media were similar; however, the signal intensity was relatively lower on R&F, owing to the accumulation of a black precipitate in the center of the colony. The PPV for Rainbow was 0.89–0.97 and for R&F 0.81–0.97 (**Table 2**). Colonies on CHROMagar formed relatively smaller diameter

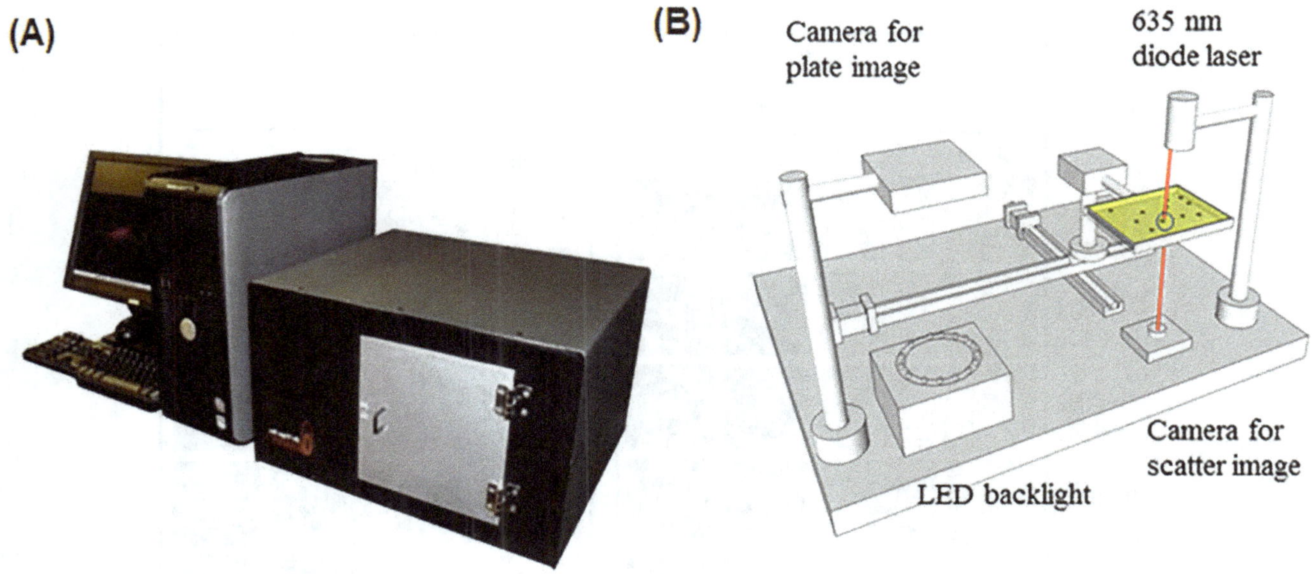

Figure 1. (A) The complete setup of the light scattering device, BARDOT (BActerial Rapid Detection using Optical scattering Technology). (B) Major components of the BARDOT system.

scatter patterns with less distinctive concentric ring structures and the PPV ranged from 0.86 to 0.94. The major drawback was that CHROMagar did not support the growth of serovar O103. This is not surprising since this medium was primarily formulated for isolation of serovar O157. Likewise, R&F *E. coli* O157:H7 was also formulated for O157:H7, thus some non-O157 serovars or strains may grow poorly or not grow at all. To further evaluate its utility for BARDOT-based detection, we excluded the antibiotic supplement to allow growth of all test serovars. Even though growth on R&F agar resulted in reasonably good discrimination (PPV = 0.81–0.97) among the seven serogroups, this agar was not examined further. Lack of the antibiotic supplement in R&F medium may obscure STEC detection due to overgrowth of background natural microbiota when tested with real-world samples. Likewise, BHI was not selected for obvious reasons since this non-selective medium will not be able to prevent overgrowth of background microbiota during real-world food sample testing. After taking all factors into consideration, it was determined that the performance of the selective media for BARDOT-based detection was SMAC>Rainbow>CHROMagar>R&F. We chose SMAC for future studies, though other media could be used in parallel to increase confidence in STEC identification. SMAC has been widely used for selective isolation of STEC from food and has been recommended by the FDA Bacteriological Analytical Manual [42], and thus, it could be used with the BARDOT system without altering established methodology in a testing laboratory.

Effect of growth media on the rate of colony growth and scatter patterns of serovars

Next, we examined colony growth and the changes in scatter patterns over time using the different selective media (**Fig 3**). Previous research suggested that bacterial growth kinetics (expressed as colony diameter) and resultant scatter patterns varied depending on media and strains tested [40,43]. To determine the correlation between colony growth on SMAC, Rainbow, CHROMagar, and R&F, the corresponding colony scatter patterns of all serovars were examined by BARDOT every 30 min from 9 h to 14 h of incubation at 37°C (**Fig 3, Fig S1-S4**). By close examination of two strains of serogroups, O157 and O26 (**Fig 3**), it was determined that the growth kinetics were generally similar on each growth medium (colony sizes reached 1.0±0.3 mm at 10–12 h of plate incubation); however, a slightly higher growth rate was achieved on SMAC. The optimum colony size selected for scatter experiments with SMAC (**Fig S1**), Rainbow (**Fig S2**), and CHROMagar (**Fig S3**) media were 1.1±0.1 mm, while colonies with smaller sizes (0.8±0.1 mm) were used with R&F medium (**Fig S4**). The smaller colony size for R&F was chosen because of the time-dependent accumulation of black pigment which blocked the interrogating laser in larger colonies (> 12 h). In general, the colonies which differed significantly from the optimum size were not selected for BARDOT analysis. The smaller colonies typically produced bright and less distinguishable patterns, while larger colonies generated images with more differential features but of low intensity.

While all representative strains exhibited consistently similar growth morphology on SMAC and Rainbow agar, a higher variability in growth rate among serogroups was observed on CHROMagar and R&F media. Therefore, we established an experimental protocol that employed size-normalized scatter patterns instead of growth-time normalized patterns. The desirable size of the colonies for most serogroups was achieved within 10–12 h of incubation at 37°C, which provided results quickly.

When the same bacterial cultures were allowed to continue to grow on the chromogenic media, the colony sizes increased, and color was produced after 18–24 h, aiding in presumptive visual identification (**Fig 4**). The O157 colonies on SMAC agar appeared as dome shaped and colorless, while non-O157 strains produced rose to pink colonies (**Fig 4, Fig S5**). On R&F agar, O157 colonies appeared dome shaped with a black precipitate, while non-O157 strains appeared green; however, the color difference between O157 and non-O157 colonies could not be easily distinguished when viewed against a white background (**Fig 4, Fig S5**). On Rainbow and CHROMagar, O157 and O111 strains produced grey to black colonies while O26, O45, O103, O121 and O145 produced pink-magenta-purple colonies

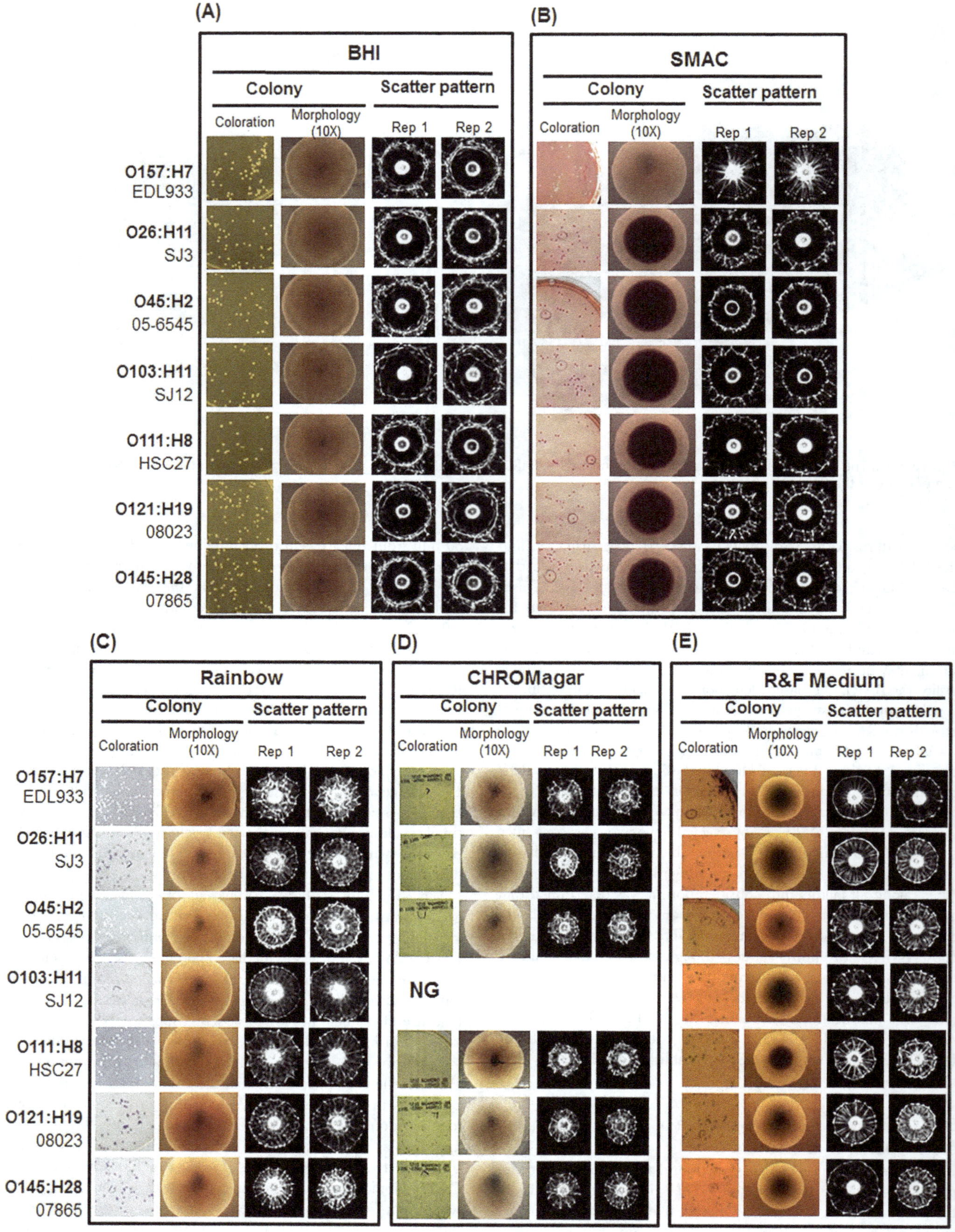

Figure 2. Representative images of colony coloration, microscopic colony morphology and scattering patterns of *E. coli* strains grown on each of the following medium: (A) BHI agar, (B) Sorbitol MacConkey agar (SMAC), (C) Rainbow, (D) CHROMagar O157, (E) R&F medium. All colony scatter images were captured at 10–12 h of incubation when colonies reached optimum size. *NG: no growth of O103 strains on CHROMagar.

Table 1. Shiga toxin-producing *Escherichia coli* strains used in this study.

Serogroup	Serotype	Strain	Source[a]	Virulence Genes		
				stx₁	*stx₂*	*eaeA*
O157	O157:H7	EDL933	Our collection	+	+	+
	O157:H7	SEA 13A53	Our collection	+	+	+
	O157:H7	SEA 13A72	Our collection	−	+	+
	O157:H7	O1	Our collection	+	+	+
	O157:H7	G5244	Our collection	+	+	+
O26	O26:H11	90.0105	Our collection	+	−	+
	O26:H11	SJ3	P. Fratamico	−	+	+
	O26:H11	00971	P. Fratamico	+	−	+
	O26:H11	05-6544	P. Fratamico	+	−	+
	O26:H11	93-3118	P. Fratamico	+	−	−
	O26:H11	94-0962	P. Fratamico	NT[b]	NT	NT
O45	O45:H2	SJ9	P. Fratamico	+	+	+
	O45:H2	05-6545	P. Fratamico	+	−	+
	O45:H2	SJ7	P. Fratamico	+	−	+
	O45:H2	SJ8	P. Fratamico	+	−	+
	O45:H2	96-3285	P. Fratamico	+	−	+
O103	O103:H2	87.1368	Our collection	+	−	−
	O103:H6	04162	P. Fratamico	+	−	+
	O103:H11	SJ12	P. Fratamico	+	−	+
	O103:H11	04-3973	P. Fratamico	+	−	+
	O103:H2	90-3128	P. Fratamico	+	−	+
O111	O111:H8	HSC27	Our collection	+	+	+
	O111:NM	SJ13	P. Fratamico	+	+	+
	O111:H8	01387	P. Fratamico	+	−	+
	O111:NM	00-4748	P. Fratamico	+	+	+
	O111:NM	98-8338	P. Fratamico	+	−	+
	O111:NM	94-0961	P. Fratamico	−	+	+
	O111:NM	96-3166	P. Fratamico	+	+	+
O121	O121:H19	08023	P. Fratamico	−	+	+
	O121:H19	SJ18	P. Fratamico	+	+	+
	O121:H19	03-2832	P. Fratamico	−	+	+
	O121:H19	97-3068	P. Fratamico	−	+	+
O145	O145:NM	SJ23	P. Fratamico	+	+	+
	O145:H28	07865	P. Fratamico	−	+	+
	O145:NM	03-4699	P. Fratamico	+	−	+
	O145:NM	94-0941	P. Fratamico	+	+	+
	O145:NM	83-75	P. Fratamico	−	+	+

[a]Source is as follows: P. Fratamico, Eastern Regional Research Center, Agricultural Research Center, Agriculture Research Service, U.S. Department of Agriculture, Wyndmoor, Pennsylvania; [b]NT: not tested

after 18 h of incubation. On CHROMagar, O157:H7 colonies (mauve-colored) could be distinguished from non-O157 STEC colonies (O111: grey-green; O26, O121 and O145: aqua); however, the colors among non-O157 STEC strains may be too close to be differentiated from each other when multiple strains are present on the same plate. Moreover, colonies on CHROMagar appeared flat with swarming properties. Thus, for all future experiments, SMAC agar was used as the best medium to acquire scatter images of STEC colonies (diameter 1.1±0.1 mm) after 10–12 h of incubation at 37°C.

Scatter image library

As indicated above, SMAC produced the best differential scatter signatures among the seven serogroups tested. Analysis of 37 strains representing all seven serogroups (4–7 strains/serogroup) generated highly reproducible scatter patterns for strains within a serogroup (**Fig 5**). Additionally, scatter patterns of 36 O157:H7 (**Fig S6**) and 11 non-O157 strains (**Fig S7**) were also generated on SMAC. Scatter images of other bacteria including *Acinetobacter baumannii*, *Citrobacter freundii*, *Klebsiella pneumo-*

Table 2. Analysis of positive predictive value (PPV) for each serovar grown on different selective media[a].

E. coli serovars	SMAC	CHROMagar	R&F	Rainbow	BHI
O103	0.91	NG	0.81	0.92	0.96
O111	0.93	0.88	0.97	0.93	0.98
O121	0.97	0.94	0.91	0.93	0.94
O145	0.91	0.86	0.93	0.89	0.93
O157	1	0.95	0.84	0.98	0.94
O26	0.95	0.92	0.91	0.94	0.89
O45	0.91	0.87	0.9	0.97	0.92

[a]Obtained by calculating the cross-validation matrix and reporting the positive predictive value [55,56]. Rainbow and SMAC agar showed the best average PPV for seven serovars tested; in particular SMAC showed 100% of classification for O157.

niae, *Pseudomonas aeruginosa* and *Shigella flexneri* that grew on SMAC were analyzed (**Fig S7**). Scatter patterns of seven serogroups of STEC strains appeared significantly different from those of the non- *E. coli* colonies on SMAC (**Fig S7**). The scatter image library consisted of about 83 strains representing all seven serogroups yielding about 3600–7000 scatter images. These images were stored in image library for use during food sample testing or mixed culture analysis. In addition, scatter image libraries for all seven serovars were also developed after growth on BHI (**Fig S8**), CHROMagar (**Fig S9**), Rainbow (**Fig S10**), and R&F (**Fig S11**) to aid in comparative analysis of any ambiguous serovars.

Mixed culture testing

To further investigate the ability of the light-scattering sensor to detect select *E. coli* serovars from a mixed culture on SMAC agar, two representative serovars (O157 and O26) were co-inoculated on the test medium and the resultant colonies at optimum sizes were analyzed by the light-scattering sensor and confirmed by multiplex PCR (mPCR) [28,44]. As expected, O157 and O26 generated unambiguous characteristic scatter patterns on SMAC when used singly or in a mixture (**Fig 6**). A typical O157 scatter pattern consisted of radial spokes extending from center to the edge, while the O26 scatter pattern consisted of two outer rings with radial spokes originating from the inner ring. These images were also verified by the image library database. The colony identity of respective serovars was also confirmed by serovar-specific mPCR (**Fig 6B**), where O157 and O26 produced amplified bands of 894 and 155 bp, respectively.

Food sample testing

Twenty-five grams of each lettuce and ground beef sample were inoculated with mixed cultures of O157 and O26 (50–100 CFU/ 25 g), enriched in modified tryptic soy broth (mTSB) with novobiocin [42] at 42°C for 10 h, plated on SMAC (at 37°C for 10.5 h), and the colonies were analyzed by BARDOT. The food inoculation experiment was repeated three times with different batches of food. Both O157 and O26 colonies on SMAC were visually indistinguishable after 10.5 h of growth; however, they produced typical scatter patterns when analyzed by BARDOT and were detected unequivocally from inoculated lettuce and ground beef samples (**Fig 7**). Representative colonies of each serovar were also picked from the plates and verified by mPCR, and the identification accuracy was estimated to be 96.6–100% (**Fig 7, Table 3**). The identification accuracy was defined as the ratio of the number of colonies positively identified with BARDOT and mPCR to the total number of colonies tested.

With lettuce testing, there were no non-O157/non-O26 background colonies on SMAC, but several background colonies were obtained from ground beef (**Fig 7B**). These background colonies also did not amplify either O157 or O26-specific genes. These data clearly show that BARDOT is capable of detecting two STEC serovars in a mixture in the presence of background microbiota in less than 24 h. Of note, none of the uninoculated food samples tested in this study contained any of the seven STEC serovars when used as controls.

Discussion

This paper is the first demonstration of the application of BARDOT to detect and differentiate colonies of seven STEC serogroups on agar plates based on colony scatter signatures. Initially four selective chromogenic media (SMAC, Rainbow, CHROMagar and R&F) were evaluated and based on the scatter pattern classification accuracy, SMAC provided the best results for STEC detection. Rainbow agar also provided high accuracy in differentiation of serogroups and may also be used for STEC detection using BARDOT. CHROMagar O157, and R&F *E. coli* O157:H7 are designed primarily for isolation of O157:H7 and may not support good growth of non-O157 STEC serovars. Moreover, scatter pattern classification accuracy values for CHROMagar O157, and R&F *E. coli* O157:H7 were slightly lower than SMAC and Rainbow, and thus they may not be suitable for BARDOT-based detection. Even though nonselective BHI agar had a very high accuracy in discriminating the seven STEC serogroups, it may not be suitable for testing of real-world food samples because of potential interference from background natural microbiota; however, BHI agar may be useful for differentiation or verification of pure cultures of STEC serovars. Recently, several new commercial selective and differential chromogenic media (ChromID O157:H7, bioMerieux; Harlequin SMAC-BCIG, Lab M; HardyCHROM E. coli O157; CHROMagar STEC, CHROMagar Microbiology [45]) have been marketed by many vendors, which could be tried with BARDOT. However, it is important to ascertain that there is no interference of the agar medium with laser propagation, since the BARDOT system generates forward scatter patterns of colonies.

We have indicated earlier that classification accuracy of colonies of different species from the same genera [37,40] or serovars from a single species [41] varies depending on the growth medium used, and this suggests that bacterial colony morphology and composition can be leveraged for accurate classification. This is possible

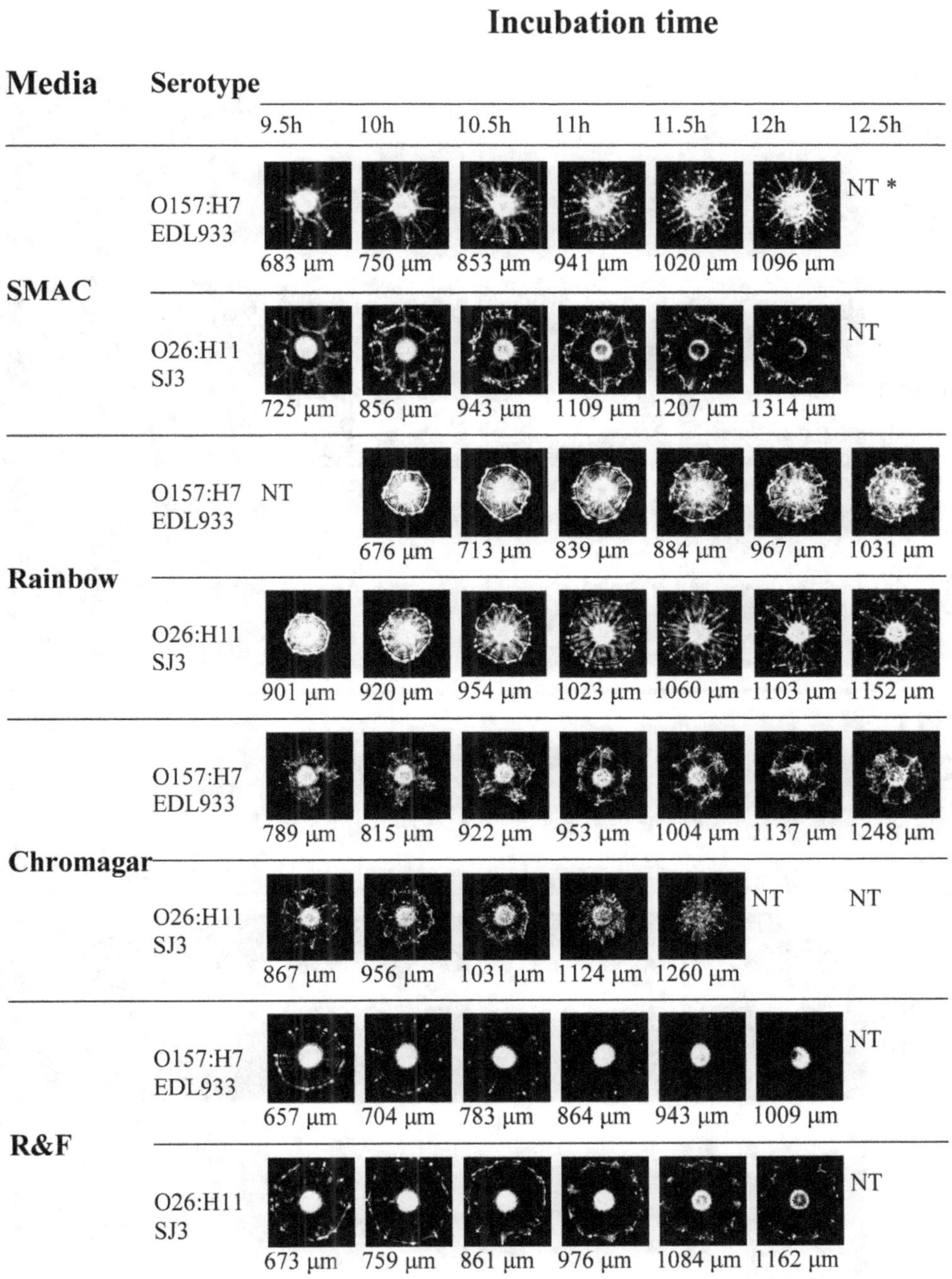

Figure 3. Effect of growth time on light-scatter images of representative O157 and non-O157 STEC strains. Colony sizes (μm) were measured within 5 min before respective scatter patterns were captured by BARDOT. *NT: not tested because no distinct scatter image could be obtained due to oversized colony (>1.2 mm).

due to the photon-cell interaction, which results in unique and reproducible scatter patterns [37,39]. The colony scatter pattern is a phenomenon that occurs due to the accumulation of the interactions of incoming photons across the depth of the colony. Their physical (color, size, shape, roughness, and thickness) or chemical (metabolic by-product composition) characteristics modify the optical amplitude and phase, which scatters into an imaging plane to create a scatterogram [43,46,47].

In addition to colony size, the height of colonies is another important physical determinant for differential scatter patterns [37,43]. We observed that elevated colonies on SMAC and Rainbow agar formed more diffused patterns, while colonies on CHROMagar appeared flat, and thus produced relatively more concentrated patterns with less distinctive ring structures (**Fig 2**), yielding a lower classification accuracy.

Chromogenic selective or differential media are integral components of classical microbiological methods for presumptive isolation of pathogens from test samples. The chromogens are produced as a result of bacterial fermentative and enzymatic activities [48,49], and thus it is speculated that differences in scatter patterns observed for different serovars are affected by the accumulation of bacterial metabolic by-products or chromogenic

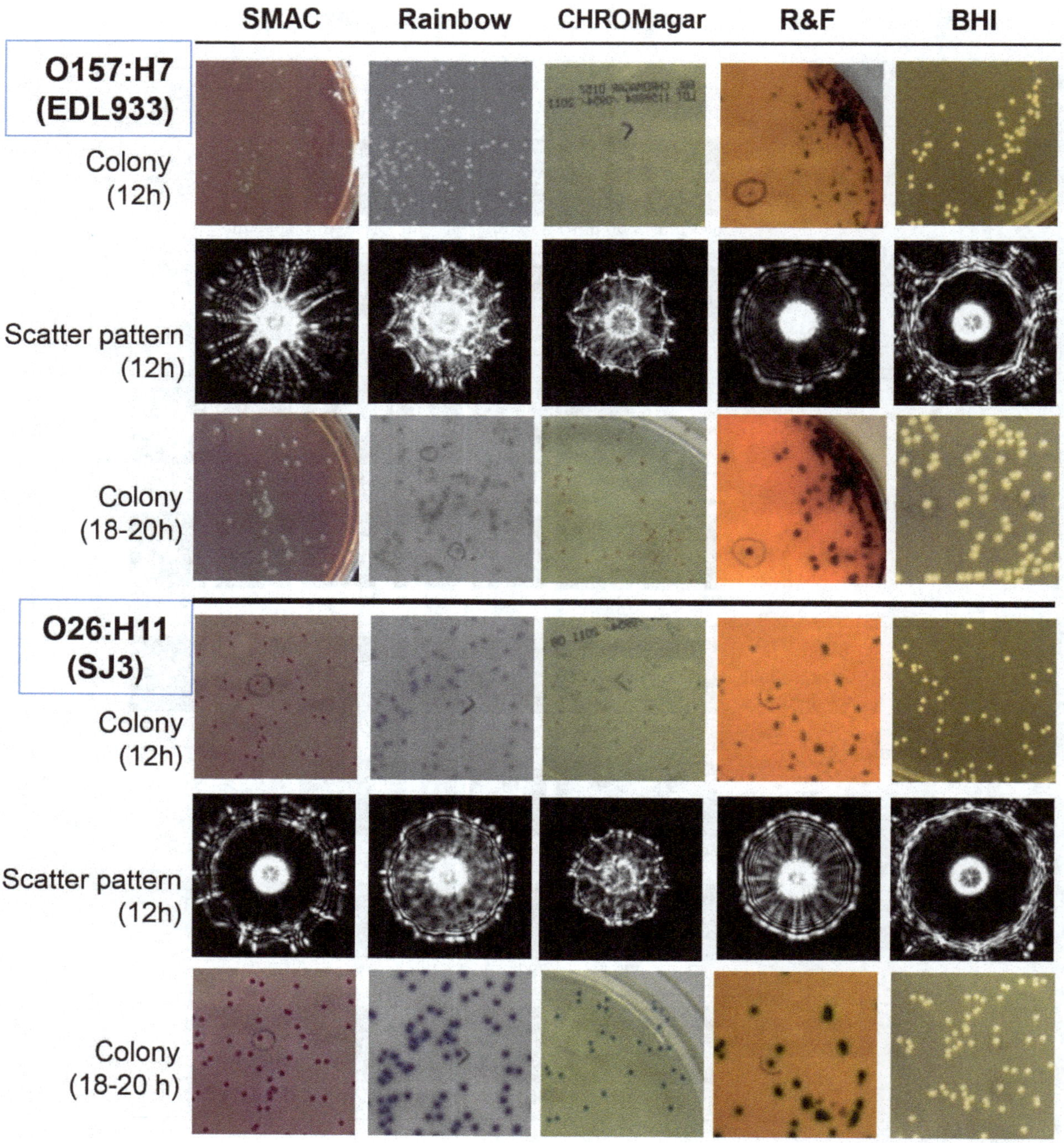

Figure 4. Chromogenic pigment production and scatter patterns of colonies of representative O157 and O26 STEC strains. Plate images and scatter patterns were captured at 10–12 h of incubation when colonies reached approximately 1 mm in diameter. Colony appearance after 18–20 h of growth was also recorded.

components [38,39]. Furthermore, the O-antigen in lipopolysaccharides (LPS) has been suggested as a possible contributing factor for colony morphology that can be interrogated by the light-scattering technology [32–34] and possibly an important discriminant for differential scatter patterns. LPS is a major component of the outer membrane of Gram-negative bacteria, and it is composed of lipid A, core oligosaccharides, and O-polysaccharides (or O-antigen). The O-(somatic) antigen is attached to the outermost domain of core oligosaccharide, while lipid A anchors to the inner core. While lipid A and core oligosaccharide are highly conserved or have limited variations, the compositional structure of O-antigens varies considerably among serogroups of pathogenic *E. coli* [50–52] and even the seven serovars of STEC [28,53] studied here. Although the size of the O-antigen is quite small (outer membrane is ~40 nm) compared to the interrogating laser wavelength used here (635 nm), the collective appearance and characteristics of the O-antigen at the surface of bacterium in a colony can provide differential scatter patterns. The H (flagellar) antigen did not appear to play any role, since scatter patterns of nonflagellated/non motile O111:NM or O145:NM strains were very similar to flagellated strains of O111:H8 or O145:H18 strains (**Fig 5**).

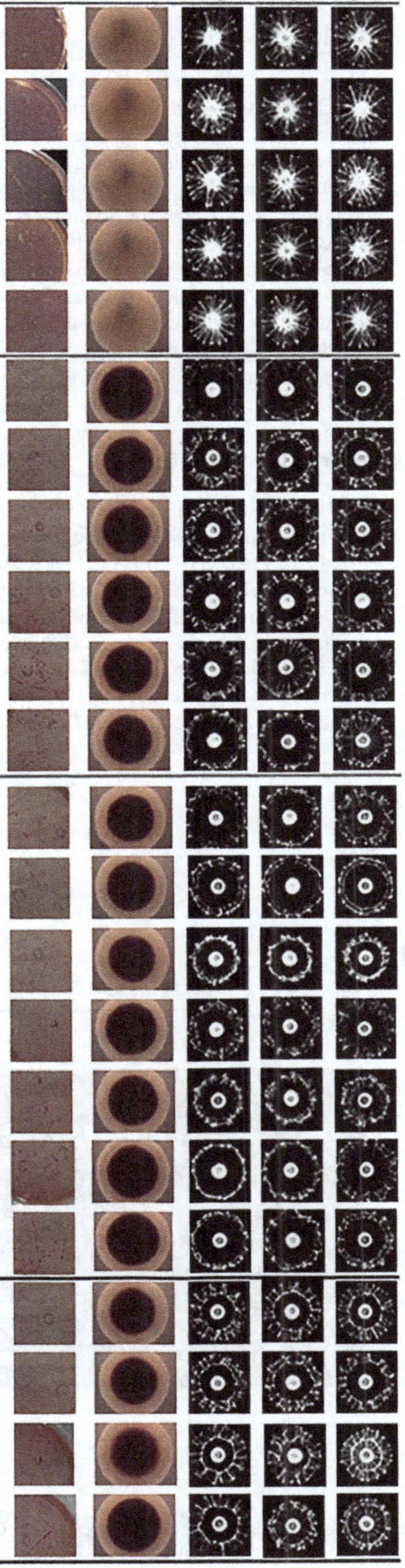

Serotype	Strain	Colony	Microcopy*	Scattering Pattern Rep 1	Rep 2	Rep 3*
O157	O157:H7 EDL933					
	O157:H7 SEA13A53					
	O157:H7 SEA13A72					
	O157:H7 O1					
	O157:H7 G5244					
O26	O26:H11 90.0105					
	O26:H11 SJ3					
	O26:H11 00971					
	O26:H11 05-6544					
	O26:H11 93-3118					
	O26:H11 94-0962					
O111	O111:H8 HSC27					
	O111:NM SJ13					
	O111:H8 01387					
	O111:NM 00-4748					
	O111:NM 98-8338					
	O111:NM 94-0961					
	O111:NM 96-3166					
O121	O121:H19 08023					
	O121:H19 SJ18					
	O121:H19 03-2832					
	O121:H19 97-3068					

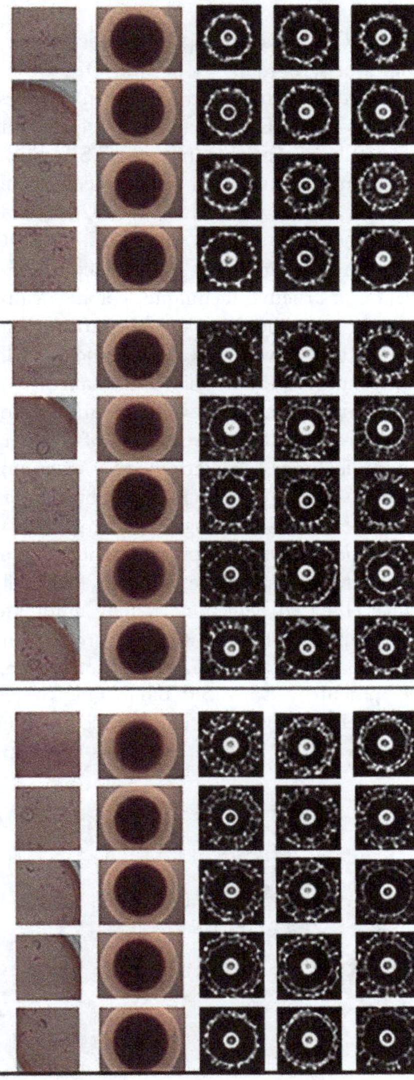

Serotype	Strain	Colony	Microscopy*	Scattering Pattern Rep 1	Rep 2	Rep 3*
O45	O45:H2 SJ9					
	O45:H2 05-6545					
	O45:H2 SJ7					
	O45:H2 SJ8					
O103	O103:H2 87.1368					
	O103:H6 04162					
	O103:H11 SJ12					
	O103:H11 04-3973					
	O103:H2 90-3128					
O145	O145:NM SJ23					
	O145:H28 07865					
	O145:NM 03-4699					
	O145:NM 94-0941					
	O145:NM 83-75					

Figure 5. Microscopic colony appearance and scatter images of colonies of STEC serogroups on sorbitol MacConkey (SMAC) agar after 10–12 h of incubation at 37°C. Three representative images for the same strains from three separate experiments are presented. *Rep 3 represents scatter images of colonies presented in this figure.

BARDOT was successful in detecting and differentiating colonies of serogroups O157 and O26 from mixed cultures and even from inoculated food systems in the presence of background microbiota. BARDOT detected these two pathogens in less than 24 h (10 h of enrichment in mTSB plus 10.5 h of on-plate incubation) in lettuce and ground beef inoculated with low levels (50–100 CFU/25g) of O157 and O26,suggesting its potential for screening of food samples for STEC. BARDOT-positive colonies were further confirmed by PCR. Since BARDOT is a noninvasive and non-destructive technique, colonies can be used for further molecular or pathophysiological characterization, if necessary.

In this study, we tested seven major STEC serovars (about 73 strains) and 10 additional miscellaneous serovars. BARDOT showed high accuracy in differentiation among the seven major STEC serovars. Continued testing of additional serovars needs to be done in order to determine any overlapping patterns among common serovars and to create a robust *E. coli* library on SMAC, which is currently in progress. The growth rate of serovars also varies depending on the strain and the medium used, which makes it difficult to identify the optimal, fit-for-all detection time for BARDOT-based detection. A fully automated system equipped with an incubator, plate handling robot, and the laser scanner would be useful. Such an automated system is currently under development by Advanced Bioimaging Systems (advancedbioimgaingsystems.com), which may be used to overcome this technical obstacle.

Conclusion

Our results demonstrate that BARDOT can detect and discriminate the colonies of seven major STEC serovars with high accuracy. Among the media tested, SMAC and Rainbow provided the best results allowing serogroup differentiation with over 90% accuracy at an early stage of colony growth when colony morphology and color are indistinguishable. BARDOT-based detection can be completed in less than 24 h, which includes sample enrichment in mTSB for 10 h followed by growth on SMAC for 10–12 h, allowing users to have access to the isolated colonies for further characterization. BARDOT could potentially be used as a real-time screening tool for on-plate differentiation of the most important STEC serogroups as they grow on selective agar plates.

Materials and Methods

Bacterial strains and culture conditions

A total of thirty-seven *E. coli* isolates belonging to serogroups O157, O26, O45, O103, O111, O121, and O145 were tested in this study (**Table 1**). In addition, 36 strains of O157:H7 (**Fig S6**), 11 miscellaneous *E. coli* strains and five other bacterial cultures including *Acinetobacter baumannii* NRRL B41237, *Citrobacter freundii* NRRL B2643, *Klebsiella pneumoniae* NRRL B41958, *Pseudomonas aeruginosa* ATCC 10145 and *Shigella flexneri* PRI 387 that grew on SMAC(**Fig S7**) were used for scatter image

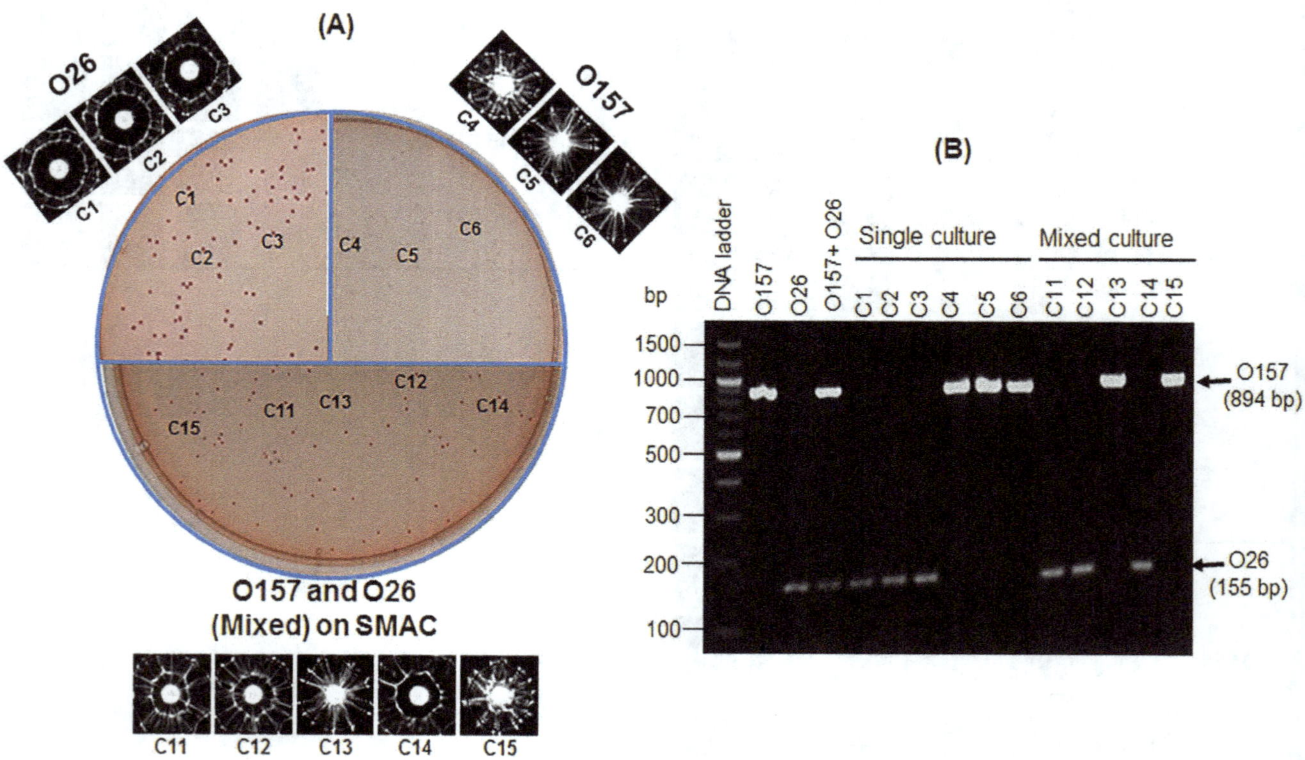

Figure 6. Light-scattering analysis and PCR confirmation of colonies of serogroup O157:H7 (EDL933) and O26:H11 (90-0105) on SMAC agar. (**A**) Scatter images of colonies of O26, O157 and the mixture of O26 and O157 grown on SMAC at 37°C for about 11 h. Representative colonies that were analyzed by multiplex PCR (mPCR) are labeled as C1-C15. (**B**). Agarose gels showing PCR amplified bands for each colony tested.

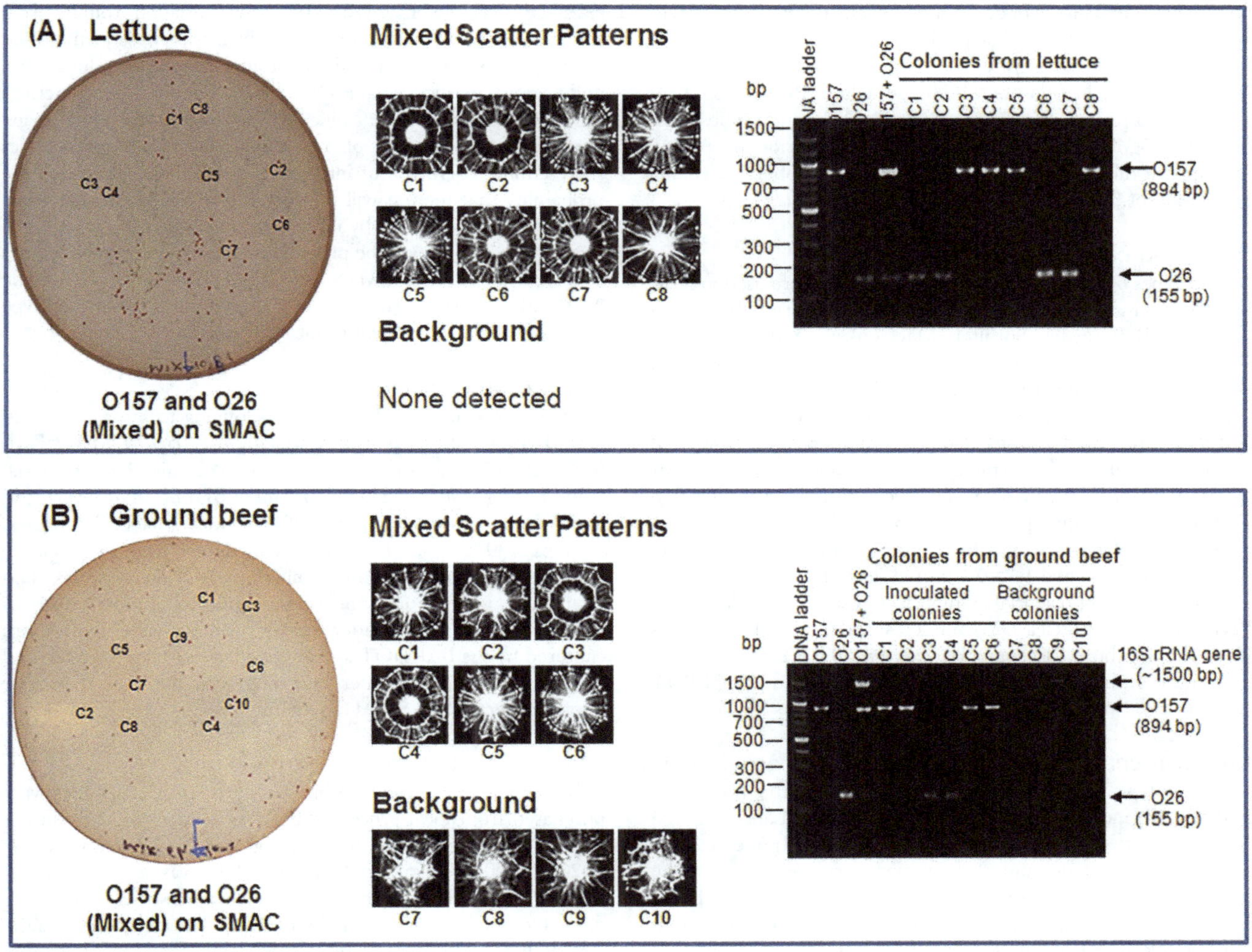

Figure 7. Application of light-scattering sensor for detection and identification of STEC O26 and O157 from inoculated (A) lettuce and (B) ground beef samples. Colonies (c1, c2...) on SMAC are first scanned with BARDOT and then analyzed by mPCR for confirmation. BARDOT accurately detected two serogroups from both food samples and confirmed by PCR. Only ground beef sample contained background non-STEC bacteria whose patterns are different from the STEC serogroups. Moreover, these colonies did not give any amplified products with serovar specific primers but amplified 16S rRNA gene.

Table 3. Differentiation of mixed cultures of *E. coli* serovars from food samples on SMAC agar based on scatter pattern.

Bacterial/Food sample[a]	No. of colony analyzed	No. of positive colony with BARDOT Library[b]		No. of positive colony with serovars-specific PCR[c]		Identification accuracy (%)[d]
		O26	O157	O26	O157	
E. coli O26 & O157 tested as mixed culture	30	15/30	15/30	15/30	14/30[e]	96.6
Lettuce with *E. coli* O26	6	6/6	0/6	6/6	0/6	100.0
Lettuce with *E. coli* O157	6	0/6	6/6	0/6	6/6	100.0
Lettuce with *E. coli* O26 & O157	12	6/12	6/12	5/12	7/12	96.6
Ground beef with *E. coli* O26 & O157	14	7/14	7/14	7/14	7/14	100.0

[a]Lettuce and ground beef samples were inoculated with 10^2CFU/25g of each *E. coli* O26 and *E. coli* O157 cells
[b]*E. coli* colonies grown on SMAC agar for 10–11 h were matched with BARDOT library containing multiple standard strains of O157 STEC and non-O157 STEC.
[c]*E. coli* serovar (O26 and O157) specific primers were used in multiplex PCR (mPCR). Prior to food sample analysis primers were validated for specificity with three standard strains of each *E. coli* O157:H7 and O26:H11. Primer sequences were adapted from reference [28].
[d]Identification accuracy measures the ratio of number of colonies correctly identified with BARDOT as well as PCR and total number of colonies analyzed. Identification of colonies with BARDOT and mPCR were performed as a blind study.
[e]One colony (#R1-3/C1) analyzed with mPCR did not produce any amplified products, however, it was identified as O157 serovar after analysis with BARDOT library.

library development. Working cultures were prepared by inoculating a loop full of frozen bacterial stocks (−80°C) into 3 ml BHI broth and incubating at 37°C for 12–15 h. Cultures were serially (10-fold) diluted in phosphate buffered saline (PBS; 1.38g/L of sodium phosphate monobasic, 2.68g/L of sodium phosphate dibasic, 8.5g/L of 0.85% sodium chloride) prior to plating appropriate dilutions on chromogenic media to obtain a colony population of 30–100 colonies per plate.

Media and phase contrast microscopy

Four types of differential chromogenic media were used to grow bacterial cultures for light-scattering experiments. The media included: BHI agar, Sorbitol MacConkey (SMAC; Becton Dickinson) agar, Rainbow Agar O157 (Biolog, Hayward, CA), BBL CHROMagar O157 (Becton Dickinson), and R&F *E. coli* O157:H7 medium (R&F Products, Downers Grove, IL). Agar plates were prepared as instructed by the manufacturer, tempered to 45°C, dispensed 20 mL/plate, cooled at room temperature for 10–20 min, and stored in a sealed plastic bag until use (used within 7–30 days) [54]. After plating appropriate dilutions of bacterial cultures, the plates were incubated at 37°C for 10–12 h or until the colony size reached 1.1±0.1 mm in diameter. The colony size and morphology of bacterial cultures were examined under a 10× PH1 objective of a Leica DMLB microscope (Leica Microsystems USA, Bannockburn, IL) equipped with a SPOT RT color camera (Diagnostic Instruments, Inc). Images were captured using SPOT Advanced software 4.6.4.2 (Diagnostic Instruments, Inc).

Light-scattering instrumentation and image acquisition

A prototype light scattering sensor known as the BARDOT system (Advanced Bioimaging Systems, West Lafayette, IN) consisting of two main functionalities was used. **Figure 1** shows instrumentation setup and diagrammatic representation of the operating principle. In brief, the standard Petri dish with the grown bacterial colony is imaged to obtain a map showing location of each colony, where the centroid locations of each colony are automatically identified. The cut-off value for absorption and circularity was set to filter the non-bacterial or doublet colonies while the colony center locations were transferred to perform the forward scattering measurement automatically. BARDOT moves the Petri dish to the respective center of the colony such that it aligns with the incoming 635 nm laser which generates the forward scattering patterns. Detailed hardware and software development and specifications were published earlier [38,39]. To build scatter image libraries, colony scatter patterns of 50–100 colonies per strain of each serogroup were collected.

Image analysis

The process of scatter-pattern analysis has been described in detail in our previous reports [55,56]. Briefly, for each individual scatter pattern characterizing a single *E. coli* colony, a total of 78 features are extracted. The quantitative pattern characteristics include 65 pseudo-Zernike orthogonal moments and 13 Haralick texture features. The features were concatenated, forming feature vectors for each colony. We used either the entire feature set (for the 7-serovar library), or the most informative features selected by a random-forest technique [57,58]. The extracted features were used to find the best combination of parameters for a Gaussian kernel-based support vector machine (SVM) classifier. All the tested classifiers were trained and their performance was evaluated using 10-times cross-validation. In every round of cross-validation, the data set was partitioned randomly into training and testing subsets. The classifiers were retrained independently on every training subset, and then the remaining testing subset was classified. The results of all the cross-validation rounds were summarized in a confusion matrix, which was subsequently used to compute sensitivity, specificity, positive predictive value (PPV), and negative predictive value (NPV) [59]. The sensitivity describes the probability that our classifier will produce a true result when used on a population of colonies also containing colonies representing a serotype of interest. The specificity illustrated the probability that the test will produce a true negative result when used on colonies formed by organisms other than the serotype of interest. The PPV gives the probability that a colony truly belongs to a serotype of interest when a BARDOT system claims so. The NPV is the probability that a colony does not represent a serotype of interest when a negative result is returned.

Mixed culture testing

One representative STEC strain belonging to serogroups O26 and O157 (*E. coli* O26:H11 90-0105 and *E. coli* O157:H7 EDL 933) were selected to prepare two-strain cocktails. Each bacterial culture was grown individually in 3 ml of BHI broth for overnight, and then equal amounts (1 ml) of each were mixed. The mixed cultures of O157 and O26 were serially diluted to the appropriate dilutions and surface-plated onto SMAC agar plates and incubated at 37°C until the colony grew to optimum sizes as described earlier. The scatter images of individual colonies were captured by the BARDOT system, and five colonies were selected for PCR confirmation after matching with the *E. coli* serovar library generated on SMAC medium.

Food sample testing

Romaine lettuce (triple washed) and ground beef samples were purchased from local grocery stores (West Lafayette, IN) on the day of the experiment. A strain of serovar O26 and O157 (O26:H11 90-0105, and O157:H7 EDL933) was used for artificial inoculation of food samples. Overnight grown cultures were diluted to obtain 5×10^2–1×10^3 CFU/mL. The cell number in the inoculum was determined by colony counts after making serial dilutions, plating onto SMAC, and incubation at 37°C for 18 h. A 100 µl-aliquot of the diluted cultures was inoculated onto a lettuce sample (25 g) to obtain inoculum levels of 50–100 CFU/25g. Inoculated samples were air-dried in a class II biosafety cabinet with a constant laminar flow at 22±2°C for 15 min to allow attachment of bacteria to leaf surfaces. After air-drying, lettuce samples were aseptically transferred into Seward filter stomacher bags (Model 400 Bags, Seward Ltd, West Sussex, UK) containing 225 ml of modified TSB (mTSB) plus 8 mg/L of novobiocin (N-1628, Sigma) [42,60]. The resulting samples were incubated at 42°C for 10 h with continuous shaking at 130 rpm. As negative controls, uninoculated samples were treated in a similar manner but using sterile PBS in place of the inoculum. The enriched samples were serially diluted and surface plated onto SMAC agar. All colonies on plates were examined by BARDOT after incubation at 37°C for 10–12 h when colonies reached appropriate sizes. Five randomly picked colonies from each plate were subjected to a multiplex polymerase chain reaction (mPCR) assay for verification of *E. coli* serovars (O157 and O26) used in the experiment.

Multiplex PCR

The identity of representative *E. coli* colonies scanned by BARDOT was further confirmed for O-antigen specific genes (**Table S1**) using an mPCR assay as described previously [28,44]. DNA samples from *E. coli* serovars were extracted using the FDA-BAM protocol for DNA template preparation for real-time PCR screening [42]. Proper positive (DNA from standard *E. coli* strains) and negative (deionized water) controls were used for each PCR reaction during validation and testing of PCR primers and colonies from mixed cultures and from food sample enrichments. As a control, amplification of the 16S rRNA gene (**Table S1**) was used to confirm background colonies obtained from ground beef samples.

Supporting Information

Figure S1 Forward-scatter images of colonies of representative strains from STEC serogroups O157, O26, O45, O103, O111, O121, and O145 grown on SMAC agar. Colony sizes are measured by light microscopy immediately before light-scatter screening, and the diameter (μm) of each colony is indicated below respective scatter images.

Figure S2 Forward-scatter images of colonies of representative strains from STEC serogroups O157, O26, O45, O103, O111, O121, and O145 grown on Rainbow agar. Colony sizes were measured by light microscopy immediately before light-scatter screening, and the diameter (μm) of each colony is indicated below respective scatter images.

Figure S3 Forward-scatter images of colonies of representative strains from STEC serogroups O157, O26, O45, O103, O111, O121, and O145 grown on CHROMagar. Colony sizes were measured by light microscopy immediately before light-scatter screening, and the diameter (μm) of each colony is indicated below respective scatter images. NG, No growth, NT, Not tested

Figure S4 Forward-scatter images of colonies of representative strains from STEC serogroups O157, O26, O45, O103, O111, O121, and O145 grown on R&F medium agar. Colony sizes were measured by light microscopy immediately before light-scatter screening, and the diameter (μm) of each colony is indicated below respective scatter images.

Figure S5 Coloration and scatter patterns of colonies of representative STEC strains from each serogroup. Scatter patterns were generated at 10–12 h of incubation when colonies reached approximately 1 mm in diameter, while plate images were captured at both 10–12 h and 18–20 h of incubation to demonstrate color change over time. * NG: no growth of O103 strains on CHROMagar. *N/A: images were not captured

Figure S6 Scatter images of *E. coli* O157:H7 strains on SMAC agar after 10–12 h of growth.

Figure S7 Scatter images of (A) *E. coli* non-O157 strains and (B) other bacterial cultures including *Acinetobacter baumannii, Citrobacter freundii, Klebsiella pneumoniae, Pseudomonas aeruginosa* and *Shigella flexneri* on SMAC agar after 10–12 h of growth.

Figure S8 Representative images of colonies on plate, light microscopic images of individual colony and scatter patterns of STEC serovars grown on BHI agar. All images were collected after about 10.5 h of incubation at 37°C. *Rep 3 represents the scatter patterns of microscopic images of colonies presented in this figure.

Figure S9 Representative images of colonies on plates, light microscopic images of individual colony and scattering patterns of STEC serovars grown on CHROMagar. All images were collected after about 10.5 h of incubation at 37°C. *Rep 3 represents the scatter patterns of microscopic images of colonies presented in this figure.

Figure S10 Representative images of colonies on plates, light microscopic images of individual colony and scatter patterns of STEC serovars grown on Rainbow agar after about 10 h of incubation at 37°C. Colony images were also captured after 18 h to illustrate visible color change. *Rep 2 represents the scatter patterns of microscopic images of colonies presented in this figure.

Figure S11 Representative images of colonies on plates, light microscopic images of individual colony and scatter patterns of STEC serovars grown on R&F O157:H7 after about 10 h of incubation at 37°C. Colony images were also captured after 18 h to illustrate visible color change. *Rep 2 represents the scatter patterns of microscopic images of colonies presented in this figure.

Table S1 Oligonucleotide primers used for detection of virulence and O-antigen genes of *E. coli* serovars.

Acknowledgments

Disclaimer: Mention of trade names or commercial products is solely for the purpose of providing specific information and does not imply recommendation or endorsement by the U.S. Department of Agriculture.

Author Contributions

Conceived and designed the experiments: AKB YT PF. Performed the experiments: YT HK AKS AA EB. Analyzed the data: BR EB AKS AKB. Contributed reagents/materials/analysis tools: PF. Contributed to the writing of the manuscript: AKB YT EB BR PF AKS.

References

1. Caro I, Mateo J, Rua J, Del Rosario Garcia-Armesto M (2011) Occurrence of *Escherichia coli* O157, O111 and O26 in raw ewe's milk and performance of two enrichment broths and two plating media used for its assessment. Int J Food Microbiol 146: 84–87.
2. Zimmerhackl LB, Rosales A, Hofer J, Riedl M, Jungraithmayr T, et al. (2010) Enterohemorrhagic *Escherichia coli* O26:H11-associated hemolytic uremic syndrome: Bacteriology and clinical presentation. Semin Thromb Hemost 36: 586–593.
3. Sekse C, O'Sullivan K, Granum PE, Rorvik LM, Wasteson Y, et al. (2009) An outbreak of *Escherichia coli* O103:H25 - bacteriological investigations and genotyping of isolates from food. Int J Food Microbiol 133: 259–264.
4. Lee JH, Hur J, Stein BD (2008) Occurrence and characteristics of enterohemorrhagic *Escherichia coli* O26 and O111 in calves associated with diarrhea. Vet J 176: 205–209.
5. Nielsen EM, Scheutz F, Torpdahl M (2006) Continuous surveillance of Shiga toxin-producing *Escherichia coli* infections by pulsed-field gel electrophoresis shows that most infections are sporadic. Foodborne Pathog Dis 3: 81–87.
6. van Duynhoven YT, Friesema IH, Schuurman T, Roovers A, van Zwet AA, et al. (2008) Prevalence, characterisation and clinical profiles of Shiga toxin-producing *Escherichia coli* in The Netherlands. Clin Microbiol Infect 14: 437–445.

7. Werber D, Beutin L, Pichner R, Stark K, Fruth A (2008) Shiga toxin-producing *Escherichia coli* serogroups in food and patients, Germany. Emerg Infect Dis 14: 1803–1806.
8. Caprioli A, Tozzi AE, Rizzoni G, Karch H (1997) Non-O157 Shiga toxin-producing *Escherichia coli* infections in Europe. Emerg Infect Dis 3: 578–579.
9. Thompson LH, Giercke S, Beaudoin C, Woodward D, Wylie JL (2005) Enhanced surveillance of non-O157 verotoxin-producing *Escherichia coli* in human stool samples from Manitoba. Can J Infect Dis Med Microbiol 16: 329–334.
10. Brooks JT, Sowers EG, Wells JG, Greene KD, Griffin PM, et al. (2005) Non-O157 Shiga toxin-producing *Escherichia coli* infections in the United States, 1983–2002. J Infect Dis 192: 1422–1429.
11. Bettelheim KA (2007) The non-O157 Shiga-toxigenic (Verocytotoxigenic) *Escherichia coli*; under-rated pathogens. Crit Rev Microbiol 33: 67–87.
12. Beutin L (2006) Emerging enterohaemorrhagic *Escherichia coli*, causes and effects of the rise of a human pathogen. J Vet Med Series B 53: 299–305.
13. Ethelberg S, Smith B, Torpdahl M, Lisby M, Boel J, et al. (2009) Outbreak of non-O157 Shiga toxin-producing *Escherichia coli* infection from consumption of beef sausage. Clin Infect Dis 48: e78–81.
14. Qin J, Cui Y, Zhao X, Rohde H, Liang T, et al. (2011) Identification of the Shiga toxin-producing *Escherichia coli* O104:H4 strain responsible for a food poisoning outbreak in Germany by PCR. J Clin Microbiol 49: 3439–3440.
15. Martin A, Beutin L (2011) Characteristics of Shiga toxin-producing *Escherichia coli* from meat and milk products of different origins and association with food producing animals as main contamination sources. Int J Food Microbiol 146: 99–104.
16. Islam MA, Mondol AS, Azmi IJ, de Boer E, Beumer RR, et al. (2010) Occurrence and characterization of Shiga toxin-producing *Escherichia coli* in raw meat, raw milk, and street vended juices in Bangladesh. Foodborne Pathog Dis 7: 1381–1385.
17. Mathusa EC, Chen YH, Enache E, Hontz L (2010) Non-O157 Shiga toxin-producing *Escherichia coli* in foods. J Food Prot 73: 1721–1736.
18. Fratamico PM, Wasilenko JL, Garman B, DeMarco DR, Varkey S, et al. (2014) Evaluation of a multiplex real-time PCR method for detecting Shiga toxin-producing *Escherichia coli* in beef and comparison to the US Department of Agriculture Food Safety and Inspection Service Microbiology Laboratory guidebook method. J Food Prot 77: 180–188.
19. USDA-FSIS (2011) Shiga toxin–producing *Escherichia coli* in certain raw beef products. Fed Regis 76: 58157–58165.
20. Zadik PM, Chapman PA, Siddons CA (1993) Use of tellurite for the selection of verocytotoxigenic *Escherichia coli* O157. J Med Microbiol 39: 155–158.
21. March SB, Ratnam S (1986) Sorbitol-MacConkey medium for detection of *Escherichia coli* O157:H7 associated with hemorrhagic colitis. J Clin Microbiol 23: 869–872.
22. Karch H, Bielaszewska M (2001) Sorbitol-fermenting Shiga toxin-producing *Escherichia coli* O157:H− strains: Epidemiology, phenotypic and molecular characteristics, and microbiological diagnosis. J Clin Microbiol 39: 2043–2049.
23. Fratamico PM, Bagi LK (2007) Comparison of methods for detection and isolation of cold- and freeze-stressed *Escherichia coli* O157:H7 in raw ground beef. J Food Prot 70: 1663–1669.
24. Posse B, De Zutter L, Heyndrickx M, Herman L (2008) Novel differential and confirmation plating media for Shiga toxin-producing *Escherichia coli* serotypes O26, O103, O111, O145 and sorbitol-positive and -negative O157. FEMS Microbiol Lett 282: 124–131.
25. Hiramatsu R, Matsumoto M, Miwa Y, Suzuki Y, Saito M, et al. (2002) Characterization of Shiga toxin-producing *Escherichia coli* O26 strains and establishment of selective isolation media for these strains. J Clin Microbiol 40: 922–925.
26. Church DL, Emshey D, Semeniuk H, Lloyd T, Pitout JD (2007) Evaluation of BBL CHROMagar O157 versus sorbitol-MacConkey medium for routine detection of *Escherichia coli* O157 in a centralized regional clinical microbiology laboratory. J Clin Microbiol 45: 3098–3100.
27. Bettelheim KA (1998) Studies of *Escherichia coli* cultured on Rainbow Agar O157 with particular reference to enterohaemorrhagic *Escherichia coli* (EHEC). Microbiol Immunol 42: 265–269.
28. DebRoy C, Roberts E, Valadez AM, Dudley EG, Cutter CN (2011) Detection of Shiga toxin-producing *Escherichia coli* O26, O45, O103, O111, O113, O121, O145, and O157 serogroups by multiplex polymerase chain reaction of the wzx gene of the O-antigen gene cluster. Foodbone Pathog Dis 8: 651–652.
29. Quinones B, Swimley MS, Narm K-E, Patel RN, Cooley MB, et al. (2012) O-antigen and virulence profiling of Shiga toxin-producing *Escherichia coli* by a rapid and cost effective DNA microarray colorimetric method. Front Cell Infect Microbiol 2.
30. Lin A, Lam N, Lee T, Clotilde LM, Kase JA, et al. (2011) Rapid O serogroup identification of the ten most clinically relevant STECs by Luminex microbead-based suspension array. J Microbiol Methods 87: 105–110.
31. Hegde NV, Praul C, Gehring A, Fratamico P, DebRoy C (2013) Rapid O serogroup identification of the six clinically relevant Shiga toxin-producing *Escherichia coli* by antibody microarray. J Microbiol Methods 93: 273–276.
32. Kjaergaard K, Schembri MA, Hasman H, Klemm P (2000) Antigen 43 from *Escherichia coli* induces inter- and intraspecies cell aggregation and changes in colony morphology of Pseudomonas fluorescens. J Bacteriol 182: 4789–4796.
33. Hasman H, Schembri MA, Klemm P (2000) Antigen 43 and type 1 fimbriae determine colony morphology of *Escherichia coli* K-12. J Bacteriol 182: 1089–1095.
34. Adamec T, Palkova Z, Forstova J (2003) Mouse polyomavirus large T antigen inhibits cell growth and alters cell and colony morphology in *Saccharomyces cerevisiae*. FEBS Lett 555: 268–273.
35. Windham WR, Yoon S-C, Ladely SR, Haley JA, Heitschmidt JW, et al. (2013) Detection by hyperspectral imaging of Shiga toxin-producing *Escherichia coli* serogroups O26, O45, O103, O111, O121, and O145 on Rainbow agar. J Food Prot 76: 1129–1136.
36. Bhunia AK (2008) Biosensors and bio-based methods for the separation and detection of foodborne pathogens. Adv Food Nutr Res 54: 1–44.
37. Banada PP, Guo S, Bayraktar B, Bae E, Rajwa B, et al. (2007) Optical forward-scattering for detection of *Listeria monocytogenes* and other *Listeria* species. Biosens Bioelectron 22: 1664–1671.
38. Banada PP, Huff K, Bae E, Rajwa B, Aroonnual A, et al. (2009) Label-free detection of multiple bacterial pathogens using light-scattering sensor. Biosens Bioelectron 24: 1685–1692.
39. Bae E, Banada PP, Huff K, Bhunia AK, Robinson JP, et al. (2007) Biophysical modeling of forward scattering from bacterial colonies using scalar diffraction theory. Appl Opt 46: 3639–3648.
40. Huff K, Aroonnual A, Littlejohn AEF, Rajwa B, Bae E, et al. (2012) Light-scattering sensor for real-time identification of *Vibrio parahaemolyticus*, *Vibrio vulnificus* and *Vibrio cholerae* colonies on solid agar plate. Microb Biotechnol 5: 607–620.
41. Singh AK, Bettasso AM, Bae E, Rajwa B, Dundar MM, et al. (2014) Laser optical sensor, a label-free on-plate *Salmonella enterica* colony detection tool. mBio 5 (1): e01019–01013.
42. FDA (2001) Bacteriological Analytical Manual Online, 8th ed AOAC International, Arlington, VA. Available: [http://www.fda.gov/Food/ScienceResearch/LaboratoryMethods/BacteriologicalAnalyticalManualBAM/default.htm];. Accessed 2014 Jan 16.
43. Bae E, Aroonnual A, Bhunia AK, Hirleman ED (2011) On the sensitivity of forward scattering patterns from bacterial colonies to media composition. J Biophoton 4: 236–243.
44. Valadez AM, Debroy C, Dudley E, Cutter CN (2011) Multiplex PCR detection of Shiga toxin-producing *Escherichia coli* strains belonging to serogroups O157, O103, O91, O113, O145, O111, and O26 experimentally inoculated in beef carcass swabs, beef trim, and ground beef. J Food Prot 74: 228–239.
45. Wylie JL, Van Caeseele P, Gilmour MW, Sitter D, Guttek C, et al. (2013) Evaluation of a new chromogenic agar medium for detection of Shiga toxin-producing *Escherichia coli* (STEC) and relative prevalences of O157 and non-O157 STEC in Manitoba, Canada. J Clin Microbiol 51: 466–471.
46. Bhunia AK, Nanduri V, Bae E, Hirleman ED (2010) Biosensors, Foodborne Pathogen Detection. In: Flickinger MC, editor. Encyclopedia of Industrial Biotechnology. Hoboken: John Wiley & Sons, Inc.
47. Bhunia AK, Bae E, Rajwa B, Robinson JP, Hirleman ED (2012) Utilization of optical forward scatter image biological database: Foodborne pathogen colony differentiation and detection. In: Yan X, Juneja VK, Fratamico PM, Smith JL, editors. Omics, Microbial Modeling and Technologies for Foodborne Pathogens. pp.553–578.
48. Guerini MN, Arthur TM, Shackelford SD, Koohmaraie M (2006) Evaluation of *Escherichia coli* O157:H7 growth media for use in test-and-hold procedures for ground beef processing. J Food Prot 69: 1007–1011.
49. Manafi M, Kremsmaier B (2001) Comparative evaluation of different chromogenic/fluorogenic media for detecting *Escherichia coli* O157:H7 in food. Int J Food Microbiol 71: 257–262.
50. Datta AK, Basu S (1999) Chemical characterization of the lipopolysaccharides from enteropathogenic *Escherichia coli* O142 and O158. Indian J Biochem Biophys 36: 55–58.
51. Raetz CR, Whitfield C (2002) Lipopolysaccharide endotoxins. Annu Rev Biochem 71: 635–700.
52. Datta AK, Basu S, Roy N (1999) Chemical and immunochemical studies of the O-antigen from enteropathogenic *Escherichia coli* O158 lipopolysaccharide. Carbohydr Res 322: 219–227.
53. Fratamico PM, Briggs CE, Needle D, Chen CY, DebRoy C (2003) Sequence of the *Escherichia coli* O121O-antigen gene cluster and detection of enterohemorrhagic *E. coli* O121 by PCR amplification of the wzx and wzy genes. J Clin Microbiol 41: 3379–3383.
54. Mialon M, Tang Y, Singh AK, Bae E, Bhunia AK (2012) Effects of preparation and storage of agar media on the sensitivity of bacterial forward scattering patterns Open J Appl Biosens 1: 24551.
55. Bayraktar B, Banada PP, Hirleman ED, Bhunia AK, Robinson JP, et al. (2006) Feature extraction from light-scatter patterns of *Listeria* colonies for identification and classification. J Biomed Optics 11: 34006.
56. Rajwa B, Dundar MM, Akova F, Bettasso A, Patsekin V, et al. (2010) Discovering the unknown: Detection of emerging pathogens using a label-free light-scattering system. Cytom Part A 77A: 1103–1112.
57. Breiman L (2001) Random forests. Mach Learn 45: 5–32.
58. Saeys Y, Inza I, Larranaga P (2007) A review of feature selection techniques in bioinformatics. Bioinformatics 23: 2507–2517.

59. Baldi P, Brunak S, Chauvin Y, Andersen CAF, Nielsen H (2000) Assessing the accuracy of prediction algorithms for classification: an overview. Bioinformatics 16: 412–424.

60. Possé B, De Zutter L, Heyndrickx M, Herman L (2008) Quantitative isolation efficiency of O26, O103, O111, O145 and O157 STEC serotypes from artificially contaminated food and cattle faeces samples using a new isolation protocol. J Appl Microbiol 105: 227–235.

8

Induction of Salivary Proteins Modifies Measures of Both Orosensory and Postingestive Feedback during Exposure to a Tannic Acid Diet

Ann-Marie Torregrossa*, Larissa Nikonova, Michelle B. Bales, Maria Villalobos Leal, James C. Smith, Robert J. Contreras, Lisa A. Eckel

Department of Psychology, Program in Neuroscience, Florida State University, Tallahassee, Florida, United States of America

Abstract

There are hundreds of proteins in saliva. Although it has long been hypothesized that these proteins modulate taste by interacting with taste receptors or taste stimuli, the functional impact of these proteins on feeding remains relatively unexplored. We have developed a new technique for saliva collection that does not interfere with daily behavioral testing and allows us to explore the relationship between feeding behavior and salivary protein expression. First, we monitored the alterations in salivary protein expression while simultaneously monitoring the animals' feeding behavior and meal patterns on a custom control diet or on the same diet mixed with 3% tannic acid. We demonstrated that six protein bands increased in density with dietary tannic acid exposure. Several of these bands were significantly correlated with behaviors thought to represent both orosensory and postingestive signaling. In a follow-up experiment, unconditioned licking to 0.01–3% tannic acid solutions was measured during a brief-access taste test before and after exposure to the tannic acid diet. In this experiment, rats with salivary proteins upregulated found the tannin solution less aversive (i.e., licked more) than those in the control condition. These data suggest a role for salivary proteins in mediating changes in both orosensory and postingestive feedback.

Editor: John I. Glendinning, Barnard College, Columbia University, United States of America

Funding: This work was funded by NIH T32 DC 000044, DK 73936, DC 004785, and DC R03 012632. The funders had no role in study design, data collection and analysis, decision to publish, or preparation of the manuscript.

Competing Interests: The authors have declared that no competing interests exist.

* Email: torregrossa@neuro.fsu.edu

Introduction

Variation in taste preferences in general, and bitter taste perception in particular, may play a key role in dietary choice, which has an uncontestable effect on human health. Bitter compounds are often thought of as aversive stimuli to be avoided [1] but are also common constituents of the omnivore diet [2]. A large number of nutritionally significant food sources contain bitter phytochemicals (e.g., broccoli [3], spinach [4]), many of which have beneficial value [3,5]. Understanding the complexity of bitter taste acceptance has been of interest to the research community for decades [6–8] and is part and parcel to the development of strategies to influence dietary choices in the service of promoting human health. Studies on bitter taste have focused mainly on the molecular identification of bitter taste receptors and their ligand-binding properties [9,10] as well as the genetic variation in such receptors [7,8,11]. In comparison, very little work has been done to investigate how salivary proteins interact with taste stimuli and alter taste sensitivity despite the fact that, under normal feeding and drinking conditions, taste compounds must inescapably mix with saliva before reaching their receptor targets. This sets the stage for potential modulation of the taste signal at its most fundamental level.

Proteomics suggest that over 1,000 different proteins are present in the saliva of healthy adults [12]. The protein content of saliva is altered under a variety of circumstances including diet composition [13,14], disease [15,16], exposure to compounds like capsaicin [17] or bitter taste stimuli [18–21]. Likewise, there is evidence that some of these proteins modulate bitter taste acceptance. For example, Kock et al. [22] introduced von Ebner's gland protein, a protein found in rat saliva, to mice that do not normally express the protein. The presence of von Ebner's gland protein altered the acceptability of the bitter stimulus denatonium benzoate. Dsamou et al. [23] determined that another salivary protein, cystatin SN, was related to variation in human sensitivity to the bitter taste of caffeine.

Most studies examining the role of salivary proteins on food intake have focused on the relationship between a class of proteins referred to as proline-rich proteins (PRPs) and a class of plant secondary compounds referred to as tannins. Tannins are polyphenolic compounds commonly consumed by both humans and non-human mammals. In the human diet, tannins are present in foods such as sorgum, tea, red wine, beans and unripe fruits. Tannins are not only associated with a sense of astringency [4,24], but several polyphenolic compounds classified as tannins activate various human bitter taste receptors, TAS2Rs [25]. In addition to their astringency and bitter taste, tannins are considered "anti-nutritional" because they can reduce non-heme iron absorption, cause loss of endogenous nitrogen, reduce digestibility and damage the kidney, liver, gastrointestinal mucosa and gastrointestinal

Table 1. Composition of the control and 3% tannic acid diets used in Experiments 1 and 2. (These diets were based on Skopec et al. [28]).

Ingredients	Control Diet (g/kg)	3% Tannic acid diet (g/kg)
Casein	200	200
DL-Methionine	3	3
Sucrose	500	500
Corn starch	150	150
Corn oil	50	50
Cellulose	50	20
Tannic acid	0	30
Mineral Mix, AIN-76 Teklad	35	35
Vitamin Mix, AIN-76	10	10
Choline bitartrate	2	2

epithelium (see [21]). Although avoidance of tannins is well documented (see [26]), no studies have addressed whether it is the taste or the postingestive effects of tannins that alter food intake. One study suggested that avoidance of high tannin diets is the result of both conditioned and unconditioned avoidance [27], however, this study could not decouple the oral and gastrointestinal effects of tannin, so the relative roles of these two sources of negative feedback remain unclear.

Salivary PRPs are considered the first line of defense against the negative consequences of ingested tannins [26]. PRPs avidly bind tannins into a complex that is stable even under the conditions of the stomach and intestine [28,29], and this complex allows the consumer to pass the tannin complex as fecal material. PRPs are not constitutively produced in rodents, as they appear to be in humans (see [30]), but can be induced by exposure to tannin containing diets or via injections of the β-agonist isoproterenol [31]. It has been demonstrated that several species of rodents decrease food intake and lose body mass when fed tannin containing diets in the absence of PRPs. In rats, food intake is reduced for several days before they resume their normal intake, presumably due to increases in PRPs [32]. In support of this hypothesis, it has been demonstrated that hamsters, which do not upregulate PRP production in response to tannin-containing diets, reduce intake on tannin diets indefinitely and lose a life-threatening amount of body mass while on the diet [32].

Although it is generally accepted that PRPs allow animals to consume tannin-containing diets, it is unclear whether the increase in diet acceptability is due to a change in the perception of the tannins in the mouth [30,33,34] or due to an ability to protect the gut from negative postingestive effects [35]. Glendinning [33] demonstrated that mice injected with isoproterenol, to increase PRP production, show an increased preference for, and intake of, tannin solutions compared to control mice via increases in both the size and number of drinking bouts (i.e. the amount of time an animal licked on the sipper tube before taking a break). These data imply a modification in the orosensory perception of the tannin solutions.

In order to better understand the role of salivary proteins on tannic acid acceptance, we conducted two experiments. In our first experiment, we monitored the alterations in salivary protein expression, while simultaneously monitoring feeding behavior, in animals consuming a control or tannic acid containing diet. In the second experiment, unconditioned licking of tannic acid solutions was measured during a series of brief-access (30-s) tests conducted before and after exposure to a tannic acid containing diet. This allowed us to isolate the contribution of orosensory signals to ongoing fluid intake and thus provided a direct measure of tannin palatability.

Methods

Experiment 1

Animals and housing. Animals (male Long-Evans rats, Charles River Breeding Laboratory, Raleigh, NC; weighing 200–240 g at study onset) were assigned to either an experimental or control group. The experimental group (n = 8) was individually housed in custom-designed Plexiglas shoebox cages. Food compartments attached to the front of each cage were equipped with infrared light emitting diodes and photo detectors. Feeding events were detected when the rat's head entered the food compartment and broke the photo beam. The time and duration of each beam break, recorded on a computer, was used to estimate meal size and rate of feeding. Rats were allowed ad lib access to food and tap water. The control group (n = 4) was housed in cages similar to the test cages but without with photo beams. The colony room was maintained at a 20±2°C with a 12:12 h light/dark cycle. All animal procedures were approved by Florida State University Animal Care and Use Committee (ACUC).

Analysis of Feeding Behavior. The start of a meal was defined as a minimum of 3 s of activity in the food cup and individual meals were considered terminated when there was no feeding activity for >5 min. Daily food intake was measured gravimetrically. Average daily meal size was defined as the total (24 h) food intake (g) divided by the number of meals consumed each day. Average daily rate of feeding was defined as the total (24 h) food intake (g) divided by the total amount of feeding activity (min).

Saliva collection. Saliva was collected from awake, trained animals. During training, each rat received 2 ml of 30 mM citric acid in 1 M sucrose. This solution, which served as an unconditioned stimulus (US), was pipetted into the mouth daily in 200 μl increments. Animals were held against the experimenter's chest with the palm of the hand while the head and mouth were stabilized by the first two fingers and the thumb. The pipette tip, which served as a conditioned stimulus (CS), was inserted into the side of the mouth and was moved over and under the tongue during CS/US pairings. The animals received 25 pairings of the US and CS across an approximately 20-min period, every day for

12 days. In this way, animals were conditioned to salivate by merely inserting the pipette into the mouth. Following training, we began collecting salivary secretions on alternate days. Saliva was gently aspirated from below and around the tongue using a 200 µl pipette fitted with a wide orifice tip. We stimulated the animals with the US several times during the saliva collection. After stimulation we allowed the rat to rest for ~60 s to minimize contamination of the saliva with the solution. We used this procedure to collect all of the saliva in Experiment 1. We now know that this intermittent stimulation is unnecessary and in Experiment 2 we were able to collect saliva from animals without the presence of the US on collection days. Both of these methods allowed us to collect uncontaminated saliva from sublingual, submandibular and parotid secretions, as all are stimulated by sweet and sour mixtures [36].

Saliva samples, ranging from 50–100 µl were immediately placed on ice in 10 µl of 10x Halt protease/phosphatase inhibitor cocktail (Thermo Scientific). All samples were then frozen at −20°C for later analysis. Saliva was collected from half of the rats on odd test days while the other half received only the citric acid/sucrose mixture and the reverse was conducted on even days. Thus, saliva was collected representing each day of the trial.

Diets. All rats were maintained on Purina 5001 and tap water ad lib until study onset at which point all rats were given a purified control diet ad lib (diet modeled after [28], Table 1). The control group was maintained on the control diet during the entire course of the experiment. The experimental group was fed the control diet for 12 days followed by the tannic acid diet for 15 days. The tannic acid diet contained 3% tannic acid (Sigma Aldrich, lot number SZBC0460V) by weight and 3% less cellulose but was otherwise identical to the control diet. The first saliva samples were collected after the animals were maintained on the control diet for 4 days.

High Performance Liquid Chromatography (HPLC) analysis of tannic acid. HPLC analysis was performed in the Florida State University Department of Biology Analytical Laboratory. A sample of the tannic acid that was used in the diet (Sigma Aldrich, lot number SZBC0460V) was dissolved in 20% acetonitrile/0.1% TFA at a concentration of 5 mg/ml. Two µl of this solution was loaded onto a C18 reversed phase column (Agilent Zorbaz 300SB-C18, 4.6×250 mm, 5 micron) equilibrated in 20% acetonitrile/0.1% TFA. Tannins were eluted with a 10 min linear gradient to 40% acetonitrile/0.1% TFA, at a flow rate of 1 ml/min and detection at 280 nm. Pentagalloyl glucose (PGG, Sigma Aldrich, lot number 063M4713V PCode 71813) was dissolved in 20% acetonitrile/0.1% TFA at a concentration of 5 mg/ml, and 0.25 µl of this solution was analyzed by reversed phase. In addition, a tannic acid sample spiked with PGG standard was analyzed to confirm the identification of PGG in the tannic acid mixture. All HPLC analyses were preformed on a Beckman System Gold HPLC equipped with a 168 diode array detector, 126-solvent delivery system, and 32 Karat software for data analysis.

Salivary protein processing. Saliva samples were defrosted and mixed with equal volumes of ice-cold 20 mM Hepes buffer, pH 7.4, supplemented with 2x Halt protease/phosphatase inhibitor cocktail (Thermo Scientific) and 2 mM phenylmethylsulfonyl fluoride on the day of processing. Samples were centrifuged at 2000xg for 6 min at 4°C to remove cells and debris. The supernatant was aspirated and was thereafter referred to as whole saliva. Total protein concentration was determined by the bicinchoninic acid (BCA) protein assay method (Pierce Protein Biology Products).

Gel electrophoresis and Western blotting. Equal volumes of saliva sample were mixed with 1/4th volume of 4x Invitrogen sample buffer with reducing agent, heated at 70°C for 10 min and resolved on a 12% SDS-PAGE (Invitrogen) with MOPS buffer. Molecular mass markers (Invitrogen, Ref LC5800, or BioRad, Ref 161-0374) were run simultaneously with the samples in each gel to calibrate molecular masses of each protein band. Gels were fixed in 40% methanol in 10% acetic acid for 30 min followed by staining with Coomassie Brilliant Blue R250 (0.1% stain in 25% methanol and 10% acetic acid) for 1 h. These gels were distained in 10% acetic acid according to previously published protocols [37,38]. Although it is usual to rinse gels with methanol/ethanol in the destaining solution, omitting these chemicals distinguishes PRPs, which stain pink-violet, from other proteins, which stain blue [37,38]. These data were used to determine which bands contained PRPs. Bands were captured using Kodak Imaging Station 440 CF (Kodak, Rochester, New York). Densitometric analysis was performed using Kodak 10 Imaging Analysis software (Kodak).

Secretory immunoglobulin A (IgA) was used as a protein loading control. Preliminary experiments demonstrated that IgA expression, in samples loaded at the same protein level, was unchanged by our treatment. Salivary IgA levels were estimated by immunoblotting using goat polyclonal antibody to rat immunoglobulin A. We used 1/10 volume of each saliva sample used for Commasie staining but without the reducing agent. Following electrophoresis, proteins were transferred to Hybond-P Western blotting membranes (VWR Scientific Product). The blots were blocked for 1-h at room temperature with 5% BSA in Tris-buffered saline containing 0.1% Tween 20 (TBST). The membranes were then incubated for 1-h at room temperature with goat anti-IgA antibody (1: 80 000) conjugated with horseradish peroxidase, (Abcam Inc. # ab97185). The immunoblotted proteins were detected using Super Signal West Dura Extended Duration Substrate (Thermo Scientific, #34076) and CL-XPosure Film (Pierce Protein Biology Products). Following development of chemiluminescence film, images of bands were captured using a Kodak Imaging Station 440 CF (Kodak, Rochester, New York). Densitometric analysis was performed using Kodak 10 Imaging Analysis software (Kodak) that measures the optical density of the immunosignal.

To quantify protein level, each gel contained several control saliva samples from untreated animals. Band intensity was normalized using the corresponding IgA protein signal and expressed as relative amount to average intensity of the control sample, which was assigned a value of 1.

Detection of glycosylated proteins. Because glycosylated PRPs are less effective at binding tannins than basic PRPs [39], we used the Pro-Q Emerald 300 Glycoprotein Gel and Blot stain Kit (Molecular Probes # P21857) to determine if the proteins were glycosylated. The kit detects as little as 0.5 ng of glycoprotein per band. Saliva samples from animals in our experimental group were tested to demonstrate the likelihood of glycosylation of each protein band. Samples (6 µg) were loaded in duplicate on a single 12% SDS/PAGE gel. After resolving the gel, it was cut in two. Each half contained several concentrations of protein collected on several days of the study from a single animal and Candy-Cane glycoprotein molecular weight standards, which include glycosylated and non-glycosylated proteins. One half was stained using Pro-Q Emerald 300 glycoprotein detection kit, which detects only glycosylated proteins. The other half was stained with Coomasie stain to detect total protein.

Protein identification. Amino-acid sequencing was performed at the Florida State University Translation Science

Laboratory. Following electrophoresis, the gels were fixed and Coomassie-stained. Protein bands of interest were excised followed by distaining, reduction, alkylation, dehydration and in-gel tryptic digestion. Tryptic digestion was conducted using the Calbiochem ProteoExtract All-in-One Trypsin Digestion Kit (Merck, Darmstadt, Germany) according to the manufacturer's instructions and using LC-MS grade solvents (Avantor Performance Materials, Center Valley, PA, USA). The digestion supernatant was stored at −80°C prior to analysis. Nanospray LC/MS^{E} was done using a Synapt G2 HD Mass Spectrometer equipped with an integrated *nano*Acquity UPLC for on-line chromatographic separation of tryptic peptides prior to MS analysis (Waters Corp., Milford, MA, USA). Samples were adjusted to 3% acetonitrile (ACN) in LC-MS grade water with 0.1% formic acid (FA) and 25 fmol/µl rabbit Phosphorylase B (PhosB, Waters Corp.) as an internal standard. Glufibrinopeptide (785.8426 m/z, Waters Corp.) was used as the lock mass (external calibrant). Instrument data acquisition parameters are provided in Table S1. Raw data were generated using MassLynx version 4.1 software (Waters Corp.) and data were processed in ProteinLynx Global SERVER version 3.0. After analysis of the protein sequences of the 14 kDa band, it was identified using the PLGS Identity search algorithm, which queried a Rattus norvegicus protein databank containing sequences from the Uniprot Protein Knowledgebase (www.uniprot.org) and the rabbit PhosB sequence. Results were validated by manual review of the raw data and results.

Statistical Analysis. Feeding data were analyzed using repeated-measures ANOVAs. To evaluate group differences in protein expression, protein levels from experimental and control animals were compared using ANOVA with diet as a between-subjects factor and time as a within-subjects factor. Significant ANOVA effects were further evaluated using Bonferoni corrected paired t-tests. Because saliva was collected from half of the rats each day, odd and even days were combined for each sampling period so that all animals were represented in the same repeated measures analysis. A linear mixed model analysis was used to explore the associations between feeding behavior and the protein measures while accounting for the correlations associated with the repeated-measures factor. We limited this analysis to the feeding behavior recorded and salivary samples collected during the first four days of tannic acid diet exposure. This time frame represents the dynamic phase when salivary proteins were upregulated and changes in feeding behavior were most pronounced. ANOVAs and post-hoc tests were conducted in Systat 12. Linear mixed models were run in SPSS 19.

Experiment 2

Animals and housing. Male Long Evans rats (n = 12) were individually housed in custom designed Plexiglas shoebox cages, equipped with a feeding niche that provided access to a spill-resistant food cup. The colony room conditions were identical to that described above. Rats were allowed ad lib access to diets (control or 3% tannic acid, lot number SZBA 3060V, Sigma) and tap water, except where otherwise noted.

Analysis of Licking Behavior. To determine whether induction of PRPs affects the rats' taste responses to tannic acid, we recorded the unconditioned licking responses to varying concentrations of tannic acid in a test chamber designed to measure solution licking (Davis MS80 Rig; Dilog Instruments and Systems, Tallahassee, FL). This apparatus consisted of a Plexiglas cage with a wire mesh floor. An opening at the front of the cage allowed access to one of ten spill-proof glass drinking tubes that reside on a sliding platform. A mechanical shutter opened and closed to allow the rat access to one of the ten tubes for a user-

Table 2. Summary of ANOVAs comparing normalized densitometry units of protein bands at each of the listed masses (kDa).

	between subjects			within subjects			interaction effects		
kDa	df	F	p	df	F	p	df	F	p
37	1,10	3.047	0.111	6,60	1.675	0.143	6,60	2.1	0.065
35	1,9	10.86	0.009*	6,54	2.9	0.016*	6,54	3.17	0.01*
25	1,10	0.54	0.49	6,60	1.79	0.116	6,60	1.92	0.084
23	1,9	16.27	0.003*	6,54	4.1	0.002*	6,54	4.6	0.001*
19	1,10	12.35	0.006*	6,60	3.26	0.0088*	6,60	3.4	0.006*
18.5	1,10	3.7	0.082	6,60	1.9	0.091	6,60	2.4	0.034*
18	1,10	12.5	0.005*	6,60	2.264	0.383	6,60	2.26	0.049*
14	1,10	17.13	0.002*	6,60	3.5	0.005*	6,60	4.2	0.001*

Analyses were conducted with experimental group (control or tannic acid diet) as the between-subjects comparison and time (days) as the within-subjects comparison. *ps<0.05.

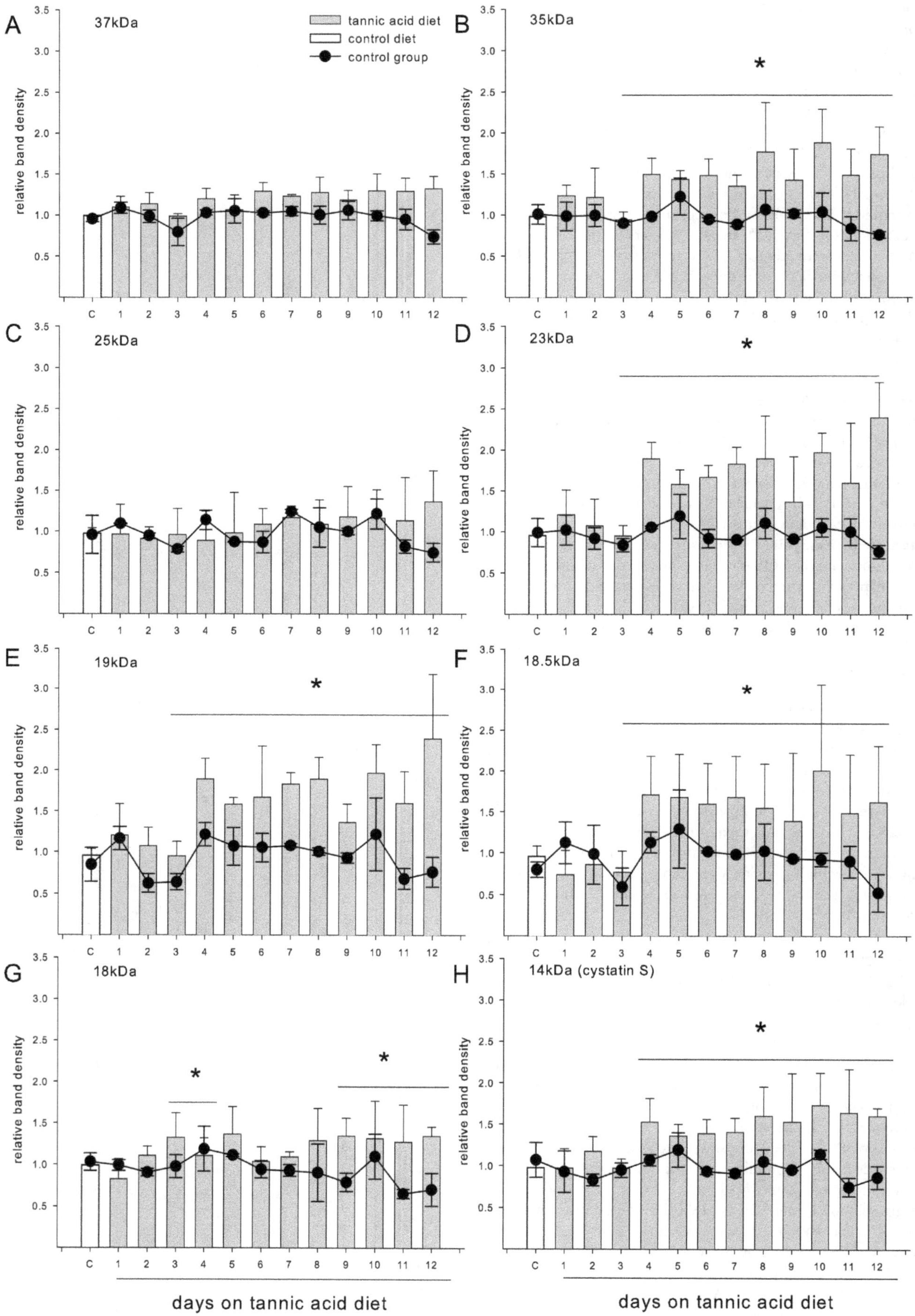
A
37kDa
tannic acid diet
control diet
control group
B
35kDa
C
25kDa
D
23kDa
E
19kDa
F
18.5kDa
G
18kDa
H
14kDa (cystatin S)
relative band density
days on tannic acid diet

Figure 1. Data are densitometry units normalized to average control diet protein expressions (set to 1) as well as IgA expression. White bars represent protein expression measured while the experimental animals were consuming the control diet (average of the final 5 days; depicted by white bars labelled "C"), and grey bars represent expression of the same protein while the experimental animals were consuming the 3% tannic acid diet. The line graphs represent the same protein densitometry measures for animals that were maintained on the control diet for the entire course of the study. *Significant within-subject difference between protein expression on the control and experimental diets ($p<0.05$, bonferoni corrected for multiple comparisons).

specified length of time. A computer controlled the movement of the platform, order of tube presentation, opening and closing of the shutter, duration of tube access and interval between tube presentations. Each individual lick was detected by a contact lickometer and recorded on a computer via DavisPro collection software (Dilog Instruments and Systems).

Rats were adapted to the test chamber and trained to drink from the sipper tubes for 4 days. On the first day of training, rats were 20-h water-deprived. The rat was presented with a single stationary bottle of 0.25 M sucrose for 30 min. On the second day, a single tube containing 0.25 M sucrose was presented again, however, the rat had to lick the tube 50 times in order for the training program to begin. At the start of the program, the shutter closed for 10 s before a new tube, containing 0.25 M sucrose, was presented. The rat was given 180 s to initiate licking and once licking was recorded the rat was given 30-s access to the tube. At the conclusion of either the 30-s access or the 180-s limit, the shutter was closed again for 10 s. Each of the 10 tubes, all containing 0.25 M sucrose, was presented 3 times. The entire training program took an average of 15 min.

During testing rats were 20-h water deprived. Rats were given varying concentrations of tannic acid (0.0, 0.011, 0.02, 0.046, 0.09, 0.187, 0.375, 0.75, 1.5, and 3%). Each bottle was presented three times per session and sessions were organized in randomized blocks. Identical to training; the rat was given 180 s to initiate licking, 30-s access once a lick was recorded and a 10-s delay between stimulus presentations.

All rats were tested in the brief-access taste test while maintained on the control diet. After initial testing, rats were assigned to either a control group (n = 6), which received only the control diet prior

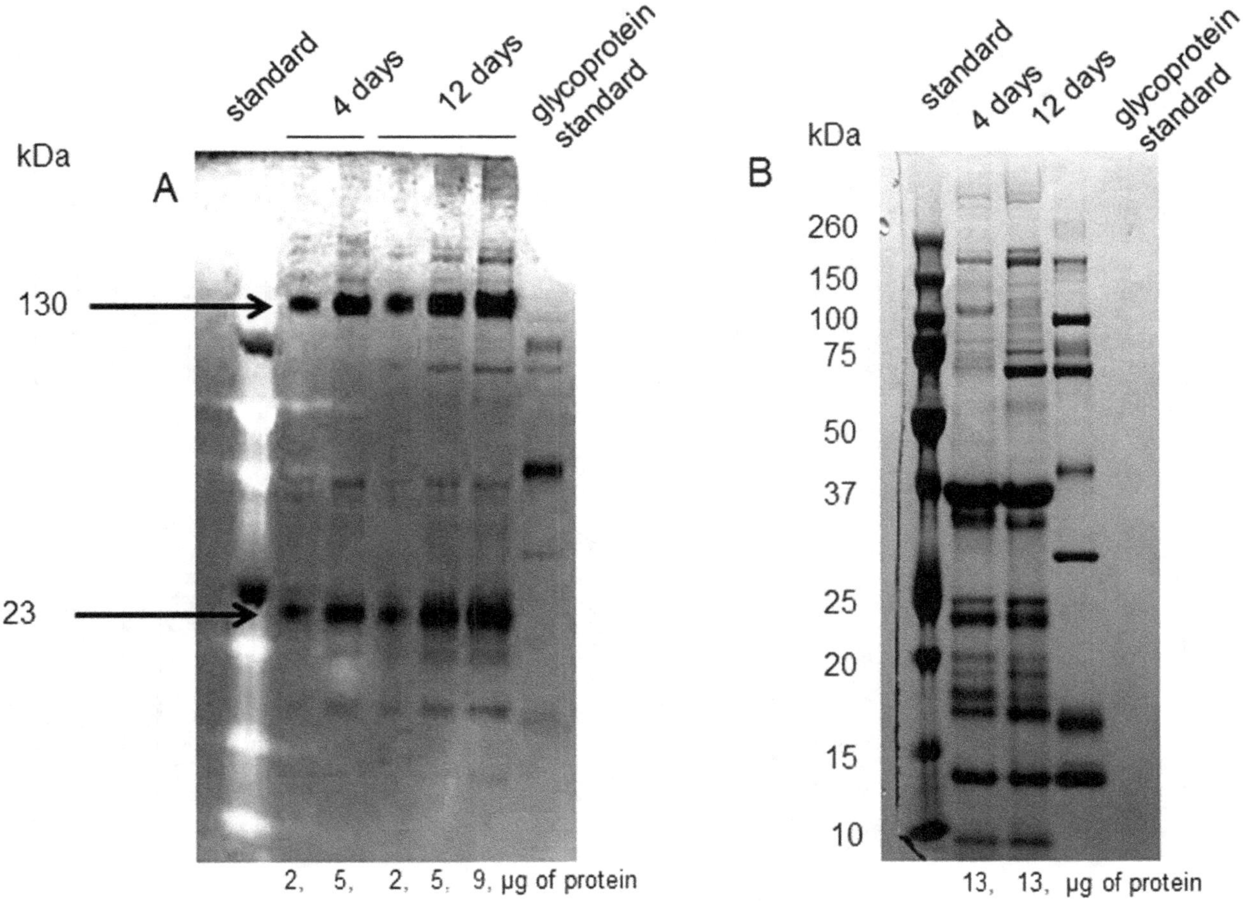

Figure 2. Representative samples of the glycosylation determination. The gel contains saliva samples from a single rat after 4 or 12 days exposure to the tannic acid diet. The samples were loaded in duplicate on the same12% SDS/PAGE. The quantity of protein loaded in each lane was varied to allow for maximal visibility of the protein band. After resolving the gel, it was cut into two pieces. Gel A was stained using Pro-Q Emerald 300 glycoprotein detection kit, which detects only glycosylated proteins. Gel B was stained with Coomassie R250 stain, which detects total proteins. Both gels contain both Candy-Cane glycoprotein molecular weight standards and Bio-Rad molecular weight standards.

10 20 30 40 50 60
MAYLLHAQLF LLTTFILVLN MRLCPVLGHF LGGIEK**SSME EEGASEALNY AVNEYNEKNS**

70 80 90 100 110 120
DLYLSRVVEV KDVQKQVVAG TK**FFFDVILG K**TICLKTQGD LTNCPLNEEA DQQEHEFCSF

130 140
VVHDIPWENY IVLLSSSCHS I

Figure 3. The sequence of rat protein cystatin S (Uniprot accession P19313). Bold regions indicate where tryptic peptides detected in proteomic analysis overlay the protein sequence.

to the second brief-access taste test, or an experimental group (n = 6), which was maintained on the 3% tannic acid diet prior to the second brief-access taste test.

Saliva collection. As described above, animals were conditioned to salivate when a pipette was inserted into their mouth. During training, animals received 5 ml of 30 mM citric acid in 1 M sucrose pipetted into the mouth daily for 14 days in 200 µl increments. Following training, conditioning was maintained by pipetting the solution into the animals' mouths once a week until the conclusion of the experiment. We found that we had no difficulty maintaining the conditioning across these time scales. Because this testing paradigm required the animals to be water

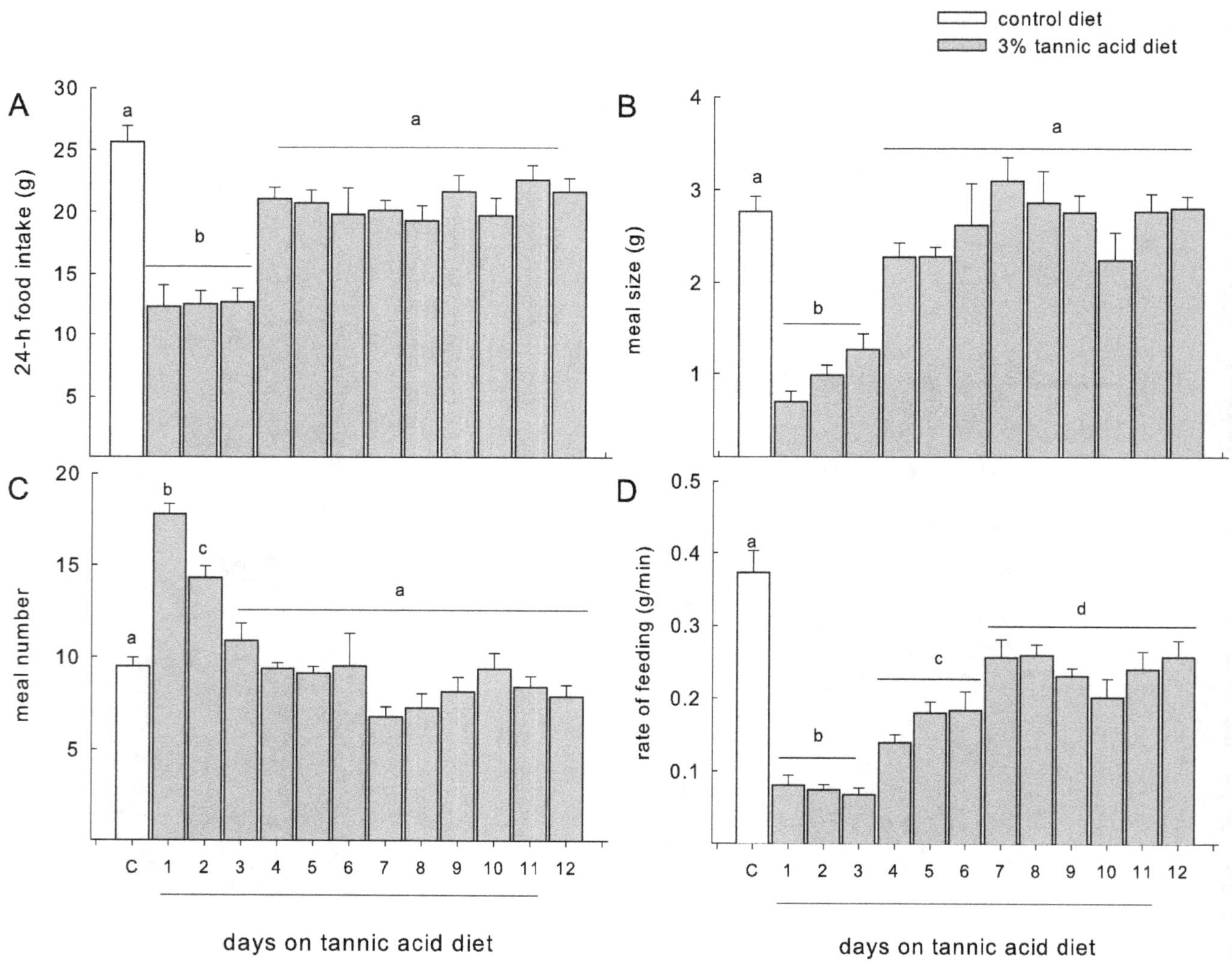

Figure 4. A–D: White bars represent feeding behaviors measured while animals were consuming the control diet; grey bars represent the same behaviors measured while animals were on the 3% tannic acid diet. The white bar labeled 'C' represents a 5-day average of behavioral measures on the control diet prior to exposure to the tannic acid diet. Food intake (A) and meal size (B) were decreased on the first 3 days of exposure to the tannic acid diet but returned to control levels by day 4. Meal number (C) was increased during the first 2 days of exposure to the tannic acid diet but returned to control-levels by day 3. Rate of feeding (D) was decreased throughout the entire exposure to the tannic acid diet buy this effect was most pronounced during the first 3 days.

deprived when saliva was collected, all saliva collection was conducted in the absence of the citric acid mixture; the conditioning alone was sufficient for the procedure. Saliva was collected the day before the brief-access test while animals were water replete and the day of the brief-access test while animals were 20-h water deprived.

Salivary protein processing. Salivary samples were processed as described above with one exception. In Experiment 1, we used IgA to confirm our total protein measures, but it was not possible to do this in the water-deprived condition. Previous studies have shown that expression of IgA is altered by water deprivation [40] as is protein concentration of saliva [41]. Because we cannot be sure that deprivation alters the expression of all proteins equally, we used a more conservative approach of analyzing the salivary protein data by t-test comparing differences in protein expression between the two test sessions (i.e. test 1 protein expression - test 2 protein expression) by treatment (control fed vs. tannin fed). Because these data do not allow an impression of relative abundance, we also present the data as corrected to the water replete expression of the same protein. We do not compare these data statistically but provide them merely to illustrate the relative abundance of the proteins.

Statistical Analysis. The behavioral data presented represent the mean number of licks to each concentration and the curves fitted to the mean number of licks to each concentration. Curves were fit to the lick data (excluding the water licking) of each individual animal using a 3-parameter logistic function: $f(x) = \frac{a}{1+10^{(\log_{10}x-c)b}}$ in which a = asymptotic lick response, excluding water; b = slope; and c = $\log_{10}$ concentration at one-half of the asymptote (i.e., EC_{50}). Licking behavior was compared by repeated-measures ANOVA and Bonferoni corrected paired t-tests. The curve parameters were compared using Bonferoni corrected paired t-tests. Curves were fit to the data and ANOVAs were conducted in Systat 12.

Results

Experiment 1

HPLC analysis of tannic acid. The area under the curve was calculated based on the chromatograms from the HPLC analysis. These data revealed that the ~67% of the area under the curve was identical to, or to the right of, the peak caused by our additional PGG marker. Larger tannin compounds are known to better interact with PRPs compared to smaller compounds [42], because PGG is a large tannin compound known to interact with PRPs, we have used PGG as a marker for size in this study. These data suggest that 67% of compounds in the tannic acid, are the same size or larger than PGG (Figure S1), therefore, we believe that the tannic acid supplied by Sigma contains large tannin compounds, which are capable of interacting with salivary proteins.

Induction of salivary proteins. In the experimental group, we saw a trend toward increased protein concentration with exposure to the tannic acid diet, but it failed to reach significance ($F_{9,63} = 2.0$, $p = 0.06$). In the control group there was no difference in the total protein concentration across time ($F_{5,20} = 1.9$, $p = 0.13$). Our method separated out 12–15 bands from each sample of saliva (Figure S2). We quantified the protein level of all the major bands identified as PRPs (37 kDa, 35 kDa, 23 kDa, 18.5 kDa and 19 kDa) and three non-PRP bands (25 kDa, 18 kDa and 14 kDa) that appeared to be altered by the tannin diet. Quantification confirmed that the density of 6 of the 8 bands was increased by tannic acid exposure. ANOVAs revealed a significant interaction between group (tannin or control treated) and time for

Table 3. Summary of linear mixed model analyses.

	meal size			number of meals			rate of feeding		
kDa	df	F	P	df	F	P	df	F	P
35	1,16	5.07	0.04*	1,16	1.01	0.33	1,15.8	3.03	0.1
23	1,16	3.33	0.09	1,16	0.06	0.8	1,15.6	4.6	0.05*
19	1,15.6	5.5	0.03*	1,16	2.9	0.11	1,16	1.85	0.2
18.5	1,16	3.04	0.01*	1,16	3.21	0.09	1,11.1	5.5	0.04*
18	1,16	1.26	0.278	1,16	0.318	0.58	1,16	0.2	0.65
14	1,16	7.4	0.02*	1,16	2.6	0.12	1,12.2	2.8	0.12

We looked for the predictive value of each of the normalized densitometry units of protein bands at each of the listed masses (kDa) on feeding behaviors. Analyses were restricted to the first four days of exposure to the tannin diet as this represented the dynamic phase over which changes in feeding behavior and salivary protein expression were observed. *ps<0.05.

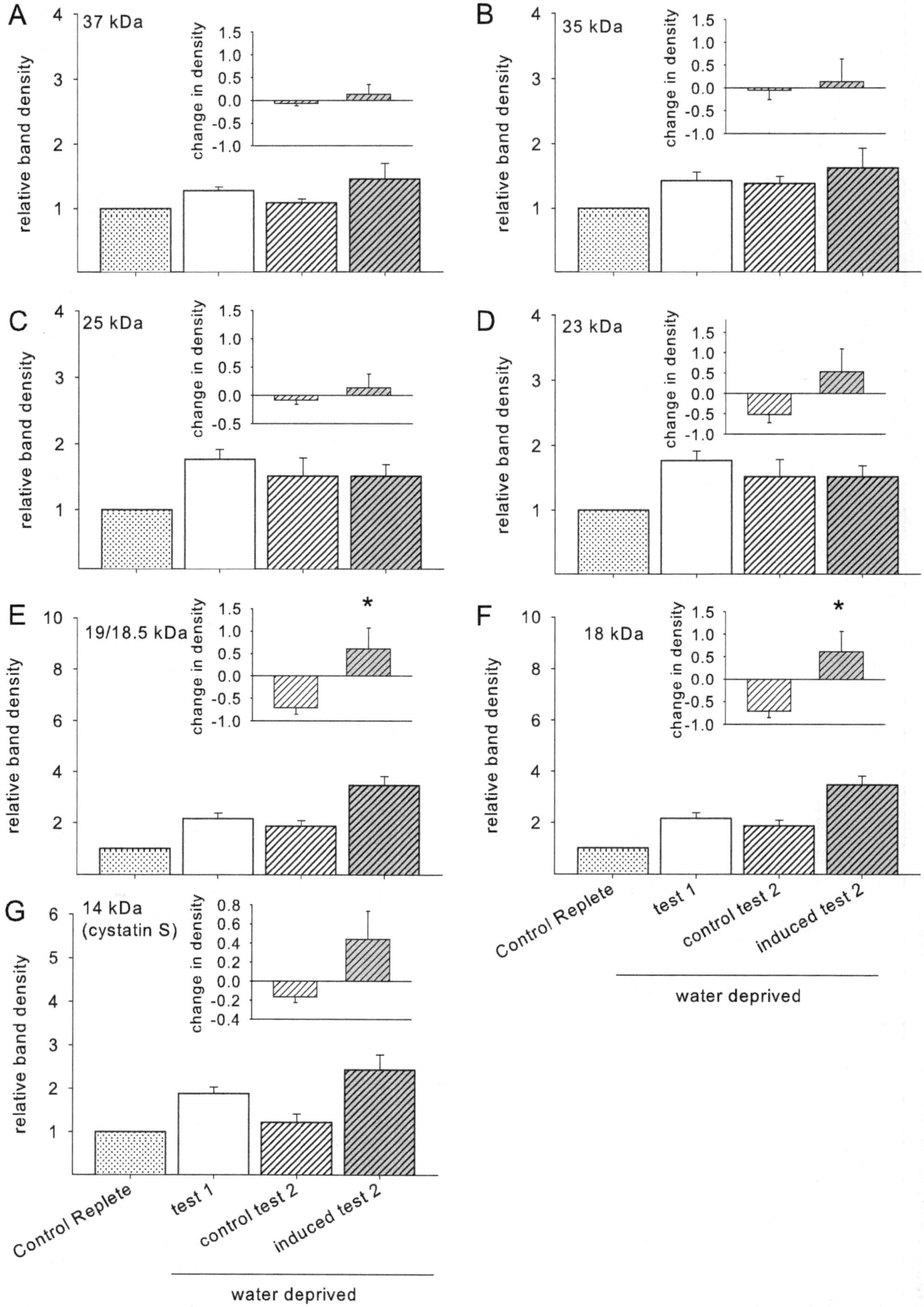
A
37 kDa
B
35 kDa
C
25 kDa
D
23 kDa
E
19/18.5 kDa
F
18 kDa
G
14 kDa
(cystatin S)
relative band density
change in density
*
Control Replete
test 1
control test 2
induced test 2
water deprived

Figure 5. Data depicted in the larger graphs are densitometry units normalized to average control (water replete) protein expressions (which are set to 1). The first bar (stippled) represents the average water replete expression of protein concentration, while all rats were fed the control diet. The data in the remainder of the bars were collected in the water-deprived condition. The white bar represents the average protein expression of all rats on the day of their first exposure to the brief-access taste test. The white bar with hash marks represents the saliva samples collected the day of the second exposure to the brief-access test by rats that were maintained on the control diet. The gray bar with hash marks represents the saliva samples collected the day of the second exposure to the brief-access test by rats that were maintained on the tannic acid diet between exposures. Statistical analyses were not preformed on these data. Total protein concentration was significantly altered by water deprivation making comparisons between samples unreliable. We have presented them only to illustrate the relative abundance of proteins across treatments. The inset graphs represent the change in densitometry units between the two test sessions (i.e. test 1 protein expression- test 2 protein expression) for the control group (white bar with hash marks) and experimental group (gray bar with hash marks). *Experimental group greater than the control group, $P<0.05$.

the PRPs at 35 kDa, 23 kDa, 18.5 kDa,19 kDa, and the non-PRPs at 18 kDa and 14 kDa, Table 2, Figure 1). Two proteins on the gel were identified as glycosylated (23 and 130 kDa), only one of these, the 23 kDa band, was significantly modified by the diet treatment (Figure 2).

Several bands seemed to be composed, to varying degrees of both PRP and non-PRP proteins as the upper portion of the band was stained pink, while the lower portion of the band was stained blue or vice versa (e.g., 23 and 18 kDa). In these cases, we could not segregate the colors during density counts. It is unsurprising to find several proteins in a single band, for example Mirels et al. [43] previously described an 18.5 kDa band isolated from rat submandibular and sublingual saliva consisting of several proteins. We were unable to determine protein sequences from the bands that were identified as proline-rich or appeared to contain some PRPs, due to the heterogeneity of sample.

We were however, able to identify the dominant protein in the 14 kDa band. This band steadily increased across days of dietary exposure and was maximally expressed by the 4th day of dietary exposure. Proteomic analysis of the 14 kDa band identified rat cystatin S (Uniprot accession P19313) as the dominant protein present. Cystatin S was identified with >95% confidence and high confidence tryptic peptides combined together provided 34% coverage of the cystatin S sequence (Figure 3), indicating that the dominant protein in the band was a cysteine protease inhibitor present in the saliva of rats and humans [44–46].

Behavioral data. For all the feeding behavior measures, we used the average of the final five days on the control diet as our

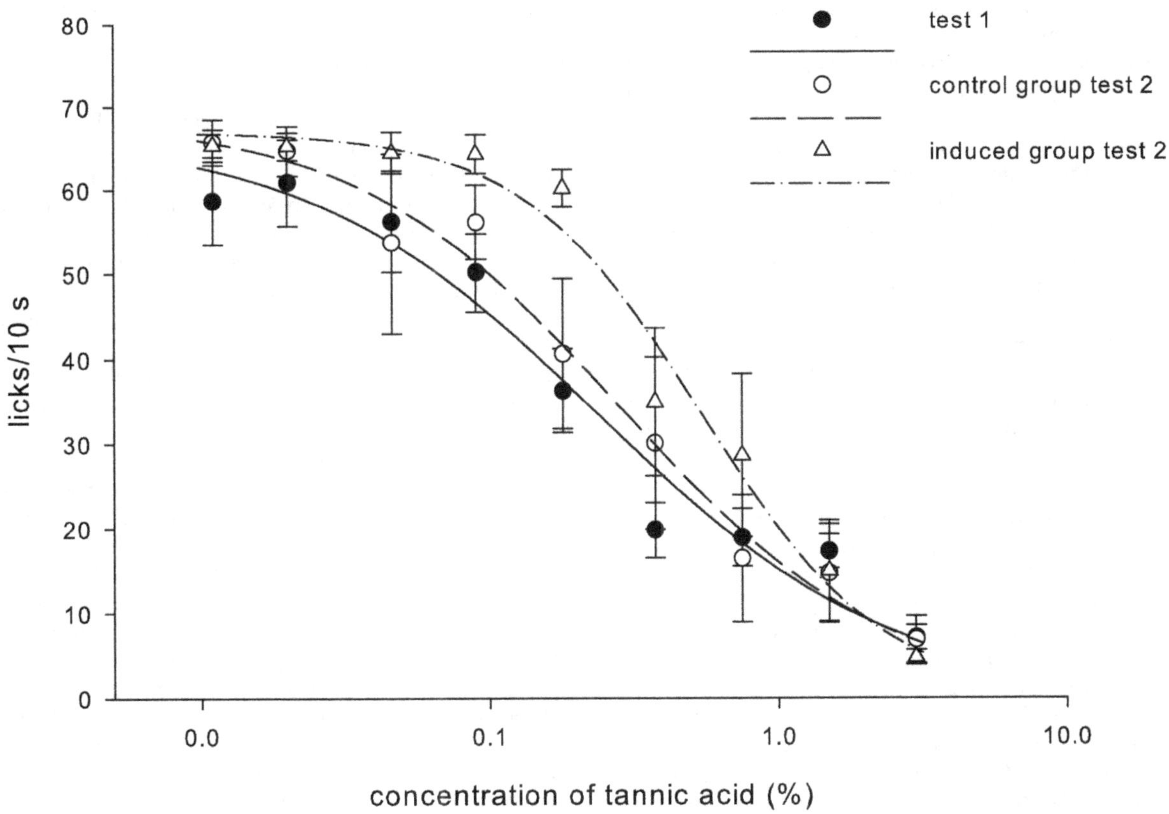

Figure 6. The closed circles represent the average licking of the two test groups during their first exposure to the brief-access test (unconditioned licking does not differ between the groups at this time point p>0.05). The open circles represent the average licking during the second exposure to the brief-access test by rats that were maintained on the control diet. The open triangles represent the average licking during the second exposure to the brief-access test by rats that were maintained on the tannic acid diet between exposures. Lines represent curves fit to the average licking behavior. Rats with an increase in the salivary protein at 19/18.5 and 18 kDa bands show a right-ward shift in the licking response curve demonstrating that they found the tannic acid less aversive in the second exposure than the first exposure, while rats maintained on the control diet did not alter their licking behavior on the second exposure.

baseline because there were no differences in 24-h food intake ($F = _{4,28} = 1.2$, $p = 0.34$), meal size ($F = _{4,28} = 0.89$, $p = 0.48$), meal number ($F = _{4,28} = 1.38$, $p = 0.27$), or rate of feeding ($F = _{4,28} = 0.23$, $p = 0.92$).

Total intake. In comparison to baseline, rats reduced total intake when fed a diet containing tannic acid ($F = _{10,70} = 12.52$, $p < 0.001$, Figure 4a). The largest reduction (~50% reduction) was seen during the first 3 days of the diet. Total food intake recovered to baseline by the fourth day.

Meal size. The reduction in total intake of the tannic acid diet was due primarily to a reduction in meal size ($F = _{10,70} = 13.23$, $p<0.001$, Figure 4b). The reduction in meal size was limited to the first three days of tannic acid diet exposure, averaging 75% less than control on the first day. During the following days the meal size returned to baseline levels. The alterations in meal size were significantly related to the expression of the 35, 19, 18.5 kDa bands and cystatin S (see Table 3), but not to the expression the 23 or 18 kDa bands (Table 3).

Meal number. Rats increased the number of meals consumed during the first 2 days of the tannic acid diet by 70% ($F = _{10,70} = 13.3$, $p<0.001$, Figure 4c) but returned quickly to baseline levels. The increase in meal number was likely acting to increase total intake in the face of the sharp decrease in meal size. These changes were uncorrelated with the increase in any of the proteins measured (Table 3).

Rate of feeding. Rats displayed a decrease in the rate of feeding while on the tannic acid diet ($F = _{10,70} = 35.84$, $p<0.001$, Figure 4d). This decrease was greatest during the first 3 days and then stabilized by day 7 at a level that was significantly lower than baseline. Alterations in rate of feeding were significantly related to the expression of the 23 and 18.5 kDa bands (Table 3), but not to the expression of the other measured protein bands (Table 3).

Body Mass. Rats lost a significant amount of body mass after the first night on the tannic acid diet (356.9±8.9 to 345.8±7.1 g, $t_7 = 4.9$, $p = 0.002$), Animals did not continue to lose significant amounts of body mass, but did decrease the rate in which they gained weight while being fed the tannic acid diet. Weight gain during the last 3 days of the control diet was 12.9 g (±1.8), however, weight gain dropped to 1.3 g (±2.0, $t_7 = 4.2$, $p = 0.004$) on the first 3 days of the tannic acid diet. The effect on body mass was, however, transient and animals had regained sufficient weight by the fourth day of the tannin treatment that they no longer differed from the last day of the control diet ($t_7 = 1.6$, $p = 0.14$).

Experiment 2

Induction of salivary proteins. As expected, salivary protein concentration was significantly increased by water deprivation ($F_{3,18} = 6.09$, $p = 0.005$) making comparisons between water replete and deprived samples unreliable. In this experiment, band densities were such that we were unable to distinguish between the 19 and 18.5 kDa bands, therefore we calculated these proteins as a single band. Since most of the proteins of interest seem to be upregulated by water deprivation alone (Figure 5), we therefore compared only the water deprived samples as described in the methods. The 19/18.5 kDa band density was significantly increased by the diet treatment compared to the control group (Figure 5, $t_{8.0} = -3.28$ $p = 0.01$) as was the non-PRP 18 kDa band ($t_{8.0} = -3.32$ $p = 0.01$). There was a non-significant trend for cystatin S to increase ($t_{8.0} = -2.13$ $p = 0.065$) and no other proteins were upregulated by the diet treatment (all p-values > 0.3).

Analysis of licking behavior. The two groups of animals did not differ in their initial licking behavior under control conditions ($F_{1,10} = 0.5$, $p = 0.49$). The rats that continued on the control diet did not alter the number of licks upon second exposure to the test paradigm (Figure 6, $F_{1,10} = 0.2$, $p = 0.67$). In contrast, rats exposed to the tannic acid diet displayed a strong tendency to increase the number of licks/10 sec ($F_{1,10} = 4.5$, $p = 0.055$). To address how the dietary treatment and subsequent salivary changes may have altered the animals' experience with the tannic acid solutions, we compared the EC_{50} of the groups between the first and second Davis Rig exposure. The EC_{50} represents lateral shifts in the curve. While the EC_{50} in the control group did not change between the first and second exposure ($t_5 = 1.4$, $p = 0.23$), there was a rightward shift of the curve in the experimental group ($t_5 = -2.8$, $p = 0.04$) indicating that the tannin was perceived as less aversive in the second licking test conducted following upregulation of salivary proteins.

Discussion

We demonstrated that the expression of six salivary proteins increased in rats exposed to a tannic acid diet and that the expression of five of these proteins, four PRPs and a non-PRP identified as cystatin S, was significantly correlated with changes in the pattern of food consumption. We also demonstrated that rats increased unconditioned licking to (and thus acceptance of) tannic acid solutions after an upsurge in salivary proteins. Taken together, our findings suggest an important role for these salivary proteins in the control of feeding behavior that is related to their ability to modulate the postingestive and orosensory feedback associated with the consumption of a tannin-rich diet.

Orosensory Function

Glendinning [33] demonstrated that injection of isoproterenol, and the resulting upregulation of salivary PRPs, increased the acceptability of tannic acid solutions in mice. Glendinning suggested that the PRPs modified the orosensory signal elicited by the tannic acid since mice with upregulated salivary PRPs licked the tannic acid solutions for a longer duration before pausing (i.e., they displayed longer drinking bouts) [33]. Our methods differed from those used by Glendinning as we measured the induction of salivary proteins while the animals consumed the tannin-rich diet in a drug-free state. This allowed us to elucidate the time-course of diet-driven production of salivary proteins. To our knowledge, our study is the first to demonstrate a relationship between salivary PRPs and tannic acid consumption in a normal feeding situation in rodents. Our work provides support for the hypothesis that salivary proteins influence the animals' orosensory response to tannic acid. This was first reflected by a change in the rate of feeding (Experiment 1), a measure indicative of palatability [47,48]. Protein expression of PRPs of 23 and 18.5 kDa were significantly correlated with an increased rate of feeding while on the tannic acid diet; these data suggest that PRPs played a role in enhancing the diet's palatability. In the brief-access taste test (Experiment 2), the stimulus concentration-lick rate response function to tannic acid solutions was shifted to the right in rats fed the tannic acid diet (Figure 6). This demonstrates that rats found tannic acid less aversive during the second exposure period compared to the first. Conversely, rats fed the control diet throughout the experiment did not alter their unconditioned licking responses during the second licking test. Thus, exposure to the tannic acid diet, not a repetition of the brief-access taste test, was responsible for the shift in licking behavior. Saliva was also collected from water-deprived rats fed the tannic acid and control diets and compared between the two dietary exposure periods for the brief-access taste tests. This analysis revealed that salivary levels of the 19 kDa and the 18/18.5 kDa mixed-protein band increased between the first and second dietary exposure period only in rats fed the tannic acid diet. Because any postingestive effects of the tannic acid solutions were minimized by the brief (30-s) access licking test, this finding suggests a role for these PRPs in the alteration of tannic acid acceptance driven primarily through orosensory control.

While it seems clear from both experiments that the salivary protein band measured at 18.5 kDa (or as 19/18.5 in Experiment 2) is correlated with orosensory acceptance, it is surprising that the 23 kDa band that was significantly predictive of orosenory acceptance in Experiment 1 did not appear to be upregulated in Experiment 2. It should be noted, however, that saliva samples were collected from water deprived animals in the second experiment and not the first, and the lot of tannic acid differed between the two experiments, perhaps these differences may offer potential explanations. Salivary levels of several proteins may be elevated by water deprivation alone (which is necessary to motivate the animals to lick potentially aversive stimuli during brief-access tests) and thus cannot be elevated further by dietary treatment. Unfortunately, due to the wide spread changes in salivary protein expression after water deprivation [41], levels of protein were not directly comparable between water deprived and replete conditions, so this supposition remains speculative. Furthermore, tannic acid is a variable stimulus, one cannot rule out differences in the composition of the stimulus may have altered the patterns of protein upregulation.

Taken together, the data from Experiment 1 on feeding behavior and Experiment 2 on brief-access licking provide evidence that PRPs were related to measures of orosensory signaling. It has been shown that PRPs bind directly to tannins (see [49]). One possibility is that once bound to a PRP, tannic acid is less able to interact with bitter taste receptor proteins and initiate the signaling cascades associated with bitter taste signaling. In this case, PRPs would exert the greatest effect and compromise orosensory signaling the most when tannic acid concentrations are relatively weak in the intermediate concentration range. Indeed, this was the case in Experiment 2 where the largest shift in licking behavior occurred at intermediate tannic acid concentrations. In this experiment, rats responded to the weakest tannic acid concentrations as similar to water and consequently salivary proteins were without effect. At the upper end of the stimulus concentration range, the tannic acid concentration may have been sufficiently strong and salivary protein levels may have been insufficient to prevent access to orosensory receptors. However, at intermediate tannic acid concentrations, PRP levels were sufficient to counteract the bitter taste of tannic acid and alter licking responses.

Postingestive feedback

Meal size is considered a measure of postingestive feedback, and it has been suggested that animals consuming a bitter compound should halt food intake before surpassing a critical threshold of the possibly toxic compound [50]. Our feeding study demonstrated that, in the presence of tannic acid, rats decreased food intake via a selective decrease in meal size. Over time, rats recovered to baseline intake by a recovery in meal size. This increase in meal size was significantly correlated with the increase in expression of several PRPs (35, 19 and 18.5 kDa) and cystatin S. Although the role of PRPs is unknown in the gut, there is evidence in the literature to suggest that PRPs may be active in the gut. Cai and colleagues [51,52] have shown that PRPs decrease the absorption of tannins across intestinal cells demonstrating that PRPs modulate interactions between tannic acid and the intestinal environment.

Our current findings suggest that additional research is needed to investigate the potential roles of PRPs and cystatin S in modulating postingestive signals arising from the consumption of bitter compounds. In this regard, previous studies have shown that activation of intestinal T2Rs, receptors that are molecularly similar to the bitter taste receptor proteins of the oral cavity, result in the release of cholecystokinin [53–55], a well described regulator of meal size [56,57]. It has been demonstrated that representative hydrolysable and condensed tannins activate specific bitter taste receptors [25], which have been shown to be present in the gut [58], perhaps the mechanism of PRP alteration of gut signaling is similar to the mechanism proposed to modify orosensory signaling. Specifically, the PRPs may bind to the tannic acid and subsequently disrupt its ability to interact with intestinal T2Rs.

The degree to which cystatin S may facilitate this process is an open question. There is some evidence that cystatins are related to bitter taste perception, however, there is no obvious mechanism for this relationship. Cystatin SN, a closely related protein to cystatin S, has been linked to the sensitivity to the bitter taste of caffeine in humans [23]. It has also been demonstrated that oral capsaicin [17] and quinine [18] stimulate the production of salivary cystatin S-like proteins suggesting that this class of proteins is generally responsive to aversive oral stimuli, but to our knowledge, this is the first suggestion that this protein is related to meal size.

Conclusions

The current findings provide the first evidence that dietary-induced expression of salivary proteins correlates with feeding behavior. Because tannic acid containing diets are not consumed by animals incapable of upregulating PRPs [32,33], we believe that the correlational relationship observed here is likely causal in nature. Our findings support and extend the work done by Glendinning [33] and Dsamou et al. [23] suggesting that salivary proteins can alter taste-guided ingestive responses. Taken together, our findings demonstrate that salivary proteins are involved in modulating both the orosensory and the postingestive feedback associated with chronic exposure to tannic acid diets. Understanding how the differential expression of these and other salivary proteins can modulate taste perception and the processing of postingestive signals represents a novel approach toward identifying individual differences in bitter taste acceptance.

Supporting Information

Figure S1 Depicts the HPLC chromatogram. The solid line represents compounds detected in the tannic acid sample (2 μl, 5 mg/ml), the dotted line represents compounds detected in the PGG sample (0.25 μl, 5 mg/ml). Analysis of area under the curve confirms that 67% of the compounds in the tannic acid are the equivalent to PGG or larger in size, i.e. has a peak that is recorded later in minutes.

Figure S2 Represents example gels of saliva samples fixed in Coomassie Brilliant Blue. Equal volumes of saliva were resolved on 12% SDS-PAGE gels. Molecular mass markers (M) are on the left hand side of each gel. Under each gel is the Western blot of secretory immunoglobulin A (IgA) for each animal. Panel A represents samples collected from a single animal in the experimental group. Five control samples were collected during control diet (C) exposure on alternating days. Six samples were collected during tannic acid (T) exposure on alternating days. Panel B represents samples collected from a single animal in the control group. Seven control samples were collected during control (C) diet exposure on alternating days.

Table S1 Liquid chromatography (LC) and mass spectrometry (MS) parameters used during protein sequencing.

Acknowledgments

We thank Fred Fletcher, Dr. Te Tang, Ross Henderson, Catherine Lambright, and Laura Martin for their excellent technical assistance, Dr. Pam Keel, Clemma Jacobsen Muller and Ginger Blonde for their assistance with the statistical analyses, Dr. Kate Calvin of the Florida State University at Translation Science Laboratory for providing proteomic analysis and Dr. Margaret Seavy of the Florida State University Department of Biology Analytical Laboratory for the HPLC analysis.

Author Contributions

Conceived and designed the experiments: A-MT LAE JCS. Performed the experiments: A-MT LN MBB MVL. Analyzed the data: A-MT LN MVL. Contributed reagents/materials/analysis tools: A-MT RJC JCS. Wrote the paper: A-MT JCS LAE RJC.

References

1. Scott TR, Mark GP (1987) The taste system encodes stimulus toxicity. Brain Research 414: 197–203.
2. John IG (1994) Is the bitter rejection response always adaptive? Physiology & Behavior 56: 1217–1227.
3. Vasanthi HR, Mukherjee S, Das DK (2009) Potential Health Benefits of Broccoli- A Chemico-Biological Overview. Mini Reviews in Medicinal Chemistry 9: 749–759.
4. Drewnowski A, Gomez-Carneros C (2000) Bitter taste, phytonutrients, and the consumer: a review. The American Journal of Clinical Nutrition 72: 1424–1435.
5. Barratt-Fornell A, Drewnowski A (2002) The Taste of Health: Nature's Bitter Gifts. Nutrition Today 37: 144–150.
6. Bartoshuk L (1979) Bitter taste of saccharin related to the genetic ability to taste the bitter substance 6-n-propylthiouracil. Science 205: 934–935.
7. Keller KL, Steinmann L, Nurse RJ, Tepper BJ (2002) Genetic taste sensitivity to 6-n-propylthiouracil influences food preference and reported intake in preschool children. Appetite 38: 3–12.
8. Tepper BJ, Ullrich NV (2002) Influence of genetic taste sensitivity to 6-n-propylthiouracil (PROP), dietary restraint and disinhibition on body mass index in middle-aged women. Physiology & Behavior 75: 305–312.
9. Adler E, Hoon MA, Mueller KL, Chandrashekar J, Ryba NJP, et al. (2000) A Novel Family of Mammalian Taste Receptors. Cell 100: 693–702.
10. Chandrashekar J, Mueller KL, Hoon MA, Adler E, Feng L, et al. (2000) T2Rs Function as Bitter Taste Receptors. Cell 100: 703–711.
11. Shi P, Zhang J, Yang H, Zhang Y-p (2003) Adaptive Diversification of Bitter Taste Receptor Genes in Mammalian Evolution. Molecular Biology and Evolution 20: 805–814.
12. Denny P, Hagen FK, Hardt M, Liao L, Yan W, et al. (2008) The Proteomes of Human Parotid and Submandibular/Sublingual Gland Salivas Collected as the Ductal Secretions. Journal of Proteome Research 7: 1994–2006.
13. Johansson G, Birkhed D (1994) Effect of a long-term change from a mixed to a lactovegetarian diet on human saliva. Archives of Oral Biology 39: 283–288.
14. Johnson DA (1983) Differences in basic proline-rich proteins in rat parotid saliva following chronic isoproterenol treatment or maintenance on a liquid diet. Archives of Oral Biology 28: 549–554.
15. Cabras T, Pisano E, Mastinu A, Denotti G, Pusceddu PP, et al. (2010) Alterations of the Salivary Secretory Peptidome Profile in Children Affected by Type 1 Diabetes. Molecular & Cellular Proteomics 9: 2099–2108.
16. Romero AC, Ibuki FK, Nogueira FN (2012) Sialic acid reduction in the saliva of streptozotocin induced diabetic rats. Archives of Oral Biology 57: 1189–1193.
17. Katsukawa H, Ninomiya Y (1999) Capsaicin Induces Cystatin S-like Substances in Submandibular Saliva of the Rat. Journal of Dental Research 78: 1609–1616.
18. Quintana M, Palicki O, Lucchi G, Ducoroy P, Chambon C, et al. (2009) Short-Term Modification of Human Salivary Proteome Induced by Two Bitter Tastants, Urea and Quinine. Chemosensory Perception 2: 133–142.
19. Costa G, Lamy E, Capela e Silva F, Andersen J, Sales Baptista E, et al. (2008) Salivary Amylase Induction by Tannin-Enriched Diets as a Possible Countermeasure Against Tannins. Journal of Chemical Ecology 34: 376–387.
20. Mehansho H, Hagerman A, Clements S, Butler L, Rogler J, et al. (1983) Modulation of proline-rich protein biosynthesis in rat parotid glands by sorghums with high tannin levels. Proceedings of the National Academy of Sciences 80: 3948–3952.
21. Mehansho H, Butler LG, Carlson DM (1987) Dietary Tannins and Salivary Proline-Rich Proteins: Interactions, Induction, and Defense Mechanisms. Annual Review of Nutrition 7: 423–440.
22. Kock K, Morley SD, Mullins JJ, Schmale H (1994) Denatonium bitter tasting among transgenic mice expressing rat von Ebner's gland protein. Physiology & Behavior 56: 1173–1177.
23. Dsamou M, Palicki O, Septier C, Chabanet C, Lucchi G, et al. (2012) Salivary Protein Profiles and Sensitivity to the Bitter Taste of Caffeine. Chemical Senses 37: 87–95.
24. Dinnella C, Recchia A, Fia G, Bertuccioli M, Monteleone E (2009) Saliva Characteristics and Individual Sensitivity to Phenolic Astringent Stimuli. Chemical Senses 34: 295–304.
25. Soares S, Kohl S, Thalmann S, Mateus N, Meyerhof W, et al. (2013) Different Phenolic Compounds Activate Distinct Human Bitter Taste Receptors. Journal of Agricultural and Food Chemistry 61: 1525–1533.
26. Shimada T (2006) Salivary Proteins as a Defense Against Dietary Tannins. Journal of Chemical Ecology 32: 1149–1163.
27. Lichtenstein G, Cassini MH (2001) Behavioral mechanisms underlaying food aversion in guinea pigs. Etologia 9: 29–34.
28. Skopec MM, Hagerman AE, Karasov WH (2004) Do Salivary Proline-Rich Proteins Counteract Dietary Hydrolyzable Tannin in Laboratory Rats? Journal of Chemical Ecology 30: 1679–1692.
29. Mitaru BN, Reichert RD, Blair R (1984) The Binding of Dietary Protein by Sorghum Tannins in the Digestive Tract of Pigs. The Journal of Nutrition 114: 1787–1796.
30. Matsuo R (2000) Role of Saliva in the Maintenance of Taste Sensitivity. Critical Reviews in Oral Biology & Medicine 11: 216–229.
31. Muenzer J, Bildstein C, Gleason M, Carlson DM (1979) Purification of proline-rich proteins from parotid glands of isoproterenol-treated rats. Journal of Biological Chemistry 254: 5623–5628.
32. Mehansho H, Ann DK, Butler LG, Rogler J, Carlson DM (1987) Induction of proline-rich proteins in hamster salivary glands by isoproterenol treatment and an unusual growth inhibition by tannins. Journal of Biological Chemistry 262: 12344–12350.
33. Glendinning JI (1992) Effect of salivary proline-rich proteins on ingestive responses to tannic acid in mice. Chemical Senses 17: 1–12.
34. Nayak A, Carpenter GH (2008) A physiological model of tea-induced astringency. Physiology & Behavior 95: 290–294.
35. Silanikove N, Perevolotsky A, Provenza FD (2001) Use of tannin-binding chemicals to assay for tannins and their negative postingestive effects in ruminants. Animal Feed Science and Technology 91: 69–81.
36. Stuchell RN, Mandel ID (1983) A Comparative Study of Salivary Lysozyme in Caries-resistant and Caries-susceptible Adults. Journal of Dental Research 62: 552–554.
37. Sarni-Manchado P, Cheynier V, Moutounet M (1998) Interactions of Grape Seed Tannins with Salivary Proteins. Journal of Agricultural and Food Chemistry 47: 42–47.
38. Beeley JA, Sweeney D, Lindsay JCB, Buchanan ML, Sarna L, et al. (1991) Sodium dodecyl sulphate-polyacrylamide gel electrophoresis of human parotid salivary proteins. ELECTROPHORESIS 12: 1032–1041.
39. Lu Y, Bennick A (1998) Interaction of tannin with human salivary proline-rich proteins. Archives of Oral Biology 43: 717–728.
40. Oliver SJ, Laing SJ, Wilson S, Bilzon JL, Walters R (2007) Salivary immunoglobulin A response at rest and after exercise following a 48 h period of fluid and/or energy restriction. British Journal of Nutrition 97: 1109–1116.
41. Walsh NP (2004) Saliva parameters as potential indices of hydration status during acute dehydration. Medicine and science in sports and exercise 36: 1535.
42. Baxter NJ, Lilley TH, Haslam E, Williamson MP (1997) Multiple Interactions between Polyphenols and a Salivary Proline-Rich Protein Repeat Result in Complexation and Precipitation†. Biochemistry 36: 5566–5577.
43. Mirels L, Miranda AJ, Ball WD (1998) Characterization of the rat salivary-gland B1-immunoreactive proteins. Biochemical Journal Pt 1: 437–444.
44. Schenkels LCPM, Veerman ECI, Nieuw Amerongen AV (1995) Biochemical Composition of Human Saliva in Relation To Other Mucosal Fluids. Critical Reviews in Oral Biology & Medicine 6: 161–175.
45. Bedi GS (1991) The effect of adrenergic agonists and antagonists on cysteine-proteinase inhibitor (cystatin) in rat saliva. Archives of Oral Biology 36: 611–618.
46. Shaw PA, Yu W-hA (2000) Autonomic regulation of cystatin S gene expression in rat submandibular glands. Autonomic Neuroscience 83: 49–57.
47. Davis JD (1973) The effectiveness of some sugars in stimulating licking behavior in the rat. Physiology & Behavior 11: 39–45.
48. Smith JC (2000) Microstructure of the rat's intake of food, sucrose and saccharin in 24-hour tests. Neuroscience & Biobehavioral Reviews 24: 199–212.
49. Bennick A (2002) Interaction of Plant Polyphenols with Salivary Proteins. Critical Reviews in Oral Biology & Medicine 13: 184–196.
50. Torregrossa A-M, Dearing MD (2009) Nutritional toxicology of mammals: regulated intake of plant secondary compounds. Functional Ecology 23: 48–56.
51. Cai K, Hagerman AE, Minto RE, Bennick A (2006) Decreased polyphenol transport across cultured intestinal cells by a salivary proline-rich protein. Biochemical Pharmacology 71: 1570–1580.
52. Cai K, Bennick A (2006) Effect of salivary proteins on the transport of tannin and quercetin across intestinal epithelial cells in culture. Biochemical Pharmacology 72: 974–980.

53. Sternini C (2007) Taste Receptors in the Gastrointestinal Tract. IV. Functional implications of bitter taste receptors in gastrointestinal chemosensing. American Journal of Physiology 295: G457–G461.
54. Jeon TI, Seo YK, Osbourne TF (2011) Gut bitter taste receptor signalling induces ABCB1 thought a mechanism involving CCK. Journal of Biochemistry 438: 33–37.
55. Chen MC, Wu SV, Reeve JR, Rozengurt E (2006) Bitter stimuli induce Ca2+ signaling and CCK release in enteroendocrine STC-1 cells: role of L-type voltage-sensitive Ca2+ channels. American journal of physiology Cell physiology 291: C726–739.
56. Woods SC, Seeley RJ, Porte D, Schwartz MW (1998) Signals That Regulate Food Intake and Energy Homeostasis. Science 280: 1378–1383.
57. Gibbs J, Young RC, Smith GP (1973) Cholecystokinin decreases food intake in rats. Journal of Comparative and Physiological Psychology 84: 488–495.
58. Rozengurt N, Wu SV, Chen MC, Huang C, Sternini C, et al. (2006) Colocalization of the alpha-subunit of gustducin with PYY and GLP-1 in L cells of human colon. Am J Physiol Gastrointest Liver Physiol 291: G792–802.

9

Modeling Tuberculosis Dynamics, Detection and Control in Cattle Herds

Mohammed El Amine Bekara[1], Aurélie Courcoul[1], Jean-Jacques Bénet[2], Benoit Durand[1]*

1 University Paris Est, Anses, Laboratory of Animal Health, Epidemiology Unit, Maisons-Alfort, France, **2** University Paris Est, National Veterinary School of Alfort (ENVA), EpiMAI Unit, Maisons-Alfort, France

Abstract

Epidemiological models are key tools for designing and evaluating detection and control strategies against animal infectious diseases. In France, after decades of decrease of bovine tuberculosis (bTB) incidence, the disease keeps circulating. Increasing prevalence levels are observed in several areas, where the detection and control strategy could be adapted. The objective of this work was to design and calibrate a model of the within-herd transmission of bTB. The proposed model is a stochastic model operating in discrete-time. Three health states were distinguished: susceptible, latent and infected. Dairy and beef herd dynamics and bTB detection and control programs were explicitly represented. Approximate Bayesian computation was used to estimate three model parameters from field data: the transmission parameter when animals are inside (β_{inside}) and outside ($\beta_{outside}$) buildings, and the duration of the latent phase. An independent dataset was used for model validation. The estimated median was 0.43 [0.16–0.84] month^{-1} for β_{inside} and 0.08 [0.01–0.32] month^{-1} for $\beta_{outside}$. The median duration of the latent period was estimated 3.5 [2–8] months. The sensitivity analysis showed only minor influences of fixed parameter values on these posterior estimates. Validation based on an independent dataset showed that in more than 80% of herds, the observed proportion of animals with detected lesions was between the 2.5% and 97.5% percentiles of the simulated distribution. In the absence of control program and once bTB has become enzootic within a herd, the median effective reproductive ratio was estimated to be 2.2 in beef herds and 1.7 in dairy herds. These low estimates are consistent with field observations of a low prevalence level in French bTB-infected herds.

Editor: Caroline Colijn, Imperial College London, United Kingdom

Funding: This work was supported by the French Ministry of Agriculture. The funder had no role in study design, data collection and analysis, decision to publish, or preparation of the manuscript.

Competing Interests: The authors have declared that no competing interests exist.

* Email: benoit.durand@anses.fr

Introduction

Bovine tuberculosis (bTB) is a chronic animal disease most often caused by *Mycobacterium bovis*, that mainly affects the respiratory system [1]. The main route of transmission of the infection between cattle is the respiratory route [2]. In France, a control program for bTB became mandatory in 1965. Detection of infected herds was based on an annual screening of animals using skin tests, and on routine inspection of carcasses at slaughter for bTB-like lesions (with subsequent isolation of *M. bovis* at the laboratory). Since 1990, the control program was reinforced by the compulsory screening (using skin tests) of animals introduced in bTB-free herds, these animals always originating from other bTB-free herds. In 1999, herd prevalence fell below 0.1% and the slaughter of all cattle in infected herds (termed below "total slaughter") was introduced in the control program. In 2001, France was declared officially free of bTB by the European Union. However, in recent years, an increase in bTB incidence has been observed in some departments. Similar trends have been observed in other European countries. In Great Britain and Ireland, the control programs became mandatory in 1950 and 1957, respectively. They were also based on an annual screening by skin test, the slaughter of positive animals and the inspection of carcasses at the slaughterhouse [3]. bTB incidence decreased in both countries, but the epidemiological situation began to deteriorate gradually from the 1980s, partly because of the existence of a wildlife reservoir in badger populations [4]. In France, such a wildlife reservoir has not been identified, although wild boars, red deer and badgers with *M. bovis* lesions have been found in several departments. Unlike France, Great Britain or Ireland, there are countries where "test and slaughter" control programs were successful in eradicating bTB: Sweden was considered bTB-free in 1958, after 40 years of this type of control program [5] (sporadic cases have been reported afterwards, the last one in 1978 [6]).

In France, data collected over 35 years, between 1965 and 2000, have shown parallel evolutions of herd management practices (with a disappearance of family farms and a professionalization of breeders) and of herd structures (with changes in herd types with a switch from dairy to beef and increasing herd sizes). Besides the effectiveness of control programs, the decrease of bTB incidence between 1965 and 2000 could be partly attributable to these changes in herd management practices and in herd structures [7].

Table 1. Description of the four datasets.

Id	Data type	Number of herds (animals)		Period (geographic origin)	Control program
		Dairy	Beef		
A	Aggregated	5 (134)		1981–1983 (Nord)	Annual screening by SITT, slaughter of all cattle if>40% of SITT-positive animals, otherwise slaughter of SITT-positive only
B	Individual	1 (60)	12 (625)	2004–2006 (Dordogne)	Biennial screening by SITT confirmed by SICCT, slaughter of SICCT-positive animals, slaughter of all cattle in case of lesions and *M. bovis* isolation
	Aggregated	9 (684)	16 (1,011)		
C	Individual	3 (142)	11 (596)	2007–2010 (Dordogne)	Annual screening by SITT with second control by γIFN[1] and confirmation by SICCT, slaughter of SICCT-positive, slaughter of all cattle in case of lesions and *M. bovis* isolation
	Aggregated	7 (530)	22 (1,344)		
D	Aggregated		29 (6,317)	2005–2009 (Côte d'Or)	Biennial screening by SICCT, slaughter of SICCT-positive animals, slaughter of all cattle in case of lesions and *M. bovis* isolation

[1]To improve the specificity of the control program C, the γIFN assay used in this control program is a combination of two tests: the PPD γIFN and the ESAT-6 γIFN. The modified γIFN test can be positive (both tests are positive), negative (both tests are negative) or divergent (the results of the two tests are discordant).

Neither ante-mortem tests [8] nor post-mortem tests [6,9] used in bTB control programs have perfect sensitivity and specificity. With the decrease of infection prevalence and because of the increase of herd sizes (multiplied on average by 3.5 between 1965 and 2000 in France [7]), ante-mortem false-positive reactions became a major problem for the surveillance and control program and its acceptability by breeders. This led to an increasing complexity of testing procedures over the past fifteen years, with combinations of several tests: single intradermal tuberculin test (SITT), single intradermal comparative cervical tuberculin test (SICCT) and gamma interferon test (γIFN). Additionally, total slaughter has been replaced in some areas by the slaughter of reactive animals only. All these adaptations allowed reducing the number of animals slaughtered due to false-positive tests, the counterpart being the burdensomeness of control programs due to prolonged restriction of cattle movements.

The failure of the eradication of bTB in France and other European countries seems therefore the result of a complex interaction between the evolution of herd management practices and herd structures, the evolution of control programs, and the implication of wildlife as a reservoir for infection in cattle.

Mathematical modelling is used for the study of complex phenomena such as the dynamics of infectious agents [10]. Diseases with a long incubation period, such as bTB, are difficult to study experimentally or in the field because of prolonged waiting times for obtaining results and the high costs of conducting experimental studies [2]. Mathematical simulation models offer the possibility to test a range of control programs in a short time and to identify the most effective one [2].

A number of mathematical models have been developed to represent the spread of bTB and assess the effectiveness of control measures, especially for wildlife (badgers, opossums and white-tailed deer) [11]. Several models have been built to simulate the dynamics of bTB within cattle herds, to quantify the importance of within-farm bTB transmission by estimating the within-herd transmission coefficient of infection [2,12–14] or to evaluate detection and control strategies against bTB [2,13,15,16].

Each of these models incorporates three processes that shape the within-herd bTB infection dynamics: (i) the natural history of the disease, (ii) husbandry practices and (iii) the surveillance and control program [15]. Because points (ii) and (iii) are specific to a particular context (geographical area and time period), the models mentioned above are difficult to extrapolate to other countries.

The aim of this study was to design, calibrate and validate a model of spread of *M. bovis* within a cattle herd. Parameter definition was designed to allow simulating various herd management practices as well as control programs of arbitrary complexity.

Materials and Methods

Ethical statement

bTB is a notifiable disease for which there are control and surveillance campaigns in France. Official methods for diagnosis of this disease are culture, PCR and histopathology. Therefore, all the datasets included in this study are issued from animals analyzed within an official context. No purpose killing of animals was performed for this study. All datasets were in complete agreement with national and European regulations. No ethical approval was necessary.

Data

Four datasets denoted A, B, C and D were used, which had been collected at different periods (between 1980 and 2010) in 3 French departments (Nord, Dordogne, and Côte d'Or). At that time and in these departments, four specific control programs were applied, also denoted A, B, C and D (Table 1).

The total number of herds in the four datasets was 115. All were submitted to a total slaughter. Out of all these 115 farms, detailed data for each animal (individual data) were available for 27 herds, namely the year of birth, the screening tests used, the date and results of these tests, the date of slaughter and the result of carcass inspection at the slaughterhouse (presence or absence of lesions). For the 88 remaining farms, we obtained a single data point aggregated at the herd level: the within-herd proportion of animals with detected lesions at total slaughter (Table 1). Dataset A was obtained from a case study conducted by Carnon [17]. The median percentage of animals with lesions per herd was 34.6% (min: 20.8%, max: 86.4%). Dataset B and C were obtained from the official veterinary services of Dordogne department. In dataset B, the median percentage of animals with lesions per herd was 6.4% (min: 0.1%, max 52%). In dataset C, it was 3.1% (min: 0.6%, max 43%). Data set D was obtained from the Alfort

National Veterinary School. The median percentage of animals with lesions per herd was 1% (min: 0.3%, max: 5%).

Model

The within-herd spread of bTB was modelled using a compartmental stochastic model operating in discrete time (Figure 1). The time step was one month. Hereafter, t represents the current time step and m the current month. Each cattle was represented by its age in years i∊A = {0,…,A_max} and its health state j∊H = {S,E,I}, with: S (susceptible): the animal is not infected, E (latent): the animal is infected but does not have lesions and does not excrete bacteria, and I (infectious): the animal is infected, has lesions and excretes bacteria. Animals were assumed to be grouped into batches according to their age class. To each age class i (i∊A) was assigned a batch denoted L(i) (with L(i)⊂A). A given batch thus contained animals of one or several age classes. In practice, these batches are often placed by farmers on distant pastures and sometimes in separate buildings, animals from distinct batches having little contact with each other.

The control program was represented by a succession of steps numbered from 1 to D_{max}. During each of these steps, biological tests were performed on the entire or part of the herd; the results of these tests determined the following step. For example, in the control program B which was applied between 2004 and 2006 in the department of Dordogne (Figure 2), the first step is the yearly screening of all animals by SITT. If one animal is positive, the second step of control program is performed two months later: positive animals of step 1 are tested by SICCT, as well as a group of randomly selected negative animals. If one animal is positive in step 2, step 3 is performed 3 months later: positive animals of step 2 are slaughtered and, when lesions are observed, bacterial cultures are performed. If one animal is positive to the bacterial culture, the total slaughter (step 4) is performed 1 month later. The status of each animal with respect to the step of the control program was represented by an integer k∊D = {0,…,D_max}, with: $k = 0$ if the animal has never been tested or always had negative test results, and $k>0$ if the animal had positive results to tests performed in step k of the control program, and negative tests thereafter.

The state of a herd at time step t was represented by a triplet$\langle X_t,y_t,z_t\rangle$, where y_t is the number of the current step of the control program ($1\leq y_t \leq D_{max}$), z_t is the date on which the biological tests associated with this step must be performed ($z_t \geq t$), and X_t is a state variable structured on age class, health status and step of the control program, which represents the state of the animals at time step t: X_t (i,j,k) represents the number of animals in age class i (i∊A), health state j (j∊H), which have the status k (k∊D) with respect to the control program.

The dynamic of infection in the herd resulted from the implementation of three sequential processes (Figure 1): the demographic process (ageing and renewal of animals), the infectious process (transmission of infection and evolution of infected animals) and the process of detection and control. A full description of the model is given in Appendix S1.

The size of the herd was assumed constant over time and the herd was assumed closed. Slaughtered animals (routine slaughter or implementation of the control program) being replaced by susceptible young animals (0–1 years old) born in the same herd. The culling rate k∊D was assumed to vary according to the month and to the age class.

We made the simplifying assumption that transmission can occur only between animals of the same batch. However, because of the ageing of animals, the composition of the batch changes every year. Animal transfers between batches then allowed the between-batch infection spread. The within-herd transmission of bTB was modelled by a frequency-dependent function. Because *M. bovis* transmission intensity was assumed to vary according to whether the animals are housed inside a stable (where the intensity of within-batch transmission is assumed to be high) or allowed to graze (where the intensity of within-batch transmission is assumed to be low), the transmission parameter (β_m) was assumed to vary according to the month. The transition from the latent (E) to the infectious (I) state was based on the transition rate α, where 1/α is the duration of the latency period in months.

A step of the control program represented the implementation of one or more biological tests, some of which potentially requiring the slaughter of the animal (for detecting lesions). Tests implemented in the context of a control program could be performed on the entire or part of the herd; the sample of tested animals depending on the results of previous steps of the control program. A step k of the control program was then represented by the quadruplet$\langle Se_k,Sp_k,M_k,Q_k\rangle$, where:

- Se_k and Sp_k are the joint sensitivity and specificity of tests (assumed independent of age and identical for animals in health states E and I)
- m_k equals 1 if the tests require the slaughter of the animal and 0 otherwise
- Q_k is a parameter structured according to age class and to the status of animals with respect to the step of the control program, which defines the sampling plan for testing animals: Q_k (i,k) is the probability that an animal is tested if it has age i and status k for the control program. This parameter verifies: $\sum_{((i,k)\in A\times D)} Q_k\ (i,k) = 1$.

The step $k = 1$ of the control program corresponded to a screening in a bTB-free herd. The steps $k>1$ corresponded to detection and control measures conducted in a herd known or suspected to be infected.

At each time step, it was further assumed that slaughterhouse surveillance allowed the detection of lesions in culled animals. This slaughterhouse surveillance combined the visual inspection of carcasses with the isolation of *M. bovis* from lesions (Figures 2 and 3).

Parameterisation

Fixed parameters. Consistent estimates of the sensitivity and specificity of diagnostic tests are found in the literature, and herd management practices were assumed homogeneous in a given region. The values of the corresponding parameters were thus fixed according to literature or based on expert opinion.

Three batches were distinguished in beef herds: young heifers (1–2 years), heifers of reproductive age (2–3 years), and cows (after the first calving at 4 years) with calves and heifers fed by their mothers (<1year). In dairy herds, animals were also separated into three batches: young heifers (<1 year), heifers of reproductive age (1–2 years), and cows (after the first calving, at 3 years).

For both types of herds, the stabling period was between November and March. Renewal and routine cull of animals was assumed to occur between January and March, animals being culled from the age of 3 years in dairy herds and from the age of 4 years in beef herds. The maximum age of the cattle (A_{max}) was set to 15 years. Other fixed parameters (culling rate, sensitivity and specificity of screening and diagnostic tests) are given in Table 2.

Month-specific transmission parameters allowed representing the difference between the stabling and grazing period, with $\beta_m = \beta_{inside}$ during the stabling period (between November and March) and $\beta_m = \beta_{outside}$ for the remainder of the year. Because of

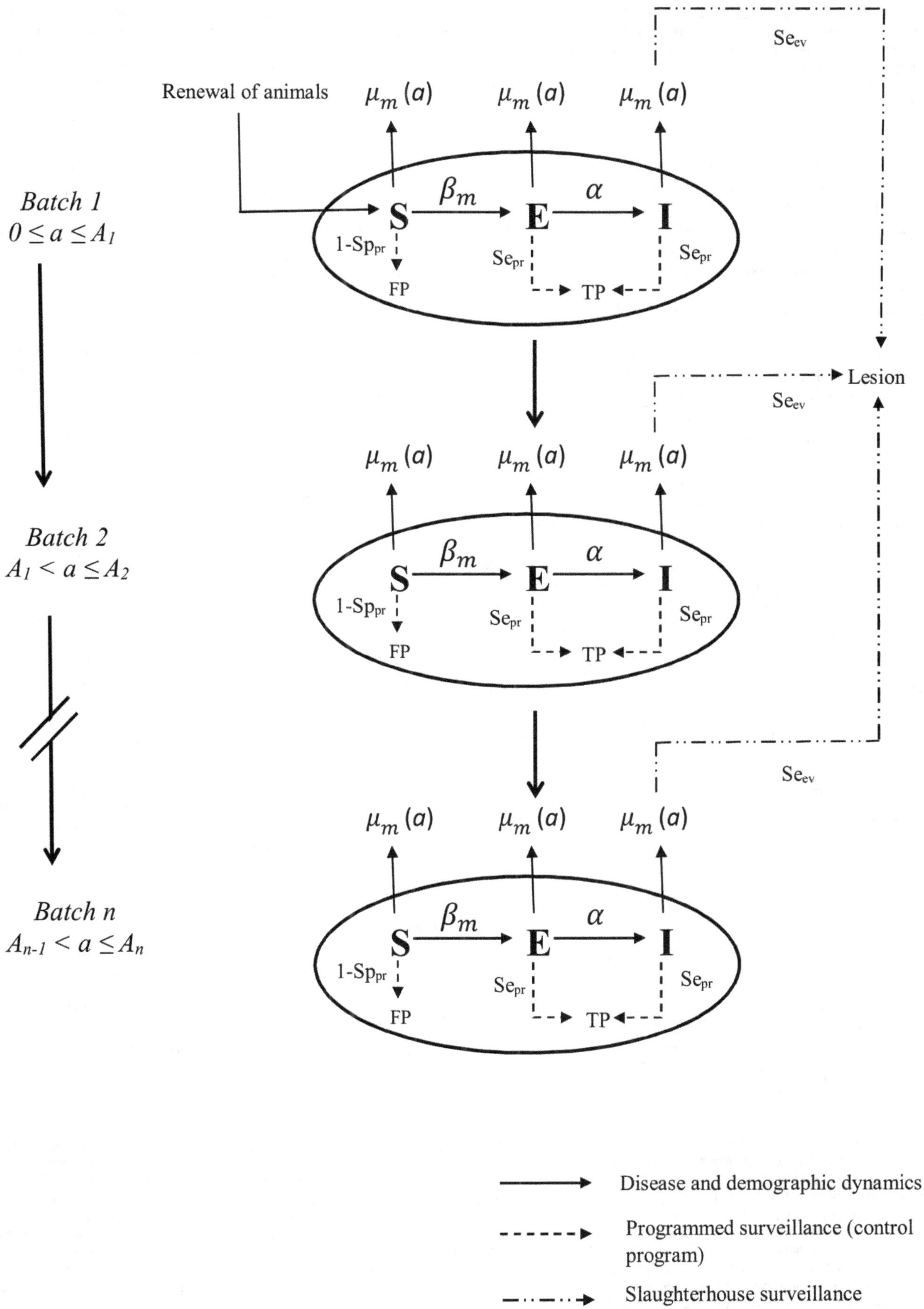
Renewal of animals
$\mu_m(a)$
Batch 1
$0 \leq a \leq A_1$
β_m
α
S
E
I
1-Sp_{pr}
Se_{pr}
FP
TP
Se_{ev}
Lesion
Batch 2
$A_1 < a \leq A_2$
Batch n
$A_{n-1} < a \leq A_n$
Disease and demographic dynamics
Programmed surveillance (control program)
Slaughterhouse surveillance

Figure 1. Schematic representation of the model of within-herd transmission of bTB by three processes: the demographic process (renewal of cattle, reform and change of batches), the infectious process (transitions between health states S: susceptible, E: latent, I: infectious) and the process of detection and control. a: age class in years; Batch: group of animals; m: month; μ_m (a): culling rate for month m and age class a; β_m: month-specific transmission coefficient; Se_{pr}: test sensitivity of step k of programmed surveillance (control program); Sp_{pr}: test specificity of step k of programmed surveillance (control program); FP: false positive; TP: true positive; Se_{ev}: sensitivity of passive surveillance at the slaughterhouse.

the close contact between dairy cows that occurs twice per day in the milking parlour, β_{inside} was used throughout the year in dairy herds for the cows' batch.

Initial conditions assumed the presence of a single infected animal in the state E. To represent the introduction of infection through contact during grazing, this animal was randomly selected among animals that had access to pasture (all batches for beef herds and the first two batches in dairy herds). Simulations were stopped when there were no more infected animals (thanks to routine cull and/or to the control program), the current step of the control program being 1 (i.e. screening in a bTB-free herd).

Parameter estimation. As estimates available in the literature are divergent or uncertain, and because many aspects of bTB pathogenesis are yet to be elucidated, three parameters were estimated from field data: α (transition rate between the health states E and I), β_{inside} (transmission parameter when animals are inside the stable) and $\beta_{outside}$ (transmission parameter when animals are grazing). Individual-level data from datasets B and C were used, corresponding to 27 herds and 1423 animals (Table 1). Control programs B (Figure 2) and C (Figure 3) were modelled according to memos of the French Ministry of Agriculture, Food and Forestry.

The ABC (Approximate Bayesian Computation) method was used to estimate the parameters (α, β_{inside} and $\beta_{outside}$). This method aims at estimating the posterior distributions of the parameters where the calculation of the likelihood is difficult or burdensome [18].

The generic form of the ABC method's "rejection algorithm" is [18]:

1- Sample parameter values θ^* from the prior distribution $\pi(\theta)$.

2- Simulate a dataset χ^* using parameter values θ^*.

3- Calculate the summary statistics for the observed data $S(\chi o)$ and simulated data $S(\chi^*)$.

4- Compare the simulated data, $S(\chi^*)$, and the observed data, $S(\chi o)$, using the distance function, d, and the tolerance ε; if $d(S(\chi_o), S(\chi^*)) \leq \varepsilon$, the value of θ^* is accepted. When $\varepsilon = 0$, the posterior distribution is exactly $\pi(\theta/S(\chi o))$, whereas when $\varepsilon \to +\infty$, the posterior distribution is equal to the prior distribution [19].

Other algorithms have been proposed for the ABC method (e.g. Markov Chain Monte Carlo or Sequential Monte Carlo). We used the rejection algorithm followed by a step of local linear regression as proposed by Beaumont et *al.* [19]. This step aims at reducing the variance of the posterior estimation in order to try to correct errors that are due to a non-zero value of the tolerance ε. A total of 100,000 simulations were performed for parameter estimation.

Prior distributions were uniform distributions U[0.027–0.50]month^{-1} for α and U [0–2]month^{-1} for β_{inside} and $\beta_{outside}$. For α, these values correspond to a period of latency between 2 and 36 months. The lower bound (2 months) is the rounded value of the lower bound (87 days) of the estimation obtained by Neill et *al.* in an experimental study [20], while the upper bound (36 months) is a rounded value of the upper bound (34 months) of the estimated duration of latency in Perez et *al.* [2]. For β_{inside} and $\beta_{outside}$, the upper bound of the prior distribution was chosen arbitrarily after having verified by simulation that, using this value, the median simulated percentage of animals with lesions at total slaughter (22% and 17% for dairy and beef farms, respectively) was significantly higher than the observed value in dataset B (6.4%).

The choice of summary statistics is a crucial step in the ABC method. This choice involves a compromise between information loss and size of the statistic [21]. Using a poorly chosen set of summary statistics can often lead to an overestimation of credible

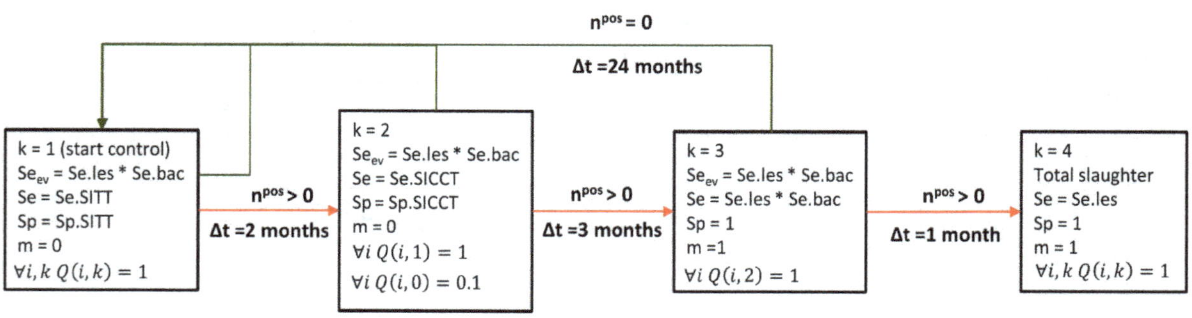

Figure 2. Control program B applied in the Dordogne department between 2004 and 2006. Step 1: biennial bTB screening using SITT (the herd being considered disease-free). All animals are tested ($\forall i,kQ(i,k) = 1$). Sensitivity (Se) and specificity (Sp): those of SITT. Transition to step 2 if an animal is positive ($n^{pos} > 0$), two months later ($\Delta t = 2$ months. Step 2: confirmation of SITT positive results using SICCT. All the positive animals of step 1 are tested (μ i Q(i,1) = 1), as well as 10% of the negative animals (μ i Q(i,1) = 1). Sensitivity (Se) and specificity (Sp): those of SICCT. Transition to step 3 if an animal is positive, three months later. Step 3: slaughter of SICCT-positive animals and isolation of *M. bovis* from lesions. All the positive animals of step 2 (μ i Q(i,2) = 1) are slaughtered (m = 1) and bacterial culture is performed from observed lesions. Sensitivity (Se): sequential combination of a visual inspection at the slaughterhouse and of a bacterial culture. Transition to step 4 if an animal is positive, 1 month later. Step 4: total slaughter. All the animals ($\forall i,kQ(i,k) = 1$) are slaughtered (m = 1). Routine detection of lesions at slaughterhouse. Sensitivity (Se_{ev}): sequential combination of a visual inspection at the slaughterhouse and of a bacterial culture. If a positive animal is thus detected, regardless of the current stage of control program, transition to step 4. See table 2 for the definition of the other parameters.

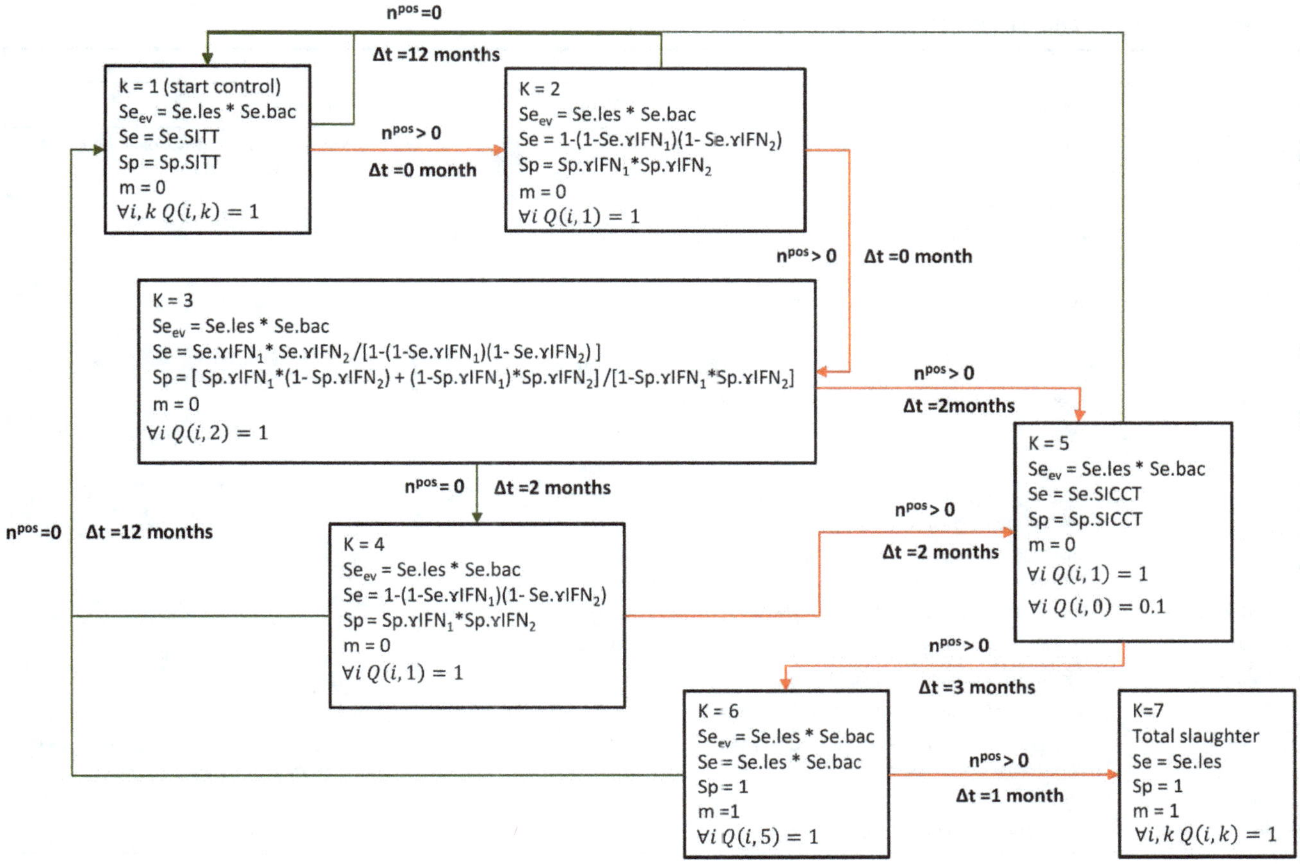

Figure 3. Control program C applied in the Dordogne department between 2007 and 2010. Step 1: yearly bTB screening using SITT (the herd being considered disease-free). All animals are tested (μ i,k Q(i,k) = 1). Sensitivity (Se) and specificity (Sp): those of SITT. Immediate transition to step 2 if an animal is positive (n^{pos}>0). Step 2: confirmation of SITT positive results using PDD γIFN (γIFN1) and ESAT-6 γIFN (γIFN2). All the positive animals of step 1 are tested (μ i Q(i,1) = 1. Sensitivity (Se) and specificity (Sp): parallel combination of both tests (positivity to any of both tests). Immediate transition to step 3 if an animal is positive; otherwise: transition to step 1. Step 3: interpretation of the positive results of step 2 as convergent (both γIFN tests are positive) or not (only one of both tests is positive). All the positive animals of step 2 (μ i Q(i,2) = 1) are concerned. Sensitivity (Se) and Specificity (Sp): sequential combination of both tests in positive animals of step 2. Transition to step 5 if an animal is positive, and to step 4 otherwise, two months later. Step 4: second confirmation of SITT positive results using PDD γIFN (γIFN1) and ESAT-6 γIFN (γIFN2). All the positive animals of step 1 are tested (μ i Q(i,1) = 1). Sensitivity (Se) and specificity (Sp): same as for step 2. Transition to step 5 if an animal is positive, two months later; otherwise: transition to step 1, 12 months later. Step 5: confirmation of SITT positive results using SICCT. All the positive animals of step 1 are tested (μ i Q(i,1) = 1), as well as 10% of the negative animals (μ i Q(i,0) = 0.1). Sensitivity (Se) and specificity (Sp): those of SICCT. Transition to step 6 if an animal is positive, three months later. Step 6: slaughter of SICCT-positive animals and isolation of *M. bovis* from lesions. All the positive animals of step 5 (μ i Q(i,5) = 1) are slaughtered (m = 1) and bacterial culture is performed from observed lesions. Sensitivity (Se): sequential combination of a visual inspection at the slaughterhouse and of a bacterial culture. Transition to step 7 if an animal is positive, 1 month later (Δt = 1 month). Step 7: total slaughter. All the animals (μ i,k Q(i,k) = 1) are slaughtered (m = 1). Routine detection of lesions at slaughterhouse. Sensitivity (Se_{ev}): sequential combination of a visual inspection at the slaughterhouse and of a bacterial culture. If a positive animal is thus detected, regardless of the current stage of control program, transition to step 7. See table 2 for the definition of the other parameters.

intervals due to the loss of information [22]. One way to capture most of the information present in the data would be to use many statistics, but the accuracy and stability of the ABC method decrease rapidly with an increasing number of summary statistics [22,23]. In order to choose the best combination of summary statistics, eight combinations (Table 3) were tested on simulated data obtained using arbitrarily fixed parameter values. The tested summary statistics combined two types of variables, the time between the last negative control and the detection of infection and the percentage of animals with detected lesions, taking into account or not the batch, the type of herd and the year. The procedure used to select the best summary statistics among the eight tested combinations is described in Appendix S2. Briefly, parameter values were set to arbitrarily chosen values and used to generate 100 simulated datasets. In a first step, one of these datasets was chosen and considered a pseudo-observation. Each set of summary statistics was then successively used to estimate the posterior distribution of the parameters, and we kept for further analysis the set of summary statistics for which the arbitrarily chosen parameter values were inside the corresponding 95% credibility interval. In a second step, the preceding procedure was successively applied to the 100 simulated datasets and we selected the set of summary statistics that maximized the proportion of cases for which the arbitrarily chosen parameter values were inside the 95% credibility interval of the posterior distribution of parameters.

The tolerance threshold ε was determined by choosing the proportion of retained simulations $p_ε$. A leave-one-out procedure was applied to a set of 100 datasets simulated using parameters (α, $β_{inside}$, $β_{outside}$) sampled from the prior distributions, to evaluate the

Table 2. Definitions and values of fixed parameters in the model.

Parameters	Description	Value	Range[1]	Reference
μ_m (*l*)	Culling rate			(Prof. Coureau, Alfort National Veterinary School, pers. Comm.)
	Dairy herd, 2000's	0.35	0.25; 0.45	
	Beef herd, 2000's	0.25	0.15; 0.35	
	All herds, 1980's	0.25		
Se.SITT	Sensitivity of single intradermal tuberculin test		0.635; 1	[8]
	1980's	0.72		
	2000's	0.839		
Sp.SITT	Specificity of single intradermal tuberculin test		0.755; 0.99	[8]
	1980's	0.988		
	2000's	0.968		
Se.SICCT	Sensitivity of single intra dermal comparative cervical tuberculin test	0.80	0.52; 1	[8]
Sp.SICCT	Specificity of single intra dermal comparative cervical tuberculin test	0.995	0.788; 1	[8]
Se.PPD γIFN	Sensitivity of gamma interferon test (PPD)	0.876	0.73; 1	[8]
Sp.PPD γIFN	Specificity of gamma interferon test (PPD)	0.966	0.850; 0.996	[8]
Se.ESAT-6 γIFN	Sensitivity of gamma interferon test (ESAT-6)	0.763	0.690; 0.836	[51]
Sp.ESAT-6 γIFN	Specificity of gamma interferon test (ESAT-6)	0.992	0.976; 1	[51]
qSICCT	Proportion of animals non-reactors to SITT tested six weeks later by SICCT	0.10	0.05; 0.15	(French Ministry of agriculture, Food and Forestry)
Se.bac	Sensitivity of bacterial culture	0.78	0.729; 0.828	[52]
Se.les	Sensitivity of visual inspection of carcass	0.50	0.255; 0.755	[6]

[1]Values used in the sensitivity analysis.

Table 3. Selection of the set of summary statistics based on simulated datasets generated using arbitrarily fixed parameter values: $\alpha = 0.083$ months, $\beta_{inside} = 0.5$, and $\beta_{inside} = 0.1$.

Id	Summary statistics	Dimension	Median [95% credible interval]			p[1]
			α	β_{inside}	$\beta_{outside}$	
A	Average percentage of animals with detected lesions[2]	1	0.72 [0.60–0.78]	0.79 [0.44–1.27]	0.61 [0,03–1,92]	–
B	Average percentage of animals with detected lesions in each batch	3	0.42 [0.00–2.43]	0.33 [0.28–0.70]	0.29 [0.00–3.9]	73%
C	Percentage of animals with detected lesions in each batch (n = 3) of each herd (n = 27)	81	0.13 [0.06–0.67]	0.35 [0.02–1.97]	0.44 [0.01–2.21]	49%
D	Same as C+percentage of herds submitted to total slaughter	82	0.97 [0.48–2.04]	0.05 [0.01–0.15]	0.03 [0.00–0.12]	–
E	Same as C+time between the last negative test and the detection of infection for each herd	108	0.29 [0.07–0.69]	0.35 [0.00–0.77]	0.07 [0.00–0.84]	32%
F	Same as E+percentage of herds submitted to total slaughter	109	0.33 [0.12–0.65]	0.29 [0.08–0.57]	0.08 [0.00–0.79]	–
G	Average percentage of animals with detected lesion for each batch, period[3] and herd type[4]; average time between the last negative test and the detection of infection for each period and herd type	16	0.26 [0.07–0.74]	0.27 [0.04–0.75]	0.07 [0.00–0.52]	71%
H	Same as G+percentage of herds submitted to total slaughter for each period and herd type	20	0.073 [0.05–0.54]	0.48 [0.03–0.76]	0.12 [0.00–0.59]	88%

[1]Proportion of cases for which each of the three arbitrarily fixed parameter values were inside the 95% credible interval of the posterior distributions (100 repetitions).
[2]For herds submitted to a total slaughter.
[3]Before 2007 (control program B) and after 2007 (control program C).
[4]Dairy of beef.

robustness of the estimates to the tolerance rate. Each of the 100 simulated datasets was successively considered a pseudo-observation and parameter values were estimated using the above procedure. A prediction error coefficient was calculated for each estimated parameter, for values of p_ε ranging from 0.1% to 5% [24]. The smallest value of p_ε for which the prediction error coefficient was stable for the three parameters (α, β_{inside}, $\beta_{outside}$) was thus selected.

We used the "abc" package of software R [25]. The function cv4abc was used to select the value for the proportion of retained simulations p_ε.

A sensitivity analysis was performed to evaluate the effect of changing the fixed parameter values (Table 2) on the estimated values of the transition rate (α) and of the transmission parameters (β_{inside} and $\beta_{outside}$). Two different values were selected for each fixed parameter (Table 2) according to literature (SITT, SICCT, γIFN and bacterial culture) or using fixed deviations (±10% or ±5%). Only first-order effects were analyzed and, for each scenario, α, β_{inside} and $\beta_{outside}$ were estimated by the ABC method, as described above. This operation was repeated 24 times (12 fixed parameters and 2 points per parameter) resulting in 24 posterior distributions for α, β_{inside} and $\beta_{outside}$. These were analysed using three generalised linear model (GLMs) (one per estimated parameter). The explanatory variables were the fixed parameters values (their deviation from their default values).

The GLMs were used to predict the effect of an increase of 5% of each fixed parameter on the average values of α, β_{inside} and $\beta_{outside}$. To identify the most influential fixed parameters, we compared the coefficient of variation of the posterior distributions (obtained using the default values of fixed parameters) with the relative error induced by a 5% change of fixed parameters, as predicted by the GLMs.

Validation

An internal validation was first performed using a leave-one-out cross-validation procedure. One hundred triples of parameter values (α, β_{inside} and $\beta_{outside}$) were randomly chosen among the 100,000 used for parameter estimation. Each was successively used to generate a dataset considered a pseudo-observation, and posterior distributions were estimated using the above procedure (without using the pseudo-observation). The reliability of the estimation procedure was quantified by the proportion of cases for which the triple (α, β_{inside} and $\beta_{outside}$) used to generate the dataset was within the 95% credible interval.

An external validation was performed to test the ability of the model to reproduce the observational data of bTB in France between 1980 and 2010, using the data that were not used for parameter estimation: dataset A, aggregated data from datasets B and C, and dataset D (Table 1). Each herd of these datasets was successively used to parameterize the model (herd size and type, control program - Figures 2, 3, S1 and S2), and the posterior distributions of parameters (α, β_{inside} and $\beta_{outside}$) were sampled to perform 1000 simulations. Those ending by a total slaughter were kept to compute the distribution of the proportion of animals with detected lesions. For each herd of the above datasets, the observed proportion was compared with the simulated distribution thus obtained. Furthermore, for dataset A, the predicted proportion of simulations ending by a total slaughter was compared with the percentage observed in the corresponding department in the 1980s: 5%.

Model exploitation

The basic reproduction ratio (R0) is used to measure the transmission potential of a disease. It is the number of secondary infections produced by an infectious animal in a fully susceptible population that is totally susceptible. This indictor is of great importance in infectious disease modelling as, when R0<1, the disease tends to vanish, whereas when R0>1, the disease tends to spread and a large epidemic may occur [26]. However, in real situations, the population is rarely entirely susceptible, mainly because of the spread of infection (and the corresponding decrease in the number of susceptible individuals). We computed the effective reproductive ratio R(t): the average number of cases secondary to an infectious case in a population consisting of susceptible and infected individuals. Two average herds, respectively representative of a French dairy herd (81 cattle) and a French beef herd (70 cattle) in the 2000s, were considered. Disease dynamics was simulated in these herds without a control program, and the distribution of the effective reproductive ratio R(t) was calculated each month after the introduction of *M. bovis*, during 360 months (twice the maximal age of cows in the model: 15 years). Details of R(t) calculation are given in Appendix S3.

Results

Parameter estimation

The procedure used to choose the set of summary statistics first led to select B, C, E, G and H, for which, when using one simulated dataset as a pseudo-observation, the arbitrarily chosen parameter values were all inside the 95% credible interval of posterior distributions of parameters (Table 3). Their dimensions varied between 3 for B and 109 for F (Table 3). Among these five sets of summary statistics, H maximized the proportion of cases (88%) where the arbitrarily fixed parameters (α, β_{inside} and $\beta_{outside}$) were all within the credible interval of 95% of posterior distributions when using the 100 simulated datasets as pseudo-observations (Table 3). This set of summary statistics was thus chosen: a combination of statistics describing the percentage of animals with detected lesions per batch and the percentage of herds with total slaughter per herd type (dairy/beef) and per period (periods where control program B and C were applied). The evolution of the values of the prediction error coefficient according to the proportion of retained simulations led to select $p_\varepsilon = 2\%$.

The median of the posterior distribution of α was 0.28 (95% credible interval [CI]: [0.13–0.56]), which corresponds to a median latency period for bTB of 3.5 months (95% CI: [2–8] months) (Figure 4). The median value of bTB transmission coefficients were 0.43 month^{-1} (95% CI [0.16–0.84] month^{-1}) inside the stable (β_{inside}) and 0.08 month^{-1} (95% CI [0.01–0.32] month^{-1}) outside the stable ($\beta_{outside}$) (Figure 4). The median of the ratio $\beta_{inside}/\beta_{outside}$ was 5 (95% CI [0.8–100]). It was>1 in 95.6% of cases (Figure 4). Negative values of Spearman's rank correlation coefficient were observed between α and β_{inside} (−0.47, p<0.0001), between α and $\beta_{outside}$ (−0.31, p<0.0001), and between β_{inside} and $\beta_{outside}$ (−0.35, p<0.0001). These negative correlations were expected, as the summary statistics (such as the proportion of animals showing lesions) may remain approximately the same if a higher value of α (i.e. a shorter latency period) is compensated by smaller values of β_{inside} and $\beta_{outside}$, or if a higher value of β_{inside} is compensated by a lower value of $\beta_{outside}$. The results of the sensitivity analysis of parameter estimates to variations of fixed parameter values are summarised in a tornado chart (Figure 5). A 5% increase in the values of the fixed parameters had limited effects on the estimation of α and $\beta_{outside}$ (Figure 5). For β_{inside}, the relative difference of the average posterior estimate greater than the coefficient of variation computed from the posterior distribution of for a single parameter: the specificity of the ESAT-6 γIFN

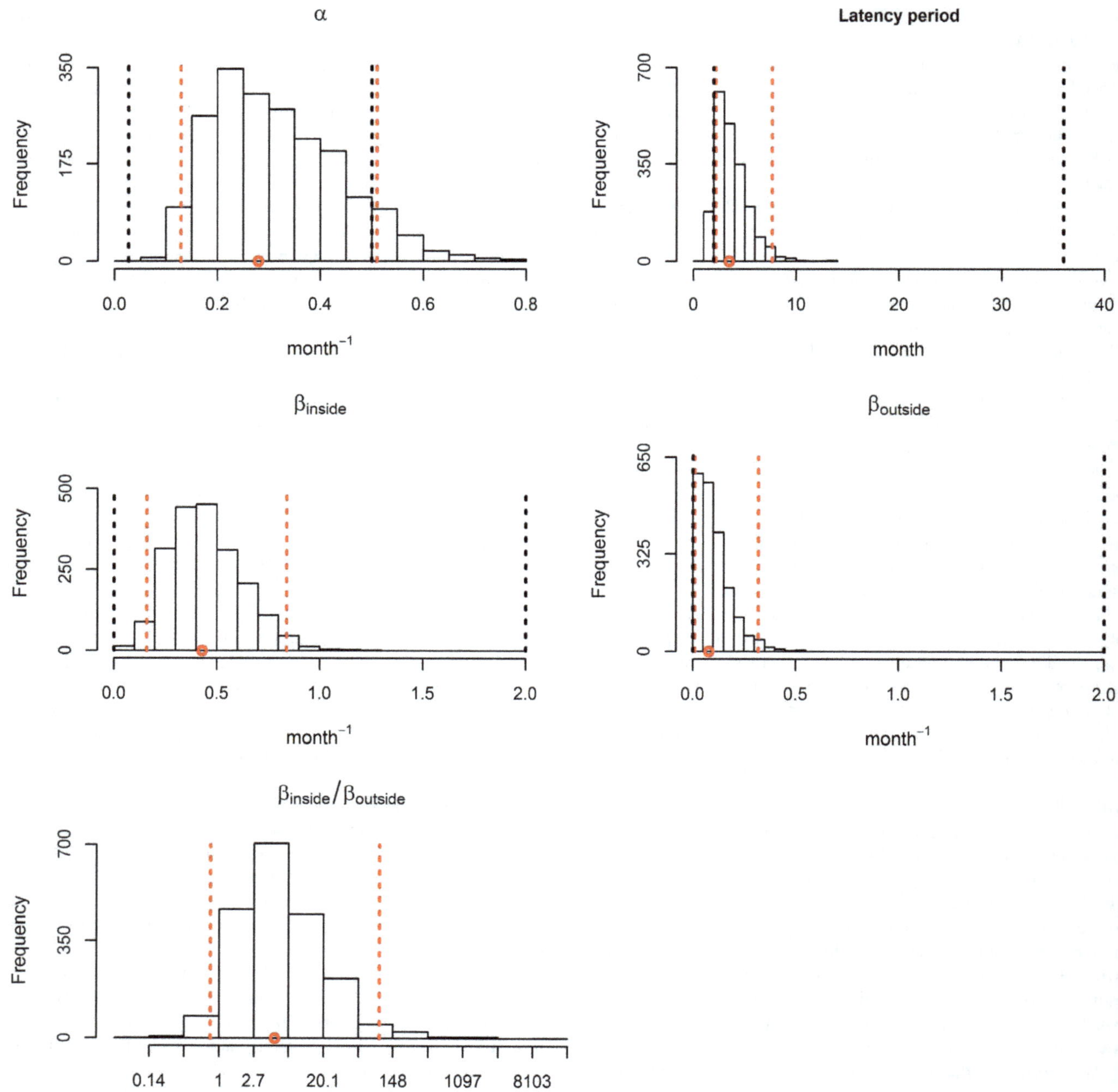

Figure 4. Posterior distribution of parameters α, β_{inside} and $\beta_{outside}$. Red dots: median value of parameter estimates; black dotted lines: lower and higher bounds of parameter prior distributions; red dotted lines: 95% credible intervals of the parameter posterior distributions. Histogram $\beta_{inside}/\beta_{outside}$ represents the value of log ratio $\beta_{inside}/\beta_{outside}$ but the x-axis values are not expressed in log.

test. A 5% increase of the specificity of the ESAT-6 γIFN test led to a 48.5% decrease of the average posterior estimate of β_{inside}.

Predicted bTB dynamics

Figure 6 and Table 4 represents the predicted bTB dynamics in two herds representing dairy farms (average size in 2000:81 animals) and beef herds (average size in 2000:70 animals) in France, with and without a control program (control program B, Table 1 and Figure 2). When the control program was simulated, after its introduction in a susceptible herd, bTB was predicted to disappear in 22% of cases in beef herds and in 17% of cases in dairy farms, thanks to routine cull: the median time from disease introduction and disease extinction was less than 10 months, in both types of herds, with or without a control program (Table 4). In most cases, *M. bovis* did not disappear from the simulated herds and the disease was predicted to be detected through passive surveillance (at slaughterhouse) (13% for beef herds and 21% for dairy farms) or through active surveillance (screening using skin tests) (65% for beef herds and 62% for dairy farms). In both cases, the median time period between the introduction of infection and total slaughter was less than 3 years in the two types of herds (Table 4). In the absence of a control program (Figure 6a and 6b), the median proportion of infected animals was predicted to increase until reaching a plateau at 61 months in beef herds and

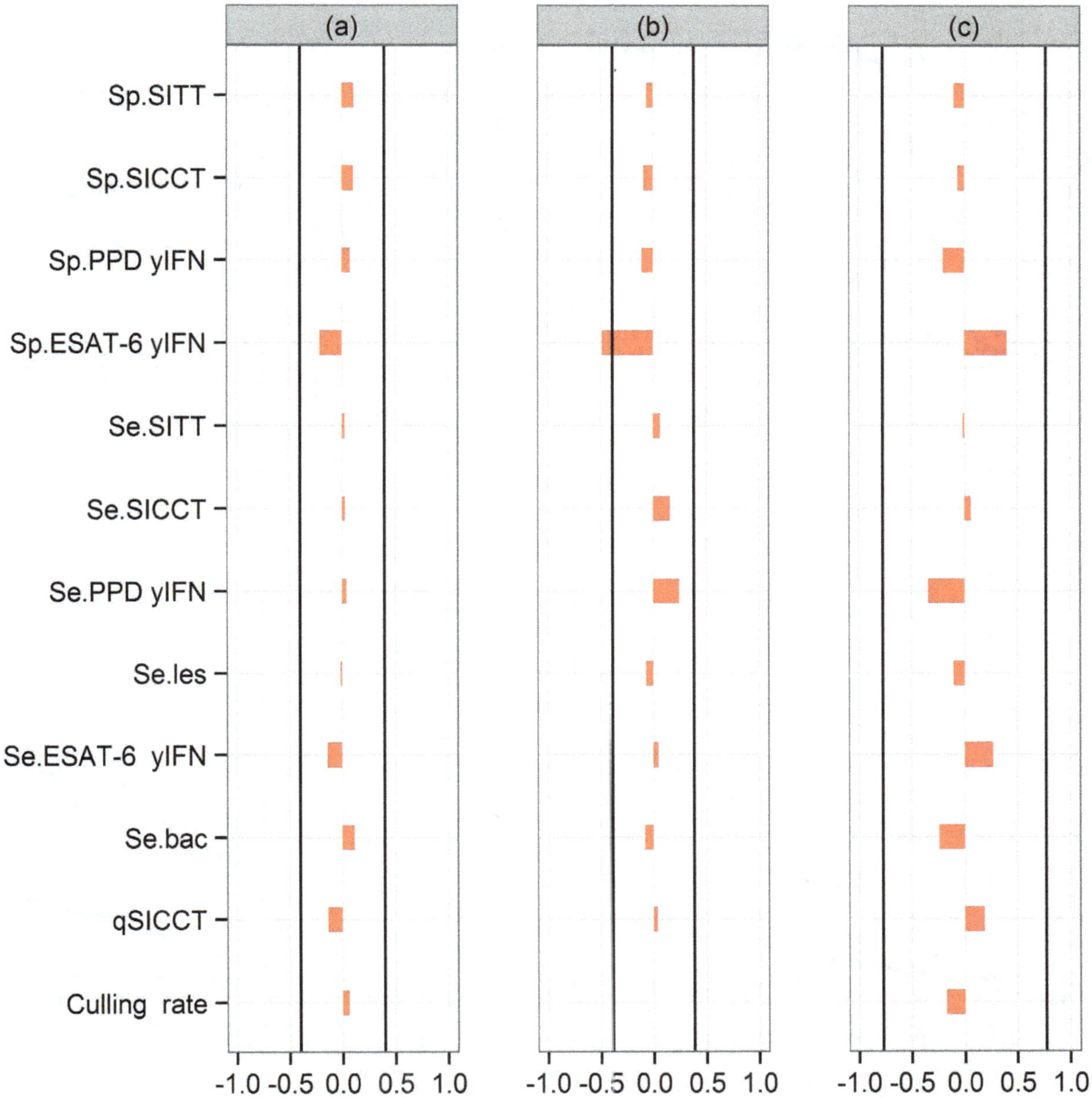

Figure 5. Impact of changes of fixed parameter values on the estimates of α, β_{inside} and $\beta_{outside}$. (a): relative error for α; (b): relative error for β_{inside}; (c): relative error for $\beta_{outside}$; black line: value of the coefficient of variation of the posterior distributions obtained when we using the default values of fixed parameters; if the relative error value is within the two black lines, the effect of fixed parameters values on parameter estimates in the model is considered limited; qSICCT: percentage of SITT-negative animals tested 6 weeks after by SICCT; see table 2 for the definition of the other parameters.

40 months in dairy herds (Figure 6a and 6b). The corresponding level of infection prevalence was predicted to be higher in beef herds (Figure 6a) than in dairy herds (Figure 6b): once reached the enzootic infection level the median prevalence of infected animals was 93% in beef farms and 53% in dairy herds. As expected, when a control program was used, the maximum percentage of infected animals was predicted to be lower in both types of herds (Figure 6c and 7d).

Validation

Internal validation showed that, for 83 of the 100 randomly selected simulations, the fixed values of the three parameters α, β_{inside} and $\beta_{outside}$, were inside the 95% credible interval of the posterior distributions.

Using dataset A, external validation showed that, in four of five herds (farms 1, 2, 3 and 4), the observed percentage of cattle with lesions was between the 2.5% and 97.5% percentiles of the simulated proportion of animals with lesions at total slaughter (Figure 7). In the fifth herd, the observed percentage of animals with lesions was very high (86.6%) and was above the 97.5% percentile of the simulated distribution (Figure 7). The proportion of simulations ending with a total slaughter varied between 3% and 7%, depending on the herd. These values are close to the proportion of 5% reported by the French Ministry of Agriculture, Food and Forestry for that department at that time.

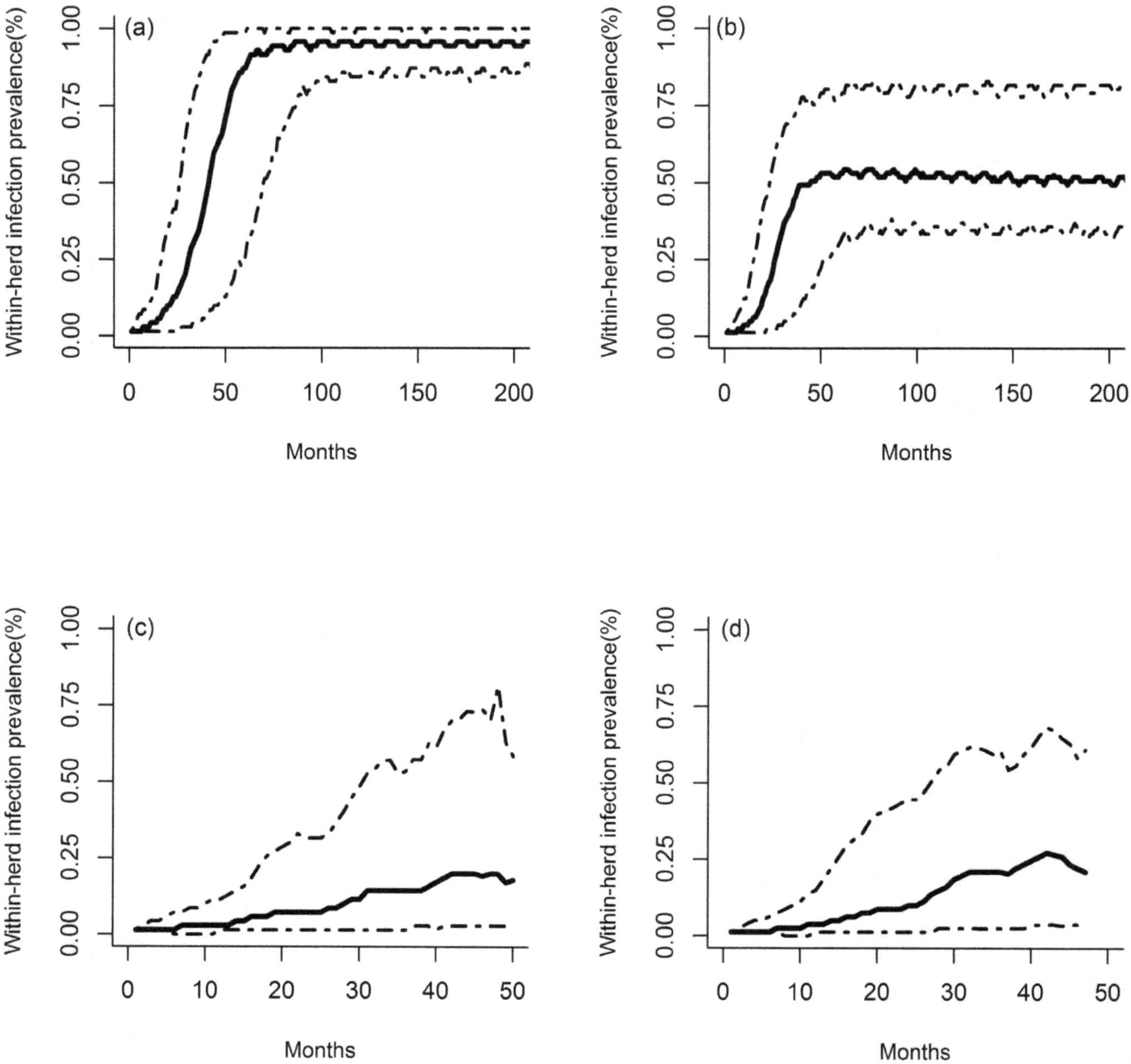

Figure 6. Monthly evolution of the simulated proportion of infected animals (animals in E or I health state; solid line: median, dashed: 2.5% and 97.5% percentiles) in standard French beef (a and c, 70 animals) and dairy (b and d, 81 animals) herds without (a and b) or with (c and d) implementation of control program B (1,000 simulations per scenario).

The observed percentage of animals with lesions was located between the 2.5% and 97.5% percentiles of the simulated proportion of animals with lesions in 92% (23 herds out of 25) and 83% (24 herds out of 29) of herds of datasets B and C, respectively. This percentage was 100% (29 herds out of 29) for dataset D.

Effective reproductive ratio

Figures 8a and 8b show the evolution of R(t) values over time. In both types of herds, the shape of the curve was similar, with an increase in the values of R(t) that reached a plateau 72 months after disease introduction in dairy herds and at 96 months after disease introduction in beef herds. After 30 simulated years, which corresponds to a situation of enzootic circulation of *M. bovis* within the herd, the value of R(t) was slightly higher for beef herds than for dairy herds. The median value and the percentiles [2.5%–97.5%] of the predicted distribution of R(t) were 2.2 [1.8–2.8] for beef herds and 1.7 [1.5–2.2] for dairy herds (Figure 8a and Figure 8b). It was higher than 1 for each of the 1,000 simulations and higher than 2 for 11% of simulations in dairy herds and 79% in beef herds (Figure 8c and Figure 8d).

Discussion

In this work, we have built a stochastic discrete-time model to simulate bTB dynamics and control in cattle herds. The model accounts for interactions among the three processes that influence the within-herd evolution of bTB: (i) the natural history of the disease (infectious process), (ii) husbandry practices (demographic

Table 4. Predicted median and percentiles [2.5%–97.5%] of the distribution of outbreak duration (in months) in standard French beef herds (70 animals) and dairy herds (81 animals) without or with control programs (1,000 simulations per scenario).

		Beef herds	Dairy herds
Time to natural extinction of infection	Without a simulated control program	7 [3–30]	8 [4–32]
	With a simulated control program		
	No detection of infection	6 [3–11]	7 [4–16]
	Infection suspected but not confirmed[1]	8 [3–25]	8 [3–23]
Time to total slaughter of the herd after infection detection by routine skin testing		24 [9–50]	23 [9–48]
Time to total slaughter of the herd after infection detection by slaughterhouse surveillance		24 [8–50]	30 [9–47]

[1]No isolation of *M. bovis*, total slaughter is thus not applied.

process) and (iii) control programs (detection and control process). The model has been designed to allow simulating control programs of arbitrary degree of complexity. Parameterization allows representing various herd types and farming practices (in particular the differences between dairy herd and beef herd management). Epidemiological parameters of the within-herd transmission of bTB (duration of the latent state, transmission parameters) were estimated using a first set and the model was validated using a second set of field data collected between 1980 and 2010. Herd management practices and bTB control programs have evolved during this period and the model could be successfully adapted by changing parameter values, suggesting a good level of genericity and an ability to simulate various herd management systems and bTB detection and control programs of arbitrary complexity. The simulated effective reproductive ratio R(t) may allow assessing the effectiveness (*i.e.* whether $R(t)<1$) of different bTB control strategies or the effect of changes in herd management practices on the bTB within-herd dynamic.

Internal validation showed a good reliability of the estimation procedure of model parameters by the ABC method. External validation showed that the model was able to reproduce field data regarding bTB collected between 1980 and 2010 in several French departments. This suggests that the transmission coefficients (β_{inside} and $\beta_{outside}$) and the duration of the latent period ($1/\alpha$) have remained roughly constant between the 1980s and today, despite changes in parameters related to herd management practices such as the culling rate, the age at culling and the herd size.

Health states used in the proposed model (susceptible, latent and infectious) are consistent with the pathology of infection. However, published models often divide the latent state into two sub-states (latent, non-skin test-responsive and latent, skin test-responsive [13–15]) and use shorter time steps (day or week). Latent non-skin test-responsive animals spend an average of four weeks in this state before developing a positive skin test reaction [13,14,27]. Conlan et *al.* [28] estimated the median period of the latent non-skin test-responsive state at 28 days. As we used a monthly time step, it was thus not necessary to represent this health state. Infectious state I was defined by the presence of detectable lesions at slaughter. The type (open or stabilised) and the location of the lesions were not taken into account. This may induce an underestimation of within-herd transmission: an animal with so-called "open tuberculosis lesions" may infect the rest of the herd in a short period of time. However, much is unclear about open tuberculosis lesions, including the probability of developing this type of lesion, its duration and its infectivity [15]. Therefore we did not incorporate the type of lesion in our model. This choice is in line with other epidemiological models of bTB [13–15].

Most of the models previously developed in the literature that simulated the within-herd spread of bTB used a single transmission parameter. In our model, we used two transmission parameters to distinguish transmission inside buildings and in pastures. Both transmission coefficients are related to herd practices, allowing to use the model for representing various farming systems by changing the grazing periods and the composition of batches. The within-herd transmission of bTB is considered higher in dairy herds than in beef herds [12]. This is attributed to a combination of several factors that contribute to the spread of infections in dairy herds such as the high contact rate, especially in the milking parlour [13], the high animal density and stress factors related to intense animal management [12,29–32]. The estimated value of β_{inside} was greater than that of $\beta_{outside}$ in 96% of cases, suggesting that the definition of two transmission coefficients allowed capturing the difference between dairy herds and beef herds in terms of within-herd transmission of bTB. Indeed, although the 95% credible intervals of the two within-herd transmission coefficients of bTB (β_{inside} and $\beta_{outside}$) overlapped, the median within-herd transmission coefficient inside the stable was 5 time as high as in the pasture: 0.43 month^{-1} [0,16–0.84] and 0.08 month^{-1} [0.01–0.32] for β_{inside} and $\beta_{outside}$, respectively. These estimated medians were consistent with the estimates of within-herd transmission of bTB in Spain proposed by Alvarez et *al.* [12], with higher transmission coefficients in dairy herds (median 0.39 month^{-1}) than in beef herds (0.19 month^{-1}). The estimated values of the transmission coefficients are also in the same range as values obtained by other studies: 0.22 month^{-1} in the study of Barlow et *al.* [13] and 0.18 months^{-1} in the study of Perez et *al.* in Argentina [2].

The only transmission route taken into account in our work is the direct transmission between animals of the same batch. Indirect transmission, the potential role of wildlife, contacts with cattle from other herds at pastures and contacts between cattle of different batches are not taken into account. In particular, between-batch disease transmission was not taken into account because we assumed that the probability of contact between animals of different batches was low: different batches of the same herd are often placed by the breeder on different and distant pastures and even sometimes in separate buildings. It should be noted that the transmission between batches does nevertheless occur in the model: as bTB is a chronic, slowly evolving disease, between-batch transmission occurs when animals are moved from one batch to another. However, the closed herd assumption would

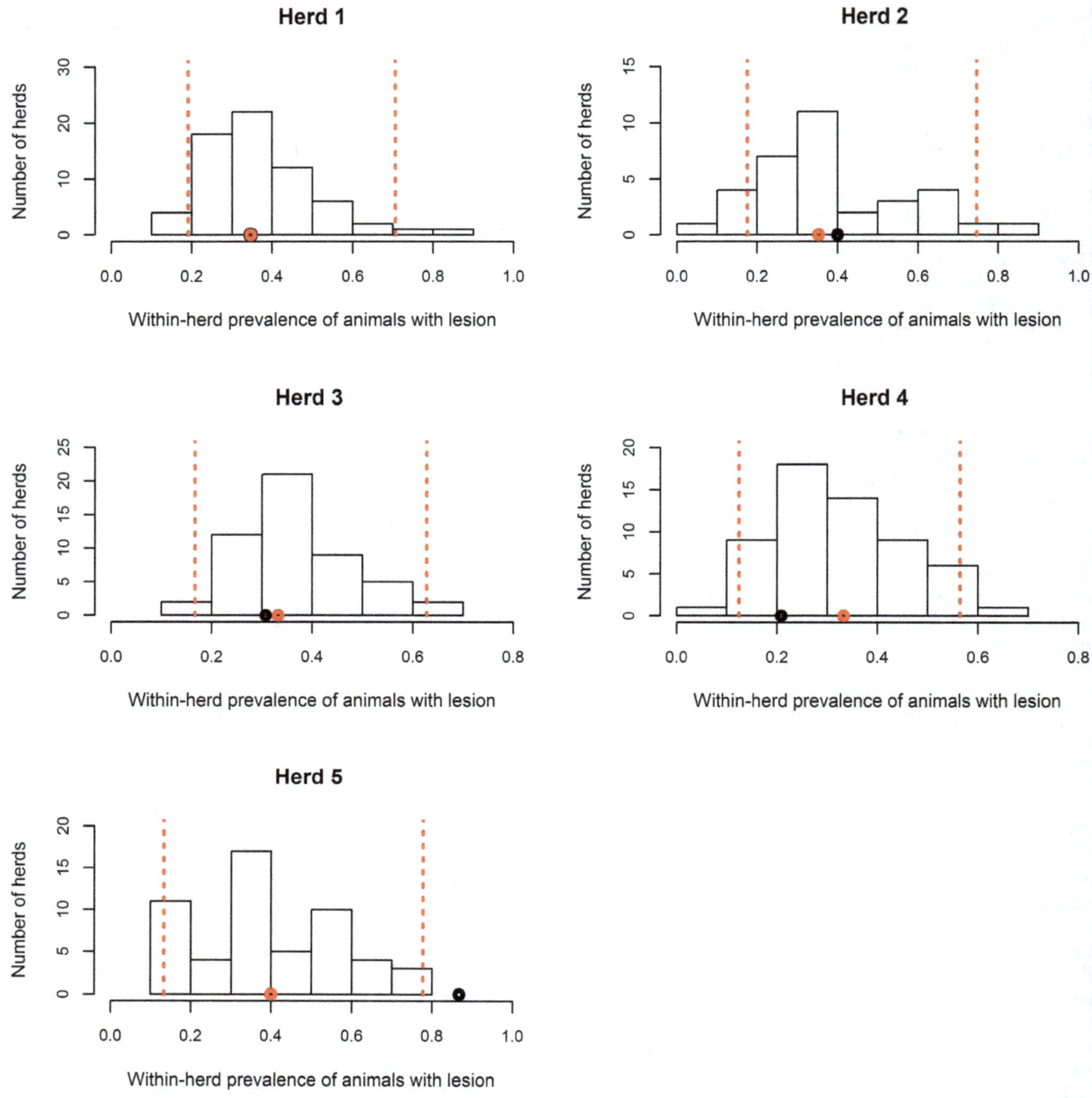

Figure 7. Observed and simulated proportions of animals with detected lesions when total slaughter is performed, for the 5 herds of dataset A. Black point: observed proportion of animals with bTB-like lesions in each herd; red point: simulated median proportion of animals with bTB-like lesions in each herd; dotted lines: 2.5% and 97.5% percentiles of the simulated distributions.

likely underestimate the persistence of *M. bovis* infection in herds, if wildlife or introduced animals can reintroduce infection [33].

The median duration of the estimated latency period (state *E*) was 3.5 months [2–8] months. This range of values is consistent with the chronic nature of bTB. However, our estimate of the latency duration was lower than the mean estimated duration of 24 months (95% confidence interval: 15–34 months) that was obtained by a simulation model of the within-herd transmission of bTB in Argentina [2]. This difference may be explained by differences among animals in the two countries, as the incubation period depends on the susceptibility of the host [34].

Model predictions for 2000 showed that the infected herds (dairy or beef) were in 15 to 20% of cases detected by slaughterhouse surveillance. This result was expected because the frequency of intradermal skin test applied in control program B was biennial. The percentage of spontaneous extinction of the disease (thanks to routine cull) was almost identical between dairy and beef herds.

When no control program was applied, simulated within-herd prevalence reached>50% in both types of farms. This simulated prevalence is high compared to the values observed in some parts of Africa and Asia (between 6% and 15%), where no control

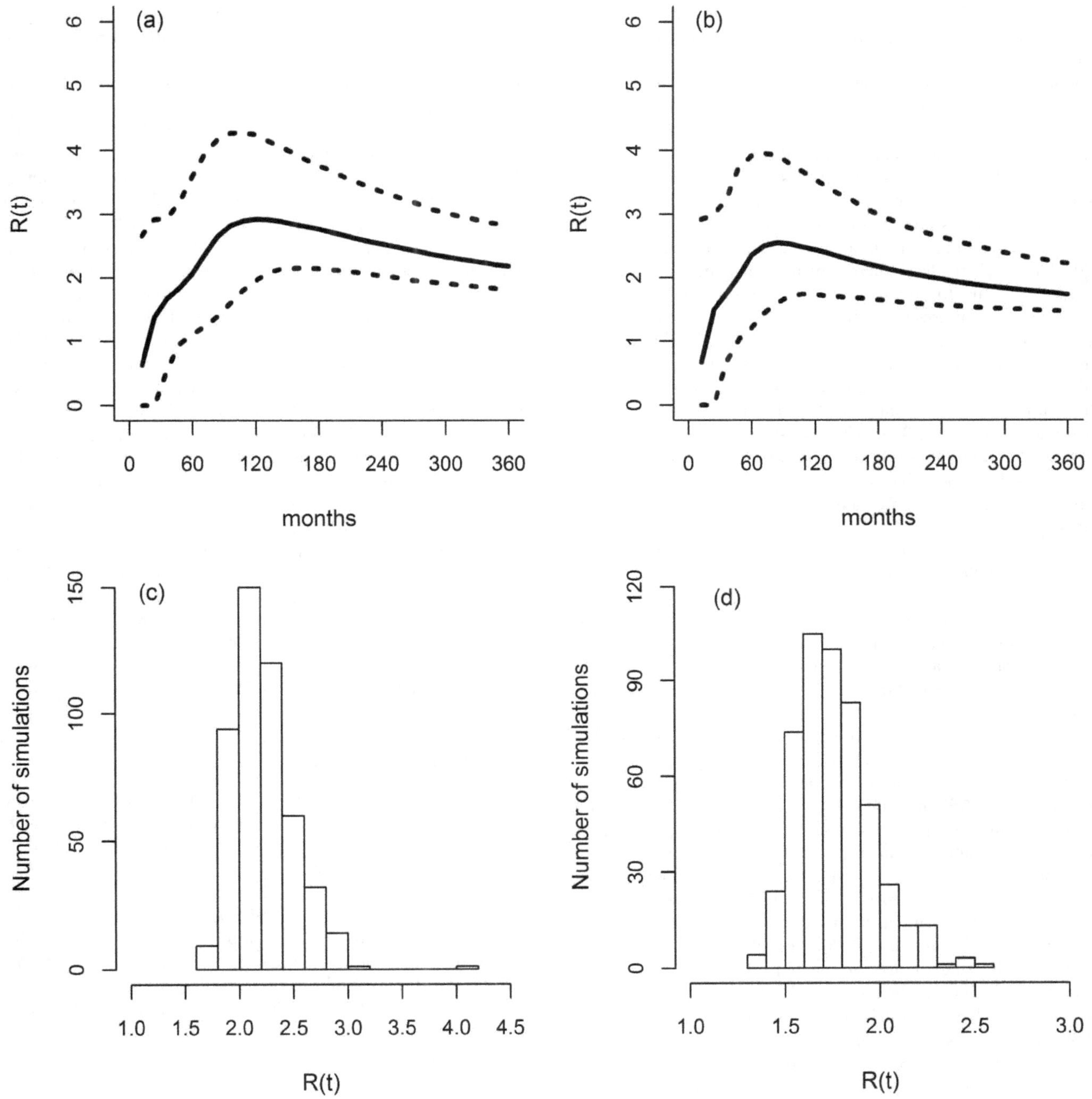

Figure 8. Monthly evolution of the simulated effective reproductive ratio R(t) (a and b), and distribution of this R(t) (c and d) when the disease has become enzootic (after 30 years) in standard French beef (a and c, 70 animals) and dairy (b and d, 81 animals) herds. Solid line: median; dashed: 2.5% and 97.5% percentiles.

program is applied [35,36]. In Africa and in Asia, most cattle are zebu (*B. indicus*) [37]. Ameni *et al.* [38] report that, under identical field husbandry conditions, a higher susceptibility to bTB was observed in Holstein cows than in zebus: (odds ratio: 2.32). In France dairy cattle are kept most of the time indoors, while beef cattle have stabling periods of approximately five months each year. Oppositely, in Africa and in Asia, cattle are most of the time kept outdoors, where contacts between animals are less intense than indoors, hence the lower observed within-herd prevalence in these regions.

The low predicted values of the effective reproductive ratio R(t) over time are consistent with field observations of a low bTB prevalence in French infected herds in the 2000s, and support the results of transmission trials indicating that cattle do not readily infect other cattle [39,40]. According to our estimation, when no control program is applied and once bTB has become enzootic within the herd, the median number of animals infected by an infectious animal is 2.2 in beef herds and 1.7 in dairy herds. This difference is due to a lower age at culling for dairy cows than for beef cows.

Several models have been proposed in the literature to simulate the dynamic of within-herd transmission of bTB: stochastic Reed-Frost model in discrete time [2,12], Reed-Frost model in continuous time [14], stochastic individual based model [15], compartmental stochastic model in continuous time [28] and compartmental stochastic model in discrete time [13,33,41]. We used a compartmental stochastic model operating in discrete time. Bovine TB health states are best represented using discrete health states (S-E-I), we thus chose to use a compartmental model. The scarcity and the discrete nature of the main simulated event which is the infection of animals (in a national survey in France between 2005 and 2007 in infected herds, the median of animals with lesion was 2), led us to use a stochastic approach rather than a deterministic approach. ABC methods are computationally cumbersome. Discrete time simulation was chosen as it appeared less computationally demanding than continuous time simulation. The duration of the time step (one month) was chosen because in literature the estimated duration of the latent state (in models with a single latent state [2] or with two states of latency [28]) was greater than one month. In addition, for the modeled screening, control and demographic processes, a one month time step also appeared satisfactory (frequency of tuberculin test, stabling period).

While this type of model is relatively easy to simulate, it is analytically difficult to manage when the number of states is high. In this case, numerical resolution by simulation is the only way to estimate the parameters [42]. The likelihood is difficult to calculate in our model, because the infection process is only partially observed (only a fraction of infectious animals is detected at the slaughterhouse, depending on the sensitivity of the visual inspection of carcasses). We thus chose to use the ABC method for the estimation of model parameters because this method does not require the calculation of the likelihood [43]. The choice of summary statistics and of the tolerance threshold are two sources of error in the ABC method [44]. To reduce errors linked to the choice of summary statistics, a preliminary step was performed in which several summary statistics were tested and compared using simulated data. Other methods have been proposed in the literature such as the algorithm developed by Barnes et *al.* [45] to choose a set of summary statistics from all possible summary statistics. This algorithm uses the mutual information as a selection tool [45]. Choosing a non-zero value for tolerance, ε, can bias the posterior estimation of the parameters [44]. To reduce errors due to non-zero values of ε, the local linear regression algorithm of the ABC method was used in our work for estimating the model parameters [19]. ABC-SMC (Sequential Monte Carlo) algorithm allows using specific methods to select the tolerance threshold [46,47]. But, according to Filippi et *al.* [48], more work needs to be done on the choice of tolerance threshold in the ABC-SMC algorithm. Besides, the use of the local linear regression algorithm is however not without problems, as the relationship between summary statistics and parameters is highly non-linear in most cases, which may bias the estimation of parameters [19].

The sensitivity analysis of a model is of great interest [42] because it helps to determine the most influential parameters. The sensitivity analysis performed here was used to independently assess the effect of fixed parameters values on the posterior parameter estimates. For practical reasons (of computation time required to perform this sensitivity analysis), the sensitivity analysis did not assess the effect of interactions among fixed parameters. Nevertheless, according to the literature, this method is the first step in exploring global associations (between the estimated and non-estimated parameters in the model), excluding interactions [49]. The results of the sensitivity analysis showed that fixed parameters have only limited effects on the posterior parameter estimates, except for the effect of the specificity of ESAT-6 γIFN test on β_{inside}. The specificity of ESAT-6 γIFN test is used in control program C (Figure 3), which includes a 2-steps confirmation of positive SITT using γIFN test (steps 2 and 3 in Figure 3). When the specificity of ESAT-6 γIFN is increased to 100% (see Table 2), the overall specificity of the 3rd step of control program C also reaches 100% (see Figure 3). Because the overall sensitivity of both γIFN-based confirmation steps is low, the time required to detect bTB increases, which induces a decrease of β_{inside} estimate.

We assumed that the sensitivity and the specificity of the screening tests were independent of cattle age. Proaño-Perez et *al.* [50] reported a negative correlation between the age of cattle and the response to avian tuberculin. This result suggests that young animals are more likely to show false positive reactions to SITT than adult animals. The impact on our results is however likely to be limited, as the sensitivity analysis showed that the specificity of screening test had a little effect on the estimated values of the epidemiological model parameters (α, β_{inside} and $\beta_{outside}$).

In conclusion, the model proposed here has been designed to be generic enough to allow simulating various herd management systems and bTB detection and control programs. Its parameters have been estimated using field data and it has been validated using an independent dataset. In the future, this model will be used to analyse the impacts of changes of control programs and of herd management practices on the dynamics of bTB in France, between the beginning of the control program (in 1965) and obtaining the bTB-free status (in 2000). Besides, it will be used to assess the effectiveness of bTB control programs, in order to identify alternative strategies to the total slaughter protocol currently applied in infected herds.

Supporting Information

Figure S1 Control program A applied in the Nord department between 1981 and 1983. Step 1: yearly bTB screening using SITT (the herd being considered disease-free). All animals are tested (μ i,k Q(i,k) = 1). Sensitivity (Se) and specificity (Sp): those of SITT. Transition to step 2 if the proportion of positive animals exceeds a predefined threshold (n^{pos}/n^{test}>P.ab), one month later (Δt = 1 months). Transition to step 3 if positive results are observed, the proportion being below the threshold. Step 2: total slaughter. All the animals (μ i,k Q(i,k) = 1)are slaughtered (m = 1). Step 3: selective slaughter. Positive animals of step 1 (μ i Q(i,1) = 1)are slaughtered (m = 1). Transition to step 1, 6 months later. See table 2 for the definition of the other parameters.

Figure S2 Control program D applied in the Côte d'Or department between 2005 and 2009. Step 1: biennial bTB screening using SICCT (the herd being considered disease-free). All animals are tested (μ i,k Q(i,k) = 1). Sensitivity (Se) and specificity (Sp): those of SICCT. Immediate transition to step 2 if non-negative results are observed (n^{pos}>0). Step 2: interpretation of SICCT non-negative results. All the positive animals of step 1 (μ i Q(i,1) = 1) are concerned. Sensitivity: for an infected animal, probability that a non-negative positive result is not doubtful (pi: probability of a doubtful SICCT result for animals in health states E or I); specificity: for a susceptible animal, probability that a non-negative SICCT result is doubtful (ps: probability of a doubtful SICCT result for animals in health state S). Transition to step 3 if all the non-negative SICCT animals are doubtful, 2 months later; otherwise: transition to step 4, 3 months later. Step 3: confirmation of the positive results of step 1 using SICCT. All the positive animals of step 1 are tested (μ i Q(i,1) = 1), as well as 10% of the negative animals (i Q(i,0) = 0.1). Sensitivity (Se) and specificity (Sp): those of SICCT. Transition to step 5 if an animal is positive, three months later; otherwise: transition to step 1. Step 4: slaughter of the positive animals of step 2 and isolation of *M. bovis* from lesions. All the positive animals of step 2 (μ i Q(i,2) = 1) are slaughtered (m = 1) and bacterial culture is performed from observed lesions. Sensitivity (Se): sequential combination of a visual inspection at the slaughterhouse and of a bacterial culture. Transition to step 6 if an animal is positive, 1 month later ($\Delta t = 1$ month). Step 5: slaughter of the positive animals of step 3 and isolation of *M. bovis* from lesions. All the positive animals of step 3 (μ i Q(i,3) = 1) are slaughtered (m = 1) and bacterial culture is performed from observed lesions. Sensitivity (Se): sequential combination of a visual inspection at the slaughterhouse and of a bacterial culture. Transition to step 6 if an animal is positive, 1 month later ($\Delta t = 1$ month). Step 6: total slaughter. All the animals (μ i,k Q(i,k) = 1) are slaughtered (m = 1). Routine detection of lesions at slaughterhouse. Sensitivity (Se_{ev}): sequential combination of a visual inspection at the slaughterhouse and of a bacterial culture. If a positive animal is thus detected, regardless of the current stage of control program, transition to step 6. See table 2 for the definition of the other parameters.

Appendix S1 Model equations.

Appendix S2 Choice of summary statistics.

Appendix S3 Effective reproductive rate R(t).

Acknowledgments

The authors would like to thank the staff of the Departmental Director of Social Cohesion and Protection of Populations (DDCSPP) of Dordogne and the Departmental Director of Protection of Populations (DDPP) of Côte d'Or, for providing data. We would also like to thank Pr. Coureau from the Alfort National Veterinary School for giving us information on herd management practices in France.

Author Contributions

Conceived and designed the experiments: JJB AC BD MEAB. Performed the experiments: AC BD MEAB. Analyzed the data: BD MEAB. Contributed reagents/materials/analysis tools: JJB BD. Contributed to the writing of the manuscript: AC BD MEAB.

References

1. Radostits OM, Blood DC, Gay CC, Arundel JH, Ikede BO, et al. (1994) Veterinary Medicine: A Textbook of the Diseases of Cattle, Sheep, Pigs, Goats and Horses. London: Bailliere Tindall. 1763 p.
2. Perez AM, Ward MP, Charmandarian A, Ritacco V (2002) Simulation model of within-herd transmission of bovine tuberculosis in Argentine dairy herds. Prev Vet Med 54: 361–372.
3. Reynolds D (2006) A review of tuberculosis science and policy in Great Britain. Vet Microbiol 112: 119–126.
4. de la Rua-Domenech R (2006) Bovine Tuberculosis in the European Union and other countries: current status, control programmes and constrains to eradication. Gov Vet J 16: 19–45.
5. Wahlstrom H, Carpenter T, Giesecke J, Andersson M, Englund L, et al. (2000) Herd-based monitoring for tuberculosis in extensive swedish deer herds by culling and meat inspection rather than by intradermal tuberculin testing. Prev Vet Med 43: 103–116.
6. Cousins DV (2001) Mycobacterium bovis infection and control in domestic livestock. Rev Sci Tech 20: 71–85.
7. Bekara ME, Azizi L, Benet JJ, Durand B (2014) Spatial-temporal Variations of Bovine Tuberculosis Incidence in France between 1965 and 2000. Transbound Emerg Dis.
8. de la Rua-Domenech R, Goodchild AT, Vordermeier HM, Hewinson RG, Christiansen KH, et al. (2006) Ante mortem diagnosis of tuberculosis in cattle: a review of the tuberculin tests, gamma-interferon assay and other ancillary diagnostic techniques. Res Vet Sci 81: 190–210.
9. Corner LA (1994) Post mortem diagnosis of Mycobacterium bovis infection in cattle. Vet Microbiol 40: 53–63.
10. de Jong MCM (1995) Mathematical modelling in veterinary epidemiology: why model building is important. Prev Vet Med 25: 183–193.
11. Smith S, Anders B (1994) Tuberculosis mastoiditis caused by Mycobacterium bovis. Pediatr Infect Dis J 13: 538–539.
12. Alvarez J, Perez AM, Bezos J, Casal C, Romero B, et al. (2012) Eradication of bovine tuberculosis at a herd-level in Madrid, Spain: study of within-herd transmission dynamics over a 12 year period. BMC Vet Res 8: 100.
13. Barlow ND, Kean JM, Hickling G, Livingstone PG, Robson AB (1997) A simulation model for the spread of bovine tuberculosis within New Zealand cattle herds. Prev Vet Med 32: 57–75.
14. Griffin JM, Williams DH, Collins JD (1999) Tuberculosis Investigation Unit, University College Dublin. Selected papers: 55–58.
15. Fischer EA, van Roermund HJ, Hemerik L, van Asseldonk MA, de Jong MC (2005) Evaluation of surveillance strategies for bovine tuberculosis (Mycobacterium bovis) using an individual based epidemiological model. Prev Vet Med 67: 283–301.
16. Kao RR, Roberts MG, Ryan TJ (1997) A model of bovine tuberculosis control in domesticated cattle herds. Proc Biol Sci 264: 1069–1076.
17. Carnon F (1985) Contribution à l'étude épidemiologique de la tuberculose bovine dans le département du Nord. Maisons-Alfort: Ecole Nationale Vétérinaire d'Alfort. 210 p.
18. Toni T, Welch D, Strelkowa N, Ipsen A, Stumpf MP (2009) Approximate Bayesian computation scheme for parameter inference and model selection in dynamical systems. J R Soc Interface 6: 187–202.
19. Beaumont MA, Zhang W, Balding DJ (2002) Approximate Bayesian computation in population genetics. Genetics 162: 2025–2035.
20. Neill SD, Hanna J, Mackie DP, Bryson TG (1992) Isolation of Mycobacterium bovis from the respiratory tracts of skin test-negative cattle. Vet Rec 131: 45–47.
21. Aeschbacher S, Beaumont MA, Futschik A (2012) A novel approach for choosing summary statistics in approximate Bayesian computation. Genetics 192: 1027–1047.
22. Csillery K, Blum MG, Gaggiotti OE, Francois O (2010) Approximate Bayesian Computation (ABC) in practice. Trends Ecol Evol 25: 410–418.
23. Beaumont MA (2010) Approximate Bayesian computation in evolution and ecology. Annual Review of Ecology, Evolution, and Systematics 41: 379–406.
24. Csilléry K, François O, Blum MGB (2012) abc: an R package for approximate Bayesian computation (ABC). Methods in Ecology and Evolution 3: 475–479.
25. R Development Core Team (2013) R: A language and environment for statistical computing. Vienna, Austria: R Foundation for Statistical Computing.
26. Anderson RM, May RM (1991) Infectious diseases of humans: dynamics and control. Oxford and New York: Oxford University Press. 768 p.
27. Kleeberg HH (1960) The tuberculin test in cattle. J South African Vet Med Assoc 31: 213–225.
28. Conlan AJ, McKinley TJ, Karolemeas K, Pollock EB, Goodchild AV, et al. (2012) Estimating the hidden burden of bovine tuberculosis in Great Britain. PLoS Comput Biol 8: e1002730.
29. Karolemeas K, McKinley TJ, Clifton-Hadley RS, Goodchild AV, Mitchell A, et al. (2011) Recurrence of bovine tuberculosis breakdowns in Great Britain: risk factors and prediction. PrevVet Med 102: 22–29.
30. Porphyre T, Stevenson MA, McKenzie J (2008) Risk factors for bovine tuberculosis in New Zealand cattle farms and their relationship with possum control strategies. PrevVet Med 86: 93–106.
31. Ramirez-Villaescusa AM, Medley GF, Mason S, Green LE (2010) Risk factors for herd breakdown with bovine tuberculosis in 148 cattle herds in the south west of England. PrevVet Med 95: 224–230.
32. Vial F, Johnston WT, Donnelly CA (2011) Local cattle and badger populations affect the risk of confirmed tuberculosis in British cattle herds. PLoS One 6: e18058.
33. Smith RL, Schukken YH, Lu Z, Mitchell RM, Grohn YT (2013) Development of a model to simulate infection dynamics of Mycobacterium bovis in cattle herds in the United States. J Am Vet Med Assoc 243: 411–423.
34. Hagan WA, Bruner DW, Gillespie JH (1973) Hagan's Infectious diseases of domestic animals: with special reference to etiology, diagnosis, and biologic therapy. Californie: Comstock Pub. Associates. 1385 p.
35. Gumi B, Schelling E, Firdessa R, Aseffa A, Tschopp R, et al. (2011) Prevalence of bovine tuberculosis in pastoral cattle herds in the Oromia region, southern Ethiopia. Trop Anim Health Prod 43: 1081–1087.
36. Thakur A, Sharma M, Katoch VC, Dhar P, Katoch RC (2010) A study on the prevalence of Bovine Tuberculosis in farmed dairy cattle in Himachal Pradesh. Vet World 3: 408–413.
37. Ameni G, Aseffa A, Engers H, Young D, Hewinson G, et al. (2006) Cattle husbandry in Ethiopia is a predominant factor affecting the pathology of bovine tuberculosis and gamma interferon responses to mycobacterial antigens. Clin Vaccine Immunol 13: 1030–1036.

38. Ameni G, Aseffa A, Engers H, Young D, Gordon S, et al. (2007) High prevalence and increased severity of pathology of bovine tuberculosis in Holsteins compared to zebu breeds under field cattle husbandry in central Ethiopia. Clin Vaccine Immunol 14: 1356–1361.
39. Costello E, Doherty ML, Monaghan ML, Quigley FC, O'Reilly PF (1998) A study of cattle-to-cattle transmission of Mycobacterium bovis infection. Vet J 155: 245–250.
40. O'Reilly LM, Costello E (1988) Bovine tuberculosis with special reference to the epidemiological significance of pulmonary lesions. Irish Veterinary News: 11–21.
41. Brooks-Pollock E, Roberts GO, Keeling MJ (2014) A dynamic model of bovine tuberculosis spread and control in Great Britain. Nature 511: 228–231.
42. Pouillot R, Dufour B, Durand B (2004) A deterministic and stochastic simulation model for intra-herd paratuberculosis transmission. Vet Res 35: 53–68.
43. Tanaka MM, Francis AR, Luciani F, Sisson SA (2006) Using approximate Bayesian computation to estimate tuberculosis transmission parameters from genotype data. Genetics 173: 1511–1520.
44. Sunnaker M, Busetto AG, Numminen E, Corander J, Foll M, et al. (2013) Approximate Bayesian computation. PLoS Comput Biol 9: e1002803.
45. Barnes C, Filippi S, Stumpf MPH, Thorne T (2012) Considerate approaches to constructing summary statistics for ABC model selection. Statistics and Computing 22: 1181–1197.
46. Del Moral P, Doucet A, Jasra A (2012) An adaptive sequential Monte Carlo method for approximate Bayesian computation. Statistics and Computing 22: 1009–1020.
47. Drovandi CC, Pettitt AN (2011) Estimation of parameters for macroparasite population evolution using approximate bayesian computation. Biometrics 67: 225–233.
48. Filippi S, Barnes CP, Cornebise J, Stumpf MP (2013) On optimality of kernels for approximate Bayesian computation using sequential Monte Carlo. Stat Appl Genet Mol Biol 12: 87–107.
49. Vose D (2000) Risk Analysis, A quantitative guide. Chichester: Wiley and Sons.752 p.
50. Proano-Perez F, Benitez-Ortiz W, Celi-Erazo M, Ron-Garrido L, Benitez-Capistros R, et al. (2009) Comparative intradermal tuberculin test in dairy cattle in the north of Ecuador and risk factors associated with bovine tuberculosis. Am J Trop Med Hyg 81: 1103–1109.
51. Pollock JM, Girvin RM, Lightbody KA, Clements RA, Neill SD, et al. (2000) Assessment of defined antigens for the diagnosis of bovine tuberculosis in skin test-reactor cattle. Vet Rec 146: 659–665.
52. Courcoul A, Moyen JL, Brugere L, Faye S, Henault S, et al. (2014) Estimation of sensitivity and specificity of bacteriology, histopathology and PCR for the confirmatory diagnosis of bovine tuberculosis using latent class analysis. PLoS One 9: e90334.

10

Macronutrient Optimization and Seasonal Diet Mixing in a Large Omnivore, the Grizzly Bear: A Geometric Analysis

Sean C. P. Coogan[1]*, David Raubenheimer[2], Gordon B. Stenhouse[3], Scott E. Nielsen[1]

1 Department of Renewable Resources, University of Alberta, Edmonton, Alberta, Canada, **2** The Charles Perkins Centre, Faculty of Veterinary Science, and School of Biological Science, University of Sydney, Sydney, Australia, **3** Grizzly Bear Program, Foothills Research Institute, Hinton, AB, Canada

Abstract

Nutrient balance is a strong determinant of animal fitness and demography. It is therefore important to understand how the compositions of available foods relate to required balance of nutrients and habitat suitability for animals in the wild. These relationships are, however, complex, particularly for omnivores that often need to compose balanced diets by combining their intake from diverse nutritionally complementary foods. Here we apply geometric models to understand how the nutritional compositions of foods available to an omnivorous member of the order Carnivora, the grizzly bear (*Ursus arctos* L.), relate to optimal macronutrient intake, and assess the seasonal nutritional constraints on the study population in west-central Alberta, Canada. The models examined the proportion of macronutrients that bears could consume by mixing their diet from food available in each season, and assessed the extent to which bears could consume the ratio of protein to non-protein energy previously demonstrated using captive bears to optimize mass gain. We found that non-selective feeding on ungulate carcasses provided a non-optimal macronutrient balance with surplus protein relative to fat and carbohydrate, reflecting adaptation to an omnivorous lifestyle, and that optimization through feeding selectively on different tissues of ungulate carcasses is unlikely. Bears were, however, able to dilute protein intake to an optimal ratio by mixing their otherwise high-protein diet with carbohydrate-rich fruit. Some individual food items were close to optimally balanced in protein to non-protein energy (e.g. *Hedysarum alpinum* roots), which may help explain their dietary prevalence. Ants may be consumed particularly as a source of lipids. Overall, our analysis showed that most food available to bears in the study area were high in protein relative to lipid or carbohydrate, suggesting the lack of non-protein energy limits the fitness (e.g. body size and reproduction) and population density of grizzly bears in this ecosystem.

Editor: Joanna E. Lambert, The University of Texas at San Antonio, United States of America

Funding: Funding for S. C. P. Coogan was provided by the Foothills Research Institute Grizzly Bear Program, Natural Sciences and Engineering Research Council (NSERC) of Canada, Alberta Innovates - Bio Solutions, and the Applied Conservation Ecology lab (http://www.ace-lab.org/). The funders had no role in study design, data collection and analysis, decision to publish, or preparation of the manuscript.

Competing Interests: The authors have declared that no competing interests exist.

* E-mail: scoogan@ualberta.ca

Introduction

A balanced macronutrient (protein, carbohydrate, and lipid) intake has been linked to many aspects of evolutionary fitness in animals, including fecundity [1], longevity [2], immune system function [3], obesity [4], sexual display [5], predation risk [6], body size and growth rate [7–8]. It may therefore be expected that animals are under strong selection for the ability to regulate the ratios of macronutrients eaten, through choosing foods that are balanced with respect to requirements or eating appropriate proportions of nutritionally complementary foods when consuming a mixed diet [9]. Laboratory studies have shown that a wide range of animals, including herbivores [7,10], omnivores [11–12] and carnivores [9,13–14] self-select specific ratios of macronutrients from nutritionally complementary foods, and that the selected ratios optimise performance [1,7–8,15]. Recent studies of primates, a group that is particularly amenable to direct observations of feeding in the field, have demonstrated that macronutrient ratios drive food selection also in the wild [16–18].

The generality, strength, and functional importance of macronutrient regulation provides a powerful framework for understanding the nutritional ecology of animals in the wild [19], and can inform management strategies for their conservation [20]. Few studies, however, have used the concepts of nutrient balance to understand the habitat requirements of animals, how they persist in natural environments in the face of temporal and spatial variation in food availability, and the nutritional constraints that limit populations. Such analyses are particularly pressing for large, vulnerable, ecologically important species that mix their diet from nutritionally diverse foods, such as omnivorous bears.

The natural diet of grizzly bears (*Ursus arctos* L.) has been well documented in parts of North America [21–25]. Being a generalist omnivore, the grizzly bear mixes its diet by consuming a variety of foods. Grizzly bear diets differ among regions, largely because of variation in food availability due to local climate and environmental factors [26], which results in individual and population level effects. For example, it has been suggested that the high fruit (carbohydrate) and low protein diet typical of grizzly bears in south-eastern British Columbia allows for a population with relatively small female bears with high body fat composition to live at high densities [27]. Much larger grizzly bears, and higher population densities, can be found in coastal areas where bears consume both fruit and salmon during the summer [28–29]. Food availability also varies temporally within grizzly bear populations, as bears consume food items that are seasonally available [21–24]. Additionally, individual grizzly bear diets can be highly variable, ranging from near complete carnivory to almost totally plant-based [25,30].

Macronutrient optimization has been documented in both captive and wild grizzly bears, which have been observed to self-select mixed diets of salmon (genus *Oncorhynchus*; a source of protein and lipid) and fruit (a source of carbohydrate) in proportions that optimized mass gain [31]. More recently, captive grizzly bears were shown to have optimized mass gain per unit energy intake on a self-selected average diet of 17% protein to 83% non-protein energy [32]. In the aforementioned study, grizzly bears prioritized a protein intake target over carbohydrate or lipid [32], which is common among terrestrial omnivores and herbivores [33]. Bears preferred lipid over carbohydrate as a non-protein energy source when optimizing protein intake. In the absence of lipid, however, bears were able to utilize carbohydrates with equal efficiency, suggesting that lipid and carbohydrate served as interchangeable non-protein-energy sources when optimizing protein intake [32].

In this paper, we used the geometric framework [8,34] to understand how seasonal food availability may constrain macro-nutrient optimization in wild grizzly bears of west-central Alberta, Canada. Grizzly bears in the study area are relatively small, and occur at low population densities [35]. Since small body size and low population density (both indicators of performance) suggest poor environmental conditions, our analysis was aimed at understanding nutritional factors that may limit population fitness (e.g. body size and reproduction). To this end, we integrated previously published data on bear diets [32] with estimates of food nutritional composition in order to examine the proportion of macronutrients that grizzly bears could consume by mixing their diet among seasonally available foods. We then assessed the degree to which, in different seasons, bears could consume the ratio of protein to non-protein energy previously demonstrated to optimize mass gain in captive bears [32].

Materials and Methods

Study area and diet

West-central Alberta, Canada, (general location 53°0'N, 117°0'W) includes portions of the eastern slopes of the Canadian Rocky Mountains and foothills. The climate is continental, with average summer temperatures ranging from 11.9°C in lower elevation montane subregions, to 9.4°C in the subalpine, while average winter temperatures are −7.8°C and −8.9°C respectively [36]. Average annual rainfall in montane regions is 464 mm and 568 mm in the subalpine [36]. The grizzly bear population in the study area (4.79 bears per 1000 km^2 [37]) resides in both mountainous and boreal foothills habitats, and large elevation gradients result in differences in resource distribution and timing of plant phenology that influence the dietary intake of bears [24,38–39].

During the post-hibernation pre-green up period (approximately late April to late May) the diet of grizzly bears in the study area is composed primarily of alpine sweetvetch (*Hedysarum alpinum*) roots and ungulates, although small mammals can make up a portion of their diet [24].Ungulate consumption is higher throughout the active season among bears living in lower elevation foothills habitats than bears residing in mountainous areas, while sweetvetch roots are consumed more heavily and for longer periods by bears in the mountains. The principal ungulate prey of grizzly bear in the study area are moose (*Alces alces*), white-tailed deer (*Odocoileus virginianus*), mule deer (*O. hemionus*), and elk (*Cervus elaphus*) [24,40]. Woodland caribou (*Rangifer tarandus caribou*) also occur in the more northerly Kakwa region of west-central Alberta. Ungulate consumption peaks in June and remains relatively high in July. Green vegetation becomes common in grizzly bear diets in June with consumption peaking in July. Commonly consumed native forbs include horsetails (*Equisetum* spp.) and cow parsnip (*Heracleum lanatum*) [24]. Forbs associated with anthropogenic disturbance (e.g., roads, oil and gas, mining, forestry, and seismic activity), such as dandelion (*Taraxacum officinale*), clover (*Trifolium* spp.), and alfalfa (*Medicago sattiva*) are also available to grizzly bears [24,38,40]. Sweetvetch root consumption is generally low during July; however, bears in the mountains continue to consume roots throughout the active season likely due to environmental gradients allowing for prolonged availability of nutritious roots and limited availability of animal-based foods [24,39]. Fruit is prominent in the diet of grizzly bears in west-central Alberta from as early as late July, with consumption peaking in September [24]. Fruit most commonly consumed by bears in the study area include russet buffaloberry (*Shepherdia canadensis*) and those of the blueberry-huckleberry complex (*Vaccinium* spp.); however, several other species are consumed in lesser quantities [24]. The consumption of green vegetation declines during the fruit season, while ungulate consumption continues for bears in the foothills, but is lower among bears in the mountains [24]. Insects, primarily ants, are consumed mostly in July and August. In late fall, approximately mid-September to mid-October, a decline in the variety of available food resources has bears consuming a diet similar to the pre-green-up period: alpine sweetvetch roots once again becomes a primary food resource, and to a lesser extent ungulates [24]. Unlike the pregreen-up period, however, fruit is also often consumed by bears in the late-fall period [24].

Macronutrient estimates

Macronutrient estimates for several food items were obtained from previous bear studies, the USDA National Nutrient Database [41], and other sources (Supporting Information S1). Chosen food items were considered generally sufficiently abundant for bears to effectively mix their diet based upon previous diet studies in the study area [24,40]. We used available carbohydrate estimates for foods only when total dietary fibre (TDF) was reported in order to more closely approximate the digestion of bears [42] and to better compare with the study of Erlenbach et al. [32] where TDF was determined via the Prosky method. Fibre estimates, however, were not often reported as TDF, and we were therefore limited by a lack of suitable available carbohydrate estimates for foods, especially vegetation. Since complete or suitable macronutrient estimates for some vegetation were unknown to us, we included vegetation proxies and combined some estimates from different sources to estimate available carbohydrate (Supporting Information S1). For example, we used celery (*Apium graveolens* var. *dulce*) as a proxy for cow parsnip because they are similar in nutrient content [43]. Limited data analysis for some grizzly bear plant foods are presented in supplementary material (Supporting Information S1) and were used to inform macronutrient estimates. We used the USDA National Nutrient Database [41] to estimate macronutrient values for some wild ungulate tissues not reported in grizzly bear literature (including brain, kidney, liver, tongue, eyeball, and bone marrow) by using estimates from both wild and domestic animals (Supporting Information S1). We note that methods of diet composition may be different among studies, nutritional composition of food available to bears may differ from published data, and that food composition varies with respect to season and environment [21,39,44].

Since grizzly bears tend to consume ungulates in their entirety with the exception of hide and large bones [28], we estimated the macronutrient content of a wholly consumed ungulates (hereinafter referred to as "non-selective consumption"; Supporting Information S1). For the first estimate, we assumed an ungulate carcass was composed of five edible components (90.2% skeletal muscle, 1% brain, 3% bone marrow, 3.8% liver, and 2% adipose tissue) as in Kuipers et al. [45]. We then averaged macronutrient estimates, including available carbohydrate, for each ungulate component per season, weighted them according to the proportion of edible carcass, and summed the components to estimate the macronutrient content of a non-selectively consumed ungulate (Supporting Information S1). Estimates for bone marrow and adipose tissue were not averaged as we used only single estimates for each component. A second estimate of non-selective ungulate consumption for moose (minus hide and injesta) was derived from Hundertmark et al. [46] (Supporting Information S1). Carbohydrate was not reported in Hundertmark et al. [46], as such we assumed available carbohydrate to be negligible. A third model of non-selective ungulate consumption was derived from McCullough and Ullrey [47] for white-tailed deer. We used data presented in Table 1 and Table 2 of McCullough and Ullrey [47] to estimate the macronutrient composition of male and female deer of three different age classes (fawn, yearling and adult) minus hide (hair and skin), hooves, and antlers (where present). Estimates from McCullough and Ullrey [47] were derived from fall and winter animals following a high food resource year and as such were in excellent body condition (high body fat). We also determined the ratio of percent crude protein to lipid of an optimally balanced non-selectively consumed ungulate on a mass basis by back-calculating from the optimal ratio of 17% protein to 83% non-protein metabolizable energy (Supporting Information S1). We considered carbohydrates to be negligible for this estimate.

Modelling approach

We used right-angled mixture triangles (RMTs) to examine the relationships between seasonal food availability to grizzly bears, macronutrient availability and macronutrient requirements [34] (see also [48]). RMTs represent 3-component (e.g. protein, fat and carbohydrate) compositions of mixtures as Cartesian points in a multi-dimensional nutrient space. We used Erlenbach et al. [32] as the basis for grizzly bear macronutrient requirements, where the ratio of 17% protein to 83% non-protein energy was considered optimal because it maximised growth efficiency. Grizzly bears also showed a strong regulatory preference for the protein intake target despite different diets, with lipid and carbohydrate being interchangeable components of non-protein energy intake [32]. Within RMTs fat and available carbohydrates were represented on the two primary (x and y) axes, and crude protein on the third, implicit, axis (the z axis). The implicit component varies inversely as distance from the origin increases [34]. Macronutrients were expressed as a percentage of total metabolizable energy (kcal) per food item (Supporting Information S1) using Atwater factors [49].

In order to examine temporal patterns in macronutrient availability, we created RMTs for four periods of the grizzly bear active season. These seasons were: 1) pre-green-up (approximately late April to late May); 2) forb and graminoid season (approximately June through July); 3) fruit season (approximately early August to mid-September); and 4) late fall (approximately mid-September to mid-October). After plotting food items, we created line segments between food points to form minimum convex polygons around the "nutrient space" potentially accessible to bears during each season. We used non-selective ungulate consumption estimates when creating nutrient space polygons in order to better approximate the nutrient space available to grizzly bears. The estimates from McCullough and Ullrey [47] were used for all seasons, but may overestimate the fat content of ungulates during pregreen-up, graminoid and forb, and berry seasons. Selective consumption of fatty ungulate components (e.g. bone, marrow and brain) were considered unlikely to contribute substantially to a balanced diet due to their size [45] and relative availability; however, we plotted macronutrient estimates of individual organs in order to illustrate the variety in nutrient composition among body parts. Small mammals were omitted from the nutrient space because they are generally a minor diet item and limited in size, although they may be a more prominent food in the diet of some bears ([24], unpublished data). In order to assess whether bears could achieve an optimal macronutrient intake, we plotted the intake target (17% protein to 83% non-protein energy) previously self-selected by captive bears, as well as the macronutrient composition of diets used to determine the intake target [32]. Overlap between the nutrient space polygon and intake target line would indicate that bears could optimize protein to non-protein energy intake by mixing their diet among seasonally available food.

Results

Pregreen-up period

RMT analysis of the macronutrient content of seasonal foods indicated that grizzly bears were unable to reach the macronutrient target of 17% protein during the pregreen-up period by mixing their diet between sweetvetch roots and whole ungulates (Fig. 1a); however, bears could come relatively close to the intake target by consuming sweetvetch root (23% protein: 77% non-protein energy), high-fat ungulates if available (28% protein: 72% non-protein energy), or a combination of the two. Alpine sweetvetch consumption would improve the macronutrient balance of bears consuming lower-fat ungulates such as our estimates for moose (53% protein: 47% non-protein energy) and average ungulate derived from Kuipers et al. [45] (70% protein: 30% non-protein energy) The carbohydrate content of brain and liver was estimated to contribute 0.5% to total metabolizable non-protein energy of an ungulate carcass based on the proportions of Kuipers et al [45]. In order for an ungulate carcass to be composed of an optimal ratio of protein to non-protein energy, it would need to have a percent mass ratio of crude protein to lipid of 0.433:1 (Supporting Information S1). Conversely, an optimal ungulate carcass would need to contain approximately 2.3 X more lipid than protein on a mass basis. These ratios are the same for both percent dry matter and percent fresh (wet) matter estimates. Alpine sweetvetch root was close to optimally balanced in protein to non-protein energy due to its relatively high carbohydrate content. Small mammals would contribute mainly protein to the diet.

Graminoid and forb season

During the graminoid and forb season, the addition of vegetation and ants to the diet allows bears to come closer to optimal protein intake by consuming a wider variety of carbohydrates and lipids (Fig. 1b). Specifically, a diet high in ants (approximately 30% protein: 70% lipid energy) would allow bears to compose a diet similar to the optimal lipid-rich diets chosen by captive bears, while some vegetation (horsetails and celery (proxy for cow parsnip)) had close to optimal ratios of macronutrients (25% protein: 75% non-protein energy, and 21% protein: 79% non-protein energy respectively). The ratio of protein to

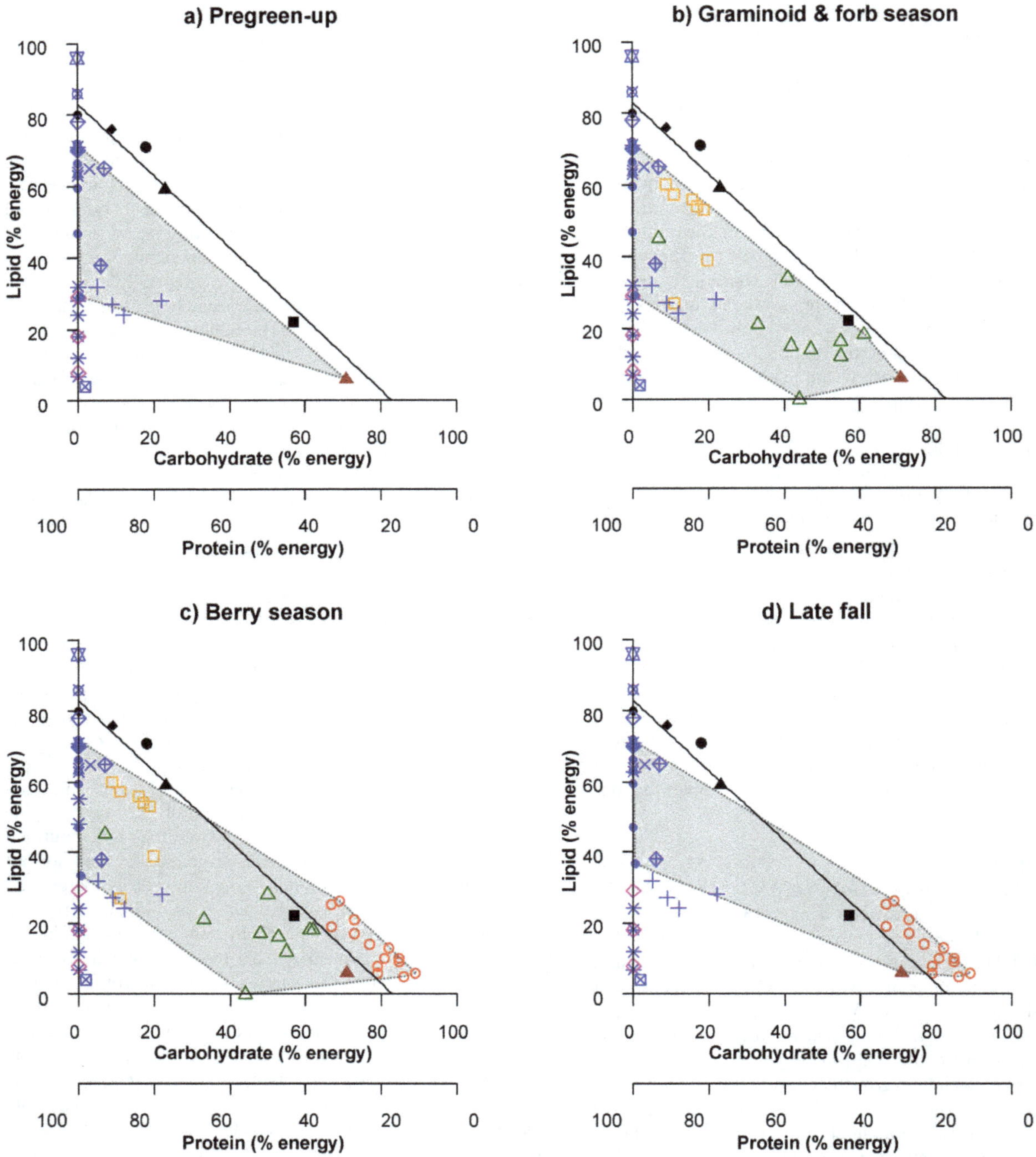

Figure 1. Right-angled mixture triangle (RMT) plots [34] **depicting the estimated macronutrient (lipid, available carbohydrate, and crude protein) content of seasonally available foods consumed by grizzly bears in west-central Alberta, given as a percentage of metabolizable energy.** Protein is represented by the third *z*-axis which varies inversely with distance from the origin. Seasons are defined based on major changes in grizzly bear diet, and include: a) pregreen-up; b) graminoid and forb season; c) berry season; and d) late fall. For reference, optimal diets self selected by captive grizzly bears [32] are shown as black symbols and marked in the legend with an asterisk (*), while the 17% protein to 83% non-protein energy intake target is shown as a black line. The grey-shaded polygon indicates the estimated nutrient space available to grizzly bears consuming seasonal foods. Overlap between the nutrient space polygon and the intake target line indicates that an optimal diet may be achieved during a season. The food items plotted do not include variation and are meant to give a general perspective.

non-protein energy in available foods is higher than optimal during this season.

Berry season

During the berry season, bears were able to optimize their macronutrient intake by mixing high-carbohydrate (67–89% metabolizable energy) fruit with all other food (ants, ungulates, sweetvetch root and green vegetation) in the nutrient space (Fig.1c). An optimal ratio of non-protein energy could be composed of a high carbohydrate/low lipid diet (approximately 78% carbohydrate and 5% lipid) to moderate carbohydrate/moderate lipid diet (approximately 33% carbohydrate and 50%

lipid). Several individual fruits were close to optimally balanced in protein to non-protein energy.

Late fall

During late fall, grizzly bears can still potentially optimize their protein to non-protein energy intake by consuming fruit with alpine sweetvetch and whole ungulates (Fig. 1d). In the absence of fruit, grizzly bears face a diet that is similar in macronutrient composition to the pregreen-up period.

Discussion

Our analysis suggests that grizzly bears in west-central Alberta optimize macronutrient intake during seasons in which fruit is available. Fruit is commonly known as an important resource for bears, and is actively sought after, forming the bulk of bear diets during late-summer and early-fall when available [24,50]. The ability of bears to optimize their macronutrient intake by consuming fruit helps explain why it is such a highly desirable food item. The timing of fruit availability is also critical: berry season coincides with the hyperphagic period in which bears attempt to accumulate sufficient fat reserves to support hibernation and female reproduction costs [51–53]. Beyond simply supplying energy to hyperphagic bears, fruit enables grizzly bears to optimize mass gain per unit energy intake. The availability of fruit, therefore, has direct implications on the reproductive success and fitness of grizzly bears in the study area.

Diet studies within the study area [24,40] report that bears in the foothills have a much more carnivorous diet than bears in the mountains where ungulates and other animals are less abundant [24]. Our analysis shows that it is unlikely for grizzly bears to be able to optimize their diet by feeding non-selectively on ungulates, given that a balanced ungulate carcass would need to contain over two times the lipid as protein. For example, assuming an average crude protein content of 20.7% (fresh weight) for a moose carcass [46] would require a lipid content of 48.3% to be optimally balanced (assuming carbohydrates to be negligible). Such a high fat content is unlikely given that the average moose carcass in the same study contained 8.8% lipid with a range of 0.3–19.4% [46]. Additionally, the majority of ungulate consumption in the study area occurs during spring [24], a time when prey tend to be lean [44,54]. However, despite not being perfectly balanced, ungulates provide more digestible protein and energy than plant-based grizzly bear foods [45]. Vegetation is complementary with ungulate consumption, in that it dilutes the level of protein in the diet and brings the diet closer to the protein intake target. This seems to be reflected in the diet of bears within the study area, which maintain the consumption of graminoids, forbs, and horsetails during periods of high ungulate intake [24]. Grizzly bears tend to gain lean mass in the spring [28] which seems consistent with a high protein diet.

Since fat-rich resources are relatively scarce in west-central Alberta, we would expect fatty ungulate tissues to be highly sought after. Selective feeding behaviour has been observed in Alaskan grizzly bears that fed on lipid-rich brain tissues and roe of spawning salmon [55]; however, as previously mentioned both wild and captive bears tend to consume ungulates in their entirety with the exception of hide and large bones [28]. It may be possible that bears in the study area selectively eat high fat ungulate tissues in order to increase their lipid intake, but presumably there are strong ecological constraints on availability to prevent bears from acquiring enough carcases to optimize their diet this way. This would be especially relevant for scavenged carcasses, as lipid rich tissue is often the first to be consumed and spoils more readily [45].

Certain individual foods were closely balanced in protein to non-protein energy, and these foods are also prominent in the grizzly bear diet. For example, celery (proxy for cow parsnip), horsetail, and dandelion were closely balanced in macronutrients. The near optimal macronutrient balance of sweetvetch root may help explain why it makes up much of the bear diet during pregreen-up and late fall [24]. Yet, despite favorable macronutrient balance, plant foods other than fruit are often low in nutrient concentration. Grizzly bears may respond to high levels of non-nutritional fibre and low macronutrient concentrations in roots, graminoids, and forbs by consuming these foods in greater quantities (a phenomenon observed in other animals [8]). Ultimately, however, grizzly bears are constrained by intake rates and stomach capacity when consuming energy- and macronutrient-dilute herbaceous foods [56]. Interestingly, for vegetation which we could estimate phenological changes in macronutrients, a decline in protein content from graminoid and forb season to berry season made these plants more closely balanced in macronutrients; however, nutrient concentration in these plants is generally lower and fibre content higher [21,23].

The macronutrient balance of ants makes them a potentially important food item for grizzly bears. Our results suggest that lipid content of ants makes them a particularly valuable food resource, because they allow bears to expand their nutrient space in the absence of high-fat ungulates and consume a diet that is close to the balance offered by preferred high-lipid diets. As well, ants have previously been suggested to provide necessary amino acids to bears on largely vegetarian diets [57]. Ants, however, are generally not heavily consumed by grizzly bears in the study area and only for a limited time [24]. Therefore, the dietary impact of ants on the study area population is likely limited.

Most food available to bears in the study area were high in protein relative to lipid or carbohydrate, and it is not unreasonable to suggest that a paucity of lipid-rich resources in part limits the study area population in terms of body size and population density relative to bears in ecosystems that provide more fatty foods (e.g., Yellowstone, and coastal British Columbia/Alaska). Yet, in the face of a suboptimal diet, generalist omnivores such as the grizzly bear may have a high capacity for capitalizing on excess nutrients in nutritionally imbalanced foods, even if it means deviating further from optimal nutrient intake [8]. One explanation for this is that a generalist species that has over-ingested a particular macronutrient has a relatively higher probability of encountering a complimentary food that enables it to correct the nutrient imbalance, thereby rendering the initial excess nutrient useable while also balancing the nutrient deficiency in the complimentary food [58]. This ability to capitalize on excess nutrients may be especially true of animals that readily store excess energy as fat [58], which likely includes grizzly bears. Given that grizzly bears tend to consume large amounts of seasonal food resources, they may be able to effectively mix their diet across longer time periods, which has been previously suggested [27], but has yet to be demonstrated.

While an optimal ratio of protein to non-protein energy could be consumed by grizzly bears in west-central Alberta, the absolute amount of food consumed would need to be adequate to support maintenance and growth. The possibility for growth is obviously not always available to bears given inter-annual variation in both ungulate densities and berry production. Other factors may limit the availability of food resources to individual grizzly bears, including sexual segregation of habitats [30]. Yet despite the challenges, years of high resource availability should be those in which bears experience the greatest growth, not solely because of increased energy availability, but also due to the increased potential for optimizing macronutrient intake through a mixed diet.

As with other wild animals [59–60], there are knowledge gaps regarding the nutritional compositions of resources consumed by grizzly bears, and, as in many nutritional ecology studies [60], protein and energy dominate the nutritional currencies used when investigating grizzly bear ecology. While such an approach is often appropriate, this work further demonstrates the importance of expanding the study of grizzly bear nutritional ecology to include other nutrients and the interactions between them. Indeed, an important priority is to extend the dimensionality of such models, to include not only macronutrients but also, for example, essential amino and fatty acids as well as micronutrients. Such studies are, of course, challenging, but we believe that the power of multi-dimensional nutritional analyses outweighs the effort [33].

Supporting Information

Supporting Information S1 Nutritional estimates and information used to model the macronutrient content of seasonal grizzly bear foods in west-central Alberta, Canada.

Acknowledgments

We thank the Academic Editor and two anonymous reviewers for providing thoughtful reviews that improved this manuscript. We also thank Joy Erlenbach and Charles Robbins for providing helpful suggestions and comments on an earlier draft of this paper.

Author Contributions

Conceived and designed the experiments: SCPC DR SEN. Performed the experiments: SCPC DR. Analyzed the data: SCPC DR. Contributed reagents/materials/analysis tools: SEN GBS. Wrote the paper: SCPC. Critically reviewed and revised the manuscript: DR GBS SEN.

References

1. Lee KP, Simpson SJ, Clissold FJ, Brooks R, Ballard JW, et al. (2008) Lifespan and reproduction in *Drosophilia*: new insights from nutritional geometry. Proc Natl Acad Sci U S A 105: 2498–2503.
2. Piper MD, Partridge WL, Raubenheimer D, Simpson SJ (2011) Dietary restriction and aging: a unifying perspective. Cellular Metab 14: 154–160.
3. Cotter SC, Simpson SJ, Raubenheimer D, Wilson K (2010) Macronutrient balance mediates trade-offs between immune function and life history traits. Funct Ecol 25: 186–198.
4. Simpson SJ, Raubenheimer D (2005) Obesity: the protein leverage hypothesis. Obes Rev 6: 133–142.
5. Maklakov AA, Simpson SJ, Zajitschek F, Hall MD, Dessmann J, et al. (2008) Sex-specific fitness effects of nutrient intake on reproduction and lifespan. Curr Biol 18: 1062–1066.
6. Hawlena D, Schmitz OJ (2010) Herbivore physiological response to predation risk and implications for ecosystem nutrient dynamics. Proc Natl Acad Sci U S A 107: 15503–15507.
7. Simpson SJ, Sibly RM, Lee KP, Behmer ST, Raubenheimer D (2004) Optimal foraging when regulating intake of multiple nutrients. Anim Behav 68: 1299–1311.
8. Raubenheimer D, Simpson SJ (1997) Integrative models of nutrient balancing: application to insects and vertebrates. Nutr Res Rev 10: 151–179.
9. Hewson-Hughes AK, Hewson-Hughes VL, Colyer A, Miller AT, McGrane SJ, et al. (2012) Geometric analysis of macronutrient selection in breeds of the domestic dog, *Canis lupus familiaris*. Behav Ecol 24: 293–304.
10. Wehi PM, Raubenheimer D, Morgan-Richards M (2013) Tolerance for nutrient imbalance in an intermittently feeding herbivorous cricket, the Wellington Tree Weta. PLoS ONE 8(12) e84641 doi: 10.1371/journal.pone.0084641.
11. Raubenheimer D, Zemke-white WL, Phillips RJ, Clements KD (2005) Algal macronutrients and food selection by the omnivorous marine fish, *Girella tricuspidata*. Ecology 86: 2601–2610.
12. Raubenheimer D, Jones SA (2006) Nutritional imbalances in an extreme generalist omnivore: tolerance and recovery through complementary food selection. Anim Behav 71: 1253–1262.
13. Hewson-Hughes AK, Hewson-Hughes VL, Colyer A, Miller AT, Hall SR, et al. (2013) Consistent proportional macronutrient intake selected by adult domestic cats (Felis catus) despite variations in macronutrient and moisture content of foods offered. J Comp Physiol B 183: 525–536 doi: 10.1007/s00360-012-0727-y
14. Mayntz D, Nielsen V, Sorensen A, Toft S, Raubenheimer D, et al. (2009) Balancing of protein and lipid intake by a mammalian carnivore, the mink, Mustela vison. Anim Behav 77: 349–355.
15. Jensen K, Mayntz D, Toft S, Clissold F, Hunt J, et al. (2012) Optimal foraging for specific nutrients in predatory beetles. Proc R Soc B doi: 10.1098/rspb.2011.2410.
16. Felton AM, Felton A, Raubenheimer D, Simpson SJ, Foley WJ, et al. (2009) Protein content of diets dictates the daily energy intake of a free-ranging primate. Behav Ecol 20: 685–690.
17. Rothman JM, Raubenheimer D, Chapman CA (2011) Nutritional geometry: gorillas prioritize non-protein energy while consuming surplus protein. Biol Lett 7: 847–849.
18. Johnson CA, Raubenheimer D, Rothman JM, Clarke D, Swedell L (2013) 30 days in the life: daily nutrient balancing in a wild chacma baboon. PLoS ONE 8: e70438. doi:10.1371/journal.pone.0070383
19. Kearney M, Simpson SJ, Raubenheimer D, Helmuth B (2010) Modelling the ecological niche from functional traits. Phil Trans R Soc B 365: 3469–3483.
20. Raubenheimer D, Simpson SJ, Tait A (2012) Match and mismatch: conservation, physiology, nutritional ecology and the timescales of biological adaptation. Phil Trans R Soc B 367: 1628–1646.
21. Hamer D, Herrero S (1987) Grizzly bear food and habitat in the front ranges of Banff National Park, Alberta. Pp. 199–213 in Bears—their Biology and Management: Proceedings of the 7th International Conference on Bear Biology and Management, Williamsburg, Va., and Plityice Lakes, Yugoslavia, February and March 1986 (P. Zager, ed.). International Association for Bear Research and Management, Washington, D.C.
22. Mattson DJ (1991) Food habits of Yellowstone grizzly bears, 1977–1987. Can J Zool 69: 1619–1629.
23. McLellan BN, Hovey FW (1995) The diet of grizzly bears in the Flathead River drainage of southeastern British Columbia. Can J Zool 73: 704–712.
24. Munro RHM, Nielsen SE, Price MH, Stenhouse GB, Boyce MS (2006) Seasonal and diel patterns of grizzly bear diet and activity in west-central Alberta. J Mammal 87: 1112–1121.
25. Edwards MA, Derocher AE, Hobson KA, Branigan M, Nagy JA (2010) Fast carnivores and slow herbivores: differential foraging strategies among grizzly bears in the Canadian Arctic. Oecologia 165: 877–889.
26. Bojarska K, Selva N (2011) Spatial patterns in brown bear *Ursus arctos* diet: the role of geographical and environmental factors. Mamm Rev 42: 120–143.
27. McLellan BN (2011) Implications of a high-energy and low-protein diet on the body composition, fitness, and competitive abilities of black (*Ursus americanus*) and grizzly (*Ursus arctos*) bears. Can J Zool 89: 546–558.
28. Hilderbrand GV, Schwartz CC, Robbins CT, Jacoby ME, Hanley TA, et al. (1999) The importance of meat, particularly salmon, to body size, population productivity, and Conservation of North American brown bears. Can J Zool 77: 132–138.
29. Hilderbrand GV, Jenkins SG, Schwartz CC, Hanley TA, Robbins CT (1999) Effect of seasonal differences in dietary meat intake on changes in body mass and composition in wild and captive brown bears. Can J Zool 77: 1623–1630.
30. Rode KD, Farley SD, Robbins CT (2006) Sexual dimorphism, reproductive strategy, and human activities determine resource use by brown bears. Ecology 87: 2636–2646.
31. Robbins CT, Fortin JK, Rode KD, Farley SD, Shipley LA, et al. (2007) Optimizing protein intake as a foraging strategy to maximize mass gain in an omnivore. Oikos 116: 1675–1682.
32. Erlenbach JA, Rode KD, Raubenheimer D, Robbins CT (2014) Macronutrient optimization and energy maximization determine diets of brown bears. J Mammal 95: 160–168.
33. Simpson SJ, Raubenheimer D (2012) The nature of nutrition: a unifying framework from animal adaptation to human obesity. Princeton: Princeton University Press. 256 p.
34. Raubenheimer D (2011) Toward a quantitative nutritional ecology: the right-angled mixture triangle. Ecol Monogr 81: 407–427.
35. Alberta Sustainable Resource Development, and Alberta Conservation Association (2010) Status of the grizzly bear (*Ursus arctos*) in Alberta: update 2010. Alberta Sustainable Resource Development. Wildlife Status Report No. 37 (Update 2010). Available: http://srd.alberta.ca/fishwildlife/speciesatrisk/DetailedStatus/Mammals/documents/Status-GrizzlyBear-inAlberta-Feb2010.pdf. Accessed 03 December 2013.
36. Beckingham JD, Corns IGW, Archibald JH (1996) Field guide to ecosites of west-central Alberta. Edmonton, Natural Resources of Canada, Canadian Forest Service, Northwest Region, Northern Forest Centre. 540 p.
37. Alberta Grizzly Bear Inventory Team (2005) 2004 population inventory and density estimates for the Alberta 3B and 4B grizzly bear management area. Alberta Sustainable Resource Development, Fish and Wildlife Division, Edmonton. Available: http://www.srd.alberta.ca/FishWildlife/WildlifeManagement/BearManagement/GrizzlyBears/documents/GrizzlyBear-DNAPopulationEstimate2004-Jul29-2005.pdf. Accessed 03 December 2013.

38. Nielsen SE, McDermid GE, Stenhouse GB, Boyce MS (2010) Dynamic wildlife habitat models: Seasonal foods and mortality risk predict occupancy-abundance and habitat selection in grizzly bears. Biol Conserv 143: 1623–1634.
39. Coogan SCP, Nielsen SE, Stenhouse GB (2012) Spatial and temporal heterogeneity creates a "brown tide" in root phenology and nutrition. ISRN Ecol 2012: 10. doi:10.5402/2012/618257
40. Cristescu B (2013) Grizzly bear response to open-pit mining in western Alberta, Canada. PhD thesis, Department of Biological Sciences, University of Alberta, Edmonton, AB, Canada. Available at: https://era.library.ualberta.ca/public/view/item/uuid:a0b36704-5571-4238-a9c9-7f7c55941ec0.
41. U. S. Department of Agriculture, Agricultural Research Service (2013) USDA National Nutrient Database for Standard Reference, Release 26. Available at: http://ndb.nal.usda.gov/. Accessed 03 December 2013.
42. Pritchard GT, Robbins CT (1990) Digestive and metabolic efficiencies of grizzly and black bears. Can J Zool 68: 1645–1651.
43. Kuhnlein HV (1990) Nutrient values in indigenous wild plant greens and roots used by the Nuxalk people of Bella Coola, British Columbia. J Food Compost Anal 3: 38–46.
44. Worden KA, Pekins PJ (1995) Seasonal change in feed intake, body composition, and metabolic rate of white-tailed deer. Can J Zool 73: 452–457.
45. Kuipers RS, Luxwolda MF, Dijck-Brouwer DAJ, Eaton SB, Crawford MA, et al. (2010) Estimated macronutrient and fatty acid intakes from an East African paleolithic diet. Brit J Nutr 104: 1666–1687 doi: 10.1017/S0007114510002679
46. Hundertmark KJ, Schwartz CC, Stephenson TA (1997) Estimation of body composition in moose. Federal Aid in Wildlife Restoration Study 1.42, Alaska Department of Fish and Game, Juneau, Alaska.
47. McCullough DR, Ullrey DE (1983) Proximate mineral and gross energy composition of white-tailed deer. J Wildl Manag 47: 430–441.
48. Raubenheimer D, Rothman JM (2013) Nutritional ecology of entomophagy in humans and other primates. Annu Rev Entomol 58: 141–160.
49. Merrill AL, Watt BK (1973) Energy value of foods: basis and derivation. Washington, DC: Agriculture Handbook 74, U.S. Government Printing Office. p 105.
50. Welch CA, Keay J, Kendall KC, Robbins CT (1997) Constraints on frugivory by bears. Ecology 78: 1105–1119.
51. Farley SD, Robbins CT (1995) Lactation, hibernation, and mass dynamics of American black and grizzly bears. Can J Zool 73: 2216–2222.
52. Hildebrand GV, Scwartz CC, Robbins CT, Hanley TA (2000) Effect of hibernation and reproductive status on body mass and condition of coastal brown bears. J Wildl Manage 64: 178–183.
53. López-Alfaro C, Robbins CT, Zedrosser A, Nielsen SE (2013) Energetics of hibernation and reproductive trade-offs in brown bears. Ecol Modell 270: 1–10.
54. Delgiudice GD, Mech LD, Seal US (1990) Effects of winter undernutrition on body composition and physiological profiles of white-tailed deer. J Wildl Manag 54: 539–550.
55. Gende SM, Quinn TP, Wilson MF (2001) Consumption choice by bears feeding on salmon. Oecologia 127: 372–382.
56. Rode KD, Robbins CT, Shipley LA (2001) Constraints on herbivory by grizzly bears. Oecologia 128: 62–71.
57. Redford KH, Dorea JG (1984) The nutritional value of invertebrates with emphasis on ants and termites as food for mammals. J Zool 203: 385–395.
58. Raubenheimer D, Simpson SJ (2004) Organismal stoichiometry: quantifying non-independence among food components. Ecology 85: 1203–1216.
59. Clements KD, Raubenheimer D, Choat JH (2009) Nutritional ecology of marine herbivorous fishes: ten years on. Funct Ecol 23: 79–92.
60. Raubenheimer D, Simpson SJ, Mayntz D (2009) Nutrition, ecology and nutritional ecology: toward an integrated framework. Funct Ecol 23: 4–16.

11

Fast Food Consumption and Gestational Diabetes Incidence in the SUN Project

Ligia J. Dominguez[1]*, Miguel A. Martínez-González[2], Francisco Javier Basterra-Gortari[2,3], Alfredo Gea[2], Mario Barbagallo[1], Maira Bes-Rastrollo[2]*

1 Geriatric Unit - Department of Internal Medicine and Specialties, University of Palermo, Palermo, Sicily, Italy, **2** Department of Preventive Medicine and Public Health, University of Navarra, Pamplona, Navarra, Spain, and CIBER Fisiopatologia de la Obesidad y Nutricion (CIBERobn), Instituto de Salud Carlos III, Madrid, Spain, **3** Department of Internal Medicine (Endocrinology), Hospital Reina Sofia, Tudela, Navarra, Spain

Abstract

Background: Gestational diabetes prevalence is increasing, mostly because obesity among women of reproductive age is continuously escalating. We aimed to investigate the incidence of gestational diabetes according to the consumption of fast food in a cohort of university graduates.

Methods: The prospective dynamic "Seguimiento Universidad de Navarra" (SUN) cohort included data of 3,048 women initially free of diabetes or previous gestational diabetes who reported at least one pregnancy between December 1999 and March 2011. Fast food consumption was assessed through a validated 136-item semi-quantitative food frequency questionnaire. Fast food was defined as the consumption of hamburgers, sausages, and pizza. Three categories of fast food were established: low (0–3 servings/month), intermediate (>3 servings/month and ≤2 servings/week) and high (>2 servings/week). Non-conditional logistic regression models were used to adjust for potential confounders.

Results: We identified 159 incident cases of gestational diabetes during follow-up. After adjusting for age, baseline body mass index, total energy intake, smoking, physical activity, family history of diabetes, cardiovascular disease/hypertension at baseline, parity, adherence to Mediterranean dietary pattern, alcohol intake, fiber intake, and sugar-sweetened soft drinks consumption, fast food consumption was significantly associated with a higher risk of incident gestational diabetes, with multivariate adjusted OR of 1.31 (95% conficence interval [CI]:0.81–2.13) and 1.86 (95% CI: 1.13–3.06) for the intermediate and high categories, respectively, versus the lowest category of baseline fast food consumption (p for linear trend: 0.007).

Conclusion: Our results suggest that pre-pregnancy higher consumption of fast food is an independent risk factor for gestational diabetes.

Editor: Rudolf Kirchmair, Medical University Innsbruck, Austria

Funding: The SUN Study has received funding from the Spanish Ministry of Health Government (current grants PI10/02658, PI10/02293, RD06/0045, G03/140 and PI13/00615), the Navarra Regional Government (45/2011) and the University of Navarra. AG is supported by a FPU fellowship from the Spanish Government. Funding sources had no role in the design, collection, analysis, and interpretation of the data; in the writing, and in the decision to submit the paper for publication.

Competing Interests: The authors have declared that no competing interests exist.

* Email: ligia.dominguez@unipa.it (LJD); mbes@unav.es (MBR)

Introduction

Gestational diabetes mellitus (GDM), traditionally defined as carbohydrate intolerance first diagnosed during pregnancy [1], has long been recognized as a risk factor for a number of unfavorable outcomes. These include short- and long-term complications for mothers (i.e., preeclampsia or eclampsia, and type 2 diabetes after delivery), and for offspring (i.e., macrosomia, increased likelihood of trauma at birth, cesarean delivery, and neonatal metabolic abnormalities, such as hypoglycemia or hyperbilirubinemia) [1,2]. GDM prevalence is increasing, mostly because obesity among women of reproductive age is continuously escalating [3–5]. It has been reported that gestational diabetes affects 1–14% of all pregnancies in the US [1], and about 2–6%of pregnancies in Europe [5]. A recent meta-analysis of RCTs suggested that interventions on glucose control/monitoring, diet, or pharmacological treatment including insulin, did not significantly reduce the risk of adverse outcomes (i.e. cesarean delivery and perinatal or neonatal death) [6]. Hence, the identification of modifiable risk factors, such as excess adiposity, decreased physical activity, and unhealthy diet for the prevention of gestational diabetes is criticalin order to avoid associated harmful outcomes [7].

Several observational studies have related some pre-pregnancy dietary factors with GDM risk. An inverse association between pre-pregnancy adherence to healthful dietary patterns and gestational diabetes incidence has been reported [8]. Low fiber intakes or high dietary glycemic index [9], high red meat/ processed meat consumptions [10], and high intakes of animal fat and cholesterol [11] have all been associated with an elevated risk of GDM.

Previous studies have suggested that Western-style fast food, which is calorically dense and usually served in large portions, is a determinant of weight gain, insulin resistance, and type 2 diabetes incidence [12,13]. However, the association of fast food consumption with GDM risk remains unknown. Therefore, we conducted the present analyses to appraise whether fast food consumption (hamburgers, sausages, and pizza) was associated with GDM risk in the SUN project ("Seguimiento Universidad de Navarra", University of Navarra Follow-up).

Materials and Methods

Study population

The SUN project is a prospective dynamic cohort study entirely composed of university graduates. The recruitment started in 1999 and it is permanently open. The design and methods utilized in the SUN study have been previously described in detail [14,15]. In brief, graduates from the University of Navarra and other Spanish universities, registered nurses and other health professionals from different Spanish provinces were invited to participate by a mailed questionnaire. The study protocol was approved by the Institutional Review Board of the University of Navarra and the initial response to the questionnaire was considered as informed consent to participate. After the baseline assessment, participants receive a follow-up questionnaire every two years on diet, lifestyle, risk factors, and medical conditions.

For the present analyses we examined the last available database as of the 1st of December 2013. From a total 13,231 women, we included 12,456 women who had answered the baseline questionnaire before the 1st of March 2011, to have enough time to answer the first follow-up questionnaire. Up to that date, 3,137 pregnant women were identified among them. Women were excluded from the analyses if they reported extremely low (below percentile 1) or high (above percentile 99) values for total energy intake (n = 67), had prevalent or previous gestational diabetes (n = 10), or had a previous diagnosis of diabetes (n = 17). Women who reported gestational diabetes in a previous pregnancy were not included in the analyses because they were thought to be more likely to have changed their diet and lifestyle during the next pregnancy to prevent recurrent gestational diabetes. The final analytic population included 3,048 pregnant women (**Fig. 1**).

Since we have excluded those pregnant women with implausible levels of total energy intake, missing data on fast food consumption (n = 40) was considered as no consumption. Those with missing values in smoking were treated as another category (current, former smoker, never smokers, and missing [n = 67]). For missing anthropometrics data we used the last value carried forward, although in this sample of the SUN Project there were no missing data for these variables.

Dietary assessment

Dietary habits at baseline were assessed by a semi-quantitative food frequency questionnaire (FFQ) with 136 items previously validated and described in detail [16,17]. The validity [18] and reproducibility [19] of this questionnaire have been also recently assessed. Updated Spanish food composition tables were used to assess nutrient intake. Nutrient scores were computed using an *ad hoc* computer software specifically developed for this aim. A trained dietitian updated the nutrient data bank using the latest available information included in food composition tables for

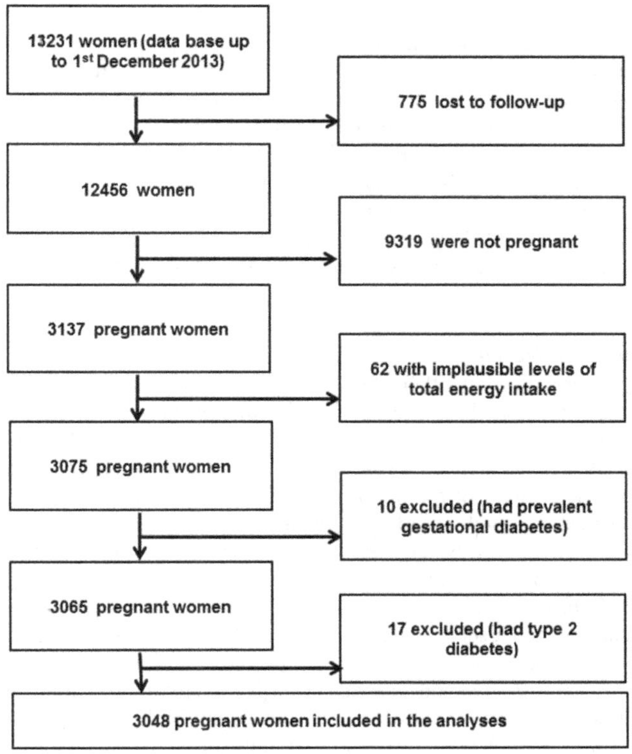

Figure 1. Flow chart depicting the selection process among participants of the SUN project to be included in the present analyses.

Spain [20,21]. Adherence to the Mediterranean food pattern was appraised using the sample-specific score proposed by Trichopoulou [22]. Fast food was defined as the consumption of hamburgers, sausages, and pizza, as previously reported [23,24]. We estimated energy adjusted fast food consumption through the residuals method [25]. Three categories of fast food (serving = 100 g) consumption were also established: low (0–3 servings/month), intermediate (>3 servings/month and ≤2 servings/week) and high (>2 servings/week).

Ascertainment of gestational diabetes

The outcome of interest was the incidence of gestational diabetes. Pregnant women identified in the SUN project (**Fig. 1**) who reported a diagnosis of GDM made by a physician in the biennial questionnaire and did not have diabetes at baseline were considered as incident cases of new-onset GDM.

We sent an additional questionnaire to participants who reported probable new onset GDM, requesting their written confirmation and date of the diagnosis of either GDM, a previous diagnosis of diabetes, their highest fasting glucose value, their first glycated haemoglobin during pregnancy, whether they had ever undergone an oral glucose tolerance test and its results, and the use during pregnancy of insulin. We also asked them to send us the medical report detailing their diagnoses. A panel of medical doctors, blinded to the information about dietary habits, used the information provided by participants (additional questions and medical reports) to classify the diagnosis or each candidate woman as an incident case of GDM or not. For the present analyses we considered only those cases of confirmed GDM. From the potential cases of GDM we had avalaible information in 98% of them. Among those with information, 80% of them were confirmed as incident cases of GDM. There is a lack of universally accepted diagnostic criteria for GDM [5]. Several different protocols are in regular use internationally, each with its own recommendations on which pregnant women should be selected for biochemical testing, how the test should be performed and what glycemic thresholds should be considered diagnostic [26]. The usual diagnosis criteria for GDM in Spain were those with 100-g oral glucose tolerance test with the cut-off points of Carpenter and Coustan [27] or the cut-off points from the National Diabetes Data Group [28] after a positive 50-g glucose challenge test.

Other covariates

Information on other covariates was assessed in the baseline questionnaire. This included socio-demographic parameters (age), anthropometric measurements (weight, body mass index [BMI]), health related habits (smoking status, physical activity, sedentary lifestyle), and clinical variables (use of medication, self-reported pregnancy, family history of diabetes, cardiovascular disease/ hypertension, parity). Age was calculated from the date of birth to the date of the questionnaire's return. Self-reported weight and BMI have previously shown a high validity in a specific study conducted in a sub-sample of this cohort [29 27]. Physical activity was assessed using a previously validated questionnaire with a Spearman correlation coefficient of 0.51 ($p<0.001$) between questionnaire information and objectively obtained measurements [30]. Physical activity was expressed in metabolic equivalent tasks (METs/weeks) as calculated from the time spent at each activity in hours per week multiplied by its typical energy expenditure [31].

Statistical analysis

Consumption frequencies of the fast food items considered (hamburgers, sausages, and pizza) were standardized, summed, and divided into categories that allowed logical cut points with a sufficient number of subjects. Means with SDs for continuous baseline characteristics and proportions for categorical characteristics were calculated by categories of fast food frequency consumption. Since the risk of gestational diabetes depends on the fact to be pregnant and not on a timely basis, we estimated the odds ratios (and 95% CIs) for each of the three categories of fast food consumption using non-conditional regression models taking as the reference category those women with the lowest fast food consumption (0–3 servings per month). For each exposure category, we fitted a crude (univariate) model, an age-adjusted model (Model 1), and multivariate models with additional adjustments (Models 2 and 3) for a priori-selected pre-pregnancy dietary and non-dietary covariables (see below). Non-conditional logistic regression models were adjusted for age, BMI (Kg/m^2), total energy intake (Kcal/day), smoking status (never, former and current smokers), physical activity (expressed in METs-h/w), family history of diabetes (yes or no), presence at baseline of cardiovascular disease or hypertension (yes or no), parity (first pregnancy/1 or 2 pregnancies before/3 or more pregnancies before), score of adherence to the Mediterranean dietary pattern (0–9 points score), and other potential dietary confounders, such as fiber intake (g/day), and sugar-sweetened soft drink consumption (ml/day). The p for trend was calculated taking the median consumption of fast food for each category and introducing this new variable as a continuous variable in the models. We evaluated the interaction between fast food consumption and sugar-sweetened soft drink consumption, physical activity, and family history of diabetes on the risk of GDM through likelihood ratio tests for each of the product-terms introduced (each at one time) in fully-adjusted models.

The analyses were performed with Stata software package version 12 (Stata Corp). All tests were two sided and statistical significance was set at the conventional cut-off of $p<0.05$.

Results

Baseline characteristics of the studied population of pregnant women in the SUN project, according to categories of fast food consumption (low to high), are shown in **Table 1.** Almost half of the participants had an intermediate consumption of fast food (>3 servings/month and ≤2 servings/week; 48%) whereas lower values (0–3 servings/week; 20%) were less frequently observed. Higher frequency of fast food consumption (>2 servings/week; 32%) was present in nearly a third of participants. The participants with a higher consumption of fast food were on average younger, more likely to be current smokers, multiparous, less physically active, less adherent to the Mediterranean dietary pattern, and also more likely to have a lower fiber intake and a higher fat intake.

During 28,064 person-year follow-up (mean follow-up: 10.2, sd: 2.9 years) 159 women reported a first diagnosis of GDM among 3,048 pregnant women of the SUN project, corresponding to 5.2% of pregnant participants. When we analyzed the association between the consumption of fast food and incident gestational diabetes during follow-up with adjustments for a set of potential dietary and non-dietary confounders (age, baseline BMI, total energy intake, smoking, physical activity, family history of diabetes, cardiovascular disease/hypertension at baseline, parity, adherence to Mediterranean dietary pattern score, fiber intake, and sugar-sweetened soft drinks consumption), we found that fast food consumption was strongly and positively associated with incident gestational diabetes risk. In fully-adjusted models, those women in the highest category of fast food consumption presented almost a twofold risk of developing GDM (adjusted OR: 1.86; 95% CI: 1.13–3.06) compared to pregnant women with the lowest fast food consumption (0–3 servings per month) (**Table 2 and Fig. 2**).The risk of incident gestational diabetes was 3.9% for those in the lowest category of fast food consumption, 4.8% for those with intermediate fast food consumption, and 6.7% for the highest category. These associations remained statistically significant after further adjustment for the presence of polycystic ovary syndrome (**Table 2**).

When we used tertiles of energy-adjusted fast food consumption the results were similar: we observed an adjusted OR of 1.82 (95% CI 1.18–2.78) for the highest versus the lowest tertile (p for trend: 0.004).

No significant interaction was observed between fast food consumption and sugar-sweetened soft drinks consumption (p for interaction: 0.645) or between fast food consumption and physical activity (p for interaction: 0.280).

When we assessed fast food consumption as a continuous variable, each additional serving (100 g) per day of fast food consumption was associated with an increased risk, although this association was not statistically significant (adjusted OR: 1.42; 95% CI: 0.76–2.63).

Several sensitivity analyses were carried out in order to appraise the robustness of our findings. This included restricting our analysis to first births from nulliparous women to reduce possible confounding by experiences from previous pregnancies. Excluding multiparous women, the results of the fully adjusted model did not change materially (highest consumption: OR 1.70 (95% CI: 1.00–2.89 for highest vs. lowest consumption; p for linear trend: 0.014). The exclusion of obese women did not either change the results of

Table 1. Characteristics of 3,048 pregnant women in the SUN cohort according to their frequency of fast food consumption.

	Fastfood consumption		
	0–3 servings*/month	**>3 servings/month and ≤2 servings/week**	**>2 servings/week**
N (%)	616 (20.2)	1461 (47.9)	971 (31.9)
Age (years)	29.3 (5.5)	28.9 (4.6)	28.6 (4.4)
Gestational diabetes (%)	3.9	4.8	6.7
Family history of diabetes (%)	10.4	11.2	9.8
Current smoking (%)	22.2	25.0	26.6
Body Mass Index (kg/m^2)	21.3 (2.6)	21.4 (2.6)	21.6 (2.7)
Nulliparous (%)	81.0	81.1	77.9
Physical activity (METs-h/week)	22.4 (23.8)	17.9 (18.2)	16.7 (19.1)
Prevalence of hypertension (%)	2.6	2.4	1.7
Prevalence of CVD (%)	0.7	0.7	0.5
Mediterranean diet score	4.6 (1.7)	4.5 (1.7)	3.9 (1.7)
Alcohol intake (g/d)	3.3 (4.9)	4.0 (5.2)	3.6 (4.7)
Fiber intake (g/d)	32.9 (17.0)	28.2 (11.7)	25.4 (10.9)
Total energy intake (kcal/d)	2479 (842)	2357 (685)	2395 (689)
Carbohydrate intake (% energy)	43.6 (8.8)	42.5 (7.2)	41.4 (6.7)
Protein intake (% energy)	18.7 (3.7)	18.6 (3.0)	18.4 (2.9)
Fat intake (% energy)	36.7 (7.9)	37.6 (6.2)	39.1 (6.1)
SFA intake (% energy)	12.0 (4.0)	12.8 (3.1)	13.5 (2.9)
MUFA intake (% energy)	16.0 (4.5)	16.2 (3.8)	16.4 (3.4)
PUFA intake (% energy)	5.4 (1.9)	5.4 (1.6)	5.7 (1.7)
Trans fatty acid intake (% energy)	0.3 (0.2)	0.4 (0.2)	0.4 (0.2)
Soft drinks (servings/week)	1.3 (2.9)	1.5 (2.4)	1.9 (2.9)

**1 serving = 100 g.*
METs: metabolic equivalent tasks; CVD: cardiovascular disease; SFA: saturated fatty acid; MUFA: monounsaturated fatty acid; PUFA: polyunsaturated fatty acid.
Values are means (SD) for age, BMI, physical activity, Mediterranean diet score, alcohol, fiber, and total energy intake.

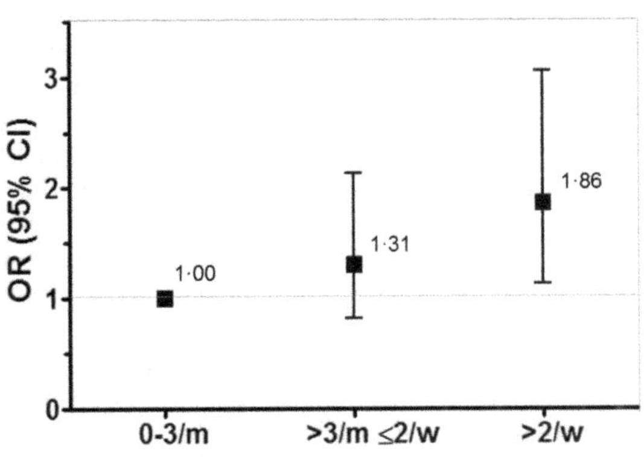

Figure 2. Odds ratio (OR) and 95% confidence interval (CI) for incident gestational diabetes according to frequency of fast food consumption in the SUN project (n = 3,048 pregnant women). Respective numbers (gestational diabetes incidence) for fast food intake of 0–3 times per month (low), >3 times a month and ≤2 times per week (intermediate), and >2 times per week (high) were 616 (24), 1,461 (70), 971 (65). Results represent fully adjusted model (age, baseline BMI, total energy intake, smoking, physical activity, family history of diabetes, cardiovascular disease/hypertension at baseline, parity, adherence to Mediterranean dietary pattern, fiber intake, alcohol intake, and sugar-sweetened soft drinks consumption).

the fully adjusted model (highest consumption: OR 1.81 (95% CI: 1.10–2.99 vs. low consumption; p for linear trend: 0.010).

To test the existence of a potential selection bias due to lost during follow-up we compared baseline characteristics between those participants included in the analyses and those lost during follow-up. There were no statistical significant differences between both groups.

Discussion

The results of the present analyses, using data from a large, well-characterized, prospective cohort of Spanish university graduates, found that among pregnant women in the cohort, a higher pre-pregnancy consumption of fast food was associated with a significantly higher risk of developing gestational diabetes. This association remained significant after several adjustments for potential confounders. Our findings are relevant in the context of a global epidemic of diabetes, which is likely driven, at least in part, by an unhealthy Westernized diet and lifestyle [32]. Fast food is a hallmark of such unhealthy diet; hence, the present results help to reinforce its harmful consequences in women of reproductive age.

It is widely accepted that one of the characteristics of normal pregnancy is a state of insulin resistance with a relative intolerance to dietary carbohydrates and a compensatory increase in insulin secretion from the beta cells in the pancreas [1,33]. The pregnancy-related insulin resistance mainly occurs after the second trimester when insulin requirements are higher. Pregnant women

Table 2. OR and 95% confidence interval of incident gestational diabetes according to fast food consumption.

	Fastfood consumption			
	0–3 servings*/month	**>3 servings/month and ≤2 servings/week**	**>2 servings/week**	**p for trend**
Cases, n/N	24/616	70/1461	65/971	
Rate	$4.11{*}10^{-3}$	$5.16{*}10^{-3}$	$7.41{*}10^{-3}$	
Model 1: OR (95% CI)	1.0 (Ref.)	1.26 (0.78–2.02)	1.80 (1.11–2.91)	0.009
Model 2: OR (95% CI)	1.0 (Ref.)	1.31 (0.81–2.12)	1.90 (1.15–3.12)	0.005
Model 3: OR (95% CI)	1.0 (Ref.)	1.31 (0.81–2.13)	1.86 (1.13–3.06)	0.007
Model 2: OR (95% CI) and PCO	1.0 (Ref.)	1.31 (0.81–2.13)	1.90 (1.16–3.13)	0.005
Model 3: OR (95% CI) and PCO	1.0 (Ref.)	1.31 (0.81–2.13)	1.86 (1.13–3.07)	0.007
Model 2: OR (95% CI) w/o multiparous	1.0 (Ref.)	1.07 (0.64–1.79)	1.71 (1.01–2.90)	0.013
Model 3: OR (95% CI) w/o multiparous	1.0 (Ref.)	1.07 (0.64–1.79)	1.70 (1.00–2.89)	0.014
Model 2: OR (95% CI) w/o obese	1.0 (Ref.)	1.25 (0.77–2.04)	1.83 (1.11–3.03)	0.008
Model 3: OR (95% CI) w/o obese	1.0 (Ref.)	1.25 (0.77–2.04)	1.81 (1.10–2.99)	0.010

The SUN project 1999–2012.
**1 serving = 100 g.*
OR: odd ratio; CI: confidence interval; Rate: crude incident gestational diabetes rate per 10,000 person-years; PCO: polycystic ovary syndrome; w/o: without.
Model 1: adjusted for age.
Model 2: model 1 plus adjustment for total energy intake, smoking, physical activity, family history of diabetes, cardiovascular disease/hypertension at baseline, parity, adherence to Mediterranean dietary pattern score, alcohol intake, fiber intake, and sugar-sweetened soft drinks consumption.
Model 3: model 2 plus adjustment for baseline BMI.

who develop gestational diabetes are assumed to have a compromised beta cell capacity unable to adapt to the increased demand of insulin due to target-organ insulin resistance. This resembles closely the pathophysiology of type 2 diabetes [34], thus, pregnancy-related metabolic challenges may unmask a predisposition to glucose metabolic disorders, which may attain hyperglycemia in the range of diabetic disease. Furthermore, gestational diabetes is a recognized risk factor for future development of type 2 diabetes [35].This and other unfavorable outcomes of gestational diabetes, from delivery complications to perinatal mortality, call for efforts to identify modifiable factors, such as an unhealthy diet, predisposing to the condition.

We found an incidence of gestational diabetes (5.8%) that was similar to that previously reported in the Nurses' Health Study (6.4%) [8]. Attempts to identify women at risk of developing gestational diabetes have been conventionally directed to socio-demographic characteristics, such as maternal weight/BMI, and family history of type 2 diabetes [1,2]. However, in the past decade, several investigations have been focused on the pregravid dietary and lifestyle factors that may contribute to such risk, in parallel with studies pointing to these factors as main drivers of type 2 diabetes epidemic. Even if former studies showed inconsistentresults on the role of total dietary fat intake and gestational diabetes risk, two recent studies taking in consideration specific types of fat concluded that higher pre-pregnancy consumptions of animal fat and cholesterol [11], and of saturated fat [36] were associated with an elevated risk of gestational diabetes. Likewise, a very recent study reported that a higher intake of animal protein, particularly red meat, was significantly associated with a greater risk of gestational diabetes. Conversely, a greater intake of vegetable protein, in particular nuts, was associated with a significantly lower risk [37]. Our findings are consistent with these studies, since the components of fast food considered in our study (hamburgers, sausages, and pizza) mainly include animal proteins and saturated fat. Our results also showed that pregnant women with a higher consumption of fast food had a lower dietary fiber intake and were less adherent to the Mediterranean dietary pattern. In accordance with our observations, previous study have reported inverse and significant associations for fiber intake [9] and adherence to healthful dietary patterns, including Mediterranean diet [8], and the risk of developing gestational diabetes.

Even if the precise molecular mechanisms are unclear, the observed associations between pre-pregnancy fast food consumption and gestational diabetes risk are biologically plausible. First, maternal pregravid BMI has been linked to gestational diabetes risk [1,2] and Western-style fast food has been identified among the greatest dietary contributors to weight gain [38]. However, our results were significant even when the data were adjusted for baseline BMI. Second, there is evidence that frequent consumption of Western-style fast food contributes to insulin resistance [12], a mechanism that is central, as mentioned above, in the development of gestational diabetes. Third, saturated fat and cholesterol, which are components of red and processed meats (part of fast food in our study), have shown to adversely affect not only insulin sensitivity but also beta cell function [39], relevant in the pathophysiology of gestational diabetes. Other components of red and processed meats, including heme iron, and nitrosamines may add to oxidative stress and beta cell damage [9].

It has been previously shown that a 'fast food' dietary pattern was associated with weight gain rate during pregnancy in a dose-dependent manner in a study conducted in Finland [40]. The result of that study is indirectly supportive of our findings. The independent association between pregravid fast food consumption and GDM incidence that we observed was present even after adjustment for baseline BMI. Indeed, we may wonder whether this association was driven by gestational weight gain among fast food eaters or by other mechanisms. Unfortunately, we do not have specific available information to track weight changes in detail throughout the gravid period of our participants and we cannot provide further specific analyses to assess whether gestational weight changes are the most important mediators of this association. However, overadjustment for intermediate mechanisms through which fast food consumption can increase the risk of GDM would be inappropriate if the aim of our analyses is to control for confounding. It is recognized that in an attempt to estimate the total effect of an exposure on some outcome, control for intermediate factors in the causal chain (that is, overadjustment) will generally bias estimates of the total effect of the exposure on the outcome [41,42].

The global epidemic of diabetes, including increasing rates of gestational diabetes [43], parallels obesity trends worldwide. These "twin epidemics" have been linked to Westernization of diet and lifestyle [32,44]. Fast food advertising and broad accessibility may have considerable influence on food choices, particularly among young people. This includes women of childbearing age, increasing their risk for gestational diabetes. In our study, women with the highest consumption of fast food were younger and more likely to have other unhealthy behaviors (i.e. sedentary, smoking, and lower adherence to Mediterranean dietary pattern). Thus, fast food consumption could be a marker of an unhealthy diet/lifestyle and not a cause of increased gestational diabetes risk. However, the multivariate analyses we present here accounted for other unhealthy behaviors, and after multiple adjustments and sensitivity analyses the consumption of fast food remained strongly significantly associated with gestational diabetes risk. Emphasis is needed to develop strategies that persuade women to optimize their diet and lifestyle before conceiving.

The present study has a number of strengths, including a large sample size with a high retention rate, prospective design, a lengthy follow-up and use of a FFQ that has been specifically and repeatedly validated in Spain [17–19]. Importantly, we were able to obtain a high degree of control for confounding, including potential lifestyle and demographic confounders, and we also controlled for overall dietary patterns. In addition, we conducted several sensitvity analyses and the results were robust. The study also has some potential limitations. Information that was self-reported and this may lead to some degree of misclassification, which most often would drive associations toward the null value. However, parameters such as self-reported weight and BMI have been previously validated in a sub-sample of this cohort [29]. The cohort is composed mostly of middle-aged, Spanish highly educated persons.Therefore the generalizability of our results must be based on common biological mechanisms instead of on statistical representativeness, and we used restriction to reduce potential confounding by disease, education, socioeconomic status, and presumed access to health care. Future studies are needed in order to test the applicability of our results in pregnant women from other populations.

Since our all participants are Spanish university graduates, we can guarantee that the vast majority of them are Caucasians and therefore, unfortunately we were not able to assess the effect of ethnicity in the association between fast food consumption and GDM.

Finally, possible concerns may arise from the use of dietary data derived from an FFQ, which may be subject to information bias. However, the FFQ used has been repeatedly validated [17–19]. Moreover, it is difficult to find a better alternative than a FFQ as an advantageous method to characterize the food habits of large samples of individuals' that need to be followed-up over long periods of time in order to rank them and assess associations with incident clinical end-points [45].

In conclusion, findings from this prospective study suggest that pre-pregnancy higher consumption of fast food (i.e. hamburgers, sausages, and pizza) is an independent risk factor for gestational diabetes. Further research to confirm these findings in other populations and to decipher underlying molecular mechanisms is warranted. Nevertheless, our results emphasize the potential importance of considering pregravid dietary recommendations for the prevention of gestational diabetes. The information on the increased gestational risk associated with fast food intake might be disseminated to women of reproductive age.

Acknowledgments

The authors thank the participants of the SUN Project for their enthusiastic collaboration.

Author Contributions

Conceived and designed the experiments: LJD MBR MAMG. Performed the experiments: MAMG FJBG MBR. Analyzed the data: MBR LJD MAMG. Contributed to the writing of the manuscript: LJD MBR MAMG MB FJBG AG. Critical revision and approval of the final version to be published: LJD MBR MAMG MB FJBG AG.

References

1. ADA (2004) Gestational diabetes mellitus. Diabetes Care (suppl 1):S88–90.
2. Bellamy L, Casas JP, Hingorani AD, Williams D (2009) Type 2 diabetes mellitus after gestational diabetes: a systematic review and meta-analysis. Lancet 373: 1773–1779.
3. Albrecht SS, Kuklina EV, Bansil P, Jamieson DJ, Whiteman MK, et al. (2010) Diabetes trends among delivery hospitalizations in the United States, 1994-2004. Diabetes Care 33: 768–773.
4. Dabelea D, Snell-Bergeon JK, Hartsfield CL, Bischoff KJ, Hamman RF, et al. (2005) Increasing prevalence of gestational diabetes mellitus(GDM) over time and by birth cohort: Kaiser Permanente of Colorado GDM Screening Program. Diabetes Care 28: 579–584.
5. Buckley BS, HarreiterJ DammP, Corcoy R, Chico A, et al, on behalf of the DALI Core Investigator Group (2012) Gestational diabetes mellitus in Europe: prevalence,current screening practice and barriers to screening. A review.Diabet Med29: 844–854.
6. Horvath K, Koch K, Jeitler K, Matyas E, Bender R, et al. (2010) Effects of treatment in women with gestational diabetes mellitus: systematic review and meta-analysis. BMJ 340:c1395.
7. Zhang C, Ning Y (2011) Effect of dietary and lifestyle factors on the risk of gestational diabetes: review of epidemiologic evidence. Am J Clin Nutr 94(suppl):1975S–1979S.
8. Tobias DK, Zhang C, Chavarro J, Bowers K, Rich-Edwards J, et al. (2012) Prepregnancy adherence to dietary patterns and lower risk of gestational diabetes mellitus. Am J ClinNutr 96: 289–295.
9. Zhang C, Liu S, Solomon CG, Hu FB (2006) Dietary fiber intake, dietary glycemic load, and the risk for gestational diabetes mellitus. DiabetesCare 29: 2223–2230.
10. Zhang C, Schulze MB, Solomon CG, Hu FB (2006) A prospective study of dietary patterns, meat intake and the risk of gestational diabetes mellitus. Diabetologia 49: 2604–2613.
11. Bowers K, Tobias DK, Yeung E, Hu FB, Zhang C (2012) A prospective study of prepregnancy dietary fat intake and risk of gestational diabetes. Am J ClinNutr 95: 446–453.
12. Pereira MA, Kartashov AI, Ebbeling CB, Van Horn L, Slattery ML, et al. (2005) Fast-food habits, weight gain, and insulinresistance (the CARDIA study): 15-year prospective analysis. Lancet 365: 36–42.
13. Odegaard AO, Koh WP, Yuan J-M, Gross MD, Pereira MA (2012) Western-Style Fast Food Intake and Cardiometabolic Risk in an Eastern Country Circulation 126: 182–188.
14. Martinez-Gonzalez MA, Sanchez-Villegas A, De Irala J, Marti A, Martinez JA (2002) Mediterranean diet and stroke: objectives and design of the SUN project. SeguimientoUniversidad de Navarra. NutrNeurosci 5: 65–73.

15. Segui-Gomez M, de la Fuente C, Vazquez Z, de Irala J, Martinez-Gonzalez MA (2006) Cohort profile: the 'Seguimiento Universidad de Navarra' (SUN) study. Int J Epidemiol 35: 1417–1422.
16. Martinez-Gonzalez MA, de la Fuente-Arrillaga C, Nunez-Cordoba JM, Basterra-Gortari FJ, Beunza JJ, et al. (2008) Adherence to Mediterranean diet and risk of developing diabetes: prospective cohort study. BMJ 336: 1348–1351.
17. Martin-Moreno JM, Boyle P, Gorgojo L, Maisonneuve P, Fernandez-Rodriguez JC, et al. (1993) Development and validation of a food frequency questionnaire in Spain. Int J Epidemiol 22: 512–519.
18. Fernandez-Ballart JD, Pinol JL, Zazpe I, Corella D, Carrasco P, et al. (2010) Relative validity of a semi-quantitative food-frequency questionnaire in an elderly Mediterranean population of Spain. Br J Nutr 103: 1808–1816.
19. de la Fuente-Arrillaga C, VazquezRuiz Z, Bes-Rastrollo M, Sampson L, Martinez-Gonzalez MA (2010) Reproducibility of an FFQ validated in Spain. Public Health Nutr13: 1364–1372.
20. Moreiras O, Carbajal A, Cabrera L, Cuadrado C (2013) Tablas de composición de alimentos [Food composition tables]. 16th ed. Madrid: Piramide.
21. Mataix Verdu J (2009) Tabla de composición de alimentos [Food composition tables]. 5th ed. Granada: Universidad de Granada.
22. Trichopoulou A, Costacou T, Bamia C, Trichopoulos D (2003) Adherence to a Mediterranean diet and survival in a Greek population. N Engl J Med 348: 2599–2608.
23. Bes-Rastrollo M, Sánchez-Villegas A, Gómez-Gracia E, Martínez JA, Pajares RM, et al. (2006) Predictors of weight gain in a Mediterranean cohort: the Seguimiento Universidad de Navarra Study. Am J Clin Nutr 83: 362–370.
24. Bes-Rastrollo M, Basterra-Gortari FJ, Sánchez-Villegas A, Marti A, Martínez JA, et al. (2010) A prospective study of eating away-from-home meals and weight gain in a Mediterranean population: the SUN (Seguimiento Universidad de Navarra) color. Public Health Nutrition 13: 1356–1363.
25. Hu FB, Stampfer MJ, Rimm E, Ascherio A, Rosner BA, et al. (1999) Dietary fat and coronary heart disease: a comparison of approaches for adjusting for total energy intake and modeling repeated dietary measurements. Am J Epidemiol 149: 531–540.
26. NICE (2008) Diabetes in Pregnancy: Management of Diabetes and its Complications from Pre-Conception to the Post-Natal Period. Clinical guideline no. 63. London: National Institute for Health and Clinical Excellence / National Collaborating Centre for Women's and Children's Health.
27. ADA (2010) Position statement. Diagnosis and classification of diabetes mellitus. Diabetes Care 33:S62–S69.
28. National Diabetes Data Group (1979) Classification and diagnosis of diabetes mellitus and other categories of glucose intolerance. Diabetes 28: 1039–1057.
29. Bes-Rastrollo M, Perez Valdivieso JR, Sanchez-Villegas A, Alonso A, Martinez-Gonzalez MA (2005) Validación del peso e índice de masa corporal auto-declarados de los participantes de una cohorte de graduados universitarios.[Validation of self-reported weight and body mass index of participants in a cohort of university graduates] Rev EspObes 3: 183–189.
30. Martinez-Gonzalez MA, Lopez-Fontana C, Varo JJ, Sanchez-Villegas A, Martinez JA (2005) Validation of the Spanish version of the physical activity questionnaire used in the Nurses' Health Study and the Health Professionals' Follow-up Study. Public Health Nutr 8: 920–927.
31. Ainsworth BE, Haskell WL, Whitt MC, Irwin ML, Swartz AM, et al. (2000) Compendium of physical activities: an update of activity codes and MET intensities. Med Sci Sports Exerc 32:S498–S504.
32. Smyth S, Heron A (2006) Diabetes and obesity: the twin epidemics. Nature Medicine 12: 75–80.
33. Buchanan TA, Xiang AH (2005) Gestational diabetes mellitus. J Clin Invest 115: 485–491.
34. Nolan CJ, Damm P, Prentki M (2011) Type 2 diabetes across generations: from pathophysiology to prevention and management. Lancet 378: 169–181.
35. ADA (2014) Standards of Medical Care in Diabetes – 2014. Diabetes Care (Suppl 1): S14–S80.
36. Park S, Kim MY, Baik SH, Woo JT, Kwon YJ, et al. (2013) Gestational diabetes is associated with high energy and saturated fat intakes and with low plasma visfatin and adiponectin levels independent of prepregnancy BMI. Eur J ClinNutr 67: 196–201.
37. Bao W, Bowers K, Tobias DK, Hu FB, Zhang C (2013)Prepregnancy dietary protein intake, major dietary protein sources, and the risk of gestational diabetes mellitus. A prospective cohort study. Diabetes Care 36: 2001–2008.
38. Mozaffarian D, Hao T, Rimm EB, Willett WC, Hu FB (2011) Changes in diet and lifestyle and long-term weight gain in women and men. N Engl J Med 364: 2392–2404.
39. Lopez S, Bermudez B, Ortega A, Varela LM, Pacheco YM, et al. (2011) Effects of meals rich in either monounsaturated or saturated fat on lipid concentrations and on insulin secretion and action in subjects with high fasting triglyceride concentrations. Am J ClinNutr 93: 494–499.
40. Uusitalo U, Arkkola T, Ovaskainen ML, Kronberg-Kippila C, Kenward MG, et al. (2009) Unhealthy dietary patterns are associated with weight gain during pregnancy among Finnish women. Public Health Nutrition 12: 2392–2399.
41. Vander Weele TJ (2009) On the relative nature of overadjustment and unnecessary adjustment. Epidemiology 20: 496–499.
42. Greenland S, Neutra R. (1980) Control of confounding in the assessment of medical technology. Int J Epidemiol 9: 361–367.
43. Lawrence JM, Contreras R, Chen W, Sacks DA (2008) Trends in the prevalence of preexisting diabetes and gestational diabetes mellitus among a racially/ethnically diverse population of pregnant women, 1999–2005. Diabetes Care 31: 899–904.
44. Pan A, Malik VS, Hu FB (2012) Exporting diabetes mellitus to Asia. The impact of Western-style fast food. Circulation 126: 163–165.
45. Willett W (1998) Nutritional epidemiology. 2nded. New York: Oxford University Press.

12

Genetic and Phenotypic Correlations between Performance Traits with Meat Quality and Carcass Characteristics in Commercial Crossbred Pigs

Younes Miar[1], Graham Plastow[1], Heather Bruce[1], Stephen Moore[1,5], Ghader Manafiazar[1], Robert Kemp[2], Patrick Charagu[3], Abe Huisman[4], Benny van Haandel[3], Chunyan Zhang[1], Robert McKay[6], Zhiquan Wang[1]*

1 Livestock Gentec Centre, Department of Agricultural, Food and Nutritional Science, University of Alberta, Edmonton, Alberta, Canada, **2** Genesus Genetics, Oakville, Manitoba, Canada, **3** Hypor Inc., Regina, Saskatchewan, Canada, **4** Research and Technology Centre, Hendrix Genetics, Boxmeer, The Netherlands, **5** Centre for Animal Science, Queensland Alliance for Agriculture & Food Innovation, University of Queensland, St Lucia, Australia, **6** McKay GENSTAT Consultants Inc., Brandon, Manitoba, Canada

Abstract

Genetic correlations between performance traits with meat quality and carcass traits were estimated on 6,408 commercial crossbred pigs with performance traits recorded in production systems with 2,100 of them having meat quality and carcass measurements. Significant fixed effects (company, sex and batch), covariates (birth weight, cold carcass weight, and age), random effects (additive, litter and maternal) were fitted in the statistical models. A series of pairwise bivariate analyses were implemented in ASREML to estimate heritability, phenotypic, and genetic correlations between performance traits (n = 9) with meat quality (n = 25) and carcass (n = 19) traits. The animals had a pedigree compromised of 9,439 animals over 15 generations. Performance traits had low-to-moderate heritabilities (±SE), ranged from 0.07±0.13 to 0.45±0.07 for weaning weight, and ultrasound backfat depth, respectively. Genetic correlations between performance and carcass traits were moderate to high. The results indicate that: (a) selection for birth weight may increase drip loss, lightness of *longissimus dorsi*, and *gluteus medius* muscles but may reduce fat depth; (b) selection for nursery weight can be valuable for increasing both quantity and quality traits; (c) selection for increased daily gain may increase the carcass weight and most of the primal cuts. These findings suggest that deterioration of pork quality may have occurred over many generations through the selection for less backfat thickness, and feed efficiency, but selection for growth had no adverse effects on pork quality. Low-to-moderate heritabilities for performance traits indicate that they could be improved using traditional selection or genomic selection. The estimated genetic parameters for performance, carcass and meat quality traits may be incorporated into the breeding programs that emphasize product quality in these Canadian swine populations.

Editor: Shuhong Zhao, Huazhong Agricultural University, China

Funding: The authors acknowledge the financial support from Natural Sciences and Engineering Research Council of Canada (NSERC): www.nserc-crsng.gc.ca; Hypor Inc.: http://www.hypor.com/; and Genesus Genetics: http://www.genesus.com/. The authors would like to extend thanks to the companies for providing the possibility and the facilities to collect the data. Except for the role of the industry staff in preparation of the manuscript as co-authors the funders had no role in study design, data collection and analysis, decision to publish, or preparation of the manuscript.

Competing Interests: The authors have declared that no competing interests exist.

* Email: Zhiquan@ualberta.ca

Introduction

Swine breeding programs have mainly focused on production efficiency to increase the leanness of the carcasses in previous decades. This has led to dramatic improvement in production efficiency including leanness and feed efficiency owing to relatively moderate-to-high heritabilities. However, the importance of meat and carcass quality is growing for pig breeders to meet processor's, packer's, and consumer's demands for better pork quality [1]. Genetic correlations between pork quality and carcass characteristics and other economic importance traits are, however, limited. Understanding of the genetic control of pork quality traits and their correlations with growth and performance traits are needed for Canadian swine populations to implement a successful breeding program that emphasizes product quality.

Meat quality traits are low-to-moderately heritable while carcass composition traits are moderate-to-highly heritable [2]. Latorre et al. [3] stated that the relationships between meat quality traits and growth traits are contradictory. Cameron [4] showed that selection for increased leanness reduced eating quality. Furthermore, weak negative genetic correlations between performance and meat quality traits have been reported and their magnitudes depend on breed [5]. Medium weight pigs at birth had a better tenderness and water holding capacity than light weight piglets but the intramuscular fat was higher in light piglets [6]. van Wijk et al. [7] stated that average daily gain was unfavorably correlated with subprimal cuts and with most meat quality traits. Jiang et al. [8] reported different breeds in Chinese swine industry had different meat quality and carcass characteristics. Various factors may influence the variance component estimates including the end-point adjustment, population size, sampling and available pedigree [9]. Phenotypic and genetic correlations between meat and carcass quality traits have been reported in our previous publication [2]. This study is a further investigation focusing on genetic and phenotypic correlations between performance traits with pork and carcass quality traits.

The objectives of this study were 1) to estimate heritabilities for various growth, and performance traits; and 2) to estimate phenotypic and genetic correlations between performance traits with pork quality and carcass traits in commercial crossbred pigs.

Methods

The hogs used in this study were cared for according to the Canadian Council on Animal Care [10] guidelines.

Animals and Management

The commercial crossbred pigs used in this study were progeny from a total of 139 sires of the Duroc boars bred to 429 F1 hybrid Landrace × Large White sows. These breeds were chosen because they are representative of a large percentage of the Canadian swine industry. They were a combination of full and half sib families representing a multi-generation family structure drawn from two breeding populations (Genesus Genetics, and Hypor Inc., Canada). Pedigree information of 15 ancestral generations comprising 9,439 individuals was available [2].

Performance Evaluation and Housing

Piglets were born over a 2-year period from 2010 to 2012. All piglets were individually tagged and weighed at birth (birth weight, **BW**), weaned at an average age of 21 days (7.5 kg), raised in a nursery for 5 to 6 weeks, and then moved to pre-grower barn for 4 weeks. During this time, both weaning weight (**WNW**) and nursery weight (NURW) were recorded. Pigs were then randomly allocated to finishing sites for 9 weeks under commercial finishing conditions with *ad libitum* access to a canola, wheat, barley, soybean diet and water [2]. Male piglets were castrated at 3 to 5 days after birth. The end body weight (**ENDW**), ultrasound backfat depth (**UFD**), ultrasound loin depth (**ULD**), and ultrasound intramuscular fat (**UIMF**) were measured at the end of finishing test with an average body weight of 115 kg. The live body weights recorded at the birth and end of finishing were used to calculate the average daily gain (**ADG**) using the following equation: ADG = (ENDW − start test weight)/Days. Feed conversion ratio (**FCR**) was calculated based on the daily feed intake recorded by electronic feeders for some animals.

Carcass and Meat Quality Measurements

Carcass and meat quality measurements have been described previously by Miar et al. [2]. Briefly, pigs were housed overnight at the abattoir (East 40 Packers, Brandon, Manitoba, Canada) with *ad libitum* access to water. Animals were slaughtered on a Federally inspected kill floor and handling of the animals upon arrival and before slaughter. Moreover, slaughter process was adhered to Government of Canada Guidelines. The average slaughter weight and age were 124 kg and 160 days, respectively. Hot carcass weight (**HCW**), cold carcass weight (**CCW**), and the carcass length (**CLEN**) were recorded according to Miar et al. [2]. Then, the carcasses were broken into the primal cuts and the loin was further broken into the front, back, 3-rib sample, 1-inch chop, and 4-rib sample. The chop removed at 3rd and 4th last rib was used to determine: (a) *longissimus dorsi* muscle area (**LEA**); (b) subcutaneous backfat depth (**FD**); (c) loin depth (**LD**); (d) texture score (**TEXS**) measured on a subjective 5-point scale (1 = extremely soft and weeping; 5 = very firm and dry; a score of 3 being normal) to determine if the loin was pale, soft and exudative (PSE); (e) subjective marbling score (**CMAR**; 1 to 6, with 0 = devoid, 1 = practically devoid, 2 = trace amount of marbling, 3 = slight, 4 = small, 5 = moderate, 6 = abundant) as determined by the National Swine Improvement Federation (NSIF) marbling charts [11] as described by Miar et al. [2].

Primal cuts of loin, ham, shoulder and belly were dissected into subprimal cuts. Untrimmed side weight (**USW**) was determined as the sum of the weights of untrimmed ham, loin, shoulder, and belly. Untrimmed shoulder (**USH**), untrimmed ham (**UHAM**) were removed from the side weight. Untrimmed loin (**ULOIN**) and belly (**UBEL**) were separated from each other. Then, subprimal cuts of ham (**THAM**), loin (**TLOIN**), picnic shoulder (**PICN**), butt (**BUTT**), belly (**TBEL**) and ribs (**RIBS**) were recorded as described by Miar et al. [2].

At the slaughterhouse, meat quality measurements were taken on *longissimus dorsi* muscle of the loin. Ultimate or 24 h pH (**PHU**), drip loss (**DL**), Minolta L*, a*, and b* (**LOINL**, **LOINA**, and **LOINB**) were taken on loin as describe by Miar et al. [2]. Minolta L*, a*, and b* measurements were taken on different muscles of ham including *gluteus medius* (**HGML**, **HGMA**, and **HGMB**), *quadriceps femoris* (**HQFL**, **HQFA**, and **HQFB**), and *iliopsoas* muscles (**HILL**, **HILA**, and **HILB**).

At the Meat Science Laboratory of University of Alberta, frozen 3-Rib and 4-Rib samples of the loin of each carcass were used to record whole loin weight (**WLW**), backfat weight (**BFW**), and rib eye weight (**REAW**) as described by Miar et al. [2]. Rib eye area was used for subsequent pork quality assays. Rib eye Minolta L*, a*, and b* values (**REAL**, **REAA**, and **REAB**) were taken using a commercial color meter (CR400, Konica-Minolta, Osaka, Japan) on a D 65 light setting which mimics daylight [2]. Cooking loss (**CL**) and shear force (**SHF**) were measured as described by Miar et al. [2]. The remainder of the loin was dissected into the muscle and fat (**RTW**), bone (**BOW**) and diaphragm.

Statistical Analyses

There were 6,408 pigs with growth and performance records with 2,100 of them having meat quality and carcass data. The significance of the fixed effects and covariates for each trait was determined using the REML procedure of ASREML 3.0 software [12]. The significance of different random terms in the model was determined by likelihood ratio test using ASREML 3.0 software [12]. The full animal model included random direct, maternal additive genetic and common environment (litter of birth) effects. Maternal genetic and common environment effects were tested separately by comparing −2 residual log likelihoods of full and reduced (excluding the random effect of interest) models having degrees of freedom equal to the number of parameters tested. The model which best fit the data was selected. Common litter effects were significant ($P<0.05$) for BW, WNW, NURW, ENDW, ADG, UFD, ULD, HCW, CCW, LEA, PH, and DL and were not significant ($P>0.05$) for most meat quality, and carcass composition traits [2]. The maternal effect was only significant ($P<0.05$) for WNW.

Genetic and phenotypic (co)variances were estimated using a pairwise bivariate animal model by ASREML 3.0 [12]. Relevant fixed and random effects for carcass and meat quality traits were described by Miar et al. [2], and for performance traits are presented in Table 1. The final animal model included linear covariates of birth weight, whole loin weight received at the Meat Science Laboratory, cold carcass weight and slaughter age. Fixed effects including company, sex, and batch (test or slaughter batch) were fitted in the final model. In addition, additive polygenic effects for all traits, random litter effect, and maternal effect for some traits were included in the final model. The model is given by:

$$y = Xb + Z_1 a + Z_2 m + Z_3 c + e,$$

where $\boldsymbol{y}$ is the vector of phenotypic measurements, $\boldsymbol{X}$ is the incidence matrix relating the fixed effects to vector $\boldsymbol{y}$, $\boldsymbol{b}$ is the vector of fixed effects, $\boldsymbol{Z}_1$ is the incidence matrix relating the phenotypic observations to the vector of polygenic (**a**) effects, $\boldsymbol{Z}_2$ is the incidence matrix relating the phenotypic observations to the vector of maternal genetic (**m**) effects, $\boldsymbol{Z}_3$ is the incidence matrix relating the phenotypic observations to the vector of common litter (**c**) effects, and **e** is the vector of random residuals.

It was assumed that random effects were independent except for the covariance between the direct and the maternal additive genetic effects. In particular, the (co)variances of random variables were as follows:

$$V\begin{pmatrix} a_1 \\ a_2 \\ m_1 \\ m_2 \\ c_1 \\ c_2 \\ e_1 \\ e_2 \end{pmatrix} = \begin{pmatrix} A\sigma^2_{a1} & A\sigma_{a12} & A\sigma_{a1m1} & A\sigma_{a1m2} & 0 & 0 & 0 & 0 \\ . & A\sigma^2_{a2} & A\sigma_{a2m1} & A\sigma_{a2m2} & 0 & 0 & 0 & 0 \\ . & . & A\sigma^2_{m1} & A\sigma_{m1m2} & 0 & 0 & 0 & 0 \\ . & . & . & A\sigma^2_{m2} & 0 & 0 & 0 & 0 \\ . & . & . & . & I\sigma^2_{c1} & I\sigma_{c1c2} & 0 & 0 \\ . & . & . & . & . & I\sigma^2_{c2} & 0 & 0 \\ . & . & . & . & . & . & I\sigma^2_{e1} & I\sigma_{e1e2} \\ . & . & . & . & . & . & . & I\sigma^2_{e2} \end{pmatrix},$$

where A is the numerator relationship matrix, I is the identity matrix, σ^2_{a1}, σ^2_{a2}, σ^2_{m1}, σ^2_{m2}, σ^2_{c1}, σ^2_{c2}, σ^2_{e1} and σ^2_{e2} are direct additive genetic variances, maternal genetic variances, common litter effect variances and residual variance for traits 1 and 2, respectively, and σ_{am} is the covariance between the direct and the maternal additive genetic effects. Variance components obtained from the bivariate analyses used to estimated heritability for each performance trait and the average estimates of corresponding pairwise bivariate analyses were reported as the heritabilities:

$$h^2 = \frac{\sigma^2_a}{\sigma^2_p}$$

A preliminary univariate animal model for each trait was performed to obtain initial values of variance parameters that were then used in subsequent bivariate analyses. Initial values of covariance parameters were obtained by multiplying their

Table 1. Significance of the fixed and random effects included in the models for the analysis of Performance Traits.

Traits	Fixed Effects				Random Effects		
	Company	Sex	Batch	BW[1]	Dam	Litter	Animal
Birth weight	**	**	**	-	NS	**	✓
Weaning weight	**	*	**	**	**	**	✓
Nursery weight	NS	**	**	**	NS	**	✓
End weight	*	**	**	-	NS	**	✓
ADG	**	**	**	-	NS	**	✓
Ultrasound backfat depth	*	**	**	-	NS	**	✓
Ultrasound loin depth	**	*	**	-	NS	**	✓
Ultrasound IMF	**	**	**	-	NS	NS	✓
Feed conversion ratio	NS	**	**	-	NS	NS	✓

**$P<0.05$; * $P<0.1$; NS: Non-significant.
[1]Birth weight.

standard deviations by their phenotypic or genetic correlations. Pairwise bivariate analyses were performed between performance traits with carcass and pork quality traits. The 2-trait individual animal model used to estimate (co)variance components, were used to calculate the phenotypic and genetic correlations as well as the heritability as implemented in ASREML 3.0 [12].

Results and Discussion

Means and standard deviations

Most of the performance, carcass and pork quality traits were recorded for all individuals within group. Means, standard deviations, number of measurements per trait, minimum and maximum for each performance trait are given in Table 2. The descriptive statistics for meat quality and carcass traits were previously reported by Miar et al. [2].

Heritabilities

Heritability estimates for performance traits with their standard errors are presented in Table 3 (diagonal elements). Univariate estimates of heritability for all traits were similar to the bivariate estimates. Moderate heritability was obtained for most of the performance traits with the estimates of 0.26, 0.24, 0.38, 0.30, 0.45, 0.38, 0.26, and 0.20 for BW, NURW, ENDW, ADG, UFD, ULD, UIMF, and FCR (Table 3). Weaning weight had a lower heritability of 0.07 in this study. These estimates were within the range (0.00–0.74) of the heritability previously reported for growth and performance traits [13,14]. Several factors influence the heritability estimates, which may include the end-point adjustment such as age or weight adjustment, sampling, population size, effect of heterosis on crossbred populations and the completeness of pedigree [9], which may result in the various estimates among the different literature. The low-to-moderate heritability estimated from this study revealed that genomic technology can play an important role for improvement of these economically important traits.

The estimated heritability for BW (0.26±0.08) in this study was higher than the estimates from many other work [13,15,16,17], but lower than the report (0.36) by Roehe et al. [18], who used two-generations of outdoor reared piglets and suggested that direct heritability estimate was substantially larger under outdoor conditions. However, the estimate from the first generation of outdoor piglets also reported by Roehe et al. [19] was lower (0.20), which is close to our estimate from the crossbred population. Another difference is that Roehe et al. [18,19] used a Bayesian method while we used an animal model. These results revealed that the breed, population structure and statistical method have an important effect on the genetic parameter estimate. The estimated heritability of WNW in this study (0.07±0.07) was in agreement with literature values [20]. The estimated maternal heritability for WNW was 0.10±0.03, which was similar to 0.17 reported by Cassady et al. [13]. Cassady et al. [13] estimated the heritability as 0.00 to 0.10 in two different genetic types. According to these studies, the maternal effect was a more important component of the genetic variation of weaning weight than the direct additive genetic effect. This may be due to effects of milk production, uterine capacity and nutrition to weaning [20]. The reports for genetic parameter estimates for NURW and ENDW are very limited, although they are important indicators to determine the production efficiency in the swine industry. The average ENDW was 110 (SD = 10) kg and this off test weight was not considered for heritability estimations in the literature. The NURW and ENDW heritability estimates were 0.24±0.16, and 0.38±0.18, respectively. The heritability for weight increased (0.07 to 0.38) from weaning to 160 days of age since the maternal genetic variance decreased as the pigs grew. This result is expected due to the separation of pigs from their dams. The common litter environment effect was fitted in the animal models for all performance traits except for UIMF and FCR.

ADG has been reported as a moderately heritable trait. The heritability estimate in this study is 0.30±0.08, which is in agreement with many other reports [14,20]. However, van Wijk et al. [7] reported a lower heritability of 0.19, which may due to the different evaluation of ADG. van Wijk et al. [7] calculated the ADG based on the carcass weight and the assumption of the same birth weight of 1.36 kg for all animals, which could narrow down the sample variance and result in the low heritability estimation. Genetic parameters for ADG were widely studied and the reported estimates vary considerably, ranging from 0.03 to 0.49 [22–26]. The heritability of UFD in this study (0.45±0.07) was in good agreement with the previous report of 0.44–0.54 [7,27]. Stewart and Schinckel [21] reviewed many papers and reported a weighted average heritability of 0.41 for backfat. The heritability estimate of ULD in the present study (0.38±0.07) was the same as the report (0.38) by Maignel et al. [28] who used the similar typical Canadian three-way cross population and sample size as our current study. However, the present estimate was slightly lower than the estimates of 0.47 and 0.48 reported by Stewart and Schinckel [21] and Ducos [29], respectively.

Marbling is one of the most important appearance factors used by consumers to perceive quality since they affect purchase decisions and satisfaction of consumption. The amount of marbling depends on implementation of different pig breeding and management techniques [23], which may be one of the reasons for the variation observed in the estimation of UIMF. The heritability of UIMF was moderate in the present study (0.26±0.06). UIMF has previously been reported to be a moderately heritable trait, ranging from 0.13 to 0.31, which was in agreement with the current result [23,30,31,32]. The estimated heritability of FCR in this study was 0.20±0.06, which was lower than the average of 0.30 reviewed by Clutter [14], which may be due to using different statistical models, breeds and sample size.

Generally, meat quality traits had low-to-moderate (0.10±0.04 to 0.39±0.06) heritabilities while carcass composition traits had moderate-to-high (0.22±0.08 to 0.63±0.04) heritabilities. The details can be found from our previous report, which was conducted in the same population [2].

Correlations among Traits

The phenotypic and genetic correlations and their standard errors are presented in Tables 3–7. Generally, almost all of the phenotypic correlations and some of the genetic correlations were significant (*P<0.05*). Although presented for completeness, phenotypic correlations will not be discussed because they are of little interpretive value.

Correlations among Growth and Performance Traits

The phenotypic and genetic correlations among growth and performance traits are presented in Table 3. Almost all of the phenotypic correlations among performance traits were significant (*P<0.05*). Genetic correlations indicated that selection for increased growth rate could increase ULD (0.31±0.13), UIMF (0.69±0.25), and UFD (0.26±0.12). Growth is in general lowly and negatively correlated with backfat thickness but favourably correlated with marbling and loin depth. The ADG and FD are the most important traits of performance testing, and the genetic correlation between them (0.01±0.14) is in the range of estimates (−0.26 to 0.55) reviewed by Clutter [14]. The wide range of

Table 2. Descriptive statistics for performance traits: number of animals per trait (n), means, SD, minimum (Min.) and maximum (Max.) values.

Traits	n	Mean	SD	Min.	Max.
Birth weight, kg	6408	1.53	0.35	0.50	2.90
Weaning weight, kg	5918	6.9	1.41	1.24	12.20
Nursery weight, kg	2262	37.58	7.70	10.00	60.00
End weight, kg	5004	109.88	10.24	67.40	147.00
ADG, g/d	4436	976.60	145.32	351.00	1492.00
Ultrasound backfat depth, mm	4810	13.73	3.17	5.20	28.70
Ultrasound loin depth, mm	4811	63.15	5.62	40.90	82.20
Ultrasound IMF	1807	1.26	0.83	0	6.60
Feed conversion ratio	708	2.64	0.30	1.55	4.06

genetic correlations between ADG and UFD reported by Clutter [14] may be due to the method of measurement, technician effect, breed differences, and sampling errors [33]. These results suggested that breeding programs aimed at improving intramuscular fat should expect improvement (higher marbling) through the selection for growth. Suzuki et al. [34] reported a low genetic correlation of 0.06 between UIMF and ADG that is lower than this study, which may be due to using the smaller samples size and purebred Duroc in their study. We highlight that the genetic correlation between ADG and ULD is a new contribution to our knowledge.

Birth weight had strong genetic correlations with ENDW (0.79±0.40) and ULD (0.75±0.36). Generally, genetic correlations of ENDW with performance traits were significant (*P<0.05*) except for the correlations with NURW and FCR. ENDW had high genetic correlations with BW (0.79±0.40), WNW (0.93±0.45), ADG (0.87±0.04), and UIMF (0.60±0.27). None of these genetic correlations were previously reported and it seems that selection for BW, WNW, and ADG will lead to increased ENDW and UIMF. Low-to-moderate correlations were found between ENDW with UFD (0.28±0.13), and ULD (0.37±0.12). Genetic correlations of ENDW with these traits were not reported in the literature. UFD had moderate genetic correlation with ULD (−0.33±0.14). This result was similar to the average value of −0.35 reported by Clutter and Brascamp [27] and −0.45 by Newcom et al. [35].

In addition, UIMF was moderately to highly correlated with NURW (0.75±0.35), ENDW (0.60±0.27), ADG (0.69±0.25), UFD (0.48±0.19), and ULD (−0.47±0.20). However, no genetic correlations were found for NURW and ENDW (−0.01±0.44) but these results confirmed that selection based on NURW would increase UIMF. These results also imply that increased backfat and decreased loin depth may be expected when selection is directed toward increased marbling. FCR was also moderately correlated with UFD (0.39±0.17), indicating that selection for lower FCR may result in greater backfat depth. Although the genetic correlation between ADG and FCR was not significant in the present study, a moderate to high and negative genetic correlation was reported by Clutter [14]. This difference may result from differences in sample size, breeds, and the feeding type. The nature of this discrepancy was not investigated further within the present study, but it warrants further examination.

Correlations between Performance and Carcass Traits. The phenotypic and genetic correlations between performance and carcass traits are presented in Tables 4–5. Almost all of the phenotypic correlations between performance and carcass traits were significant (*P<0.05*). Although, pork quality importance is increasing, pig breeders are only paid for carcass yield. Results of genetic correlations indicated that selection for BW would reduce the amount of backfat depth (−0.69±0.30), which was different from the report by Fix et al. [36] who demonstrated no significant (*P>0.05*) genetic correlation between BW and FD. The differences may be due to different statistical models.

However, selection for WNW and NURW would increase loin depth because of their moderate to high genetic correlations (0.39±0.14 and 0.69±0.27), respectively. To our knowledge, these estimates in the present study are a new contribution to the literature. Weaning weight had low genetic correlations with THAM, TBEL, and PICN (0.17±0.08, 0.19±0.05, and 0.27±0.13, respectively). Nursery weight was highly correlated with subprimal cuts including TBEL (0.91±0.11), PICN (0.94±0.13), BUTT (0.94±0.17), and RIBS (0.94±0.32). This implies that selection for high nursery weight will also lead to increased belly, picnic shoulder, and butt muscle yield. This study also indicates that the NURW should be recorded in pig breeding programs as an indicator trait for subprimal cuts selection. However, no genetic correlations for WNW and NURW with carcass traits were found in the literature.

Average daily gain is one of the most important traits of selection in the pig breeding programs. Based on the estimates of this study, genetic correlations between ADG and carcass yield were moderate to high, and selection on ADG would have favorable effects on carcass yield. In general, growth is moderately to highly correlated (averaging 0.47) with primal and subprimal cut weights. These results indicated that selection for higher growth could have an increasing effect on the most valuable primal and subprimal weights. However, our results were not in agreement with van Wijk et al. [7] who reported adverse effects (on an average of −0.29) of growth on some primal and subprimal weights. The discrepancy might be due to the different genetic background, less pedigree information, and smaller sample size in their study. In addition, growth is highly correlated to HCW (0.75±0.28) and CCW (0.78±0.27), which were not reported previously.

This study revealed that ultrasound measurements of backfat thickness, marbling score, and loin depth have moderate to strong genetic correlations with their corresponding measurements of carcass merit. The weakest genetic correlation (0.39±0.12) between ultrasound measures and their corresponding carcass

Table 3. Estimates of genetic (below diagonal), phenotypic (above diagonal) correlations, heritabilities (diagonal) and their standard error of estimates among performance traits.

Traits[1]	BW	WNW	NURW	ENDW	ADG	UFD	ULD	UIMF	FCR
BW	*0.26±0.08*	**0.69±0.06**[2]	**0.47±0.03**	**0.25±0.04**	**0.42±0.04**	−0.05±0.04	**0.10±0.04**	**0.13±0.05**	–
WNW	−0.00±0.74	*0.07±0.07*	**0.19±0.03**	**0.31±0.02**	**0.22±0.08**	**0.26±0.02**	**0.16±0.02**	**0.25±0.06**	–
NURW	−0.05±0.74	0.02±0.83	*0.24±0.16*	**0.50±0.03**	**0.52±0.03**	**0.26±0.02**	**0.18±0.04**	**0.47±0.06**	–
ENDW	**0.79±0.40**	**0.93±0.45**	−0.01±0.44	*0.38±0.08*	**0.80±0.01**	**0.31±0.02**	**0.41±0.02**	**0.36±0.04**	**0.33±0.04**
ADG	−0.68±0.70	0.06±0.67	−0.03±0.45	**0.87±0.04**	*0.30±0.08*	**0.27±0.02**	**0.31±0.02**	**0.32±0.03**	**0.31±0.04**
UFD	−0.36±0.40	0.03±0.83	−0.47±0.86	**0.28±0.13**	**0.26±0.12**	*0.45±0.07*	**0.08±0.02**	**0.34±0.04**	**0.28±0.04**
ULD	**0.75±0.36**	0.04±0.79	−0.48±0.49	**0.37±0.12**	**0.31±0.13**	**−0.33±0.14**	*0.38±0.07*	0.10±0.07	**0.21±0.05**
UIMF	0.33±0.39	0.00±0.72	**0.75±0.35**	**0.60±0.27**	**0.69±0.25**	**0.48±0.19**	**−0.47±0.20**	*0.26±0.06*	–
FCR	–	–	–	0.04±0.21	−0.19±0.20	**0.39±0.17**	0.05±0.21	–	*0.20±0.06*

[1]**BW** = Birth weight (kg); **WNW** = Weaning weigh (kg); **NURW** = Nursery weight (kg); **ENDW** = End weight (kg); **ADG** = Average daily gain (g/d); **UFD** = Ultrasound backfat depth (mm); **ULD** = Ultrasound loin depth (mm); **UIMF** = Ultrasound IMF; **FCR** = Feed conversion ratio.
[2]The significant correlations are bolded ($P<0.05$).

measurements was observed between ULD and LD. This may be due to the difficulty of ultrasonic measurement of loin depth compared to backfat depth and marbling. Ultrasound backfat depth was correlated with UBEL (0.29±0.13), TBEL (0.29±0.13), and PICN (0.29±0.14). Again, to our knowledge, these estimates are new and imply that selection against ultrasound backfat depth would not necessarily reduce belly and picnic shoulder weights.

Low genetic correlations were estimated for ULD with HCW (0.20±0.10), USW (0.26±0.13), UHAM (0.29±0.13), ULOIN (0.26±0.13), PICN (0.23±0.11), and BUTT (0.34±0.13). These new results indicated that selection for high ultrasound loin depth may result in higher carcass, primal and subprimal yield including ham, loin, picnic shoulder and butt weight. High genetic correlations were also found between UIMF with TBEL (0.75±0.22), PICN (0.77±0.25), and BUTT (0.82±0.22). These imply that selection for high UIMF results in high trimmed belly, picnic shoulder and butt weight. This may be due to similar pattern of intramuscular fat deposition in these subprimal cuts. Feed conversion ratio was only correlated with TLOIN, indicating that selection for low FCR has no significant effect on carcass traits except of TLOIN (0.44±0.26). However, these results need to be further confirmed in a larger sample with FCR records.

Correlations between Performance and Meat Quality Traits. The phenotypic and genetic correlations between performance and meat quality traits are presented in Tables 6–7. Almost all of the phenotypic correlations between performance and meat quality traits were significant ($P<0.05$). However, a few significant ($P<0.05$) genetic correlations were found that can explain the hypothesis of negative effect of selection for performance traits on pork quality.

Several novel aspects were derived from this study in terms of the genetic correlation of birth weight, weaning weight, and nursery weight with pork quality. High genetic correlations were observed between BW with LOINL (0.76±0.37), LOINB (0.86±0.43), HGML (0.80±0.31), and DL (0.93±0.42). These results imply that selection for birth weight may increase drip loss, which could result in lighter color of loin *longissimus dorsi*, and ham *gluteus medius* muscles. No genetic correlations between BW and meat quality traits were found in the published literature. However, selection for high WNW does not affect pork quality but may increase the REAW (0.20±0.07), RTW (0.34±0.14), and BOW (0.46±0.17). These results indicate that selection for WNW will have no negative effects on pork quality. Moderate to high genetic antagonism was observed between NURW with CL (−0.51±0.24), and HGML (−0.69±0.35), which were also novel in this study. These results indicate that selection for high nursery weight will result in low cooking loss and lighter color of ham *gluteus medius*. However, NURW had low-to-moderate and favorable genetic correlations with other pork quality traits, indicating that selection for NURW does not have adverse effects on pork quality according to our study. The high genetic correlation found between NURW and BFW, indicating that selection for NURW will increase the backfat weight of rib eye area muscle.

Average daily gain, which is one of the main selection criteria, had no genetic correlations with all of the pork quality traits except for BOW and RTW, indicating that deterioration of pork quality was not occurring through selection for increasing ADG in these two populations. This is different to the report by van Wijk et al. [7] who showed unfavorable strong genetic correlations between growth rate and pork quality traits. However, De Vries et al. [5] and Hermesch et al. [37] reported no genetic correlation between growth and pork quality traits, which are similar to our results. In addition, ADG was correlated with RTW (0.32±0.16), and BOW

Table 4. Estimates of phenotypic correlations and their standard error of estimates between carcass and performance traits.

Traits[1]	**BW**	**WNW**	**NURW**	**ADG**	**UFD**	**ULD**	**UIMF**	**FCR**
HCW	0.02±0.05	0.04±0.05	−0.03±0.04	**0.37±0.02**[2]	**0.14±0.03**	**0.16±0.03**	**0.40±0.05**	**0.41±0.05**
CCW	0.02±0.05	0.04±0.05	−0.03±0.05	**0.37±0.02**	**0.13±0.03**	**0.16±0.03**	**0.40±0.05**	**0.41±0.05**
FD	−0.06±0.05	−0.07±0.04	**0.28±0.06**	**0.34±0.03**	**0.37±0.03**	**0.16±0.04**	−0.05±0.04	**0.32±0.05**
LD	0.07±0.04	**−0.09±0.04**	0.06±0.06	**0.32±0.03**	**−0.06±0.03**	**0.15±0.03**	0.03±0.04	−0.09±0.06
CLEN	0.00±0.05	0.01±0.05	**0.19±0.08**	**0.36±0.05**	**0.09±0.04**	**0.15±0.07**	0.04±0.05	−0.09±0.07
LEA	−0.01±0.05	−0.02±0.04	−0.00±0.04	**0.07±0.03**	**−0.10±0.03**	**0.12±0.03**	**0.32±0.06**	**0.27±0.07**
TEXS	**0.18±0.07**	−0.05±0.04	**0.41±0.08**	**0.32±0.03**	**0.17±0.05**	**0.19±0.05**	0.04±0.04	0.04±0.05
CMAR	0.05±0.05	−0.03±0.06	**0.36±0.09**	**0.33±0.03**	**0.15±0.05**	**0.17±0.05**	0.00±0.04	**0.12±0.05**
USW	0.02±0.05	0.04±0.05	**0.19±0.08**	**0.39±0.04**	**0.19±0.05**	**0.26±0.06**	0.04±0.04	0.09±0.07
UHAM	0.10±0.06	0.03±0.05	**0.37±0.09**	**0.34±0.05**	**0.26±0.07**	**0.31±0.07**	0.05±0.04	0.02±0.07
ULOIN	0.01±0.05	−0.01±0.05	**0.27±0.09**	**0.35±0.05**	**0.22±0.06**	**0.28±0.07**	0.02±0.04	0.14±0.08
USH	**0.12±0.06**	**0.09±0.04**	**0.36±0.10**	**0.36±0.05**	**0.24±0.08**	**0.29±0.07**	0.01±0.04	0.09±0.07
UBEL	0.07±0.06	−0.02±0.05	**0.37±0.10**	**0.35±0.05**	**0.33±0.07**	**0.30±0.07**	0.03±0.04	**0.18±0.07**
THAM	**0.17±0.05**	**0.17±0.04**	**0.35±0.10**	**0.35±0.05**	**0.23±0.08**	**0.28±0.08**	0.00±0.04	0.02±0.09
TLOIN	0.03±0.06	−0.01±0.05	**0.33±0.10**	**0.34±0.05**	**0.19±0.08**	**0.28±0.08**	0.04±0.04	0.03±0.10
TBEL	**0.24±0.05**	**0.14±0.04**	**0.53±0.04**	**0.29±0.04**	**0.33±0.07**	**0.32±0.07**	**0.18±0.04**	**0.26±0.08**
PICN	**0.35±0.06**	**0.12±0.05**	**0.42±0.06**	**0.28±0.04**	**0.33±0.07**	**0.29±0.07**	**0.11±0.04**	0.06±0.07
BUTT	**0.39±0.07**	**0.11±0.04**	**0.43±0.06**	**0.31±0.05**	**0.30±0.07**	**0.28±0.07**	**0.11±0.04**	−0.02±0.06
RIBS	**0.54±0.09**	**0.16±0.07**	**0.40±0.09**	**0.32±0.05**	**0.32±0.07**	**0.29±0.07**	**0.22±0.07**	0.06±0.07

[1]**BW** = Birth weight (kg); **WNW** = Weaning weigh (kg); **NURW** = Nursery weight (kg); **ENDW** = End weight (kg); **ADG** = Average daily gain (g/d); **UFD** = Ultrasound backfat depth (mm); **ULD** = Ultrasound loin depth (mm); **UIMF** = Ultrasound IMF; **FCR** = Feed conversion ratio; **HCW** = Hot carcass weight (kg); **CCW** = Cold carcass weight (kg); **FD** = Backfat depth (mm); **LD** = Loin depth (mm); **CLEN** = Carcass length (cm); **LEA** = *Longissimus dorsi* muscle area (cm^2); **TEXS** = Texture score; **CMAR** = Carcass marbling score; **USW** = Untrimmed side weight (kg); **UHAM** = Untrimmed ham weight (kg); **ULOIN** = Untrimmed loin weight (kg); **USH** = Untrimmed shoulder weight (kg); **UBEL** = Untrimmed belly weight (kg); **THAM** = Trimmed ham weight (kg); **TLOIN** = Trimmed loin weight (kg); **TBEL** = Trimmed belly weight (kg); **PICN** = Trimmed picnic shoulder weight (kg); **BUTT** = Butt shoulder weight (kg); **RIBS** = Ribs weight (kg).

[2]The significant correlations are bolded ($P<0.05$).

Table 5. Estimates of genetic correlations and their standard error of estimates between carcass and performance traits.

Traits[1]	BW	WNW	NURW	ADG	UFD	ULD	UIMF	FCR
HCW	0.19±0.84	−0.06±0.13	−0.94±0.89	**0.75±0.28**[2]	0.11±0.34	**0.20±0.10**	0.47±0.41	0.15±0.28
CCW	0.40±0.74	−0.07±0.12	−0.93±0.89	**0.78±0.27**	0.05±0.33	0.39±0.30	0.54±0.40	0.15±0.27
FD	**−0.69±0.30**	−0.85±0.68	−0.18±0.40	0.01±0.14	**0.53±0.12**	0.10±0.13	−0.22±0.28	0.20±0.20
LD	0.32±0.26	**0.39±0.14**	**0.69±0.27**	−0.10±0.13	−0.02±0.12	**0.39±0.12**	0.16±0.24	0.30±0.20
CLEN	0.18±0.59	−0.07±0.13	−0.18±0.33	**0.44±0.14**	0.05±0.14	0.10±0.13	0.15±0.23	−0.21±0.18
LEA	−0.25±0.73	−0.08±0.14	0.80±0.71	0.10±0.27	0.12±0.30	0.47±0.27	0.57±0.38	0.33±0.24
TEXS	−0.34±0.48	0.11±0.26	−0.29±0.42	−0.36±0.20	0.09±0.20	−0.24±0.20	−0.64±0.48	−0.03±0.33
CMAR	−0.38±0.34	−0.09±0.12	−0.32±0.31	0.05±0.15	−0.16±0.14	−0.09±0.14	**0.59±0.28**	0.38±0.23
USW	−0.19±0.26	−0.08±0.13	−0.10±0.33	**0.43±0.14**	0.09±0.14	**0.26±0.13**	0.24±0.24	0.18±0.17
UHAM	−0.18±0.26	−0.06±0.13	0.01±0.31	**0.34±0.14**	0.11±0.14	**0.29±0.13**	0.30±0.24	0.15±0.18
ULOIN	−0.25±0.19	−0.11±0.11	−0.01±0.26	0.13±0.13	0.14±0.13	**0.26±0.13**	0.17±0.19	0.34±0.18
USH	0.01±0.25	0.16±0.12	0.01±0.27	**0.35±0.14**	−0.09±0.14	0.17±0.13	−0.06±0.22	0.17±0.18
UBEL	−0.25±0.24	−0.17±0.12	0.10±0.28	**0.48±0.14**	**0.29±0.13**	0.21±0.13	0.18±0.23	0.21±0.18
THAM	0.22±0.18	**0.17±0.08**	0.12±0.21	**0.25±0.12**	−0.04±0.11	0.13±0.10	0.05±0.15	0.09±0.20
TLOIN	−0.24±0.22	−0.12±0.12	−0.01±0.27	0.18±0.16	0.06±0.15	0.14±0.14	0.22±0.21	**0.44±0.26**
TBEL	0.16±0.22	**0.19±0.05**	**0.91±0.11**	**0.77±0.07**	**0.29±0.13**	0.19±0.13	**0.75±0.22**	0.32±0.20
PICN	0.40±0.25	**0.27±0.13**	**0.94±0.13**	**0.79±0.08**	**0.29±0.14**	**0.23±0.11**	**0.77±0.25**	0.17±0.19
BUTT	0.50±0.30	0.26±0.16	**0.94±0.17**	**0.74±0.10**	−0.15±0.16	**0.34±0.13**	**0.82±0.22**	0.07±0.18
RIBS	0.45±0.47	0.29±0.22	**0.94±0.32**	**0.73±0.12**	−0.22±0.20	0.23±0.17	0.62±0.41	0.00±0.21

[1]See Table 4 for trait abbreviation definitions.
[2]The significant correlations are bolded ($P<0.05$).

Table 6. Estimates of phenotypic correlations and their standard error of estimates between meat quality and performance traits.

Traits[1]	BW	WNW	NURW	ADG	UFD	ULD	UIMF	FCR
WLW	**0.48±0.08**[2]	**0.11±0.04**	**0.36±0.08**	**0.33±0.05**	**0.32±0.07**	**0.28±0.06**	**0.06±0.03**	0.09±0.07
REAW	**0.53±0.09**	**0.26±0.04**	**0.41±0.09**	**0.33±0.05**	**0.21±0.08**	**0.24±0.07**	**−0.16±0.04**	−0.10±0.06
BFW	**0.40±0.11**	**0.12±0.05**	**0.41±0.08**	**0.34±0.05**	0.31±0.54	**0.26±0.08**	**0.19±0.04**	**0.38±0.06**
RTW	**0.51±0.10**	**0.24±0.04**	**0.42±0.09**	**0.34±0.05**	**0.20±0.09**	**0.27±0.08**	0.00±0.04	**−0.19±0.06**
BOW	**0.50±0.10**	**0.18±0.04**	**0.41±0.09**	**0.33±0.05**	**0.26±0.08**	**0.27±0.08**	−0.07±0.04	**−0.18±0.06**
CL	0.04±0.04	−0.07±0.04	0.15±0.09	**0.33±0.03**	**−0.06±0.03**	**0.12±0.04**	−0.06±0.04	−0.01±0.06
REAL	−0.08±0.05	**−0.14±0.04**	**0.23±0.09**	**0.32±0.03**	**0.12±0.04**	0.06±0.05	**0.21±0.04**	0.07±0.06
REAA	**0.15±0.05**	**0.14±0.04**	**0.18±0.04**	0.02±0.03	**0.11±0.03**	**−0.06±0.03**	**0.22±0.05**	**0.21±0.08**
REAB	**0.13±0.05**	−0.03±0.04	**0.43±0.08**	**0.33±0.03**	**0.19±0.04**	0.11±0.06	**0.29±0.04**	**0.14±0.06**
SHF	−0.06±0.04	−0.03±0.04	−0.02±0.05	**0.30±0.04**	**−0.11±0.03**	−0.02±0.03	**−0.15±0.04**	−0.06±0.06
LOINL	**0.16±0.05**	0.00±0.04	**0.26±0.08**	**0.33±0.03**	**0.15±0.03**	**0.13±0.04**	−0.03±0.04	**0.12±0.06**
LOINA	**0.15±0.05**	0.03±0.04	**0.37±0.08**	**0.33±0.03**	**0.11±0.04**	**0.13±0.05**	−0.06±0.04	0.06±0.06
LOINB	**0.18±0.04**	0.03±0.04	**0.36±0.08**	**0.33±0.03**	**0.18±0.04**	**0.17±0.05**	−0.03±0.04	**0.14±0.06**
PHU	−0.03±0.04	−0.01±0.04	0.01±0.04	0.03±0.03	−0.02±0.03	−0.04±0.03	0.05±0.04	−0.01±0.06
HGML	**0.15±0.04**	0.01±0.04	**0.25±0.09**	**0.32±0.03**	0.00±0.04	0.07±0.04	0.04±0.04	0.03±0.06
HGMA	**0.15±0.05**	0.01±0.04	**0.30±0.10**	**0.32±0.03**	**0.11±0.05**	**0.13±0.05**	−0.06±0.04	0.02±0.06
HGMB	**0.10±0.05**	0.03±0.04	**0.41±0.08**	**0.33±0.03**	**0.10±0.04**	**0.15±0.05**	0.02±0.04	0.00±0.06
HQFL	0.04±0.05	−0.02±0.04	**0.25±0.07**	**0.33±0.03**	**0.06±0.03**	**0.08±0.04**	−0.03±0.04	0.06±0.06
HQFA	0.04±0.04	0.02±0.04	**0.34±0.08**	**0.33±0.03**	**0.10±0.04**	0.09±0.05	0.05±0.04	−0.08±0.05
HQFB	0.08±0.05	0.00±0.04	**0.42±0.06**	**0.33±0.03**	**0.12±0.04**	**0.13±0.05**	0.06±0.04	−0.00±0.06
HILL	**0.11±0.04**	0.01±0.04	**0.18±0.08**	**0.33±0.03**	**0.13±0.03**	**0.10±0.04**	0.03±0.04	0.03±0.06
HILA	0.07±0.04	0.03±0.04	**0.36±0.08**	**0.33±0.03**	0.05±0.04	**0.11±0.05**	0.01±0.04	0.04±0.06
HILB	**0.11±0.05**	−0.01±0.04	**0.30±0.09**	**0.32±0.03**	**0.14±0.04**	**0.13±0.05**	0.03±0.04	0.04±0.06
DL	**0.14±0.04**	0.02±0.04	−0.07±0.04	−0.02±0.03	**−0.06±0.03**	0.01±0.03	0.02±0.05	0.11±0.08

[1] **BW** = Birth weight (kg); **WNW** = Weaning weigh (kg); **NURW** = Nursery weight (kg); **ADG** = Average daily gain (g/d); **UFD** = Ultrasound backfat depth (mm); **ULD** = Ultrasound loin depth (mm); **UIMF** = Ultrasound IMF; **FCR** = Feed conversion ratio; **WLW** = Whole loin weight (kg); **REAW** = Rib eye weight (kg); **BFW** = Backfat thickness weight (kg); **RTW** = Rib trim weight (kg); **BOW** = Bone/Neural weight (kg); **CL** = Cooking loss (%); **REAL** = Minolta L* rib eye area; **REAA** = Minolta a* rib eye area; **REAB** = Minolta b* rib eye area; **SHF** = Shear force (newton); **LOINL** = Minolta L* loin; **LOINA** = Minolta a* loin; **LOINB** = Minolta b* loin; **PHU** = pH ultimate; **HGML** = Minolta L* ham *gluteus medius*; **HGMA** = Minolta a* ham *gluteus medius*; **HGMB** = Minolta b* ham *gluteus medius*; **HQFL** = Minolta L* ham *quadriceps femoris*; **HQFA** = Minolta a* ham *quadriceps femoris*; **HQFB** = Minolta b* ham *quadriceps femoris*; **HILL** = Minolta L* ham *iliopsoas*; **HILA** = Minolta a* ham *iliopsoas*; **HILB** = Minolta b* ham *iliopsoas*; **DL** = Drip loss (%).

[2] The significant correlations are bolded ($P<0.05$).

Table 7. Estimates of genetic correlations and their standard error of estimates between meat quality and performance traits.

Traits[1]	BW	WNW	NURW	ADG	UFD	ULD	UIMF	FCR
WLW	0.41±0.25	**0.20±0.07**[2]	**0.80±0.18**	**0.52±0.13**	0.19±0.15	**0.42±0.13**	0.21±0.25	−0.05±0.24
REAW	0.43±0.31	**0.33±0.12**	−0.24±0.29	0.17±0.16	**−0.75±0.11**	**0.66±0.10**	−0.39±0.25	0.13±0.23
BFW	−0.33±0.27	0.08±0.14	**0.67±0.31**	−0.15±0.16	**0.89±0.05**	−0.17±0.14	0.36±0.23	0.24±0.19
RTW	−0.02±0.28	**0.34±0.14**	−0.09±0.40	**0.32±0.16**	**−0.66±0.11**	0.24±0.15	0.02±0.28	−0.28±0.22
BOW	0.09±0.34	**0.46±0.17**	−0.66±0.49	**0.43±0.19**	**−0.45±0.17**	**−0.36±0.18**	0.28±0.38	−0.33±0.26
CL	0.05±0.31	−0.02±0.18	**−0.51±0.24**	0.25±0.15	**−0.41±0.13**	0.11±0.15	**−0.67±0.26**	0.08±0.25
REAL	−0.11±0.25	−0.14±0.14	−0.10±0.22	0.02±0.14	**0.24±0.12**	0.04±0.13	**0.63±0.22**	0.29±0.20
REAA	0.63±0.44	0.22±0.13	−0.22±0.73	−0.14±0.18	0.05±0.17	−0.07±0.17	0.36±0.27	−0.07±0.22
REAB	0.36±0.34	0.03±0.15	0.23±0.23	−0.01±0.14	**0.24±0.12**	−0.14±0.12	**0.77±0.18**	0.18±0.22
SHF	−0.14±0.26	−0.04±0.13	−0.17±0.20	0.10±0.14	−0.14±0.12	−0.15±0.12	−0.30±0.23	−0.09±0.23
LOINL	**0.76±0.37**	−0.22±0.15	−0.06±0.41	0.08±0.14	0.12±0.13	0.20±0.13	−0.43±0.26	**0.43±0.19**
LOINA	0.50±0.34	−0.02±0.15	0.29±0.25	−0.00±0.14	−0.12±0.12	−0.12±0.12	−0.35±0.25	−0.18±0.21
LOINB	**0.86±0.43**	−0.17±0.17	0.41±0.26	0.11±0.16	0.05±0.14	0.11±0.15	−0.33±0.28	0.32±0.24
PHU	0.11±0.71	0.06±0.14	0.40±0.90	0.19±0.24	−0.43±0.25	**−0.49±0.24**	**0.73±0.37**	−0.30±0.30
HGML	**0.80±0.31**	−0.12±0.17	**−0.69±0.35**	0.00±0.16	−0.25±0.14	−0.13±0.14	0.42±0.29	0.30±0.23
HGMA	0.44±0.32	−0.00±0.15	−0.40±0.26	−0.20±0.13	0.05±0.12	−0.10±0.12	−0.23±0.26	−0.29±0.19
HGMB	0.79±0.49	−0.24±0.24	−0.11±0.65	−0.13±0.20	−0.18±0.19	−0.15±0.18	**0.73±0.36**	0.22±0.29
HQFL	0.02±0.33	−0.18±0.18	0.06±0.39	−0.07±0.16	−0.05±0.14	0.19±0.14	−0.24±0.31	0.15±0.23
HQFA	−0.40±0.30	−0.10±0.16	0.53±0.46	0.03±0.15	0.15±0.13	−0.09±0.13	0.14±0.29	−0.25±0.21
HQFB	−0.24±0.40	−0.30±0.24	−0.19±0.23	0.03±0.19	0.15±0.17	0.12±0.18	0.45±0.39	−0.03±0.28
HILL	0.41±0.28	−0.07±0.14	−0.01±0.25	0.22±0.14	**0.34±0.13**	0.10±0.13	0.28±0.24	0.20±0.22
HILA	0.37±0.29	0.28±0.17	0.21±0.35	−0.15±0.16	−0.01±0.14	0.01±0.14	−0.19±0.30	−0.29±0.22
HILB	0.45±0.30	−0.06±0.16	−0.11±0.26	0.16±0.15	**0.33±0.14**	0.08±0.14	0.34±0.26	−0.08±0.24
DL	**0.93±0.42**	0.07±0.13	−0.92±0.91	0.07±0.22	−0.15±0.21	−0.09±0.21	−0.25±0.34	0.13±0.27

[1]See Table 6 for trait abbreviation definitions.
[2] The significant correlations are bolded (*P*<*0.05*).

(0.43±0.19) of rib eye area, which are also novel in this study. Ultrasound backfat depth was negatively correlated to REAW (−0.75±0.11), RTW (−0.66±0.11), BOW (−0.45±0.17), and CL (−0.41±0.13) but positively correlated to BFW (0.89±0.05). Low to moderate genetic correlations were also found between UFD with REAL (0.24±0.12), REAB (0.24±0.12), HILL (0.34±0.13), and HILB (0.33±0.14). These results indicate that selection for leaner carcass will not affect pork quality traits except for cooking loss and rib eye weight (Table 7). Most of the color traits were favorably correlated with UFD except for the lightness and yellowness of *iliopsoas* muscle of ham.

Unfavorable moderate genetic correlation was observed between ULD and PHU (−0.49±0.24). This was also different to the genetic correlation between carcass loin depth and pH observed by van Wijk et al. [7]. This might be due to the different method of loin depth measurement, genetic background, less pedigree information, and smaller sample size in their study. This indicates that single-trait selection on ultrasound loin depth may lead to undesirable lower pH pork. However, this result was similar to the genetic correlation between carcass loin depth and pH in this population [2]. Ultrasound loin depth was also correlated to REAW (0.66±0.10) and BOW (−0.36±0.18), which were not reported before. Unfavorable strong genetic correlations were obtained between UIMF with PHU (0.73±0.37), REAB (0.77±0.18), and HGMB (0.73±0.36). This indicates that selection on ultrasound intramuscular fat may lead to undesirable higher pH of meat with darker color. However, cooking loss was negatively correlated to UIMF (−0.67±0.26), indicating that increased UIMF will result in decreased cooking loss. Feed conversion ratio was only correlated with LOINL, indicating that selection for low FCR does not change pork quality except of lightness of loin (0.43±0.19). Genetic correlations between FCR and pork quality traits obtained in this study may be biased due to the small dataset available for FCR.

Some of the estimates herein are new contributions to the genetic correlations between performance traits with carcass and pork quality traits. Novel results from this study showed the nursery weight is an important trait and selection for NURW will have significant effects on carcass and pork quality traits through indirect selection. Novel genetic correlations in this study indicate that selection for birth weight, weaning weight, and growth may increase market weight, ultrasound loin depth, and ultrasound intramuscular fat. Favorable correlations were found between both weaning and nursery weight with loin depth. However, selection for nursery weight would lead to increased belly, picnic shoulder, and butt muscles yield, which were dissimilar with weaning weight. Birth weight has adverse effects on pork quality traits that may lead to undesirable higher drip loss pork with paler color but no adverse effect was found between weaning weight and pork quality. In addition, favorable genetic correlation was observed between nursery weight and pork quality, showing that selection for nursery weight may lead to increased carcass yield with no adverse effect on pork quality except for *gluteus medius* lightness. Therefore, selection for nursery weight can be valuable for increasing market weight and loin depth without adverse effects on pork quality traits.

Novel genetic correlations were obtained between growth and most valuable primal, subprimal, cold and hot carcass weight. These results indicate that selection for growth traits will increase carcass yield, which was dissimilar to selection for ultrasound loin depth. It was concluded that single-trait selection on ultrasound loin depth might lead to undesirable lower pH pork. However, no genetic effect was observed on water holding capacity. Therefore, selection for ADG can be valuable for increasing both carcass weight, primal and subprimal cuts weights. Selection for intramuscular fat may increase belly, picnic shoulder, butt weights, backfat thickness and reduce ultrasound loin depth and cooking loss with undesirable higher pH of meat with darker color. In addition, novel results show that selection for lower FCR may reduce backfat depth with no adverse consequences on pork quality traits except for paler loin, and selection for leaner carcass may affect pork quality traits including cooking loss and lightness of ham.

Implications

Meat quality and carcass yield are important traits for the pork industry with consumers paying more attention to quality as well as value. Measurements of carcass and pork quality traits are difficult and expensive and can only be performed post-mortem. Genetic improvement of these traits is possible through indirect selection on performance traits, which requires knowledge of genetic parameters for these traits. However, the estimates of genetic correlations between carcass and pork quality with performance traits are limited despite its importance because the lack of measurement records of carcass and pork quality traits. In addition, segregation of the alleles from major loci is affecting the variation of pork quality traits in certain populations [38]. Therefore, understanding of genetic parameters for performance, pork quality, and carcass traits is essential for Canadian swine populations to implement efficient selection programs that emphasize product quality.

Genetic parameters obtained herein are valuable for the design of a breeding program emphasizing product quality in Canadian swine population. The low-to-moderate heritabilities of performance traits indicated that they could be improved using traditional breeding methods or genomic selection. Selection for high birth weight would have unfavorable consequences on pork quality traits including undesirable higher drip loss pork with paler color. It was concluded that selection for nursery weight would increase both quantity and quality traits. Furthermore, selection for ADG is also favorable for increasing carcass weight, primal and subprimal cuts weights with no adverse effects on pork quality. However, selection for intramuscular fat may affect pork quality traits but selection for FCR may reduce the lightness of loin. These results imply that selection for leaner carcass may affect cooking loss and lightness of ham. Although, these results indicated that deterioration of pork quality may have occurred over many generations through the selection for lower backfat thickness, and feed efficiency, but selection for growth had no adverse effects on pork quality traits. The genetic parameters identified here are valuable for understanding the biology of these traits making it possible to improve them simultaneously resulting in high quality product produced more efficiently and at lower cost.

Author Contributions

Conceived and designed the experiments: ZW GP SM. Performed the experiments: YM HB CZ. Analyzed the data: YM GM ZW. Contributed reagents/materials/analysis tools: RK PC AH BvH RM. Wrote the paper: YM ZW GP.

References

1. Dransfield E, Ngapo TM, Nielson AN, Bredahl L, Sjödén PO, et al. (2005) Consumer choice and suggested price for pork as influenced by its appearance, taste and information concerning country of origin and organic pig production. Meat Sci 69: 61–70.

2. Miar Y, Plastow GS, Bruce HL, Moore SS, Manafiazar G, et al. (2014) Genetic and Phenotypic Parameters for Carcass and Meat Quality Traits in Commercial Crossbred Pigs. J Anim Sci 92: 2869–2884.
3. Latorre MA, Pomar C, Faucitano L, Gariépy C, Methot S (2008) The relationship within and between production performance and meat quality characteristics in pigs from three different genetic lines. Livest Sci 115: 258–267.
4. Cameron ND (1990) Genetic and phenotypic parameters for carcass traits, meat and eating quality traits in pigs. Livest Prod Sci 26: 119–135.
5. De Vries AG, van der Wal PG, Long T, Eikelenboom G, Merks JWM (1994) Genetic parameters of pork quality and production traits in Yorkshire populations. Livest Prod Sci 40: 277–289.
6. Rehfeldt C, Tuchscherer A, Hartung M, Kuhn G (2008) A second look at the influence of birth weight on carcass and meat quality in pigs. Meat Sci 78: 170–175.
7. van Wijk HJ, Arts DJG, Matthews JO, Webster M, Ducro BJ, et al. (2005) Genetic parameters for carcass composition and pork quality estimated in a commercial production chain. J Anim Sci 83: 324–333.
8. Jiang YZ, Zhu L, Tang GQ, Li MZ, Jiang AA, et al. (2012) Carcass and meat quality traits of four commercial pig crossbreeds in China. Genet Mol Res 11: 4447–4455.
9. Miar Y, Plastow GS, Bruce HL, Moore SS, Durunna ON, et al. (2014) Genetic and Phenotypic Parameters Estimation for Ultrasound and Carcass Merit traits in Crossbred Beef Cattle. Can J Anim Sci 94: 273–280.
10. Canadian Council on Animal Care (1993) Guide to the Care and Use of Experimental Animals. Vol. 1. Olfert ED, Cross BM, McWilliams AA, ed. Can Counc Anim Care, Ottawa, Ontario, Canada.
11. National Swine Improvement Federation (1997) Guidelines for uniform swine improvement programs. http://www.nsif.com.
12. Gilmour AR, Gogel BJ, Cullis BR, Thompson R (2009) ASReml User Guide Release 3.0. VSN International Ltd., Hemel Hempstead, UK.
13. Cassady JP, Young LD, Leymaster KA (2002) Heterosis and recombination effects on pig growth and carcass traits. J Anim Sci 80: 2286–2302.
14. Clutter AC (2011) Genetics of performance traits, In: The Genetics of the Pigs. Rothschild MF, Rubinsky A, ed. CAB Int, New York, NY. p. 325–354.
15. Roehe R (1999) Genetic determination of individual birth weight and its association with sow productivity traits using Bayesian analyses. J Anim Sci 77: 330–343.
16. Knol EF, Leenhouwers JI, van der Lende T (2002) Genetic aspects of piglet survival. Livest Prod Sci 78: 47–55.
17. Arango J, Misztal I, Tsuruta S, Culbertson M, Holl JW, et al. (2006) Genetic study of individual preweaning mortality and birth weight in Large White piglets using threshold-linear models. Livest Sci 101: 208–218.
18. Roehe R, Shrestha NP, Mekkawy W, Baxter EM, Knap PW, et al. (2010) Genetic parameters of piglet survival and birth weight from a two-generation crossbreeding experiment under outdoor conditions designed to disentangle direct and maternal effects. J Anim Sci 88: 1276–1285.
19. Roehe R, Shrestha NP, Mekkawya W, Baxter EM, Knap PW, et al. (2009) Genetic analyses of piglet survival and individual birth weight on first generation data of a selection experiment for piglet survival under outdoor conditions. Livest Sci 121: 173–181.
20. Kaufmann D, Hofer A, Bidanel JP, Kunzi N (2008) Genetic parameters for individual birth and weaning weight and for litter size of Large White pigs. J Anim Breed Genet 117: 121–128.
21. Stewart TS, Schinckel AP (1991) Genetic parameters for swine growth and carcass traits, In: L. D.Young (ed.) Genetics of Swine. USDA-ARS, Roman L. Hruska U.S. Meat Animal Research Center, Clay Center, NE. p 77.
22. Cameron ND, Curran MK, Thompson R (1988) Estimation of sire with feeding regime interaction in pigs. Anim Prod 46: 87–95.
23. Lo LL, McLaren DG, McKeith FK, Fernando FL, Novakofski J (1992) Genetic analysis of growth, real time ultrasound, carcass and pork quality traits in Duroc and Landrace pigs: II. Heritabilities and correlations. J Anim Sci 70: 2357–2396.
24. Gilbert H, Bidanel, Gruand J, Caritez, Billon Y, et al. (2007) Genetic parameters for residual feed intake in growing pigs, with emphasis on genetic relationships with carcass and meat quality traits. J Anim Sci 85: 3182–3188.
25. Hoque MA, Kadowaki H, Shibata T, Oikawa T, Suzuki K (2007) Genetic parameters for measures of the efficiency of gain of boars and the genetic relationships with its component traits in Duroc pigs. J Anim Sci 85: 1873–1879.
26. Cai W, Casey DS, Dekkers JCM (2008) Selection response and genetic parameters for residual feed intake in Yorkshire swine. J Anim Sci 86: 287–298.
27. Clutter AC, Brascamp EW (1998) Genetics of performance traits, In: The Genetics of the Pig. Rothschild MF, Ruvinsky A, ed. CAB Int., Oxford, U.K. p. 427–462.
28. Maignel L, Daigle JP, Gariépy C, Wilson D, Sullivan B (2010) Prediction of intramuscular fat in live pigs using ultrasound technology and potential use in selection. In: Proceedings of 9th World Congress on Genetics Applied to Livestock Production, Leipzig, Germany.
29. Ducos A (1994) Paramètres génétiques des caractères de production chez le porc. Mise au point bibliographique Techni-porc 17: 35–67.
30. Schwab CR, Baas TJ, Stalder KJ, Nettleton D (2009) Results from six generations of selection for intramuscular fat in Duroc swine using real-time ultrasound. I. Direct and correlated phenotypic responses to selection. J Anim Sci 87: 2774–2780.
31. Gibson JP, Aker C, Ball R (1998) Levels of genetic variation for growth, carcass and meat quality traits of purebred pigs. In Proc. 6th World Cong. Genet. Appl Livest Prod, Armidale, Australia. 23: 499–502.
32. Sonesson AK, de Greef KH, Meuwissen THE (1998) Genetic parameters and trends of meat quality, carcass composition and performance traits in two selected lines of large white pigs. Livest Prod Sci 57: 23–32.
33. Koots KR, Gibson JP (1994) How precise are genetic correlation estimates? In Proc. 5th World Cong. Genet. Appl Livest Prod 18: 353–360.
34. Suzuki K, Irie M, Kadowaki H, Shibata T, Kumagai M, et al. (2005) Genetic parameter estimates of meat quality traits in Duroc pigs selected for average daily gain, longissimus muscle area, backfat thickness, and intramuscular fat content. J Anim Sci 83: 2058–2065.
35. Newcom DW, Baas TJ, Mabry JW, Goodwin RN (2002) Genetic Parameters for pork carcass components. J Anim Sci 80: 3099–3106.
36. Fix JS, Cassady JP, Herring WO, Holl JW, Culbertson MS, et al. (2010) Effect of piglet birth weight on body weight, growth, backfat, and longissimus muscle area of commercial market swine. Livest Sci 127: 51–59.
37. Hermesch S, Luxford BG, Graser HU (2000) Genetic parameters for lean meat yield, meat quality, reproduction and feed efficiency traits for Australian pigs. 2. Genetic relationships between production, carcass and meat quality traits. Livest Prod Sci 65: 249–259.
38. Ciobanu D, Lonergan SM, Huff-Lonergan EJ (2011) Genetics of meat quality and carcass traits, In: The Genetics of the Pigs. Rothschild MF, Rubinsky A, ed. CAB Int, New York, NY. p. 355–389.

13

Towards the Determination of *Mytilus edulis* Food Preferences Using the Dynamic Energy Budget (DEB) Theory

Coralie Picoche[1]*, Romain Le Gendre[1¤], Jonathan Flye-Sainte-Marie[2], Sylvaine Françoise[1], Frank Maheux[1], Benjamin Simon[1], Aline Gangnery[1]

1 Laboratoire Environnement Ressources de Normandie, IFREMER, Port en Bessin, France, **2** Université de Bretagne Occidentale, Institut Universitaire Européen de la Mer, Laboratoire des sciences de l'Environnement Marin (LEMAR), UMR 6539 CNRS/UBO/IRD/IFREMER, Plouzané, France

Abstract

The blue mussel, *Mytilus edulis*, is a commercially important species, with production based on both fisheries and aquaculture. Dynamic Energy Budget (DEB) models have been extensively applied to study its energetics but such applications require a deep understanding of its nutrition, from filtration to assimilation. Being filter feeders, mussels show multiple responses to temporal fluctuations in their food and environment, raising questions that can be investigated by modeling. To provide a better insight into mussel–environment interactions, an experiment was conducted in one of the main French growing zones (Utah Beach, Normandy). Mussel growth was monitored monthly for 18 months, with a large number of environmental descriptors measured in parallel. Food proxies such as chlorophyll *a*, particulate organic carbon and phytoplankton were also sampled, in addition to non-nutritious particles. High-frequency physical data recording (*e.g.*, water temperature, immersion duration) completed the habitat description. Measures revealed an increase in dry flesh mass during the first year, followed by a high mass loss, which could not be completely explained by the DEB model using raw external signals. We propose two methods that reconstruct food from shell length and dry flesh mass variations. The former depends on the inversion of the growth equation while the latter is based on iterative simulations. Assemblages of food proxies are then related to reconstructed food input, with a special focus on plankton species. A characteristic contribution is attributed to these sources to estimate nutritional values for mussels. *M. edulis* shows no preference between most plankton life history traits. Selection is based on the size of the ingested particles, which is modified by the volume and social behavior of plankton species. This finding reveals the importance of diet diversity and both passive and active selections, and confirms the need to adjust DEB models to different populations and sites.

Editor: Adam J. Munn, The University of Wollongong, Australia

Funding: This work was achieved with the financial fundings of BlueDEB and OGIVE projects. BlueDEB was supported by the French Norwegian Foundation, Basse Normandie region and Hordaland County Council. OGIVE is supported by the European Fund for Fisheries, Seine-Normandie Water Agency, Basse Normandie region and the departments of Manche and Calvados. The funders had no role in study design, data collection and analysis, decision to publish, or preparation of the manuscript.

Competing Interests: The authors have declared that no competing interests exist.

* Email: cpicoche@gmail.com

¤ Current address: Unité Lagons, Ecosystèmes et Aquaculture Durable, IFREMER, Nouméa, New-Caledonia

Introduction

The blue mussel *Mytilus edulis* is common in Europe and North America and has been consumed by man for centuries. Aquaculture can be traced back to the 13th century and now exceeds fishing due to its stability and the possibility it offers to regulate harvests. Production has been increasing for the last 50 years in response to the rise in mussel consumption and trade. This economic significance has drawn attention to *M. edulis*. Understanding the behavior and physiological responses of this species may help maximize its productivity through optimization of rearing strategies. Several models have been developed to describe mussel growth in relation to the environment. The Dynamic Energy Budget [1] theory has been the most successful of these models to date [2].

DEB models allow the quantitative description of energy acquisition and use in living systems. These models quantify energy fluxes through organisms, from energy uptake to its allocation to growth, maintenance and reproduction. As for other bivalve species [3], one of the difficulties in applying DEB models to *M. edulis* growth is to link trophic resources available in the environment with energy uptake (assimilation). In order to solve this problem, various modeling strategies have been used: the first and simplest of these consists in re-estimating the food-ingestion parameters for each studied location [4], [5]; this has allowed the DEB model to be adapted for low [6], [7] or high [8] seston conditions, for example. Different food proxies have also been tested. Chlorophyll *a* (chl a) has often been used, either as a raw input [9] or a refined input taking into account Chl a/C ratio [10]. Phytoplankton also gives good results [11], as does total particulate matter (TPM) [12]. Nevertheless, no consensus has been reached when comparing all these quantifiers [12]. In order to develop a more generic approach, other authors formalized more detailed processes for food ingestion that could incorporate several food proxies [13].

Knowledge is also needed about mussel feeding processes. Physiological aspects of food uptake have been thoroughly studied [14], [15], [16], [17], but data on the differential effects of food quality on growth are scarce. Recent studies tend to indicate that mass growth is significantly affected by diet quantity and quality [18], and that mussels may even modify their feeding behavior according to local food composition [19]. Until now, investigation focused on food physical properties, such as size, that could affect feeding behavior [20]. New techniques are being developed that give more detailed insight into the diet of *M. edulis* [21], [22], [23], [24] in terms of *e.g.*, types of food, phytoplankton species and diversity. Results are presently contradictory, however, even for the most generic points such as the comparative roles of diatoms and dinoflagellates [21], or the effect of particulate matter and other food sources (*e.g.*, detritus) [25]. This is partly due to local variability and lack of knowledge about feeding mechanisms. In the present work, we suggest that the DEB model can provide this type of information, as well as benefit from such data.

Inversing the model makes food reconstruction possible from growth observations. This has been done for several bivalves using different approaches: shell length can be mathematically related to ambient food using DEB assumptions [26]; successive approximates can be made for food [27] and the fit of different simulations obtained with different food proxies can be used as an indicator of their accuracy [12]. All these methods have their advantages and drawbacks and, until now, have focused on global food quantifiers. Here, we compare these three approaches at the scale of the phytoplankton species. This article is thus structured in three main steps: (1) we test two existing parameter sets for mussels, each representing a different way of studying food; (2) we then develop and apply our own food reconstruction methods and (3) use results to deduce general properties for food quality assessment.

Materials and Methods

Study area

Mussels were raised on the French coast of the English Channel in the western part of the Bay of Seine, northwest of the Bay of Veys and south of Utah Beach (49°24.369′N/1°09.230′W) (Fig. 1). The Bay of Veys covers 37 km^2 and has a semi-diurnal macrotidal regime with maximum amplitudes ranging from 2.5 to 7 m during neap and spring tides respectively. Freshwater inputs enter this area from the Carentan and Isigny channels, supplied by four rivers, dominated by the Vire, which contributes up to 40% of total flow [28]. Jouenne *et al.* [29], [30] described the primary production dynamics at different timescales in this bay. This small catchment area is characterized by relatively high chl a content and low turbidity compared with other estuaries, making it an intermediately productive ecosystem. Nutrient deficiency is debated: while some authors consider that their input is sufficient in the Bay of Veys [30], others hypothesize that nitrogen might be limiting during spring [10]. Anthropogenic activities seem more important than climatic conditions in explaining temporal variability in ecosystem functioning. There is a significant level of shellfish farming in this area: cultured *Crassostrea gigas* amounted to 2262 tons on Utah Beach in 2006, accounting for 14% of oyster production in whole of the Bay of Veys; *M. edulis*, at about 1332 t, represented about 85% of total mussel production in this area.

Field measurements

Mussel seed used for the experiment was collected during spring 2009 in La Plaine-sur-Mer (French Atlantic coast), and first transferred to pregrowing structures in Agon (west coast of Normandy). Pregrown mussels (20.99±1.85 mm and 0.79±0.04 g) were finally installed on Utah Beach in mid-September 2009. This site is located at around 1 km offshore and could be accessed from land at low tide for mussel sampling and by sea for hydrological measurements at high tide. Tide variation in this area led to daily emersion of the mussels lasting around 39±5% of the day. All structures were located on private sites lent by professional oyster or mussel farmers. These sites are usually used for shellfish farming and the experiment was therefore not considered to alter the environment, flora or fauna. Mussels were put in 18 plastic baskets (35 cm in height and a triangular section of side 20 cm). The baskets were installed on the middle height of 3 adjacent poles at a rate of 6 baskets per pole. Poles were separated by about 1 meter. They are the common rearing structure used for mussel culture in Normandy. Sixty mussels were placed in each half-basket, giving an initial available volume of 50 cm^3 per individual. Ninety-six individuals were separated in 9 specific nets for individual shell length monitoring. These nets were distributed in 3 baskets at a rate of 3 nets per basket. Baskets were installed on a fourth adjacent pole. Monthly sampling began in January 2010 and continued for 18 months. Each sampling date comprised two sets of measurements: one from mussels that were alive throughout the study and one from mussels that were sacrificed. In the first set, the shell length (L in mm) of the 96 identified mussels was determined *in situ* using a manual caliper (FACOM, accuracy: 0.02 mm), allowing the acquisition of individual trajectories. For the second set, the content of one randomly selected basket was sampled at each date and brought back to the laboratory. Forty of the live mussels were randomly selected, measured using a digital caliper (MITUTOYO, accuracy: 0.02 mm) and sacrificed in order to separate flesh and shell. Dry flesh mass (DFM) was measured after a complete freeze-drying cycle (METTLER TOLEDO Balance, accuracy: 1 mg). Based on the assumption that average flesh mass is proportional to cubed mussel length (eq. 1), masses were corrected for size differences on the basis of the length obtained from the individual monitoring [31].

$$M_t = a_t L_t^3 \tag{1}$$

where M_t is the reconstructed flesh mass, L_t is the measured length from the non-destructive sampling at date t and a_t is the coefficient relating length and mass, calculated with the destructive sampling. An example of such relation between mass and length is given in Fig. S1. This is different from the DEB formulation relating length and mass with a constant parameter set (eq. 13 in Text S1). Here, a_t is recalculated at each sampling date.

The two sets of mussels, corresponding to two different processes, were necessary because of the invertebrate nature of the mussels. Neither body length, nor flesh mass can be accessed without killing the animal. However, individuals should not be killed as their continuous monitoring alone can accurately assess growth. Indeed, the use of different individuals at each sampling date may introduce a bias: two different basket samples can show growth variations that should not be taken into account in the model. As a consequence, we used a first set of sacrificed mussels to calculate a proxy of the relation between shell length and flesh mass. We then used the shell length, the only measurement that we could obtain from the second set of non-sacrificed mussels, to

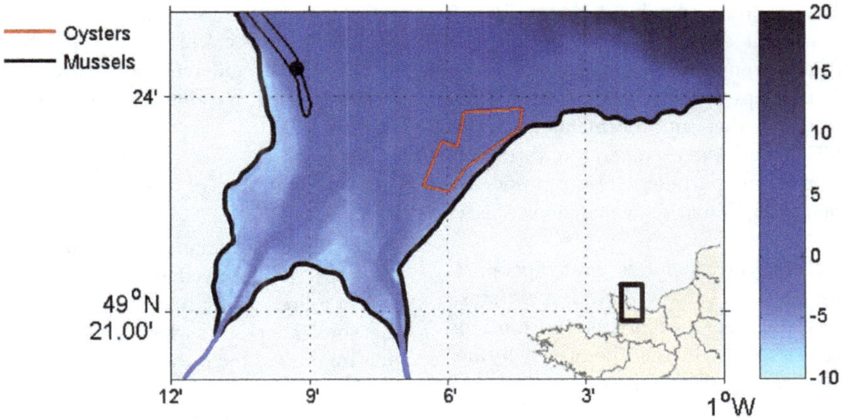

Figure 1. Location of the study area in the Bay of Veys.

reconstruct the dry flesh mass of the individuals. As a consequence, the dry flesh masses that are used as inputs in the model are a proxy of the masses of the same individuals at each sampling date.

Hydrological data (water temperature, water depth and salinity) were continuously recorded with an autonomous NKE data logger STPSO2-SI placed in a basket. Two data loggers were specifically dedicated to the experiment, used in rotation and changed every month. Observations were checked for outliers or drift, cleaned when necessary and filtered to account for immersed values only. As a consequence, temperature measurements were used only when they corresponded to immersion time. Metrological verifications were made before each deployment in the field. The frequency of data acquisition was set at 10 minutes.

Hydrobiological parameters were assessed fortnightly for a total of 33 sampling dates over 18 months. All water samplings were performed from the boat within the two hours around high tide. For nutrients (ammonia NH_4^+, silicates $Si(OH)_4$, phosphates PO_4^{3-} and nitrates-nitrites NO_2+NO_3^-), samples were taken 1 m below the surface using a Niskin bottle. Pre-filtrations were made on board with a 48 µm mesh for all nutrients plus a 0.45 µm mesh for silicates. Back in the laboratory, analyses were done with a Technicon Autoanalyzer III, according to the method described in [32]. For the other parameters, water samplings were performed by hand at around 50 cm below the surface. Particulate matter samples were filtered in duplicate through pre-combusted (450°C for 1 h) and pre-weighed Whatman GF/F filters, rinsed with distilled water to remove salts and stored at −20°C until analysis. Filters were dried at 70°C for at least 2 h and weighed for total particulate matter (TPM, mg dry mass l^{-1}). Inorganic matter (PIM, mg ash dry mass l^{-1}) was given by the mass of ash remaining after burning at 450°C for 5 h. Organic matter (POM, mg ash free dry mass l^{-1}) was given by losses at ignition. PIM and POM values are available from February to October 2010. In order to estimate trophic resources potentially available for mussels, phytoplankton biomass (chl a and pheopigment concentrations, µg l^{-1}) and composition (cell abundances of micro-, nano- and picoplankton, cell number l^{-1}) and particulate organic carbon (POC) and nitrogen (PON) were determined. For chl a and pheopigments, samples were filtered in duplicate through Whatman GF/F filters, which were frozen at −80°C for up to a month. Pigments were extracted in 90% acetone for 12 h and analyzed with the Lorenzen spectrophotometric method described by [33]. For POC and PON determination, water samples were filtered in duplicate through Whatman GF/F filters, rinsed with sodium sulfate and analyzed with a CHN analyzer according to [33]. Additional filtrations were also made for blank materials [33]. Water samples were fixed in a Lugol's solution for phytoplankton determination. The portion of phytoplankton between 20 and 200 µm in size was identified and counted in 10 ml tanks with the Ütermohl method [34] using a phase-contrast inverted microscope (Olympus IMT2 or IX71). The same analyst conducted the identification process for the entire experiment in order to maintain a consistent account of species evolution. Accuracy started at the family level and could reach species or groups of species depending on the plankton morphology. In agreement with the analyst, the level of detail was coarser in the post-processing than during the experiment: 53 out of the 77 initially identified groups of plankton were finally used. This approach discarded potential mistakes in the identification process. For pico- and nanoeukaryotes, as well as the bacteria *Synechococcus* and *Cryptophyceae*, water samples of 1 ml were fixed in 1.8 ml cryotubes with electron microscopy grade glutaraldehyde at a final concentration of 1% (vol/vol) and immediately stored in liquid nitrogen for a few months [35]. Samples were then counted by flow cytometry according to [36].

Finally, hourly rainfall measurements, wind direction and velocity and irradiance were provided by Météo France for the Sainte-Marie-Du-Mont station, located 6 km southwest of our sampling site.

Dynamic Energy Budget model

The model used in this study is based on the Dynamic Energy Budget (DEB) theory [1]. This model quantifies growth and energy allocated to reserves, structure and reproduction as a function of two forcing variables: water temperature and food availability. This type of model has been widely applied to the study of bivalve energetics [3], [4], [6], [10] and has been used to predict *M. edulis* growth and reproduction [5], [7], [9], [12], [13]. The main equations are given in Text S1. Implementation was taken from Rosland *et al.* [6], including a possible decrease in somatic mass during starvation (eq. 12 in Text S1), and adapted to take into account additions and adjustments concerning food assimilation and energy processing from Saraiva *et al.* [13] (eq. 1 to 4 in Text S1). Briefly, the model describes the energetics of an individual through the dynamics of three state variables: reserves (E), structure (V) and energy allocated to reproduction (E_R). Energy is taken from the environment and fuels the reserve compartment (eq. 1 to 6 in Text S1). A constant fraction κ of this energy is allocated to somatic maintenance and structural growth and the remaining 1-κ is allocated to maturity maintenance, development (in juveniles) and reproduction (in adults) (eq. 7 to 10 in Text S1). The energy content of the reproductive buffer is liberated at spawning. In the present application, spawning dates are forced and correspond to drops in dry flesh mass (DFM) [6]. Such a formulation is less flexible than an implementation based on gonado-somatic index (GSI) and water temperature thresholds [5] but was chosen for simplicity purposes. The reproductive buffer is assumed to be totally emptied at spawning, according to Sprung *et al.* [37].

The Arrhenius law was used to correct all rates for temperature. Main parameter values are given in Table 1. Recent food intake developments were included, requiring a calibration based on the carbon content of the particles [13]. In the absence of further knowledge, a conversion-to-carbon factor λ was added and calibrated for each food source (eq.1 in Text S1); some conversion factors are shown in Table 2. Additionally, due the same lack of knowledge, assimilation efficiency γ was assumed to be constant and equal to 0.75 [6].

Simulation and validation

Simulations were run with Matlab (Matlab R2012b), using the implementation of Rosland et al. [6]. Input daily temperature was the daily average of water temperature, measured during immersion time. Daily available food was linearly interpolated from the fortnightly observations. Chl a, abundance of micro-, nanophytoplankton and even smaller species like bacteria or *Synechococcus* (alone or as a group), POC and TPM were tested as model inputs one after the other. Composite variables were also tested by balancing chl a or phytoplankton abundance with the corresponding richness (number of species) or evenness (calculated as the ratio of the Shannon diversity index and the natural logarithm of the number of species). To account for inedible material, PIM was approximated as 80% of TPM. This is the maximum ratio of PIM to TPM that was measured during the experiment and was used to reduce assimilation [13]. Initial mass was the average mussel mass at the beginning of the experiment. Shell length was calculated accordingly.

The effect of different food sources on growth was assessed by deviation d (eq. 2). This calculates the distance to mass measures.

$$d = \sum \frac{|M_{obs,t} - M_{sim,t}|}{M_{obs,t}} \quad (2)$$

where d is the deviation of the simulation, and $M_{obs,t}$ and $M_{sim,t}$ are the respective observed and simulated DFM at observation time t.

A non-linear optimisation method (Nelder-Mead) was applied in the auto-calibration, which searched iteratively for the λ values that minimised the deviation d.

Food reconstruction

An inverse method was used to assess the quality of our food sources. Shell length and DFM were used to compute the corresponding functional response over the 18-month experiment. This response is taken as a function of both food availability and digestibility.

The first step was to reconstruct the evolution of the functional response over time from individual shell length time series, using a reversed DEB model as described in [38]. Briefly, temperature and shell length are taken as inputs of this reversed model to calculate the corresponding functional response. Different individual measurements of length are averaged and interpolated using a spline function so that the reversed model applies on the same daily time step as the standard one. The reconstructed functional response is based on the same equations and is therefore theoretically exact.

An iterative method was then used to compute a functional response corresponding to mass variation. The functional response was used with the modeling of Rosland *et al.* [6] (eq. 5 and 6 in Text S1) including the non-food related parameters that have been described by Saraiva *et al.* [13]. An initial functional response was built to vary randomly between 0 and 1. This was then used as an

Table 1. DEB parameters and values.

Symbol	Description	Value	Unit
TA	Arrhenius temperature	7022	K
$[\dot{p}_M]$	Volume-specific maintenance costs	11.6	J d^{-1} cm^{-3}
$[E_m]$	Maximum storage density	1438	J cm^{-3}
$[E_G]$	Specific cost for structure	5993	J cm^{-3}
κ	Fraction of reserves spent on somatic growth and maintenance	0.67	-
δ	Shape parameter	0.297	
$\{\dot{C}_{Rm}\}$	Maximum surface area specific clearance rate	96	L d^{-1} cm^{-2}
$\{\dot{J}_a F\}$	Algal max. s.a. specific filtration rate	0.00048	mol C $d^{-1} m^{-2}$
$\{\dot{J}_i F\}$	Inorganic material max. s.a. specific filtration rate	3.5	g d^{-1} cm^{-2}
ρ_a	Algal binding probability	0.99	-
ρ_i	Inorganic material binding probability	0.4	-
$\dot{J}_a I$	Algal max. ingestion rate	13000	mol C d^{-1}
$\dot{J}_i I$	Inorganic material maximum ingestion rate	0.11	g d^{-1}
C	Conversion factor	697000	mol J^{-1}
AE	Assimilation efficiency	0.75	-

Values were taken from Saraiva (2011a) and adapted to allow different food proxies.

Table 2. Food proxy calibration and use in the model.

Food source	Conversion parameter	Deviation (%)
Chl a	7.9×10^{-6} mol C.(μg Chl a)$^{-1}$	23.2
Chl a × richness	4.6×10^{-7} mol C.(μg Chl a)$^{-1}$	21.2
POC	8.3×10^{-8} mol C.(μg C)$^{-1}$	37.7
Phytoplankton	3.6×10^{-6} mol C.(Cell)$^{-1}$	35.8
Chaetoceros	1.8×10^{-9} mol C.(Cell)$^{-1}$	18.6

Food proxies had to be converted to mol C to adapt them to the rest of the model. Deviation corresponds to the relative difference between simulated and observed DFM, as described in eq. 2.

input for the simulation, skipping food ingestion and assimilation to affect growth directly. To do this, the classic DEB formulation was used ([6]), adjusting the maximum assimilation rate with the functional response term. Simulated growth was then compared with observed growth. For each time step between first and last sampling dates, the functional response was respectively increased or decreased as long as the simulated mass was below or above observed mass within a 1% range, and functional response was above 0. These stringent conditions ensured that variations were respected over time while maintaining a physiological sense. A functional response above 1 may indicate a bad parameter value for the maximum assimilation rate, which was expected from the results of the first simulations. On the contrary, a negative functional response can only indicate "negative" assimilation, which does not make sense.

Both reconstructed functional responses were then scaled by their maximum to vary between 0 and 1, and smoothed with a 4-day moving average to remove modeling bias.

Food quality assessment

The contribution of each food source was evaluated for each sampling date after being transformed with a Holling-type II function (eq. 3).

$$T_{i,t}=\frac{F_{i,t}}{F_{i,t}+c_i} \tag{3}$$

where $T_{i,t}$ is the transformed food source F_i at time t and c_i is a scaling coefficient, linked to saturation or satiation. This parameter regulates food absorption.

This transformation was meant to avoid signal distortion and to homogenize units between different food sources (phytoplankton abundance may vary between 0 and 10^6). It remains close to the usual DEB model formulation and helps to scale different food values. The same scaling constant was used for both functional responses (length and DFM) as mussels ingest food in the same way, with possibly different allocation. Values of both signals were similarly extracted. A linear combination of processed food measures was then used as a proxy for functional response signals. Each sampling date is thus characterized by a system of two equations (eq. 4).

$$\begin{cases}\sum_i a_i\frac{F_{i,t}}{F_{i,t}+c_i}=f_{l,t}\\ \sum_i b_i\frac{F_{i,t}}{F_{i,t}+c_i}=f_{m,t}\end{cases} \tag{4}$$

Where a_i and b_i represent the contribution of the food source F_i to growth in length or mass, respectively, and c_i is the scaling coefficient, which should be understood in this context as an index of the quantity of available food above which the contribution to total food input is maximal. It can be seen as the intensity with which mussels react to food presence: a lower c_i helps reaching a_i and b_i with lower food concentrations. f_l and f_m are the functional responses corresponding to length and mass, respectively.

Thirty-three sampling dates were available, which gave 66 equations. Each food source needed to be described by 3 parameters (a_i, b_i and c_i). An identifiability analysis ([39], used in [40], [41], [42]) showed that all three of these parameters could not be determined at the same time with a sufficient number of plankton species to study the ecological characteristics (see Text S2, Fig. S2 and S3 for more details about model assessment). c_i parameters were thus fixed, corresponding, for each species, to the median value of the abundance when the species was present in the field. This is close to the value that is obtained for X_k with the DEB model when using a single plankton species as the food input. The number of species for which a_i and b_i can be calculated is a trade-off between the condition index of the matrix model (indicating the quality of the formulation) and the final model error: in our study, 30 plankton species or groups of species was the maximum we could take into account while maintaining a reasonable condition index (3.3×10^3). These were chosen as the most abundant species that were also large enough to be efficiently retained [20].

Resolution was performed with Matlab's active-set sequential quadratic programming under constraints (Matlab R2012b). Plankton species used in hatchery were assumed to have a positive impact on growth (a_i and b_i are positive for *Chaetoceros, Skeletonema costatum, and Naviculaceae* for instance [43]). Initial a_i and b_i followed a uniform random distribution between -1 and 1, complying with the above constraints.

a_i and b_i were then transformed according to eq. 5 to represent relative contributions to total diet value.

$$w_i=\frac{x_i}{\sum_{j=1}^{n}|x_j|}*100 \tag{5}$$

where w_i is the relative contribution of the food source i corresponding to the coefficient x_i (a_i or b_i) and n is the total number of food sources.

Statistical analysis

Relative contributions of each plankton species to total diet value were linked with plankton characteristics. Several databases

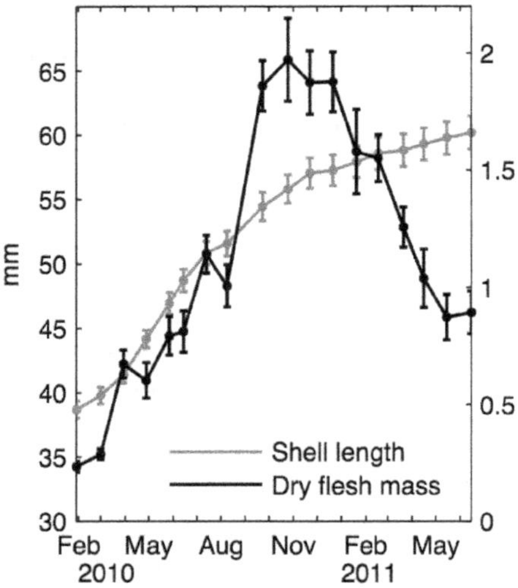

Figure 2. Observed mussel growth during the experiment. Shell length (grey) and dry flesh mass (DFM) (black) mean values and deviations correspond to monitoring with sacrifices, corrected for sampling bias.

([44], [45], [46] and M. Schapira's personal atlas) were collated and completed with data from the literature (see Table S1). Family was the first classification criterion, separating diatoms, dinoflagellates and others. Among diatoms, pennate and centric species were differentiated. Biovolume, surface area and their ratio were taken from [46], using the median value of the observations in our study area. The difference between smaller and larger species was qualitatively assessed by the plankton analyst to account for local variability. Biovolume and area were then log-10 transformed. Cell shape was also extracted from [46], using the conventions in [47]. Habitat values classified plankton according to their preference for coastal or pelagic areas ([28], [45]). Habitat was turned into an ordinal variable ranging from 1 to 3, 1 characterizing species that are specifically found in a coastal brackish environment, including those coming from freshwater inputs and 3 characterizing species that could mostly be found in the ocean. This was decided using classifications by [48], [49], [50] and [51] and evaluation of salinity and eutrophication tolerance. Plankton social behavior qualifies colony frequency. For some species, this has been quantified as the mean number of cells per colony. When this number is below 1, the species is considered as single. Above, it is considered colony forming.

Explanatory variables were chosen based on a stepwise approach using the AIC relative change as the selection criterion (LinearModel.stepwise routine in Matlab 2012b). For contribution based on DFM, social behavior and biovolume were the only relevant parameters while contributions based on length were influenced by social behavior only. To be consistent, an ANCOVA (analysis of covariance) was performed for both relative contributions, taking into account both explanatory variables.

Results

Mussel growth

Out of the 96 individually-monitored mussels, 22 individuals died during the experiment and shell-length measures of 18 individuals decreased at least once during the experiment. These trajectories were removed before data processing. Monitoring data obtained with and without sacrifice were consistent.

Mussel growth is shown on Fig. 2. During the experiment, shell length increased from 36 to 60 mm. Maximum relative length increase took place in April 2010 with a 7% gain. Shell length increased by 1.7 mm per month during 2010, while 2011 was characterized by a length gain of around 0.45 mm per month. Mass observations can be divided into two main periods: 2010 was characterized by a mass gain followed by a period of loss during year 2011. DFM increased by 1.7 g between February and October 2010. This high growth mainly took place during March, with a growth rate of +13 mg d^{-1} and between August and September (+19 mg d^{-1}). Mass was then stable until the end of the year. DFM was halved between January and May 2011.

Mussel length and mass growth were uncoupled: periods of maximum growth did not occur at the same time for shell length and flesh. In addition, the drop in flesh mass was obviously not reflected by shell length.

Environmental conditions

Variations of the main environmental descriptors over the studied period are shown in Fig. 3. During 2010, water temperature (Fig. 3A) varied between 3°C in February and 21°C at the beginning of July. During 2011, it varied between 4.4°C at the end of January and 17.6°C at the beginning of June. Average temperature from February to mid-June was 9.4°C in 2010 vs. 10.8°C in 2011. Water temperature varied 1.1±0.6°C within a day, with a minimum variation of 0.2°C and a maximum of 3.3°C, which is low enough to consider temperature to be constant over a day in the DEB model. Rainfall, irradiance and nutrient concentration dynamics (Fig. 3B) were not significantly different between the two years (Kolmogorov-Smirnov test, $p>0.05$) and patterns were consistent with previous records on this point.

Chl a dynamics can be divided into two periods (Fig. 3C). In 2010, two peaks appeared, in mid-March (16.5 μg L^{-1}) and mid-June (8.9 μg L^{-1}), followed by a longer period with a chl a level stabilized around 3 μg L^{-1} for a month at the end of summer. It reached its minimum value of 0.6 μg L^{-1} in December. Conversely, the first six months of 2011 were marked by a low chl a concentration for this period of the year. It only reached a maximum of 3.1 μg L^{-1} at the beginning of May and therefore showed a low spring plankton biomass. Between February and June, chl a was on average 66% higher in 2010 than in 2011. The maximum difference was in the intensity of the spring bloom.

Nanoeukaryote and phytoplankton dynamics were similar to one another (Fig. 3D). Nano- and microplankton abundance were low during the first four months, then tripled in mid-June 2010 to reach almost 5×10^6 C L^{-1} and nearly 2×10^6 C L^{-1} respectively. End of summer and autumn were also characterized by two smaller peaks of abundance. Winter had a low concentration of microorganisms. In 2011, phytoplankton growth resumed in April, resulting in a 13-fold increase in biomass. Nanoeukaryote abundance began increasing significantly from mid-May. Nanoeukaryotes were more abundant in 2010 than in 2011 throughout the common experiment period. Picoplankton abundance was about one order of magnitude higher than nanoeukaryote abundance but seemed to follow the same patterns. It reached a peak in July 2010 and remained high until November. After a sharp decrease, it bloomed again from April 2011, with values comparable to those observed in 2010. Overall, it may represent 86% of total chl a production. No difference was significant between the two years for the picoplankton populations.

Richness varied between 11 and 31 species in 2010, with a median value around 20, while it varied between 7 and 20 in 2011 with a median value of 14 and a standard deviation around 2.9 for both periods. It was positively correlated with abundance

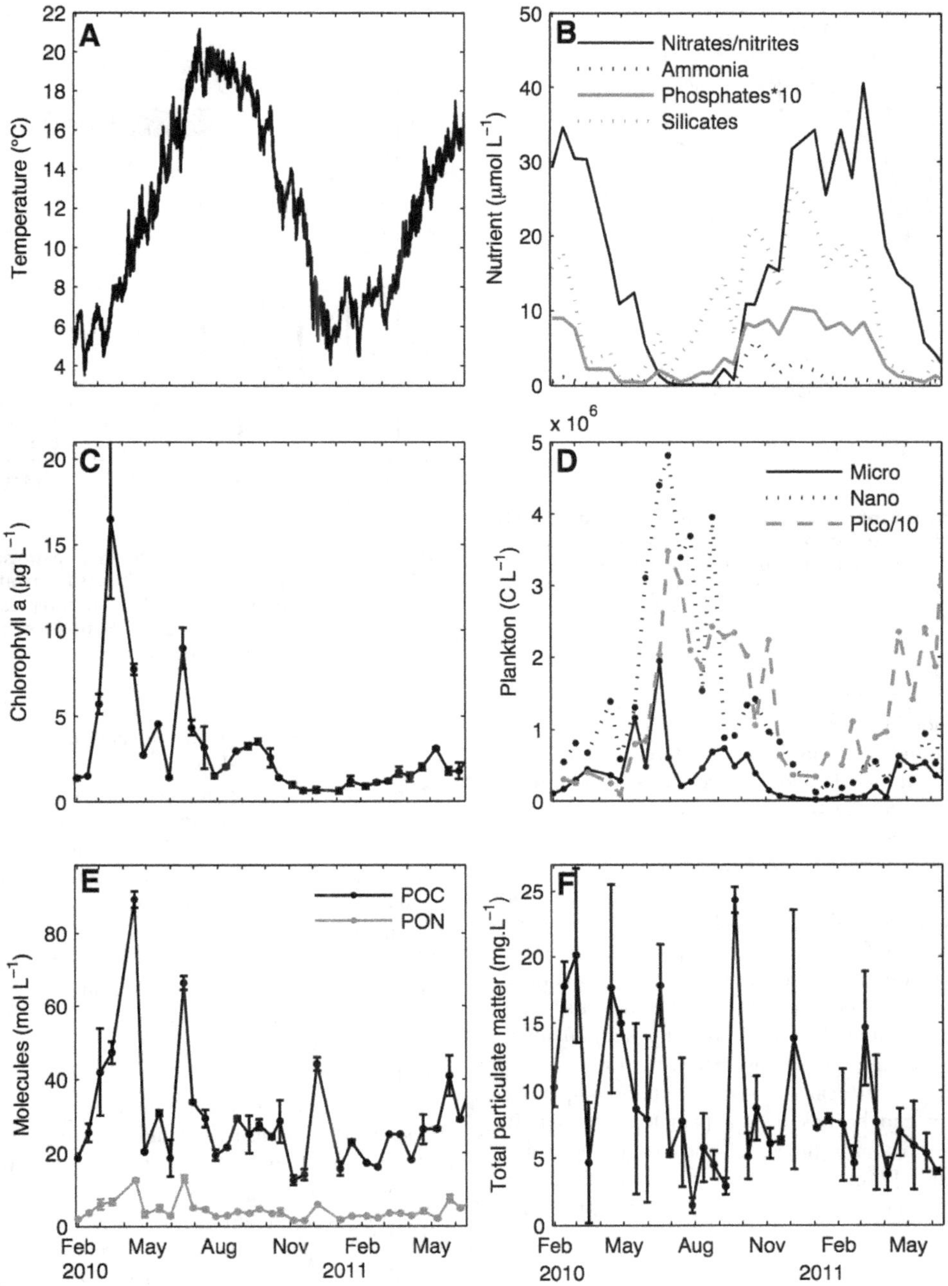

Figure 3. Observed environmental descriptors during the experiment. Average daily sea water temperature (A), nutrients (B), chlorophyll a (C), abundance of different sizes of plankton (D), particular organic carbon and nitrogen (E) and total particulate matter (F) were measured in 2010 and 2011.

($R^2 = 0.31$, $p = 0.08$). Evenness varied between 0.27 and 0.86 with a deviation of 0.17 in 2010, and varied between 0.33 and 0.74 with a deviation of 0.13 in 2011; it was negatively correlated with total abundance ($R^2 = -0.64$, $p < 0.05$). Chl a concentration could be related to these dynamics. The first chl a peak cannot be totally explained by phytoplankton or nanoeukaryote abundance but is confirmed by pheopigment concentration on the next sampling date. Phytoplankton counts explain the dynamics of last two blooms. In July, *Asterionellopsis glacialis* accounted for 76% of the total phytoplankton bloom while *Chaetoceros* amounted to 77% of the September phytoplankton biomass.

Chemical compounds did not vary as much between the two years as the variables mentioned above (Fig. 3E). POC ranged between 12.6 and 89.6 mol C L^{-1} during 2010, and between 16.1 and 40.9 mol C L^{-1} during 2011. PON ranged between 1.6 and 13.0 mol N L^{-1} during 2010, and between 1.7 and 7.4 mol N L^{-1} during 2011. Considering only the February–June period to compare the two years, there was a 33% decrease in POC and PON in 2011. This is only half the difference in chl a between 2010 and 2011. POC and PON are not only due to algal presence but also to detritus and river inputs.

Water quality was also impacted by TPM (Fig. 3F) as part of it is inorganic and may decrease food quality ([13]). TPM was highly

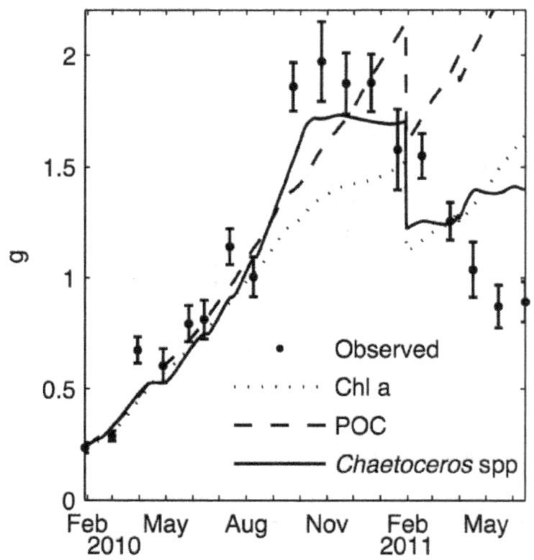

Figure 4. Comparisons of observed and modeled dry flesh mass (DFM) with different food inputs. Observations (dots) and DEB simulations (lines) are based on *in situ* measurements of food sources, with chl a (dashed line), POC (dotted line) and *Chaetoceros* spp. separately (solid line). The latter produced the best fit.

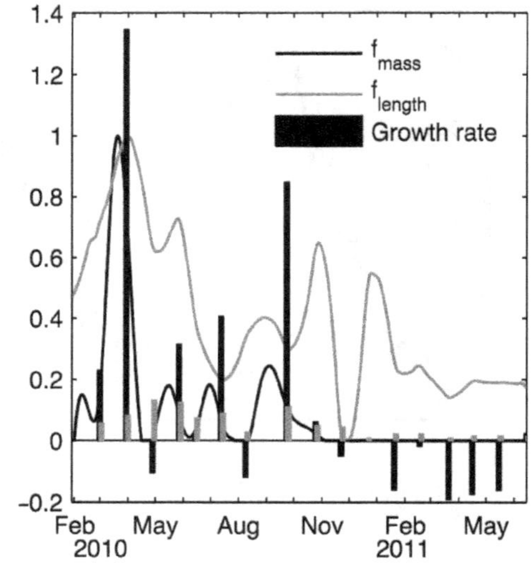

Figure 5. Comparisons of functional responses obtained with shell length (grey) and DFM (black) variation (see text for functional response computation). Bars represent the daily relative growth rates between two points. Both functional responses were standardized to vary between 0 and 1.

variable (CV = 63%), ranging from 1.49 mg L^{-1} in July 2010 to 24.3 mg L^{-1} two months later. 2011 showed less extremes with only one peak around 14.6 mg L^{-1} in March. The lower concentrations observed in 2011 should nevertheless be interpreted with caution as the strong northeasterly wind that predominated during this period may have suspended many more particles than the levels recorded at low frequency.

Relating food abundance and growth patterns is a first step towards simulations. Usual food proxies such as chl a and plankton abundance decreased in 2011, which can partly explain the observed mass loss. However, mass gain timing in 2010 cannot be totally explained by these food sources. Indeed, the first mass increase in March 2010 cannot be related to plankton abundance, but can be related to a chl a peak. Conversely, the extent of the mass gain in September 2010 cannot be related to a comparable chl a increase but it can be linked to a planktonic bloom. In contrast, the plankton bloom in June 2010 was not related to any great increase in mass. From the other point of view, POC and PON do not decrease enough in 2011 to totally explain the mass loss.

DEB model

The first simulations with the DEB model did not provide satisfactory results, especially when chl a and POC were used as food proxies, as shown on Fig. 4 and Table 2. The model failed to represent both mass gain and loss. The two steep slopes of the growth curve in March and August 2010 could not be reproduced and led to underestimates of DFM at the end of the growth season and during winter. On the contrary, food was always sufficient in 2011 to allow growth or, at least, to avoid the mass loss observed in the field. A different set of parameters (from [6] and [13]) may lead to different decrease due to spawning. The most satisfactory results were obtained using the *Chaetoceros* genus alone, which cannot represent the reality of mussel nutrition. However, when chl a was balanced by species richness, the second best fit was obtained with a total deviation of 21%; these contrasting results led us to consider the plankton species in more detail.

Figure 5 shows the functional responses computed with the reverse DEB model and compared to length and mass growth rates. Length and DFM do not show the same patterns, as their increase and decrease do not match.

Figure 6 shows the difference between observed and simulated DFM, using the corresponding reconstructed functional response. This highlights problems in the parameter sets that could not be totally remediated by adjusting food input. Food availability is not the only explanation of these variations, as a functional response of more than one is necessary to reach the masses observed in 2010. This is especially true in March where the simulated functional response can reach 8. Mass loss was underestimated when no food was input in 2011.

Food quality

Table 3 shows the contributions of the 30 different plankton species to the reconstructed function responses based on length and soft tissue growth. Of the tested plankton groups 77% were diatoms.

Relative contribution coefficients associated with DFM/length variations ranged from 0.076/0.065 for *Ditylum* spp. to −0.113/−0.087 for *Phaeocystis* spp; 57% of them were positive. Contributions obtained with shell lengths or DFM were not significantly different (Kolmogorov-Smirnov test, $p>0.05$). Consensus on the sign of the contributions was 73%. Species ranking was similar for length and DFM.

Cerataulina spp., *Euglenaceae, Guinardia striata* and *Thalassiosiraceae* play a positive role in growth in terms of mass but not in terms of length. On the contrary, *Bacillariaceae*, *Plagiogramma* spp, *Rhizosolenia setigera*, *R. pungens* and *Thalassionema nitzschioides* seem to have a positive effect on growth in terms of length, but not in terms of mass.

Both distributions were normal (Shapiro-Wilk test, $p>0.05$), enabling the use of the ANCOVA method. Social behavior has a significant effect on food quality, related to DFM (ANCOVA, $F_{1,27} = 2.9$, $p<0.01$), while this effect is unclear for length-related coefficients (ANCOVA, $F_{1,27} = 2.8$, $p = 0.11$). When plankton species tend to form colonies, mussel affinity decreases (Fig. 7A). Biovolume was not deemed significant in either group of contributions (ANCOVA, $F_{1,27} = 2.2$, $p = 0.15$ for DFM and

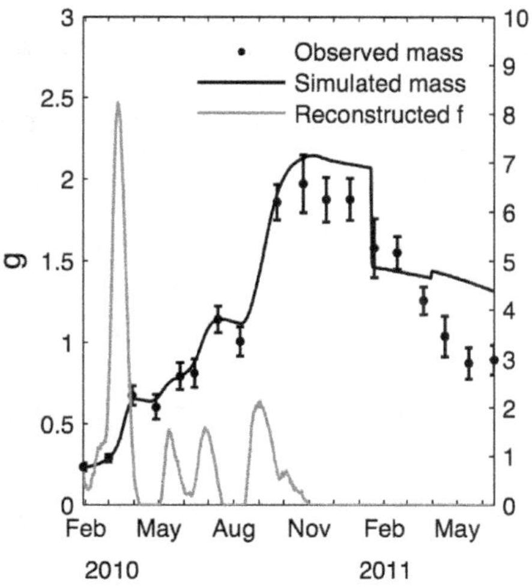

Figure 6. Comparisons of observed and modeled DFM with the reconstructed functional response. Functional response without standardization (grey) was obtained with DFM observations. Simulated DFM is shown by solid lines, observations are shown by dots.

$F_{1,27} = 0.4$, $p = 0.53$ for length). However, a slight effect can be seen, as mussels seem to grow better on larger cells (Fig. 7B). Shape effect was not significant in the analysis; however, it can be seen that large species with low contributions are all cylindrical. Among the positive contributions, 23% of plankton groups are cylinder-shaped, but these account for 46% of negative contributions. When this cylindrical shape is excluded from the analysis, size effect is significant at the 0.1 level.

Discussion

DEB performance

Mussel flesh and shell length variations reflect the ecosystem dynamics and seem to magnify them. The first mass increase (+135% in March and +85% at the end of summer) was higher than observed elsewhere for intertidal mussels, even on larger individuals [9], [52], [53]. Maximum mass at the end of the summer was surprisingly high for mussels of this size and age [4], [31], [54]. Relative gain remained coherent as it was still lower than values obtained with continuously immersed mussels [7], [55]. In all these cases, mass gain was observed much later in the year, with the more favorable climatic conditions. Total mass loss (58%) recorded in 2011 was among the highest values obtained during starvation studies [5], [6], [31].

The DEB model, as it is presently parameterized, is not able to reproduce these observations. Different parameter sets and food proxies have been tried but it has not been possible to obtain less than a 20% deviation in mass simulation, except when the input was made up of *Chaetoceros* spp only. However, diet diversity clearly improves the fit of the simulation to the observations when chl a was balanced by species richness (Table 2). These contrasted results are the first step towards a more specific analysis of the different plankton species.

More importantly, bias was always the same at the beginning of the simulation, underestimating mass during 2010. In 2011, only a total absence of food could lead to mass loss. Furthermore, while simulations were more satisfactory with the set of parameters from [13] for the first year, the one from [6] was more efficient at modeling the mass loss in 2011. When trying to avoid this problem by reconstructing the functional response, we found values over 7 for the beginning of 2010. Cardoso *et al.* [27] were faced with the same problems with *Macoma balthica* modeling, leading to functional responses higher than 1. We can conclude, as they did, that work is still needed on parameterization. δ and X_k are already known to depend on study site [5], [6] but other parameters may also be sensitive to phytoplankton ecotypes. We should therefore focus more on variations than on values.

Model quality is also problematic in recent works on *M. edulis*: while shell length is often correctly reproduced, this is not the case for DFM [7], [8] although mussel flesh is the most important aspect from an economic production viewpoint. The higher variability of flesh mass is mostly due to the losses that cannot be reproduced in shell length variation as this is an exoskeleton that is made of metabolically inert material. Gamete and reserve loss can be modeled with DEB theory, but structural loss cannot be modeled without altering the relationship between length and somatic energy [6]. This is due to the fact that we only have access to shell length and not body length. Studies have found no correlation between flesh and shell growth, even when both are increasing [12], [56]. This is partly due to differences in timing: shell length growth may precede soft tissue growth ([57], our data set) or succeed it [56]. Shell material is different from soft tissues and part of it comes from non-metabolic sources [58], [59]. This explains observed shell growth during starvation periods [60]. For the moment, the DEB model assumes that shell length is directly linked to structural flesh growth but, if this correlation does not always hold, other parameters will also need to be re-evaluated to obtain further knowledge about the species (*e.g.*, investment ratio κ). This also calls into question the use of shell length alone in functional response computation, as it can lead to the overestimation of ambient food conditions [26]. On the contrary, a comparison of both length and mass should be performed before conclusions are drawn. This is all the more difficult as shell length monitoring is preferable to avoid sampling bias that could emerge from the killing of animals to measure body length and dry flesh mass

Food preferences

The first DEB modeling led us to choose several food quantifiers to test. We focused on phytoplankton abundance which was the closest available approximate of primary production. Chl a is commonly used, but its production inside each cell depends on varying environmental conditions [61]. POC and POM are composite elements that may overestimate available food [53]. Finally, Bracken *et al.* have found that mussels might depend more on phytoplankton than on other organic elements [62]. Plankton abundance was also the most flexible variable, allowing for several levels of detail. Pre-processing included the use of a transformation to homogenize values, which can be highly variable. We chose a Holling-type II transformation (eq. 3) mostly for its physiological grounding and closeness to the DEB formulation.

It is difficult to compare our plankton dataset with others in the literature because plankton assemblages and successions are highly variable. However, some species seem to bring about a consensus. For instance, our results agree with [24], showing that *Leptocylindrus* is not ingested by mussels, while *Pleurosigma* and *Gyrosigma* spp. are preferentially ingested and *Nitzschia longissima* and *Thalassiosiraceae* may have neutral roles.

Underlying patterns appeared among food preferences. Free-living cells seem to have a positive effect on mussel growth. Even if not significant in our dataset, a preference for larger species may be another component of food quality. Both characteristics may tend towards a passive selectivity, relying both on physical and chemical properties. Size is important, as put forward by [63], who

Table 3. Phytoplankton groups and contributions for flesh- and length-based growth.

Plankton group	Contribution to flesh growth (%)	Contribution to shell length growth (%)
Asterionellopsis glacialis	4.4	3.2
Bacillariaceae	−1.8	0.4
Biddulphia spp.	1.3	2.4
Cerataulina spp.	0.2	−1.3
Chaetoceros spp.	0.01	0.01
Ciliophora	3.5	4.1
Cryptophyceae	2.7	6.2
Dactyliosolen fragilissimus	−1.2	−5.2
Ditylum spp.	7.6	6.5
Euglenaceae	3.0	−2.1
Guinardia delicatula	−7.7	−5.1
Guinardia striata	2.5	−0.4
Gymnodiniaceae+Gymnodinium spp.	4.3	4.3
Leptocylindrus spp.	−4.5	−1.6
Melosiraceae	−5.3	−7.2
Navicula+Fallacia+Haslea+Lyrella+Petroneis spp.	1.4	1.3
Nitzschia longissima	−3.3	−2.2
Odontella spp.	−0.2	−2.5
Paralia sulcata	−4.9	−1.1
Plagiogramma spp.	−5.1	4.4
Pleurosigma+Gyrosigma spp.	4.1	5.7
Phaeocystis spp.	−11.3	−8.7
Prorocentrum spp.	4.2	3.2
Pseudo-nitzschia spp.	1.7	4.7
Rhizosolenia imbricata+styliformis	4.9	3.2
Rhizosolenia setigera+pungens	−5.5	1.7
Scrippsiella+Ensiculifera+Pentapharsodinium+Bysmatrum spp.	−3.5	−6.9
Skeletonema costatum	0.01	0.01
Thalassionema nitzschioides	−1.5	1.1
Thalassiosiracaea	2.0	−3.4

Groups were determined as described in the Material and Methods. Coefficients represent the contributions of each group to the total functional response of the DEB model, given by variation in length or DFM.

used the relative amount of small planktonic species as a depletion indicator because it is the only part of plankton that cannot be affected by bivalve consumption. Following [63] and [20], picoplankton was ignored and addition of nanoplankton to our model did not improve the fit. Even when targeting species in an accurate size range according to [20], smaller species were still less important for mussel growth. Cell size is modified by the ability to form a colony, increasing the actual volume that is filtered by mussels in the field. Our results could therefore be seen as contradictory.

The mechanism behind size preference needs to be clarified, as variability in retention efficiency cannot be attributed to larger species size only [20]. Colonies, which rely on other chemical components to bind themselves together, may overload the digestive system or the ciliary-gill pump, or may clog the gills [53]; this would trigger the ejection of pseudofaeces and/or feces consisting of undigested material [17]. Such a mechanism could explain the food assimilation decrease and mass loss, and seems all the more probable as *Phaeocystis* spp., forming colonies surrounded by an organic mucilage that can decrease clearance rate [64], are identified as the worst food source in our dataset. The potential role of shape also needs to be investigated.

Other plankton life history traits were not considered to make significant contributions to food quality, which may indicate the importance of a diverse diet. Regarding plankton ecological niche, Rouillon *et al.* [21] found more tychopelagic species in mussel stomachs than in ambient water, and Lefebvre *et al.* [65] showed that oyster growth in the Bay of Veys was dependent on microphytobenthos. Toupoint *et al.* [66] pointed out that pelagic cues overwhelmed biofilm ones, at least for mussel settlement. Our study cannot settle this argument, as few benthic species were found in our dataset and no biofilms could be observed at our sampling site. These films may not settle because of water mixing and sampling during flood tide leads to a bias towards pelagic species.

No preference was found for diatoms or dinoflagellates. The proportion of diatoms in food sources match that observed in the whole dataset. Previous studies are contradictory: some insist on

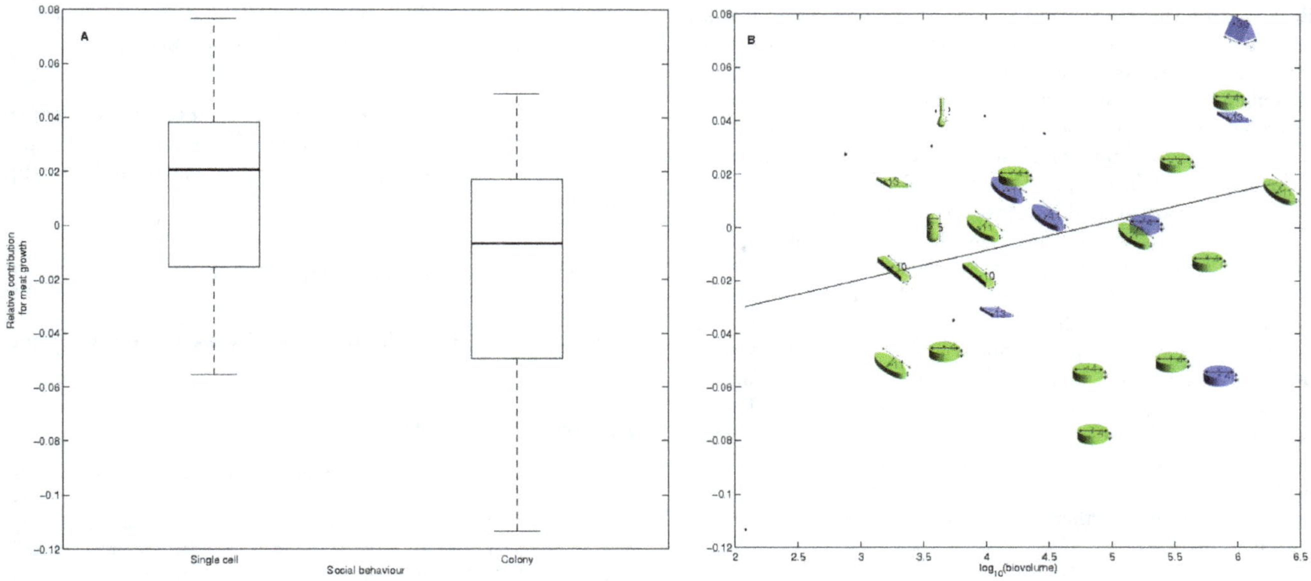

Figure 7. Effect of social behaviour (A) and biovolume (B) on mussel preference for plankton species. In the second panel, shapes correspond to the shape classification of each species, according to [47]. Blue color indicates that a species is free-living; green color indicates that it tends to form colonies. Black dots correspond to species with no defined shape.

the importance of diatoms in mussel diet [22], [67] while others emphasize the increase of dinoflagellates in the mussel diet compared with available species [68]; this has been discussed at length by Rouillon *et al.* [21]. Currently, our dataset can only show that both these groups are consumed and can play both positive and negative roles in food quality. Mussels may be sensitive to finer characteristics and/or may favor diversity [69].

Other characteristics that could have been investigated in our dataset include: how stickiness, electrostatic charge, mucopolysaccharides affect capture efficiency [17], and how morphology impacts palatability and digestibility [15]. Protein, carbohydrate and lipid contents are the key to assessing food effect on mussel growth by changing its composition [18] and even metabolism and reproductive cycle [70], [19]. Plankton composition is, however, too variable, and time- and site-dependent [14], [43], [62] to use values from the literature. Work on these aspects remains to be done and would certainly help in the search to find a structure behind our local species results. Once again, variability is high and the species that can be found in our area are certainly missing from the nearby sea [71] or will be in the coming years [30].

Finally, there are other food sources that have not been investigated and have already been found in the mussel diet: zooplankton [72], crustaceans, cnidarians, nematodes [22] and detritus [25] also contribute to the organic matter that can be ingested. Recent results tend to show that all of these sources are less influential than diatoms [23], but spatial and temporal variability would likely moderate any general conclusion [12].

Until now, we have tried to explain mass gain and loss with an emphasis on food availability and quality. Metabolism may have been altered by a significant switch between abundance and restriction. The former may have led to a decrease in growth efficiency that worsened the effect of restriction [73]. A high concentration of PIM may have altered assimilation efficiency while food was already low in quantity and quality for mussels. However, two other, non-exclusive, explanations should be considered but cannot be proven with our dataset.

The reproductive cycle must have played a key role in mass regulation [54]. We cannot differentiate the loss due to starvation from that due to spawning. These must have coexisted as spawning alone cannot explain the mass loss in its entirety. Gonadosomatic ratio, although very variable, rarely reaches 55% [74], [75], [76], and recent studies tend to show that *M. edulis* might invest less in reproduction than was previously thought [13]. No mass recovery was recorded for 5 months, contrary to what is usually observed after spawning [56]. Conversely, this mass drop is too sharp to be due to metabolism alone.

Mussels have multiple and contradictory reproductive strategies depending on environmental conditions [19], [77], [78]. According to mussel farmers working in the study area, climatic conditions were very favorable to spawning in 2011. Metabolism might change during spawning time and requires more energy [79] or energy in a different form [24], which could have worsened mass loss that year. Loss of mass due to spawning in the DEB model depends on several parameters: allocation parameter κ, spawning efficiency and percentage of gametes left in the reproductive compartment after spawning. The latter has been discussed: mussels can spawn completely [37] or partially [76]. Furthermore, the use of GSI and temperature thresholds was not successful in reproducing growth and led to incoherent patterns (*e.g.* up to 5 or 6 spawning dates in 2010 at times where the actual reproduction cycle was not completed). This was not the main point of our study, which is why we decided, like [7] and [12], to empty the gonads at a fixed spawning date. Without further organ differentiation, it would have been presumptuous to model a reproductive cycle for our experiment, which is why this explanation has not been developed further; knowledge is still required in this area and needs to be improved.

The possibility of infection must also be presented. During 2010, the presence of *Mytilicola intestinalis* was recorded on Utah

Beach. Although infestation level was ranked low, there is still a possibility that the parasite developed and infected mussels in our experiments. Digestive disruptions may have resulted, decreasing assimilation efficiency; maintenance costs may also have been increased by the presence of a parasite. This could lead to differences in the physiological parameters describing mussel growth and explain the problems in DEB simulations that were observed even when food input was reconstructed.

To conclude, this article highlights the difficulty of representing different mussel growth patterns with a model smoothing tendency. Work needs to be done on DEB parameterization for *M. edulis* in this area. In the absence of further information, functional response reconstruction enabled us to get over the problem while still taking into account other environmental elements. This led to the selection of the preferred species that mussels have in the environments and to the identification of some patterns. A size gradient is noticeable in our dataset. Mussels tend to grow better on larger, single species. Plankton composition now needs to be studied further in order to relate it to mussel growth and investment.

Supporting Information

Figure S1 Comparisons of observed and modeled DFM as a function of cubed length.

Figure S2 Example of an eigenvector contribution to the model coefficients for the smallest eigenvalue, using a model optimizing the scaling coefficient c_i and simultaneous contributions of a_i and b_i.

Figure S3 Evolution of the parameter identifiability with the number of species taken into account. The condition number of the Hessian matrix of the model cost function (in grey) is related to the convergence rate of the model. The fit is measured by the mean square model error (in black).

Table S1 Plankton ecological characteristics. Family affiliation and social behavior are from [44]. Position in the water column is mostly from [45] and [28]. Habitats are from [48], [49], [50] and [51]. Biovolumes are from [46].

Text S1 Main DEB model equations.

Text S2 Analysis of the food quality assessment model.

Acknowledgments

The idea of this study originates from the BlueDEB project coordinated by Marianne Alunno-Bruscia and Øivind Strand. We are grateful to Mr Clouet for providing and storing young mussels in La-Plaine-sur-Mer and the Lefebvre company for loaning a part of their farming area for their rearing. We thank Aurore Lejolivet, Charlotte Mary and Sophie Parrad for their help on the field site and for taking care of our mussels, dead or alive; Xavier Philippon for CHN analyses; and Olivier Pierre-Duplessix and Emilie Rabiller for hydrological analyses. We would also like to thank Banyuls Oceanologic Observatory for the cytometry analyses. The data could not have been so fully understood without Mathilde Schapira's invaluable plankton atlas. English assistance was provided by Helen McCombie. Finally, we are especially grateful to both our reviewers for their insightful comments that have greatly improved this paper.

Author Contributions

Conceived and designed the experiments: AG FM BS. Performed the experiments: FM BS SF. Analyzed the data: CP JFSM AG RLG. Contributed reagents/materials/analysis tools: JFSM CP RLG AG. Wrote the paper: CP AG RLG.

References

1. Kooijman SALM (2010) Dynamic Energy Budget theory for metabolic organisation. Cambridge University Press. 532 pp. ISBN 9780521131919.
2. Beadman HA, Willows RI, Kaiser MJ (2002) Potential applications of mussel modeling. Helgol Mar Res 56: 76–85.
3. van der Veer HW, Cardoso JFMF, van der Meer J (2006) The estimation of DEB parameters for various Northeast Atlantic bivalve species. J Sea Res 56(2): 107–124.
4. Troost TA, Wijsman JWM, Saraiva S, Freitas V (2010) Modeling shellfish growth with Dynamic Energy Budget (DEB) models: an application for cockles and mussels in the Oosterschelde (SW Netherlands). Phil Trans R Soc B (365): 3567–3577.
5. Thomas Y, Mazurié J, Alunno-Bruscia M, Bacher C, Bouget JF, et al. (2011) Modelling spatio-temporal variability of *Mytilus edulis* (L.) growth by forcing a dynamic energy budget model with satellite-derived environmental data. J Sea Res 66(4): 308–317.
6. Rosland R, Strand Ø, Alunno-Bruscia M, Bacher C, Strohmeier T (2009) Applying Dynamic Energy Budget (DEB) theory to simulate growth and bio-energetics of blue mussels under low seston conditions. J Sea Res 62(2–3): 49–61.
7. Duarte P, Fernández-Reiriz MJ, Labarta U (2012) Modelling mussel growth in ecosystems with low suspended matter loads using a Dynamic Energy Budget approach. J Sea Res 67: 44–57.
8. Saraiva S, van der Meer J, Kooijman SALM, Witbaard R, Philippart CJM, et al. (2012) Validation of a Dynamic Energy Budget (DEB) model for the blue mussel *Mytilus edulis*. Mar Ecol Prog Ser 463: 141–158.
9. Dabrowski T, Lyons K, Curé M, Berry A, Nolan G (2013) Numerical modelling of spatio-temporal variability of growth of *Mytilus edulis* (L.) and influence of its cultivation on ecosystem functioning. J Sea Res 76: 5–21.
10. Grangeré K, Ménesguen A, Lefebvre S, Bacher C, Pouvreau S (2009) Modelling the influence of environmental factors on the physiological status of the Pacific oyster *Crassostrea gigas* in an estuarine embayment; The Baie des Veys (France). J Sea Res 62: 147–158.
11. Bourlès Y, Alunno-Bruscia M, Pouvreau S, Tollu G, Leguay D, et al. (2009) Modelling growth and reproduction of the Pacific oyster *Crassostrea gigas*: Advances in the oyster-DEB model through application to a coastal pond. J Sea Res 62 (2–3): 62–71.
12. Handå A, Alver M, Edvardsen CV, Halstensen S, Olsen AJ, et al. (2011) Growth of farmed blue mussels (*Mytilus edulis* L.) in a Norwegian coastal area; comparison of food proxies by DEB modeling. J Sea Res 66: 297–307.
13. Saraiva S, van der Meer J, Kooijman S, Sousa T (2011a) DEB parameters estimation for *Mytilus edulis*. J Sea Res 66: 289–296.
14. Widdows J, Fieth P, Worrall CM (1979) Relationships between Seston, Available Food and Feeding Activity in the Common Mussel *Mytilus edulis*. Mar Biol 50: 195–207.
15. Bougrier S, Hawkins AJS, Héral M (1997) Preingestive selection of different microalgal mixtures in *Crassostrea gigas* and *Mytilus edulis*, analysed by flow cytometry. Aquaculture 150: 123–134.
16. Saurel C, Gascoigne JC, Palmer MR, Kaiser MJ (2007) In situ Mussel Feeding Behavior in Relation to Multiple Environmental Factors: Regulation through Food Concentration and Tidal Conditions. Limnol Oceanogr 52(5): 1919–1929.
17. Riisgård HU, Egede PP, Saavedra IB (2011). Feeding Behaviour of the Mussel, *Mytilus edulis*: New Observations, with a Minireview of Current Knowledge. J Mar Biol DOI: 10.1155/2011/312459.
18. Pleissner D, Eriksen NT, Lundgreen K, Riisgård HU (2012) Biomass Composition of Blue Mussels, *Mytilus edulis*, is Affected by Living Site and Species of Ingested Microalgae. ISRN Zool doi:10.5402/2012/902152
19. Toupoint N, Gilmore-Solomon L, Bourque F, Myrand B, Pernet F, et al. (2012a) Match/mismatch between the *Mytilus edulis* larval supply and seston quality: effect on recruitment. Ecology 93(8): 1922–1934.
20. Strohmeier T, Strand Ø, Alunno-Bruscia M, Duinker A, Cranford PJ (2012) Variability in particle retention efficiency by the mussel *Mytilus edulis*. J Exp Mar Bio Ecol 412: 96–102.
21. Rouillon G, Guerra Rivas J, Ochoa N, Navarro E (2005) Phytoplankton composition of the stomach contents of the mussel *Mytilus edulis* L. from two populations: comparison with its food supply. J Shellfish Res 24(1): 5–14.
22. Maloy AP, Nelle P, Culloty SC, Slater JW, Harrod C (2013) Identifying trophic variation in a marine suspension feeder: DNA- and stable isotope-based dietary analysis in *Mytilus* spp. Mar Biol 160(2): 479–490.
23. Pernet F, Malet N, Pastoureaud A, Vaquer A, Quéré C., et al. (2012) Marine diatoms sustain growth of bivalves in a Mediterranean lagoon. J Sea Res 68: 20–32.

24. Lauringson V, Kotta J, Orav-Kotta H, Kaljurand K (2014) Diet of mussels *Mytilus trossulus* and *Dreissena polymorpha* in a brackish nontidal environment. Mar Ecol 35(1): 56–66.
25. Rodhouse PG, Roden CM, Burnell GM, Hensey MP, McMahon T (1984) Food resource, gametogenesis and growth of *Mytilus edulis* on the shore and in suspended culture: Killary Harbour, Ireland. J Mar Biol Assoc UK 64(3): 513–529.
26. Freitas V, Cardoso JFMF, Santos S, Campos J, Drent J, et al. (2009) Reconstruction of food conditions for Northeast Atlantic bivalve species based on Dynamic Energy Budgets. J Sea Res 62: 75–82.
27. Cardoso JFMF, Witte JIJ, van der Veer HW (2006) Intra- and interspecies comparison of energy flow in bivalve species in Dutch coastal waters by means of the Dynamic Energy Budget (DEB) theory. J Sea Res 56: 182–197.
28. Ubertini M, Lefebvre S, Gangnery A, Grangeré K, Le Gendre R, et al. (2012) Spatial Variability of Benthic-Pelagic Coupling in an Estuary Ecosystem: Consequences for Microphytobenthos Resuspension Phenomenon. PLoS ONE 7(8): e44155. doi:10.1371/journal.pone.0044155.
29. Jouenne F, Lefebvre S, Véron B, Lagadeuc Y (2005) Biological and physicochemical factors controlling short-term variability in phytoplankton primary production and photosynthetic parameters in a macrotidal ecosystem (eastern English Channel). Estuar Coast Shelf Sci 65: 421–439.
30. Jouenne F, Lefebvre S, Véron B, Lagadeuc Y (2007) Phytoplankton community structure and primary production in small intertidal estuarine-bay ecosystem (eastern English Channel, France). Mar Biol 151: 805–825.
31. Bayne BL, Worrall CM (1980) Growth and production of mussels *Mytilus edulis* from two populations. Mar Ecol Prog Ser 3: 317–328.
32. Aminot A, Kérouel R (2007) Dosage automatique des nutriments dans les eaux marines. Ed. Ifremer, 336 p.
33. Aminot A, Kérouel R (2004) Hydrologie des écosystèmes marins. Paramètres et analyses. Ed. Ifremer, 336p.
34. Utermöhl H (1958) Zur vervolkommung der quantativen phytoplankton methodik. Int Ver Theoret Angew Limnol 9: 1–38.
35. Vaulot D, Courties C, Partensky F (1989) A simple method to preserve oceanic phytoplankton for flow cytometric analyses. Cytometry, 10: 629–635.
36. Marie D, Partensky F, Jacquet S, Vaulot D (1997) Enumeration and cell cycle analysis of natural populations of marine picoplankton by flow cytometry using the nucleic acid stain SyBR Green I. Appl Environ Microbiol. 63: 186–193.
37. Sprung M (1983) Reproduction and fecundity of the mussel *Mytilus edulis* at Helgoland (North Sea). Helgol Mar Res 36: 243–255.
38. Flye Sainte Marie J, Alunno-Bruscia M, Gangnery A, Rannou E, Rosland R, et al. (2009). Individual mussel growth model using DEB (Dynamic Energy Budget) theory: revisiting the DEB parameter values for *Mytilus edulis*. Aquaculture Europe 2009, Trondheim, 14–17 August 2010.
39. Thacker WC (1989) The role of the Hessian matrix in fitting models to measurements. J Geophys Res 94: 6177–6196.
40. Fenner K, Losch M, Schröter J, Wenzel M (2001) Testing a marine ecosystem model: sensitivity analysis and parameter optimization. J Mar Syst 28: 45–63.
41. Faugeras B, Lévy M, Mémery L, Verron J, Blum J, et al. (2003) Can biogeochemical fluxes be recovered from nitrates and chlorophyll data? A case study assimilating data in the Northwestern Mediterranean Sea at the JGOFS-DYFAMED station. J Mar Syst 40: 99–125.
42. Dueri S, Faugeras B, Maury O (2012) Modelling the skipjack tuna dynamics in the Indian Ocean with APECOSM-E – Part 2: Parameter estimation and sensitivity analysis. Ecol Model 245: 55–64.
43. Leonardos N, Lucas IAN (2000) The nutritional value of algae grown under different culture conditions for Mytilus edulis L. larvae. Aquaculture 182: 301–315.
44. Horner RA (2002) A taxonomic guide to some common marine phytoplankton. Bristol: Biopress. 195p.
45. Guilloux L, Rigaut-Jalabert F, Jouenne F, Ristori S, Viprey M, et al. (2013) An annotated checklist of Marine Phytoplankton taxa at the SOMLIT-Astan time series off Roscoff (Western English Channel, France): data collected from 2000 to 2010. Cah Biol Mar 54: 247–256.
46. Leblanc K, Aristegui J, Armand L, Assmy P, Beker B, et al. (2012) A global diatom database – abundance, biovolume and biomass in the world ocean. Earth Syst Sci Data 4(1): 149–165.
47. Sun J, Liu D (2003) Geometric models for calculating cell biovolume and surface area for phytoplankton. J Plankton Res 25(11): 1331–1346.
48. Marshall HG, Burchardt L (2004) Phytoplankton composition within the tidal freshwater-oligohaline regions of the Rappahannock and Pamunkey Rivers in Virginia. Castanea 69(4): 272–283.
49. Marshall HG, Lacouture RV, Buchanan C, Johnson JM (2006) Phytoplankton assemblages associated with water quality and salinity regions in Chesapeake Bay, USA. Estuar Coast Shel Sci 69(1–2): 10–18.
50. Brand LE (1984) The salinity tolerance of forty-six marine phytoplankton isolates. Estuar Coast Shelf Sci 18(5): 543–556.
51. Jiang H (1996) Diatoms from the surface sediments of the Skagerrak and the Kattegat and their relationship to the spatial changes of environmental variables. J Biogeogr 23(2): 129–137.
52. de Zwaan A, Zandee DI (1972) Body distribution and seasonal changes in the glycogen content of the common sea mussel *Mytilus edulis*. Comp Biochem Physiol 43(A): 53–58.
53. Smaal AC, Vonck APMA (1997) Seasonal variation in C, N and P budgets and tissue composition of the mussel *Mytilus edulis*. Mar Ecol Prog Ser 153: 167–179.
54. Garen P, Robert S, Bougrier S (2004) Comparison of growth of mussel, *Mytilus edulis*, on longline, pole and bottom culture sites in the Pertuis Breton, France. Aquaculture 232: 511–524.
55. Dare PJ, Edwards DB (1975) Seasonal changes in flesh mass and biochemical composition of mussels (*Mytilus edulis* L.) in the Conwy estuary, North Wales. J exp Mar Biol Ecol 18: 89–97.
56. Hilbish TJ (1986) Growth trajectories of shell and soft tissue in bivalves: seasonal variation in *Mytilus edulis* L. J exp Mar Biol Ecol 96: 103–113.
57. Kautsky N (1982) Quantitative Studies on Gonad Cycle, Fecundity, Reproductive Output and Recruitment in a Baltic *Mytilus edulis* Population. Mar Biol 68: 143–160.
58. Tanaka N, Monaghan MC, Rye DM (1986) Contribution of metabolic carbon to mollusc and barnacle shell carbonate. Nature 320: 520–523.
59. Gillikin DP, Lorrain A, Bouillon S, Willenz P, Dehairs F (2006) Stable carbon isotopic composition of *Mytilus edulis* shells: relation to metabolism, salinity, $\delta^{13}C_{DIC}$ and phytoplankton. Org Geochem 37: 1371–1382.
60. Palmer AR (1981) Do carbonate skeletons limit the rate of body growth? Nature 292: 150–152.
61. Behrenfeld MJ, Halsey KH, Milligan AJ (2008b) Evolved physiological responses of phytoplankton to their integrated growth environment. Phil Trans R Soc B 363: 2687–2703.
62. Bracken MES, Menge BA, Foley MM, Sorte CJB, Lubchenco J, Schiel DR (2012) Mussel selectivity for high-quality food drives carbon inputs into open-coast intertidal ecosystems. Mar Ecol Prog Ser 459: 53–62.
63. Cranford PJ, Hargrave B, Li W (2009) No mussel is an island. ICES insight 46, 44–49.
64. Smaal AC, Twisk F (1997) Filtration and absorption of *Phaeocystis* cf. *globosa* by the mussel *Mytilus edulis* L. J Exp Mar Biol Ecol 209: 33–46.
65. Lefebvre S, Harma C, Blin JL (2009) Trophic typology of coastal ecosystems based on $\delta^{13}C$ and $\delta^{15}N$ ratios in an opportunistic suspension feeder. Mar Ecol Prog Ser 390: 27–37.
66. Toupoint N, Mohit V, Linossier I, Bourgougnon N, Myrand B, et al. (2012b) Effect of biofilm age on settlement of *Mytilus edulis*. Biofouling 28(9): 985–1001.
67. Pronker AE, Nevejan NM, Peene F, Geisjen P, Sorgeloos P (2007) Hatchery broodstock conditioning of the blue mussel *Mytilus edulis* (Linnaeus 1758). Part I. Impact of different micro-algae mixtures on broodstock performance. Aquacult Int 16(4): 297–307.
68. Trottet A, Roy S, Tamigneaux E, Lovejoy C, Tremblay R (2008) Impact of suspended mussels (*Mytilus edulis* L.) on plankton communities in a Magdalen Islands lagoon (Québec, Canada): A mesocosm approach. J exp Mar Biol Ecol 365: 103–115.
69. Strömgren T, Cary C (1984) Growth in length of *Mytilus edulis* L. fed on different algal diets. J Exp Mar Bio Ecol 76: 23:34.
70. Fearman JA, Bolch CJS, Moltschaniwskyj NA (2009) Energy Storage and Reproduction in Mussels, *Mytilus galloprovincialis*: The Influence of Diet Quality. J shellfish Res 28(2): 305–312.
71. Masquelier S, Foulon E, Jouenne F, Ferréol M, Brussaard CPD, et al. (2011) Distribution of eukaryotic plankton in the English Channel and the North Sea in summer. J Sea Res 66: 111–122.
72. Lehane C, Davenport J (2006) A 15-month study of zooplankton ingestion by farmed mussels (*Mytilus edulis*) in Bantry Bay, Southwest Ireland. Estuar Coast Shelf Sci 67: 645–652.
73. Bayne BL (1973) Physiological changes in *Mytilus edulis* L. induced by temperature and nutritive stress. J Mar Biol Ass UK 53: 39–58.
74. Toro JE, Thompson RJ, Innes DJ (2002) Reproductive isolation and reproductive output in two sympatric mussel species (*Mytilus edulis*, *M. trossulus*) and their hybrids from Newfoundland. Mar Biol 141: 897–909.
75. Doherty SD, Brophy D, Gosling E (2009) Synchronous reproduction may facilitate introgression in a hybrid mussel (*Mytilus*) population. J exp Mar Biol Ecol 378: 1–7.
76. Cardoso JFMF, Dekker R, Witte JIJ, van der Veer HW (2007) Is reproductive failure responsible for reduced recruitment of intertidal *Mytilus edulis* L. in the western Dutch Wadden Sea? Mar Biodivers 37(2): 83–92.
77. Newell RIE, Hilbish TJ, Koehn RK, Newell CJ (1982) Temporal variation in the reproductive cycle of *Mytilus edulis* L. (bivalvia, mytilidae) from localities on the East coast of the United States. Biol Bull 162: 299–310.
78. Thorarinsdóttir GG, Gunnarsson K (2003) Reproductive cycles of *Mytilus edulis* L. on the west and east coasts of Iceland. Polar Res 22(2): 217–223.
79. Hagger JA, Lowe D, Dissanayake A, Jones MB, Galloway TS (2010) The influence of seasonality on biomarker responses in *Mytilus edulis*. Ecotoxicology 19: 953–962.

14

Genome-Wide Association Studies Using Haplotypes and Individual SNPs in Simmental Cattle

Yang Wu[1], Huizhong Fan[1], Yanhui Wang[1], Lupei Zhang[1], Xue Gao[1], Yan Chen[1], Junya Li[1], HongYan Ren[2]*, Huijiang Gao[1]*

1 Institute of Animal Science, Chinese Academy of Agricultural Science, Beijing, China, **2** Department of life sciences, National Natural Science Foundation of China, Beijing, China

Abstract

Recent advances in high-throughput genotyping technologies have provided the opportunity to map genes using associations between complex traits and markers. Genome-wide association studies (GWAS) based on either a single marker or haplotype have identified genetic variants and underlying genetic mechanisms of quantitative traits. Prompted by the achievements of studies examining economic traits in cattle and to verify the consistency of these two methods using real data, the current study was conducted to construct the haplotype structure in the bovine genome and to detect relevant genes genuinely affecting a carcass trait and a meat quality trait. Using the Illumina BovineHD BeadChip, 942 young bulls with genotyping data were introduced as a reference population to identify the genes in the beef cattle genome significantly associated with foreshank weight and triglyceride levels. In total, 92,553 haplotype blocks were detected in the genome. The regions of high linkage disequilibrium extended up to approximately 200 kb, and the size of haplotype blocks ranged from 22 bp to 199,266 bp. Additionally, the individual SNP analysis and the haplotype-based analysis detected similar regions and common SNPs for these two representative traits. A total of 12 and 7 SNPs in the bovine genome were significantly associated with foreshank weight and triglyceride levels, respectively. By comparison, 4 and 5 haplotype blocks containing the majority of significant SNPs were strongly associated with foreshank weight and triglyceride levels, respectively. In addition, 36 SNPs with high linkage disequilibrium were detected in the GNAQ gene, a potential hotspot that may play a crucial role for regulating carcass trait components.

Editor: Zhongxue Chen, Indiana University Bloomington, United States of America

Funding: This work was supported by the Cattle Breeding Innovative Research Team (cxgc-ias-03), the 12th "Five-Year" National Science and Technology Support Project (2011BAD28B04) basic research fund program, Chinese Academy of Agricultural Sciences Fundamental Research Budget Increment Project (2013ZL031), National High Technology Research and Development Program of China (863 Program 2013AA102505-4) and National Natural Science Foundations of China (31372294). The funders had no role in study design, data collection and analysis, decision to publish, or preparation of the manuscript.

Competing Interests: The authors have declared that no competing interests exist.

* Email: gaohj111@sina.com (HG); renhy@nsfc.gov.cn (HR)

Introduction

Single nucleotide polymorphisms (SNPs) are the genetic variant most commonly used in association studies. Successful attempts using genome-wide association studies (GWAS) to examine human diseases [1], especially for those studies using a case-control design, have made GWAS based on a single marker a widely accepted approach for gene detection in general. Inspired by this, subsequent large GWAS have been conducted focused mainly on complex traits, such as genetic defects and disease resistance or susceptibility [2]. These studies not only expanded applications of genome-wide molecular markers to marker-assisted selection but also provided important information for elaboration of the genetic mechanisms of these traits. Recent GWAS have explored economically important traits and breed characteristics of major livestock species [3,4]. Thus, a wide range of successful applications of GWAS to animal breeding and genetics has been reported and many genes or markers affecting economic traits in animals have been identified. In beef cattle, for instance Japanese black cattle [5], Korean Hanwoo cattle [6], Korean beef cattle [7], and Australian taurine and indicine cattle [8], GWAS detected genetic variations associated with carcass and meat quantitative traits. Many significant main effects of SNPs were identified via simple linear regression and stepwise regression procedures. With more advanced genome sequencing and high-throughput SNP genotyping technologies, GWAS with individual markers will more efficiently and reliably determine underlying genetic mechanisms.

As specific sets of alleles observed on a single chromosome or part of a chromosome, haplotypes are inherited together with little chance of contemporary recombination. Numerous inherent merits have made haplotypes an integral part of genetic variants and available as super alleles. Recently, haplotypes have been identified that confer high susceptibility for schizophrenia [9], nicotine dependence [10], macular degeneration [11], and recurrent laryngeal neuropathy in horses [12]. Moreover, some studies [13,14] assert that the analysis of haplotypes with the grouping and interaction of several variants is superior to any individual SNP analysis technique. Indeed, compared with individual SNP-based association studies, the use of multi-allelic haplotypes has significantly improved the power and robustness of association studies [15–17].

However, methodologies are always accompanied by drawbacks. For single marker analysis, only a small fraction of the genetic variation in quantitative traits can be explained using significant SNPs. One reason for this limitation is that the effects of individual SNPs are too small to pass the stringent significance criterion. Another reason is incomplete linkage disequilibrium (LD) between the genotyped SNPs and casual variants [18]. Haplotype-based GWAS are often hampered by the prohibitive time and costs required for haplotype inference [19]. Additionally, haplotype block structure and phase are rarely observed in genotyping data and may be subject to errors when inferred using statistical methods [20]. Moreover, when a block of genome contains a large number of haplotypes, the increased degrees of freedom within the block of the genome can erode statistical power [19].

Although haplotype association analysis has been conducted for many years using the human genome [21], little is known about the performance of this type of analysis in livestock. Indeed, the haplotype block structure and its distribution in the genome of cattle, especially studies based on high density SNPs, have been rarely reported [22]. Thus, the current study was performed to construct the haplotype structure in the bovine genome and to detect the relevant genes genuinely affecting a carcass trait component and meat quality trait.

Results

Haplotype blocks

We found that the whole cattle genome was partitioned into 92,553 haplotype blocks. The largest haplotype block consisted of 116 SNPs, the smallest block contained only 2 SNPs, and the average size of a block was 5.69. These haplotype blocks covered a total of 526,822 SNPs from the high density chips. The regions of high LD extended to approximately 200 kb, and the size of the haplotype blocks ranged from 22 bp to 199,266 bp. These haplotype blocks covered 1,620,979 bp of genetic information in the bovine genome. As depicted in Figure 1, the haplotype blocks were not evenly distributed. Instead, haplotype blocks were likely distributed according to the length of each chromosome and the density of the markers. The large number of haplotypes verified the existence of high LD in the BovineHD chip and validated the merits of haplotype analysis.

Population stratification assessment

Using a portion of the SNPs, we constructed and plotted the population structure based on the results of a principal component analysis (PCA). As illustrated in Figure 2, the structure of this population was drawn based on the top three eigenvectors using principal component 1 (PC1), principal component 2 (PC2), and principal component 3 (PC3). The three major distributed sectors indicate apparent population stratification in the reference samples, making a population stratification correction prerequisite in this analysis. The population stratification may have occurred because the cattle used in this study were collected from different farms and had different genetic backgrounds. In Figure 3, the kinship among individuals calculated using the classical equation from Vanden [23] is plotted, clearly illustrating the genetic relationships within the reference population.

Significant SNPs

The profiles of P values (in terms of –log[p]) of all tested SNPs for the foreshank weight and the triglyceride levels are shown in Figures 4A and 4B, respectively. The details of the genomically significant SNPs detected using the single marker analysis for the two investigated traits are presented in Table 1 and Table 2, including their heritability, their positions in the genome, the nearest known genes, and the raw P values. The total number of significant SNPs identified using the single marker regression model was 12 and 7 for the corresponding two traits, foreshank weight and triglyceride levels, respectively. Specifically, for the association analysis using the weight of foreshank, all of the 12 significant SNPs were distributed closely in terms of physical distance, from 54.1 Mb to 54.5 Mb in BTA 8. These SNPs were mainly possessed by or adjacent to genes GNAQ and CEP78. Additionally, the total heritability obtained by all 12 significant markers was 58.36. For the association analysis using the triglyceride levels, 7 significant SNPs were located in close proximity to one another, from 95 Mb to 97 Mb in BTA 5, and they are found in the adjacent genes GRIN2B and ATF7IP. The heritability explained by the 7 significant SNPs was 32.96. The quantile–quantile (Q–Q) plots for the test statistics using a mixed linear model (MLM) shown in Figures 5A and 5B indicate that there is no inflation of statistics or overall systematic bias caused by the population stratification. That is, the observed test statistics generally agreed with the expected values; however, the values for the significant SNPs were above the expected values, which markedly surpassed the genome-wide significance level.

Significant Haplotypes

In addition to the single marker analysis, Manhattan plots of the P value for each SNP against the genomic coordinates of each block were adopted to illustrate the results. Because there were no issues with overlap, the physical location of the first SNP was used to plot the graph. The P values of all tested haplotype blocks for foreshank weight and triglyceride levels are also shown in Figures 4C and 4D, respectively. The details of the genomically significant haplotype blocks detected using the haplotype-based method for the two target traits are also shown in Tables 3 and 4, including the starting and ending positions in the genome of the haplotype blocks, the number of SNPs they contain, the nearest known genes, and the raw P values. A total of 4 and 5 significant haplotype blocks were identified using a haplotype regression model for the corresponding traits of foreshank weights and triglyceride levels, respectively. Consistent with the results using the single marker analysis, all 4 significant haplotypes consistently converged on BTA 8 for the association analysis with foreshank weight. Two genes (GNAQ and CEP78) already detected in the single marker analysis and one gene (MGC134066) newly identified in the haplotype-based analysis constituted the associated gene information for foreshank weight. For the association analysis with the triglyceride levels trait, all 5 significant haplotypes were located in a similar region on BTA 5 and closely related to two genes (gene GRIN2B and ATF7IP). Most of the significant SNP regions detected using the individual SNP analysis were also identified in the haplotype-based analysis, suggesting strong LD among the detected SNPs. To test this hypothesis, we selected the significant SNPs and created the linkage map depicted in Figure 6. The majority of the SNPs were in high LD with other significant SNPs, and some pairs of significant SNPs were in complete LD. For the association analysis with foreshank weight, a region of nearly 0.1 Mb was strongly associated with the target trait and was located in the GNAQ gene, which is important in growth and development. Thus, we utilized the 36 SNPs contained in this region to infer the LD level and to estimate the combination of the superior haplotype, as shown in Figure 7. The Q–Q plots for the test statistics from the general linear model (GLM) shown in

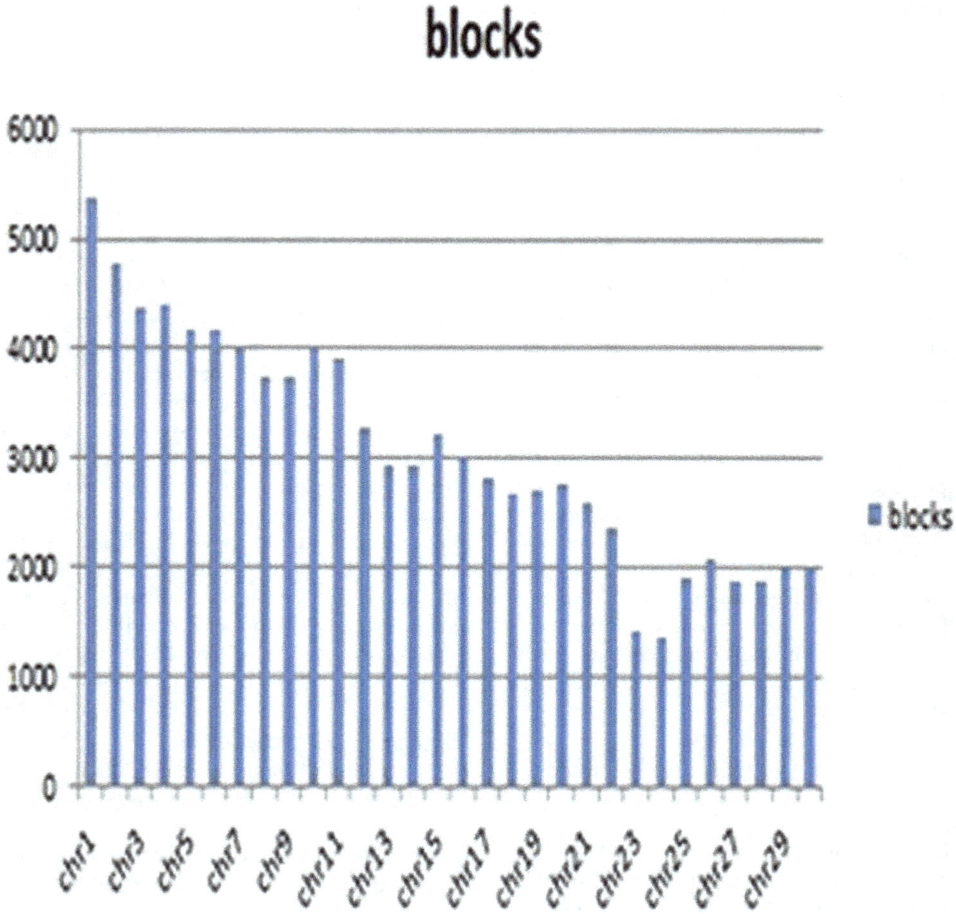

Figure 1. Number of haplotype blocks per chromosome.

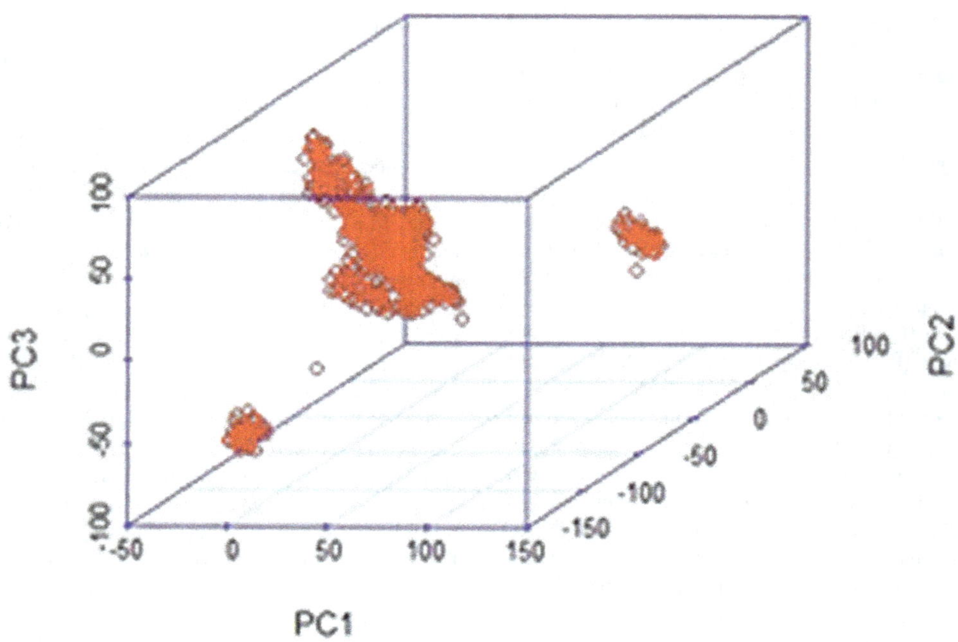

Figure 2. Population structure map drawn from the first three principal components. Using the R package, three principal components of markers for each individual are used to show the population stratification of the reference population.

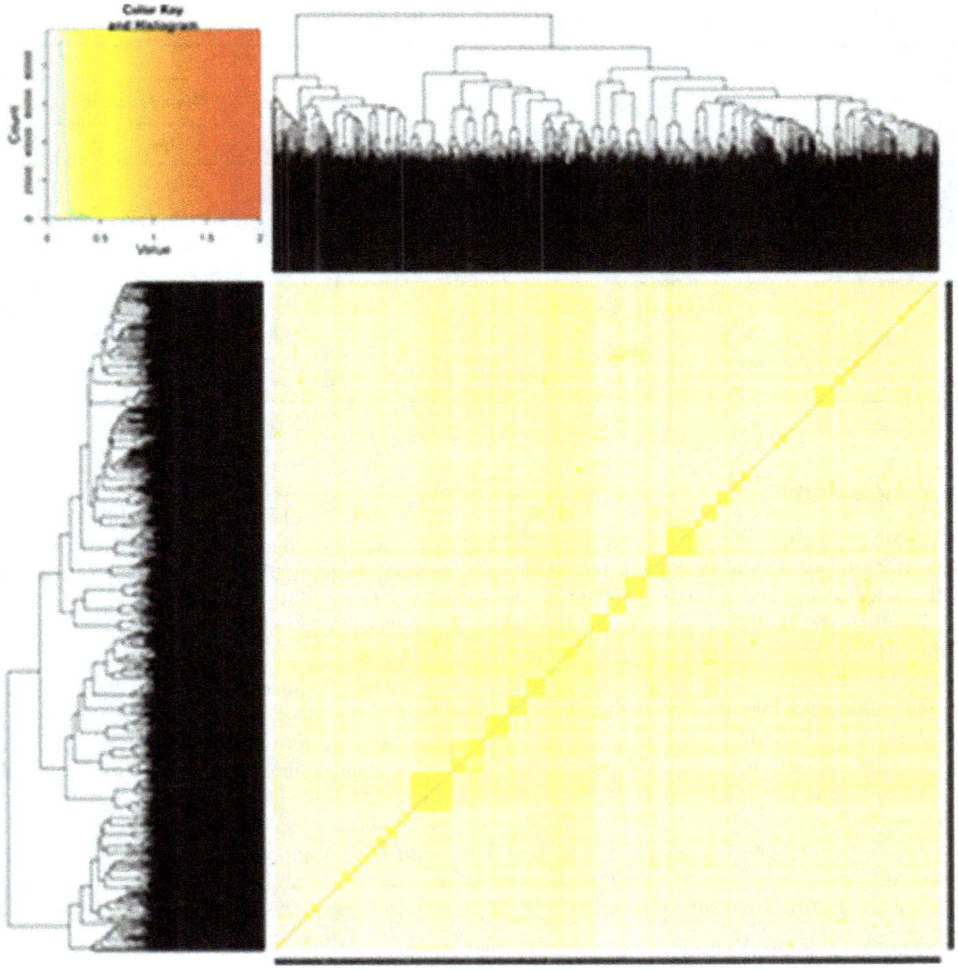

Figure 3. Kinship among individuals in the reference population.

Figures 5C and 5D suggest that there is no inflation of statistics or overall systematic bias caused by population stratification in the haplotype-based analysis.

Table 1. Associated SNPs and nearby candidate genes for foreshank weight.

SNP	Chr	Position	P value	Heritability	Nearest gene	
					Name	Distance (bp)
BovineHD0800016290	8	54140695	1.33E-08	4.34	GNAQ	Within
BovineHD0800016379	8	54381564	1.01E-07	5.33	CEP78	52101
BovineHD0800016396	8	54443407	1.73E-07	4.48	CEP78	Within
BovineHD0800016286	8	54131549	2.00E-07	4.10	GNAQ	Within
BovineHD0800016392	8	54435508	2.06E-07	4.10	CEP78	Within
BovineHD0800016404	8	54465071	2.06E-07	4.48	CEP78	Within
BovineHD0800016406	8	54473267	2.06E-07	4.48	CEP78	4742
BovineHD0800016302	8	54167336	2.52E-07	4.82	GNAQ	Within
BovineHD0800016349	8	54281748	2.52E-07	9.08	GNAQ	1090
BovineHD0800016353	8	54291081	2.52E-07	3.97	GNAQ	10423
BovineHD0800016309	8	54183380	9.21E-07	4.59	GNAQ	Within
BovineHD0800016317	8	54204895	9.21E-07	4.59	GNAQ	Within

Table 2. Associated SNPs and nearby candidate genes for triglyceride levels.

SNP	Chr.	Position	P value	Heritability	Nearest gene	
					Name	Distance (bp)
BovineHD0500027280	5	96135744	6.18E-08	5.01	GRIN2B	273060
BovineHD0500027277	5	96120620	1.36E-07	4.39	ATF7IP	261657
BovineHD0500027310	5	96183375	1.88E-07	4.89	GRIN2B	225429
BovineHD0500027268	5	96080574	1.95E-07	5.14	ATF7IP	221611
BovineHD0500027313	5	96185924	2.97E-07	4.67	GRIN2B	222880
BovineHD0500027311	5	96184216	8.09E-07	4.18	GRIN2B	224588
BovineHD0500027272	5	96090773	8.53E-07	4.68	ATF7IP	231810

Discussion and Conclusions

In this study, both the individual marker analysis and the haplotype-based method identified significant associations of two quantitative traits with comparable genomic regions. However, the distributions of the P values along the genome were slightly different between the two methods. Some associations were detected using only the individual marker analysis, whereas others were found using only the haplotype-based analysis. Some inconsistencies were observed between the two methods, suggesting that the efficiency of the method may be highly dependent upon the nature of the data. Interestingly, most of the previous studies restricted their comparisons of the performance of different methods to a small subset of the genome. Our data showed that there was no apparent difference between the two methods in terms of test statistic values determined from Manhattan plots, especially for those results that were significant. However, a greater number of significant variables were detected by the single marker analysis than by the haplotype-based method. In this latter method, because of the close linkages between consecutive SNPs potentially located in the same regions, the effects were combined collectively into blocks, reducing the number of significant associations.

Recently, the detection of genes has revealed numerous genetic explanations of economic traits in beef cattle. In the present study, a carcass trait, foreshank weight, was significantly associated with 12 SNPs and 4 haplotypes located in an area of approximately 54 Mb on BTA 8. This result is consistent with those of previous studies examining the genetic associations of a carcass trait in commercial Angus cattle [24], the body weights of African cattle [25], and the average daily weight gain in Angus cattle [26]. These studies all reported significant quantitative trait loci (QTL) peaking

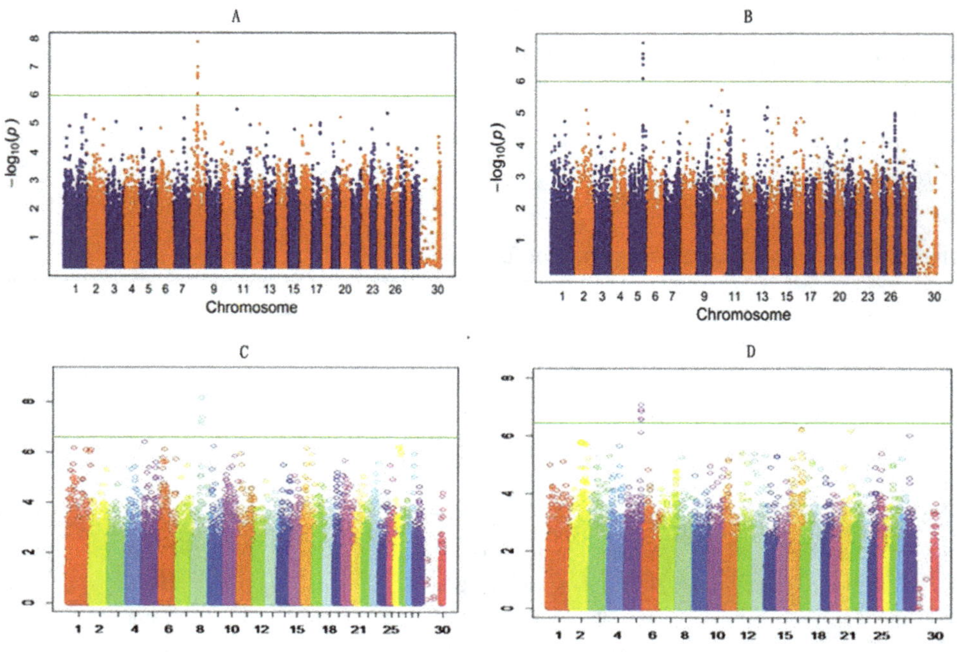

Figure 4. Manhattan plots of genome-wide association studies for two target traits. A and B are the plots for foreshank weight and triglyceride levels in the single marker analysis, respectively. C and D are the plots for foreshank weight and triglyceride levels in the haplotype analysis, respectively. Chromosome 1–30 is shown separated by colors, and marker positions are indicated by the ticks on the horizontal axis. In each plot, the genome-wide significance level is shown as a horizontal reference line. The single marker results for both traits show several overlapping SNPs in each map, and this apparent overlap may easily lead to misunderstandings. These SNPs are actually located within close physical proximity, and the P values are nearly the same or even identical.

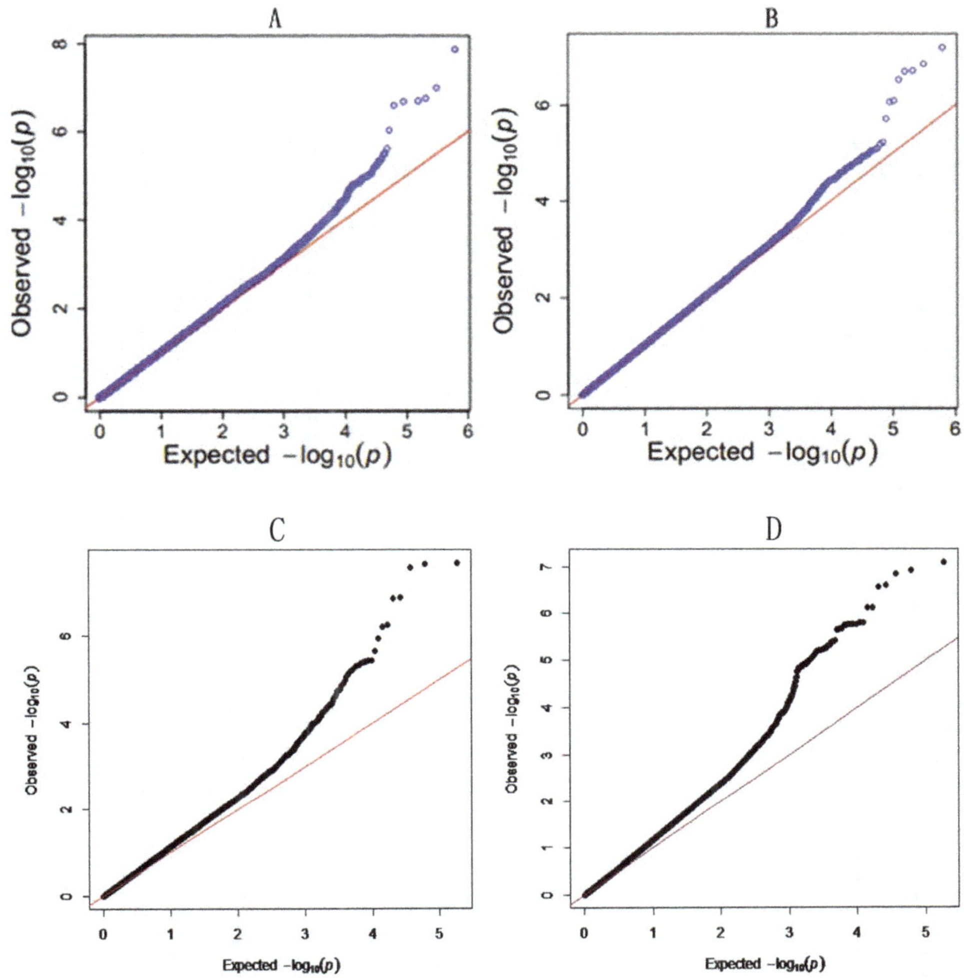

Figure 5. Quantile–quantile (Q–Q) plots of the genome-wide association studies. This result shows the Q–Q plots of the observed P values versus the expected P values under the null hypothesis that there was no association.

at a similar area, 51 Mb to 55 Mb on BTA 8. The GNAQ protein reportedly participates in GTPase activity, skeletal system development, regulation of catenin importation into the nucleus, and the negative regulation of protein kinase activity. The CEP78 protein is localized in the centrosome and MGC134066 is a transmembrane protein. All of these proteins potentially regulate the growth of cattle and thus their body weights. The triglycerides examined in the present study were significantly associated with 7 SNPs and 5 haplotypes within a physical distance of approximately 96 Mb on BTA 5. Although we did not detect major regulatory fatty acid genes, such as CAST and CAPN1, in our analysis and neither method directly localized the results to a specific gene, our results were consistent with those of previous studies in terms of the levels of certain special fatty acids, for instance, the discovery of the genomic associations of trans-vaccenic acid in a Charolais × Holstein crossbred population [27], sirloin fat depth in a commercial Angus-cross population [28], and fat thickness at the twelfth rib in hybrid steers [29]. All of the above analyses mapped the associated QTL in a similar area, including the study that detected the nearby PPARA gene, which reportedly greatly influences the metabolism of fatty acids [28,30].

To further eliminate potential associations due to population structure, we fitted the first three principal components derived from all the SNP genotypes as covariates to capture false associations attributable to population structure. This analysis sacrificed statistical power for mutations with effects confounded by population structure. In previous studies that did not incorporate the population structure into the analysis, the P value was often overestimated and the Q–Q plots markedly deviated from the expectation. For a haplotype-based analysis, it is unrealistic to incorporate the kinship matrix using the MLM because the complex indicator variables may decrease the accuracy of equation and even lead to a result that deviates from the original definition of kinship. In addition, the large sample size would create a huge computational burden for the mixed model analysis because the computing time increases cubically with a large number of individuals. In terms of the MLM, some studies [31] assert that the statistical model proposed by Zhang [32] has higher statistical power than approaches that consider population structure only or those that consider both population structure and individual relationships without grouping. Our results verify this assertion and find that the statistical power is closely related to the definition of the groups.

Although QTL mapping for economically important traits in domestic animals has already achieved remarkable results, only a small percent of the genetic variation has been captured because of the low density of the markers. GWAS, which utilize high-density SNPs, provide a new way to confront this issue. With the

Table 3. Associated haplotype blocks and nearby candidate genes for foreshank weight.

NSNP	Chr	Start	End	SNP1	SNP2	P value	Cover	Nearest gene	
							Sig SNP	Name	Distance (bp)
7	8	54443407	54467908	BovineHD0800016396	BovineHD0800016405	6.69E-09	Y	CEP78	Within
7	8	59583900	59617549	BovineHD0800017790	BovineHD0800017800	4.03E-08	N	MGC134066	3252
6	8	54284149	54351569	BovineHD0800016350	Hapmap49140-BTA-38265	5.93E-08	Y	GNAQ	3491
9	8	54194680	54233883	BovineHD0800016313	BovineHD0800016327	7.52E-08	Y	GNAQ	Within

Table 4. Associated haplotype blocks and nearby candidate genes for triglyceride levels.

NSNP	Chr	Start	End	SNP1	SNP2	P value	Cover	Nearest gene	
							Sig SNP	Name	Distance (bp)
28	5	96135744	96177119	BovineHD0500027280	BovineHD0500027309	8.25E-08	Y	GRIN2B	273060
2	5	96183375	96184216	BovineHD0500027310	BovineHD0500027311	1.23E-07	Y	GRIN2B	225429
9	5	96069476	96093159	BovineHD0500027264	BovineHD0500027274	1.43E-07	Y	ATF7IP	210513
2	5	96185924	96186658	BovineHD0500027313	BovineHD0500027314	2.58E-07	Y	GRIN2B	222880
4	5	96112564	96128475	BovineHD0500027275	BovineHD0500027279	2.77E-07	N	ATF7IP	253601

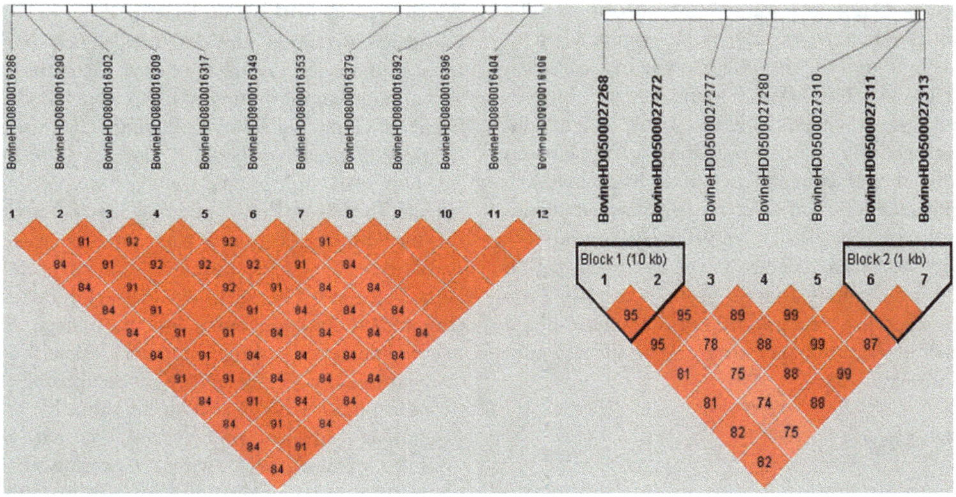

Figure 6. The extent of linkage disequilibrium among the 12 significant SNPs for foreshank weight and the 7 significant SNPs for triglyceride levels.

imputation strategy, using lower density markers may offer a few advantages with respect to lower costs. However, that strategy would introduce an additional imputation error rate in the already high false discovery rates that exist for association studies. In current GWAS, how to best reduce the data dimension is a thorny problem. When markers are divided into many blocks based on their LD levels, a block or group of markers is considered as one super marker. Only effects of the marker groups are estimated and tested, efficiently avoiding the little knowledge about the interactions between markers. This solution substantially reduces the data dimension and makes it possible to detect the interactions (epispastic effects) at the gene level. Hu et al [33] established a new method for analyzing large datasets, developing a bin model to predict genomic values based on an infinitesimal model. Nevertheless, haplotype blocks are natural choices as grouping markers in the bin model compared with the rigid definition of evenly distributed blocks. Theoretically, multiple traits can be analyzed simultaneously in a single model; however, traits were examined separately in the present study due to the lack of an accurate model. Many studies have proven the superiority of multiple trait association studies over association studies using individual traits [34–36]. Even so, there is no consensus on a consistent model that might further improve multiple trait GWAS [37].

In summary, this is the first broad application of the GWAS method using single marker-based and haplotype-based analyses, as well as haplotype construction, in Simmental cattle. We partitioned the whole cattle genome into 92,553 haplotype blocks

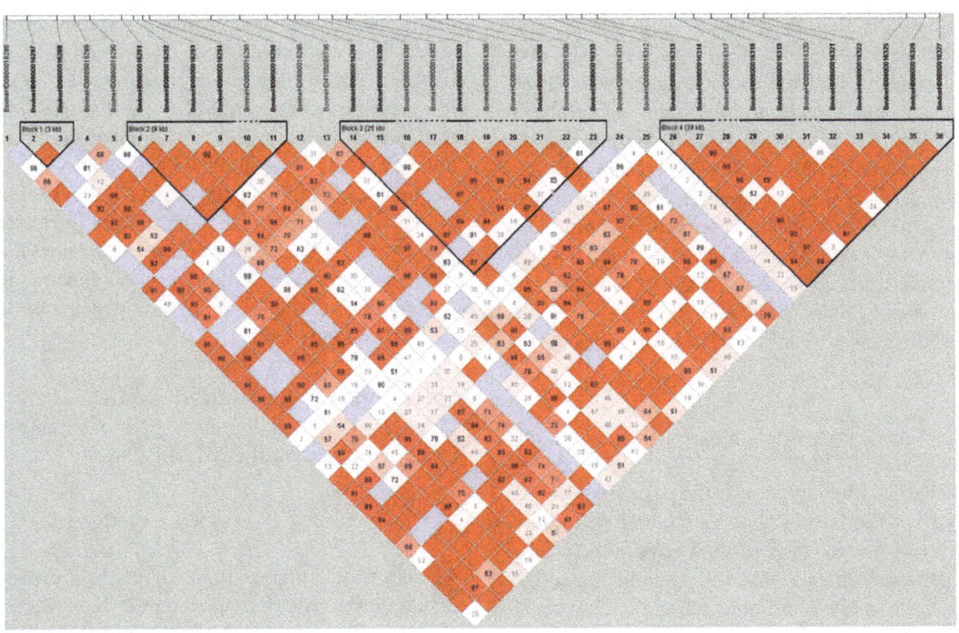

Figure 7. Potential haplotype structure of the hotspot area for influencing the carcass weight component. A total of 36 SNPs constitute this strong linkage disequilibrium region in chromosome 8. Solid lines mark the identified block.

using the standard expectation–maximum (EM) algorithm. The results showed that the regions of high LD extended up to approximately 200 kb and that the size of haplotype blocks ranged from 22 bp to 199,266 kb. The GWAS found 12 and 7 SNPs significantly genomically associated with foreshank weight and triglyceride levels, respectively. By contrast, the haplotype-based association found that 4 and 5 haplotype blocks contained the majority of the significant SNPs that were strongly associated with foreshank weight and triglyceride levels, respectively. In addition, 2 and 3 genes, respectively, were detected in the significant region and might be responsible for the variation of the two traits.

In conclusion, this study provides important information on the genetic mechanisms of two traits in beef cattle and on the structure of the genome in Simmental cattle.

Materials and Methods

Ethics statement

All animal procedures were conducted with strict adherence to the guidelines proposed by the Chinese Council on Animal care, and all protocols were approved by the Science Research Department of the Institute of Animal Science at the Chinese Academy of Agricultural Sciences (Beijing, China). Samples were collected during regular quarantine inspections on the farms. The farm owners approved the use of the animals and private land for this study.

Animal resources and phenotypes

The training population consisted of 942 young Simmental bulls born in 2008–2011 and is part of a resource population established in Inner Mongolia. Each individual was observed and measured for growth and developmental traits until they were slaughtered when they were 16 to 18 months old. During slaughter, carcass traits and meat quality traits were measured according to the Institutional Meat Purchase Specifications for fresh beef guidelines. The two target traits were measured as follows. After removing the exposed fat and tendons, the weight of foreshank was determined for the high quality meat, which was kept fresh and intact, from the elbow to the wrist while maintaining strict compliance with the rules stated in GB/T 27643-2011. For triglyceride levels, samples were taken in accordance with GB/T 2223-2008 from the loin eye muscle and extracted according to the procedure described by Sukhija (1998). Subsequently, the triglyceride samples were analyzed using gas chromatography (gas chromatograph, GC-2014 CAFsc, Shimadzu Scientific Instruments) under the following conditions: the temperature of the inlet was 220°C. The oven was heated up to 250°C at a rate of 5°C per min and then maintained at 220°C. Each analysis took 20 min. After collecting the original data, fixed effects, including years, farm, and month of birth, were corrected in advance using the following equation:

$$y_{ijkm} = u + \mathrm{Farm}_i + \mathrm{Month}_j + \mathrm{Year}_k + e_{ijkm} \tag{1}$$

where $\boldsymbol{y_{ijkm}}$ is the vector of phenotype, $\boldsymbol{u}$ is the population mean, $\mathbf{Farm_i}$ is the category of the farm where the animal was raised, $\mathbf{Month_j}$ is the number of months after birth, $\mathbf{Year_k}$ is the year of slaughter, $\boldsymbol{e_{ijkm}}$ is the random residual. The residual $\boldsymbol{e_{ijkm}}$ was subsequently used for the study examining the genomic associations with SNPs and haplotypes.

Genotyping and quality control

Semen or blood samples were collected during the regular quarantine inspection of the farms. Genomic DNA was extracted from blood samples using a TIANamp Blood DNA Kit (Tiangen Biotech Company limited, Beijing, Chain), and DNA with an A260/280 ratio between 1.8 and 2.0 were subjected to further analysis. All individuals were genotyped using the Illumina BovineSNP BeadChip containing 774,660 SNPs. The mean value of the distance between each marker was 3.43 kb, and the variance value of the distance between each marker was 19.19 Mb. The genotyping platform adopted in this study was Illumina's Infinium II Assay (Illumina Inc., San Diego, CA, USA). Samples were genotyped using Illumina's BeadStudio data analysis software, and SNP chips were scanned using iScan and analyzed using Infinium GenomeStudio (Illumina Inc.).

Prior to statistical analysis, the SNP data were pre-processed and the following SNPS were removed: SNPs with call rates less than 90%, minor allele frequencies less than 5%, genotype appearances in less than five individuals, and marked departure from the Hardy-Weinberg equilibrium (with lower than 10^{-6} probability). Moreover, individuals with more than 10% missing genotypes or those above a 2% Mendelian error rate for SNP genotypes were excluded. Thus, a total of 942 individuals and 631,396 SNPs remained in the sample for the subsequent analysis.

Haplotype block partitioning algorithms

The history of recombination between a pair of SNPs can be estimated with the use of the normalized measure of allelic association, D' [38]. Using the definition given by Gabriel [39], the pairs were considered in "strong LD" if the one-sided upper 95% confidence boundary of D' was >0.98 (that is, consistent with no historical recombination) and the lower boundary was above 0.7 [39]. If the D' for a pair of SNPs was lower than 0.7, then the next haplotype block began. That is to say, only nearby SNPs with continuous combinations were included in a haplotype block, and few SNPs having low LD with adjacent markers were omitted in the haplotype-based association study. After the detection of haplotype blocks, haplotypes and their frequencies for an individual were obtained with the standard expectation–maximum (EM) [40] algorithm. Specifically, the EM iteration alternates between performing an expectation (E) step, which creates a function for the expectation of the log-likelihood evaluated using the current estimate for the haplotype and its frequency, and a maximization (M) step, which computes haplotype and its frequency maximizing the expected log-likelihood found on the E step. These parameter-estimates are then used to determine the distribution of the latent variables in the next E step. The reference threshold of SNPs within a close linkage haplotype and the partitioning standard can be founded in the user manual of the PLINK software [41].

Single-marker association studies

Association data for each SNP via regression analysis were presented based on the MLM below:

$$y^* = \mathrm{X}b_i + Qv + \mathrm{Zu} + \mathrm{e} \tag{2}$$

where $\mathbf{y^*}$ is the adjusted phenotype, $\mathbf{b_i}$ is the regression coefficient of phenotype on SNP genotypes, $\mathbf{X}$ is the vector of the SNP genotype indicators and takes values 0, 1, or 2 corresponding to the three genotypes 11, 12 and 22, $\mathbf{v}$ is the effect of population structure, $\mathbf{Q}$ is the corresponding principal components matrix, $\mathbf{u}$ is the vector of the residual polygenetic effects with $\mathbf{u \sim N(0, K}\sigma_a^2\mathbf{)}$

(where **K** is the genetic relationship calculated by the markers, σ_a^2 is the additive variance), **Z** is the corresponding matrix, and **e** is the vector of residual errors with $\mathbf{e}\sim\mathbf{N}(\mathbf{0},\ \mathbf{I}\sigma_e^2)$. The population structure was quantified using the first three eigenvectors as covariates in this model. A t-test statistic was used to determine the significance of each SNP and was calculated as follows:

$$t_i = \frac{|\hat{b}_i|}{\sqrt{V(\hat{b}_i)}} \tag{3}$$

where $\hat{b}_i$ is the estimate of b and the corresponding variance $V(\hat{b}_i)$ can be obtained via mixed model equations (MME). For both analyses, the Bonferroni method was adopted to adjust for multiple testing from the number of SNP loci detected. A SNP was considered significant at the genome level if the raw P value was less than 0.05/N, where N is the number of SNP loci tested in analyses. However, with 631,396 markers, the Bonferroni correction was too stringent for the potential associated SNPs. Thus, in the single marker analyses, the significance threshold for the P value was set at 1.0×10^{-6}. The significance threshold for the P value of the haplotype was set based on the equation at 5.4×10^{-7} (0.05/92,553).

Haplotype-based association studies

Different from the single marker analysis, a GLM was adopted to perform the regression analysis in the haplotype-based association studies as shown below:

$$y^* = Xb_i + Qv + e \tag{4}$$

where $\mathbf{y^*}$ is the adjusted phenotype, $\mathbf{b_i}$ is the regression coefficient of phenotype on haplotype block, **X** is the vector of the corresponding haplotype indicators, **v** is the effect of population structure, **Q** is the corresponding principal components matrix and **e** is the vector of residual errors with $\mathbf{e}\sim\mathbf{N}(\mathbf{0},\ \mathbf{I}\sigma_e^2)$. Based on equation (4), the t-test statistic was also used for the significance test. An MLM was not adopted here mainly because of the complicated process for attaining the genetic relationship constructed by the haplotypes. Moreover, rarely seen haplotypes and individuals with low frequency were eliminated before the association study to avoid an adverse impact on the significance test.

Author Contributions

Conceived and designed the experiments: HJG HYR JYL. Performed the experiments: YW HZF. Analyzed the data: YW YHW. Contributed reagents/materials/analysis tools: XG YC LPZ. Contributed to the writing of the manuscript: YW HZF.

References

1. Donnelly P (2008) Progress and challenges in genome-wide association studies in humans. Nature 456: 728–731.
2. Hirschhorn JN, Daly MJ (2005) Genome-wide association studies for common diseases and complex traits. Nat Rev Genet 6: 95–108.
3. Zhang H, Wang Z, Wang S, Li H (2012) Progress of genome wide association study in domestic animals. Journal of Animal Science and Biotechnology 3: 26.
4. Barsh GS, Copenhaver GP, Gibson G, Williams SM (2012) Guidelines for Genome-Wide Association Studies. PLoS Genet 8: e1002812.
5. Nishimura S, Watanabe T, Mizoshita K, Tatsuda K, Fujita T, et al. (2012) Genome-wide association study identified three major QTL for carcass weight including the PLAG1-CHCHD7 QTN for stature in Japanese Black cattle. BMC Genetics 13: 40.
6. Alam M, Lee YM, Park BL, Kim JH (2010) A whole genome association study to detect single nucleotide polymorphisms for carcass traits in hanwoo populations. Asian-Australasian Journal of Animal Sciences 23: 417–424.
7. Kim Y, Ryu J, Woo J, Kim JB, Kim CY, et al. (2011) Genome-wide association study reveals five nucleotide sequence variants for carcass traits in beef cattle. Animal Genetics 42: 361–365.
8. Bolormaa S, Neto LRP, Zhang YD, Bunch RJ, Harrison BE, et al. (2011) A genome-wide association study of meat and carcass traits in Australian cattle. Journal of Animal Science 89: 2297–2309.
9. Beuten J, Payne TJ, Ma JZ, Li MD (2005) Significant Association of Catechol-O-Methyltransferase (COMT) Haplotypes with Nicotine Dependence in Male and Female Smokers of Two Ethnic Populations. Neuropsychopharmacology 31: 675–684.
10. Bray NJ, Buckland PR, Williams NM, Williams HJ, Norton N, et al. (2003) A Haplotype Implicated in Schizophrenia Susceptibility Is Associated with Reduced COMT Expression in Human Brain. The American Journal of Human Genetics 73: 152–161.
11. Hageman GS, Anderson DH, Johnson LV, Hancox LS, Taiber AJ, et al. (2005) A common haplotype in the complement regulatory gene factor H (HF1/CFH) predisposes individuals to age-related macular degeneration. Proceedings of the National Academy of Sciences of the United States of America 102: 7227–7232.
12. Dupuis M-C, Zhang Z, Druet T, Denoix J-M, Charlier C, et al. (2011) Results of a haplotype-based GWAS for recurrent laryngeal neuropathy in the horse. Mammalian Genome 22: 613–620.
13. Zhao H, Pfeiffer R, Gail MH (2003) Haplotype analysis in population genetics and association studies. Pharmacogenomics 4: 171–178.
14. Morris RW, Kaplan NL (2002) On the advantage of haplotype analysis in the presence of multiple disease susceptibility alleles. Genetic Epidemiology 23: 221–233.
15. Hayes BJ, Chamberlain AJ, Mcpartlan H, Macleod I, Sethuraman L, et al. (2007) Accuracy of marker-assisted selection with single markers and marker haplotypes in cattle. Genetics Research 89: 215–220.
16. Calus M, Meuwissen T, Windig J, Knol E, Schrooten C, et al. (2009) Effects of the number of markers per haplotype and clustering of haplotypes on the accuracy of QTL mapping and prediction of genomic breeding values. Genetics Selection Evolution 41: 11.
17. Grapes L, Dekkers JCM, Rothschild MF, Fernando RL (2004) Comparing Linkage Disequilibrium-Based Methods for Fine Mapping Quantitative Trait Loci. Genetics 166: 1561–1570.
18. Yang J, Benyamin B, McEvoy BP, Gordon S, Henders AK, et al. (2010) Common SNPs explain a large proportion of the heritability for human height. Nat Genet 42: 565–569.
19. Shim H, Chun H, Engelman C, Payseur B (2009) Genome-wide association studies using single-nucleotide polymorphisms versus haplotypes: an empirical comparison with data from the North American Rheumatoid Arthritis Consortium. BMC Proceedings 3: S35.
20. Niu T (2004) Algorithms for inferring haplotypes. Genetic Epidemiology 27: 334–347.
21. Jiang H, Orr A, Guernsey DL, Robitaille J, Asselin G, et al. (2009) Application of Homozygosity Haplotype Analysis to Genetic Mapping with High-Density SNP Genotype Data. PLoS ONE 4: e5280.
22. Villa-Angulo R, Matukumalli L, Gill C, Choi J, Van Tassell C, et al. (2009) High-resolution haplotype block structure in the cattle genome. BMC Genetics 10: 19.
23. VanRaden PM (2007) Efficient Methods to Compute Genomic Predictions. Journal of Dairy Science 91: 4414–4423.
24. McClure MC, Morsci NS, Schnabel RD, Kim JW, Yao P, et al. (2010) A genome scan for quantitative trait loci influencing carcass, post-natal growth and reproductive traits in commercial Angus cattle. Animal Genetics 41: 597–607.
25. Hanotte O, Ronin Y, Agaba M, Nilsson P, Gelhaus A, et al. (2003) Mapping of quantitative trait loci controlling trypanotolerance in a cross of tolerant West African N'Dama and susceptible East African Boran cattle. Proceedings of the National Academy of Sciences 100: 7443–7448.
26. Rolf MM, Taylor JF, Schnabel RD, McKay SD, McClure MC, et al. (2012) Genome-wide association analysis for feed efficiency in Angus cattle. Animal Genetics 43: 367–374.
27. Gutiérrez-Gil B, Wiener P, Richardson RI, Wood JD, Williams JL (2010) Identification of QTL with effects on fatty acid composition of meat in a Charolais x Holstein cross population. Meat Science 85: 721–729.
28. Gill JL, Bishop SC, McCorquodale C, Williams JL, Wiener P (2010) Associations between single nucleotide polymorphisms in multiple candidate genes and carcass and meat quality traits in a commercial Angus-cross population. Meat Science 86: 985–993.
29. Nalaila SM, Stothard P, Moore SS, Li C, Wang Z (2012) Whole-genome QTL scan for ultrasound and carcass merit traits in beef cattle using Bayesian shrinkage method. Journal of Animal Breeding and Genetics 129: 107–119.
30. Szczerbal I, Lin L, Stachowiak M, Chmurzynska A, Mackowski M, et al. (2007) Cytogenetic mapping of DGAT1, PPARA, ADIPOR1 and CREB genes in the pig. Journal of Applied Genetics 48: 73–76.
31. Zhou Z, Sheng X, Zhang Z, Zhao K, Zhu L, et al. (2010) Differential Genetic Regulation of Canine Hip Dysplasia and Osteoarthritis. PLoS ONE 5: e13219.

32. Zhang Z, Ersoz E, Lai C-Q, Todhunter RJ, Tiwari HK, et al. (2010) Mixed linear model approach adapted for genome-wide association studies. Nat Genet 42: 355–360.
33. Hu Z, Wang Z, Xu S (2012) An Infinitesimal Model for Quantitative Trait Genomic Value Prediction. PLoS ONE 7: e41336.
34. Lange C, Whittaker JC (2001) Mapping Quantitative Trait Loci Using Generalized Estimating Equations. Genetics 159: 1325–1337.
35. Huang J, Jiang Y (2003) Genetic Linkage Analysis of a Dichotomous Trait Incorporating a Tightly Linked Quantitative Trait in Affected Sib Pairs. The American Journal of Human Genetics 72: 949–960.
36. Allison DB, Thiel B, St. Jean P, Elston RC, Infante MC, et al. (1998) Multiple Phenotype Modeling in Gene-Mapping Studies of Quantitative Traits: Power Advantages. The American Journal of Human Genetics 63: 1190–1201.
37. Shriner D (2012) Moving towards system genetics through multiple trait analysis in genome-wide association studies. Frontiers in Genetics 3.
38. Daly MJ, Rioux JD, Schaffner SF, Hudson TJ, Lander ES (2001) High-resolution haplotype structure in the human genome. Nat Genet 29: 229–232.
39. Gabriel SB, Schaffner SF, Nguyen H, Moore JM, Roy J, et al. (2002) The Structure of Haplotype Blocks in the Human Genome. Science 296: 2225–2229.
40. Excoffier L, Slatkin M (1995) Maximum-likelihood estimation of molecular haplotype frequencies in a diploid population. Molecular Biology and Evolution 12: 921–927.
41. Purcell S, Neale B, Todd-Brown K, Thomas L, Ferreira M, et al. (2007) PLINK: a tool set for whole-genome association and population-based linkage analyses. American Journal of Human Genetics 81: 559–575.

15

Coexistence of Fish Species in a Large Lowland River: Food Niche Partitioning between Small-Sized Percids, Cyprinids and Sticklebacks in Submersed Macrophytes

Małgorzata Dukowska*, Maria Grzybkowska

Department of Ecology and Vertebrate Zoology, Faculty of Biology and Environmental Protection, University of Łódź, Łódź, Poland

Abstract

In the spring and summer of each year, large patches of submersed aquatic macrophytes overgrow the bottom of the alluvial Warta River downstream of a large dam reservoir owing to water management practices. Environmental variables, macroinvertebrates (zoobenthos and epiphytic fauna, zooplankton) and fish abundance and biomass were assessed at this biologically productive habitat to learn intraseasonal dynamics of food types, and their occurrence in the gut contents of small-sized roach, dace, perch, ruffe and three-spined stickleback. Gut fullness coefficient, niche breadth and niche overlap indicated how the fishes coexist in the macrophytes. Chironomidae dominated in the diet of the percids. However, ruffe consumed mostly benthic chironomids, while perch epiphytic chironomids and zooplankton. The diet of dace resembled that in fast flowing water although this rheophilic species occurred at unusual density there. The generalist roach displayed the lowest gut fullness coefficient values and widest niche breadth; consequently, intraspecific rather than interspecific competition decided the fate of roach. Three-spined stickleback differed from the other fishes by consuming epiphytic simuliids and fish eggs. The diet overlap between fishes reaching higher gut fullness coefficient values was rather low when the food associated with the submersed aquatic macrophytes was most abundant; this is congruent with the niche overlap hypothesis that maximal tolerable niche overlap can be higher in less intensely competitive conditions.

Editor: Tomoya Iwata, University of Yamanashi, Japan

Funding: This work was supported by a grant of the University of Lodz No 505/424. The funder had no role in study design, data collection and analysis, decision to publish, or preparation of the manuscript.

Competing Interests: The authors have declared that no competing interests exist.

* Email: mdukow@biol.uni.lodz.pl

Introduction

Dams usually affect downstream characteristics, like flow regimes, river-channel geomorphology, water and sediment quality, aquatic environment and biota [1–3]. The effects of the dam related river management practice may be evident for many kilometers of downstream reaches; one such effect is the development of submersed aquatic macrophytes (SAM) [4,5]. The main factors and processes controlling macrophyte status in lowland rivers are discharge and/or current velocity, light, substrate and nutrients, while the role of the first two is of most fundamental importance, as these hydrological parameters control instream macrophyte colonization, establishment and persistence [6]. The presence of SAM may be considered as a very important component of riverine biota, causing an increase in habitat structural complexity in alluvial lotic ecosystems. The water plants serve as a substrate for epiphyton, constituting a rich foraging habitat for macroinvertebrates [7], shelter against predation, heterogeneous substrate for co-existence and, to a small extent, a direct, food source [8–10]. Besides, the submersed plants' morphological characteristics (size, number and orientation of leaves and steams) influence both invertebrate [8,10] and fish distribution [11–13]. Thus SAM may support a high density of small fish individuals, because submersed plant beds offer protection from predators by hindering predators' foraging activities [14]. The foraging activity of vertebrate predators may decline monotonically with increasing habitat complexity [15].

At the river bed macrophyte patches, fish may exploit prey types from three ecological formations: zooplankton (especially numerous below dam reservoirs), fauna dwelling on the surface of vegetation (epiphytic fauna, mainly several taxa of Chironomidae and Simuliidae) and benthos. Submersed plants create favourable conditions for pelophilous forms like most of Oligochaeta and Chironomidae by extensive particle trapping and accumulation of a fine-grained, nutrient enriching sediment [16–18]. Thus the development of SAM on the alluvial bed river attracts many small fish individuals. Being a little competitive, the coexistence of these species is possible if there are differences in their responses to limiting resources. The species-specific differences that allow such coexistence can be considered as species' niche with four major axes: resources, predators, space and time [19,20].

Untypical, but abundant development of SAM has been observed in the large lowland alluvial Warta River downstream of the Jeziorsko Reservoir every year as an effect of a low discharge in late spring and summer [10]. Every early autumn large volumes of water start to be released through the reservoir dam sluices, and the SAM habitat is torn out of the bottom or gets inundated with the bottom substrate [3,10]. The trophic relationships among this rich but temporary habitat have been investigated with regard to the primary and secondary invertebrate consumers (gathering collectors, scrapers and predators) and the tertiary consumer of three-spined stickleback (*Gasterosteus aculeatus* L.), as well as percids [7,18,21,22].

For a long time every year, however, the Jeziorsko tailwater has been dominated by cyprinids [3,22–25], many small individuals of which were also foraging in the tailwater's SAM. The trophic impact of the fishes on this habitat has not been investigated, although we have long expected that all types of the rich food resources connected with the SAM (zoobenthos, epiphytic fauna and zooplankton) are exploited by these (and other) fishes. Consequently, the main objective of the present study was to identify patterns in the feeding of the five predominant fish species occurring in that area (roach, dace, perch, ruffe and three-spined stickleback), in order to evaluate their trophic niches' breadths and overlaps in relation to resources, time and space. To this end, we investigated in detail the gut contents and intraseasonal changes in the diet of these five fish species there.

Study area

The Warta River rises 380 meters above sea level, is 808 km long and empties into the Oder River at 13 meters above sea level. Its catchment area is ca. 53 710 km^2 and its slope ranges from 2.0–1.0‰ in the upper course, and from 0.3–0.1‰ in the middle and lower courses [26]. The study site was established in this lowland alluvial river about 1.5 km downstream of the dam of the large Jeziorsko Reservoir, whose maximal surface area is 42.3 km^2 (Fig. 1). At the investigated site, the Warta River is about 60 m wide, with a maximum depth of 2.5 m in the erosion zone.

During sampling in 2004, similarly as in a few former years, the discharge of the Warta River below the dam was quite different in comparison with the natural, upstream reach, especially in summer, when its flow stabilized at a much lower level than in other seasons. One consequence of this phenomenon was the appearance of submersed macrophytes, which started to spread each year from the summer of 1992 along a short stretch of the tailwater [3,27]. Detailed site descriptions can be found in Grzybkowska et al. [10,28].

Material and Methods

The sampling was conducted in 2004, 18 years after the reservoir started functioning routinely and 10 years after the construction of a hydroelectric plant. In the investigated reach, large patches of *Potamogeton pectinatus* L. and small patches of *Potamogeton lucens* L. gradually developed since late spring through late summer in the transitional riverbed zone, which is located between the depositional zone, close to a bank, and the midriver channel (Fig. 1). The percentage of river bottom covered by macrophytes, samples of particulate organic matter and inorganic substrate, macrophytes, zoobenthos and epiphytic fauna, zooplankton, and fish, were collected, at the same time, within an area sized 40 m by 2.5 m, and extending along the bank and along the transitional zone. The area was randomly selected within the zone. The samples were obtained twice a month from May through late August. As a result, nine samples of each biotic and abiotic component were collected.

On each sampling occasion each sample of benthos (containing benthic invertebrates, particulate organic and inorganic matter) consisted of five subsamples (each subsample covered 100 cm^2 of stream-bed area collected with a tabular sampler of a catching area of 10 cm^2). The sampling places were uniformly distributed within the sampled area. The invertebrates of the samples were sorted from the detritus and benthic sediments by hand and preserved in 10% formalin. All invertebrates from these quantitative samples were counted and their wet weight (w.w.) assessed; these data were used to estimate the biomass of zoobenthos. Most invertebrates were classified to the lowest taxonomic level of the dominant macrobenthic group, while chironomids were identified to the species level when possible. As the exact identification on the basis of their larvae was often impossible, we reared their immature stages in the laboratory from additional qualitative samples taken each time in order to obtain larval and pupal skins, and imagines.

These samples were also used to determine the organic matter content in the bottom sediment. For this purpose a 1 mm mesh sieve was used to separate benthic particulate organic matter (BPOM) into:>1 mm (coarse – BCPOM) and <1 mm (fine – BFPOM) [29]. Next, the benthic organic matter was dried at 60°C for two days, weighed, ashed at 600°C for two hours and reweighed. A more detailed description of these methods can be found in Grzybkowska et al. [10], Grzybkowska & Dukowska [27].

To estimate the amount of dry weight of plants growing in the study site, a special frame (0.5×0.7 m) was placed on the riverine bottom and all the *Potamogeton* within the frame was collected. This procedure was repeated three times on each sampling occasion. In the laboratory, the pondweeds were dried for 24 hours at 65°C to estimate their dry weight (d.w.).

Five subsamples of the epiphytic fauna settled on *Potamogeton* were collected on each sampling occasion. Each of the subsamples consisted of three fragments of stems (about 20 cm long, on average) of the plants cut off under the water surface, stored in plastic containers, and preserved in 10% formalin in the fields. In the laboratory, the plant material was removed from the containers and the invertebrates were washed off the plants, sorted by hand, identified to the species level when possible, counted, had their wet weight assessed. The obtained data were recalculated to estimate the biomass of epiphytic invertebrates per 1 m^2 of *Potamogeton* covering the riverine bottom on given sampling occasions.

To evaluate the density of zooplankton (mainly Cladocera), 0.03 m^3 samples of river water were filtered through a planktonic net, of 50 μm mesh size, and preserved in formalin with riverine water in the fields. In the laboratory, individuals were identified to the species level and counted. The biomass of the zooplankton was estimated on the basis of suitable equations [30].

To assess fish density and gut contents, fish were caught in the sampled area using an electric current of 220 V and 3 A supplied from a backpack battery generator. A single pass CPUE sampling was carried out, which consisted in one person wading against the water current with an anode dipnet and another one with a bucket for collecting stunned fish along the longitudinal axis of the sampled area. The sampling period was 15 minutes on each occasion. As the equipment was battery-powered fish were not scared by noise, hence no barrier preventing fish from escaping was necessary. Immediately after the capture, fish were anaesthetised (MS-222, tricaine methanesulfonate) and then preserved in 4% formalin. The field studies did not involve endangered or protected species. The Polish Angling Association in Konin (a tenant of the water body, director Jerzy Olejnik, 1 Wyspiańskiego Str., 62–510 Konin) issued the permit to conduct the field study (see Fig. 1 for details of the study area location). Electrofishing was performed with the license No 1180/01 for the operation of electric fishing tools, and the other procedures were conducted under the permission No 219/2011 to perform experiments on animals, issued by the University of Lodz, and the individual

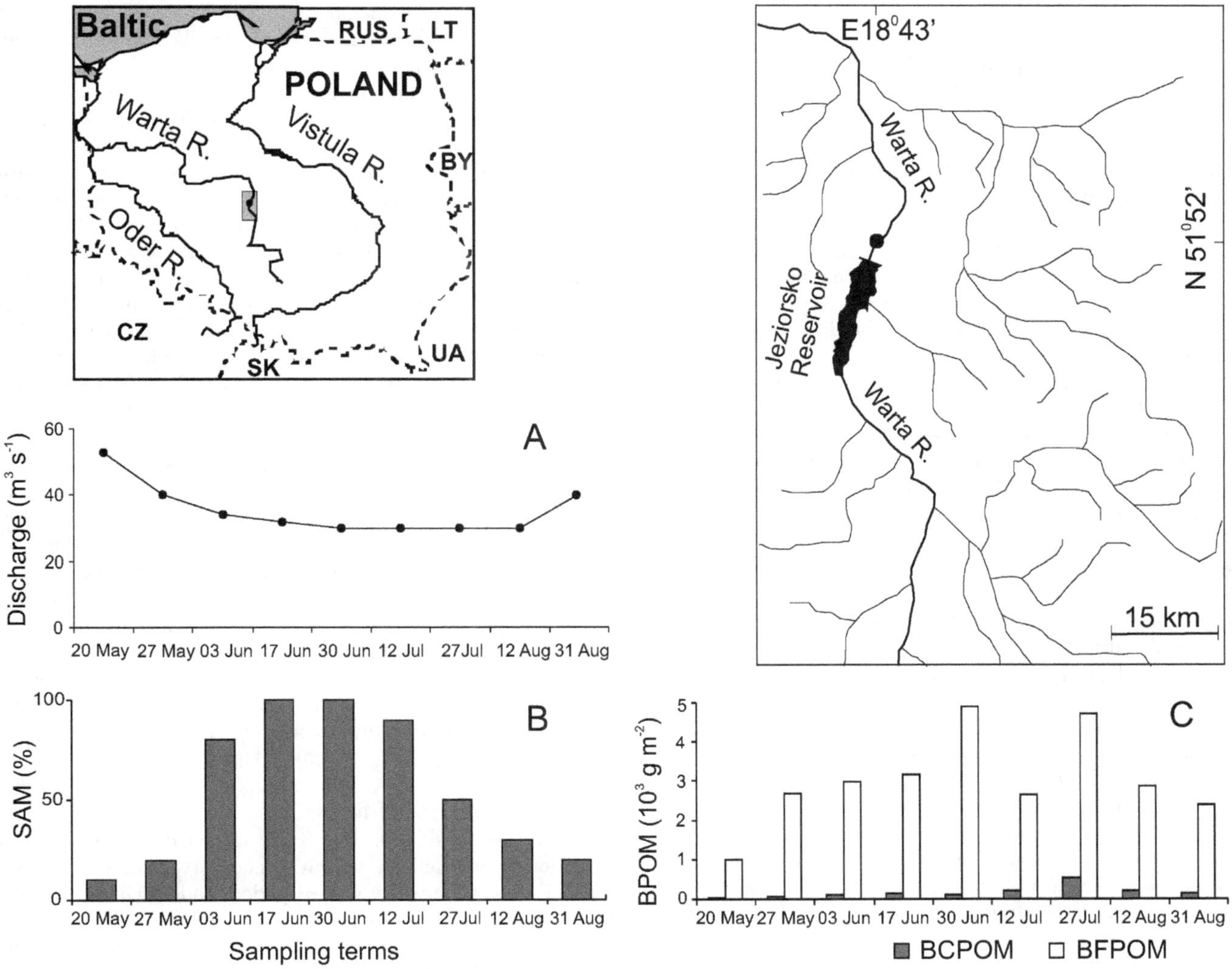

Figure 1. Study area with the marked sampling site in the tailwater of the Jeziorsko Reservoir on the Warta River. Parameters of the site over the study period: A. discharge; B. SAM -% of river bottom covered by hydrophytes; C. BFPOM and BCPOM, two fractions of benthic particulate organic matter (details in the text).

licence No 6/2006 to perform experiments on animals according to the Law on the protection of animals and the recommendations of the ICLAS.

In the laboratory, the total length (TL) of each analysed fish specimen was measured to the nearest 1 mm, and weighed to the nearest 0.1 g. The gut contents of all investigated individuals (n = 242) were analysed using a stereomicroscope and microscope. Prey types from the whole gut length, after identification to the lowest possible taxonomic category, were counted and weighed (w.w.), except zooplankton, the biomass of which was estimated in the same way as described above.

The gut fullness coefficient (FC) was calculated by the formula [31]:

$$FC = \frac{a}{b} \times 100$$

where:

a – total gut content weight (g)

b – weight of fish (g)

Niche breadth (B_n) was calculated using Levins' index:

$$B_n = \frac{1}{\sum p_j^2}$$

where:

B_n – Levins' measure of niche breadth

p_j – proportion of food type j

n – number of possible food types.

We standardized the trophic niche values (ranging from 0 to 1) using the Hurlbert formula [32]:

$$B_A = \frac{B_n \ 1}{n-1}$$

where:

B_A – Levins' standardized niche breadth

B_n – Levins' measure of niche breadth

n – number of possible food types.

The interspecific diet overlap among the investigated species was calculated using the Schoener overlap index [33]:

$$C_{xy} = 1 - 0.5\left(\sum_i |P_{xi} - P_{yi}|\right)$$

where:

C_{xy} – is the overlap index ranging from 0 (no overlap) to 1 (complete overlap)

P_{xi} – is the proportion of food type i of species x

P_{yi} – is the proportion of food type i of species y

It is worth noting that $C_{xy}>0.6$ is considered biologically significant [34].

The cluster analysis was also applied for identifying fish species' groups with similar gut contents.

The Kruskal-Wallis test and the post-hoc Dunn test in the STATISTICA software package, v. 10 [35,36] were applied to compare the percentage of the most frequent food items in the diet, the gut fullness coefficient, as well as diet niche breadth, to determine whether significant changes during the investigated period occurred. The significance level of the tests was $\alpha = 0.05$.

Results

Intraseasonal dynamics of environmental parameters of the SAM habitat

The development of macrophytes started in late May. It gradually intensified the cumulation of benthic fine particulate organic matter on the bottom, which strengthened the possibilities of the development of pelophilous zoobenthos. The highest biomass values of *P. pectinatus* (over 210 g d.w. m^{-2}) and the highest density of BFPOM were recorded during the second half of June 2004; at that time the macrophytes were also covered with filaments of green algae *Cladophora glomerata* (L.) Kutz. The intraseasonal dynamics of the above characteristics are presented in Fig. 1. Inorganic substratum was mostly fine and coarse sand, as well as some gravel.

Fish assemblage attributes

Over the investigated period the total of 14 fish species inhabiting *Potamogeton* patches in the SAM habitat were captured. The dominant species was perch (*Perca fluviatilis* L.), constituting 32.7% of the total fish density and 23.0% of their total biomass. In order of their decreasing importance in total fish biomass, the following species were: dace (*Leuciscus leuciscus* (L.) and roach (*Rutilus rutilus* (L.)), 38.2% and 12.1% of the biomass and 15.5% and 18.2% of the density, respectively. In turn ruffe (*Gymnocephalus cernuus* (L.)), accounted for 9.1% of the biomass and 11.8% of the density, while three-spined stickleback (*Gasterosteus aculeatus* L.) reached 4.0% of the biomass and 11.8% of the density. Spined loach (*Cobitis taenia* L.), gudgeon (*Gobio gobio* (L.) and ide (*Leuciscus idus* (L.), were captured less frequently, constituting with other fish species 13.6% of the biomass and 10.0% of the density (Fig. 2).

All guts of the analysed individuals of the five species were filled to various extent (n = 242). The characteristics of the fish are presented in Table 1.

Food resources associated with SAM

Microcrustaceans. Over the whole investigated period Cladocera dominated in water column, reaching 99% of the zooplankton biomass of all investigated periods. Copepoda were very scarce, with the maximum in late August. The maximum values of cladoceran biomass were recorded in August due to the presence of large-sized predator *Leptodora kindtii* (Focke) (49.7% of the total cladoceran biomass during the study period). The most numerous specimens in water column were the small sized species of *Chydorus sphaericus* (O. F. Müller) (which constituted only 15.1% of zooplankton biomass over the investigated period), *Bosmina* spp. (17.1%) and large size taxa, *Daphnia* spp. (17.2%) (Fig. 2).

Epiphytic and benthic fauna connected with *Potamogeton*. Simuliids dominated among the macrophytes, amounting to 84.7% of the biomass of the total epiphytic fauna, but were abundant only till late June. Different seasonal dynamics was showed by chironomids (14.1% of total epiphytic fauna biomass), which reached the highest biomass in June and July but occurred throughout the study period. Main chironomid species, on *Potamogeton*, were: *Cricotopus sylvestris* (Fabricius) (Orthocladiinae), and *Parachironomus gracilior* (Kieffer) (Chironominae-Chironomini). Other epiphytic invertebrates (including *Hydra* sp.) occurred rarely (1.2%) (Fig. 2).

Chironomidae dominated in the benthos over the whole investigated period, reaching 83.7% of total benthic invertebrate biomass, and their abundance decreased over time. The dominant chironomids in benthos were represented by *Chironomus riparius* Meigen, *Dicrotendipes nervosus* (Staeger), *Glyptotendipes cauliginellus* (Kieffer) and *Polypedilum* spp. (Chironominae-Chironomini), as well as *Cricotopus bicinctus* (Meigen) (Orthocladiinae) and *Paratanytarsus* (Tanytarsini). Oligochaeta (9.3%) were present at the same level over the whole studied period, while Trichoptera (4.1%, mainly *Hydropsyche* spp.) were present mostly in May. The macrophyte bed was also inhabited by *Hydra* sp. (1.2%), especially in May and June (Fig. 2).

Trophic attributes of fish

Fish associated with the SAM exploited five main food categories: zooplankton (mainly Cladocera), benthos (Chironomidae during the whole studied period, and Trichoptera at the beginning of the investigated period), epiphyton (Chironomidae and Simuliidae), plants, detritus with algae, including the filamentous ones (Fig. 3).

In dace, Cladocera occurred on six of the seven sampling occasions on which the fish species was recorded. However, the biomass of Cladocera first rapidly increased to mid June, when they became dominant, and then decreased to none in late July. Both epiphytic and benthic chironomids became the first/second most important food category of dace in July. It is worth noting that dace also exploited imagines from the water surface. Three-spined stickleback consumed mainly Cladocera in May, which were replaced by Simuliidae in June. Benthic Chironomidae were the second/third most important food category in May and June but almost completely dominated the diet of this species in July. In ruffe, benthic chironomids were the main food category consumed on all sampling occasions, except late May and early July, when Trichoptera dominated instead. Epiphytic chironomids appeared in ruffe's diet since late June. Cladocerans and epiphytic chironomids dominated the diet of perch to a similar extent on most of the sampling occasions, although copepods became a subdominant and trichopterans a decisive dominant on one occasion each. In turn in roach, plants were the dominant food component on the first and a subdominant on all other sampling occasions. Cladocera were the main food type on three sampling occasions, in July and August. Detritus and algae were present during the whole study period (Fig. 3).

From the point of view of given food categories, in the course of the whole investigated period, the main component of roach diet were plants (about 28.2% of gut contents), while for other species it was the accessory food (Kruskal-Wallis test, $H = 178.49$, $p<$

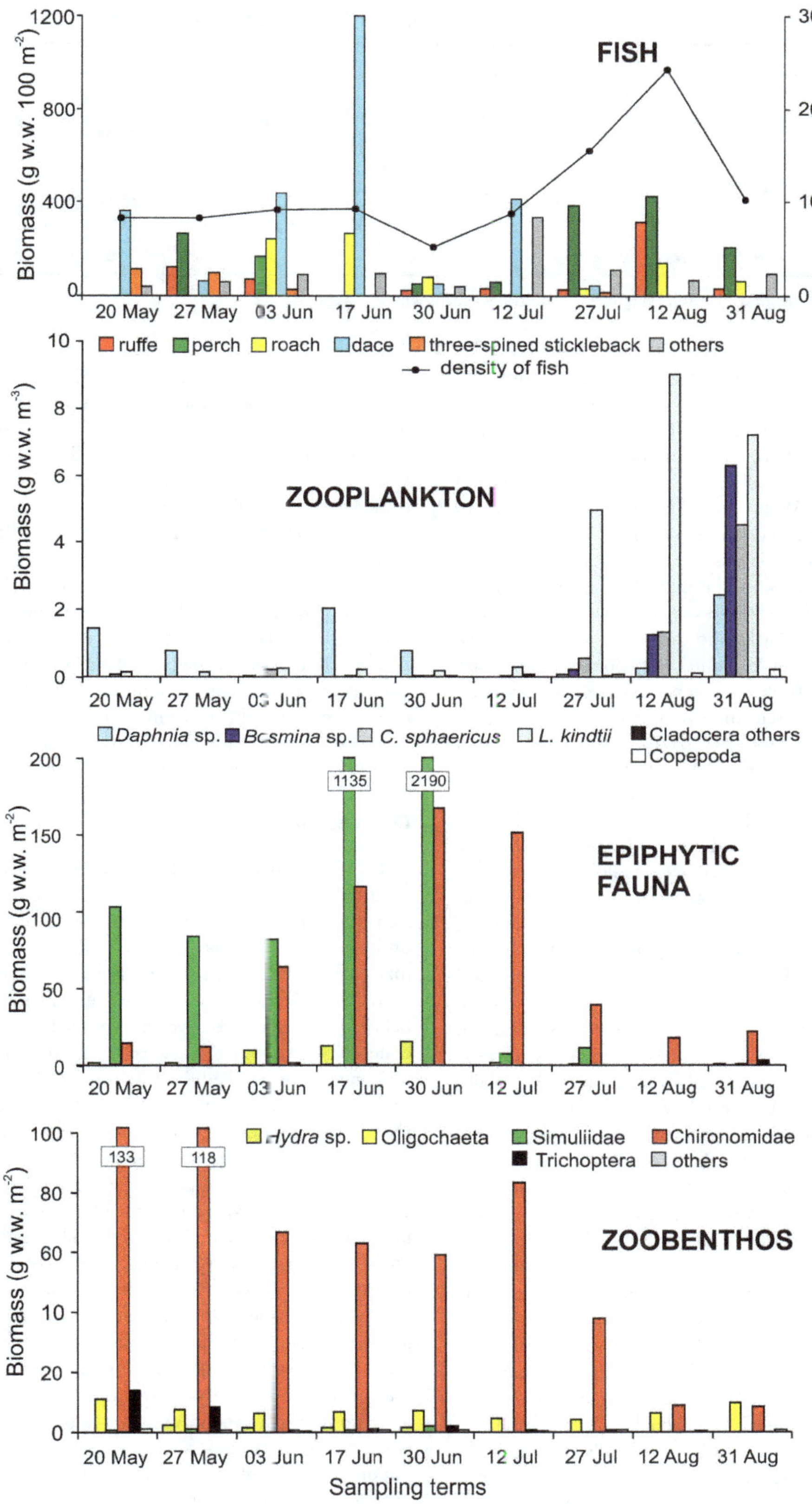

Figure 2. Fish and their food resources. Intraseasonal dynamics of biomass and density of fish and of their food resources (zooplankton, epiphytic fauna and zoobenthos) over the study period.

Table 1. Characteristics of analysed fish specimens in the SAM habitat of the Warta River, Poland.

Fish species	N		B (g)	TL (mm)	FC
Gymnocephalus cernuus (L.) (ruffe)	41	mean R	2.7 0.8–16.0	63 44–113	2.4 0.6–7.3
Perca fluviatilis L. (perch)	55	mean R	3.3 0.8–14.2	66 41–102	0.8 0.1–4.9
Rutilus rutilus (L.) (roach)	76	mean R	1.8 0.13–44.2	56 24–147	0.4 0.03–1.5
Leuciscus leuciscus (L.) (dace)	37	mean R	16.6 10.8–29.3	116 100–136	1.0 0.1–2.1
Gasterosteus aculeatus L. (three-spined stickleback)	33	mean R	2.4 0.3–4.2	54 31–70	4.1 0.5–7.2

N – number of specimens, B – biomass, TL – total length, FC – gut fullness coefficient, R – range of values.

0.0001), among which higher percentages of SAM (about 4%) were recorded for dace.

Chironomidae were consumed by all fish during the whole studied period; these dipterans, living in the bottom, were the main food of ruffe and statistically more important than those of other fish species (Kruskal-Wallis test, $H = 108.51$, $p<0.0001$). In turn, epiphytic chironomid taxa were consumed by perch more than by other fishes (Kruskal-Wallis test, $H = 57.87$, $p<0.0001$). Other dipterans, Simuliidae, were the main food category (about 26.8% of gut contents) only for three-spined stickleback (Kruskal-Wallis test, $H = 33.92$, $p<0.0001$), and to a lesser extent, for dace and perch (about 6% of gut contents). Trichoptera (large size larvae represented by *Hydropsyche*) were exploited to a greater extent by dace, ruffe and perch, than by roach and three-spined stickleback (Kruskal-Wallis test, $H = 61.16$, $p<0.0001$); perch consumed *Hydropsyche* larvae at a lower level than dace (post-hoc Dunn test, $p<0.036$). Detritus with algae was the main component in the gut contents of roach and dace and statistically different than of the other studied fishes (Kruskal-Wallis test, $H = 142.24$, $p<0.0001$). Cladocerans were exploited by all fish; the lowest biomass of this prey was recorded in ruffe guts (Kruskal-Wallis test, $H = 28.03$, $p<0.0001$). Other microcrustaceans, Copepoda, were an important diet component for perch only (Kruskal-Wallis test, $H = 60.08$, $p<0.0001$). Complementary food types (included in the "others" category) were ephemeropterans, other insects and *Asellus aquaticus* (Isopoda), as well as ostracods.

Over the investigated season, the fullness coefficients of these five analysed fish species were statistically different (Kruskal-Wallis test, $H = 130.58$, $p<0.0001$). As showed by the post-hoc Dunn test the differences did not exist only between ruffe and three-spined stickleback and between perch and dace. Moreover, for the two last species the highest variability in FC values was noted: for perch from 0.25 at the end of August to 2.8 at the end of June, while for dace from 0.5 at the end of July to 2.8 at the end of May. However, the lowest variability was observed for roach: from 0.3 at the end of August to 0.6 in the middle of June. For the whole studied period, the highest FC values were noted for three-spined stickleback (at the beginning of June) (Fig. 3).

The diet compositions of the five fish species were analyzed using hierarchical cluster analysis, which distinguished three feeding groups: 1) three-spined stickleback which consumed epiphytic simuliids (main prey), and occasionally fish eggs, 2) roach, feeding mainly on plant materials, detritus and algae, zooplankton, and Chironomidae as an important complementary food category, 3) dace, perch and ruffe, which ate mainly animal materials (aquatic and terrestrial invertebrates) (Fig. 4).

Niche breadths (Levins' index) of these species were statistically different (Kruskal-Wallis test, $H = 125.02$, $p<0.0001$) and varied seasonally. On each sampling occasion when roach and ruffe occurred, the niche breadth of the former was always much wider than of the latter (Fig. 5A). The evaluation of niche breadth revealed a less diverse diet of typical benthic fishes, such as ruffe, while the most diverse diet was in the case of roach. As regards niche breadths, three non-hierarchical groups of species (Kruskal-Wallis test, post hoc Dunn test, $H = 77.015$, $p<0.0001$) were distinguished: the first group was roach, the second group were dace and perch, and the third were ruffe and three-spined stickleback (Fig. 5A and B).

The Schoener interspecific diet overlap index did not differ between cyprinids, percids and three-spined stickleback over the studied period. However, this index varied seasonally, reaching the highest value between ruffe and dace (0.78 at the end of May when both species exerted pressure on the *Hydropsyche*) while the lowest ones were attained a few times: between roach and other fish (4 times lower or equal to 0.2) and between three-spined stickleback and other species (also 4 times lower, Fig. 6).

Discussion

Submersed aquatic macrophytes in large rivers

In the two recent decades, the bed zone between the bank and midriver channel of the tailwater stretch of the Warta River has undergone a seasonal regime shift from an alluvial to a macrophyte-dominated system. Such processes also took place in many other impacted large rivers. As this phenomenon is usually believed to exert negative environmental impacts, attempts to counteract it, using various methods, particularly artificial flooding, were applied in these rivers [37]. SAMs are rather undesirable elements in large rivers because they modify the in-river environment mainly by altering river flows, and by decreasing the depth of trapping sediments, which is also beneficial for large populations of pelophilous macrobenthic fauna. However, SAMs are the excellent surface for epiphyton. Some groups of invertebrates, represented by grazers, like snails, macrocrustaceans and cladoceran zooplankters, are able to protect aquatic macrophytes by removing epiphytes and phytoplanktonic algae. The plants themselves help the process of defense because they are a source of biochemical compounds that, on one hand, negatively affect the growth of algae (allelopathy), but, on the other hand, may attract grazers. Many fish species occupying this rich habitat also positively affect SAMs as main predators foraging on epiphytic invertebrates. Consequently, these vertebrates are an important part of a complex network of relations between nutrients, phytoplankton, epiphytes, herbivorous invertebrates and benthos [38–40].

Fish foraging among vascular plants

From the beginning of the functioning of the Jeziorsko Reservoir (1986) in the Warta River downstream from its dam the diversity of fish declined regularly, while the number of these

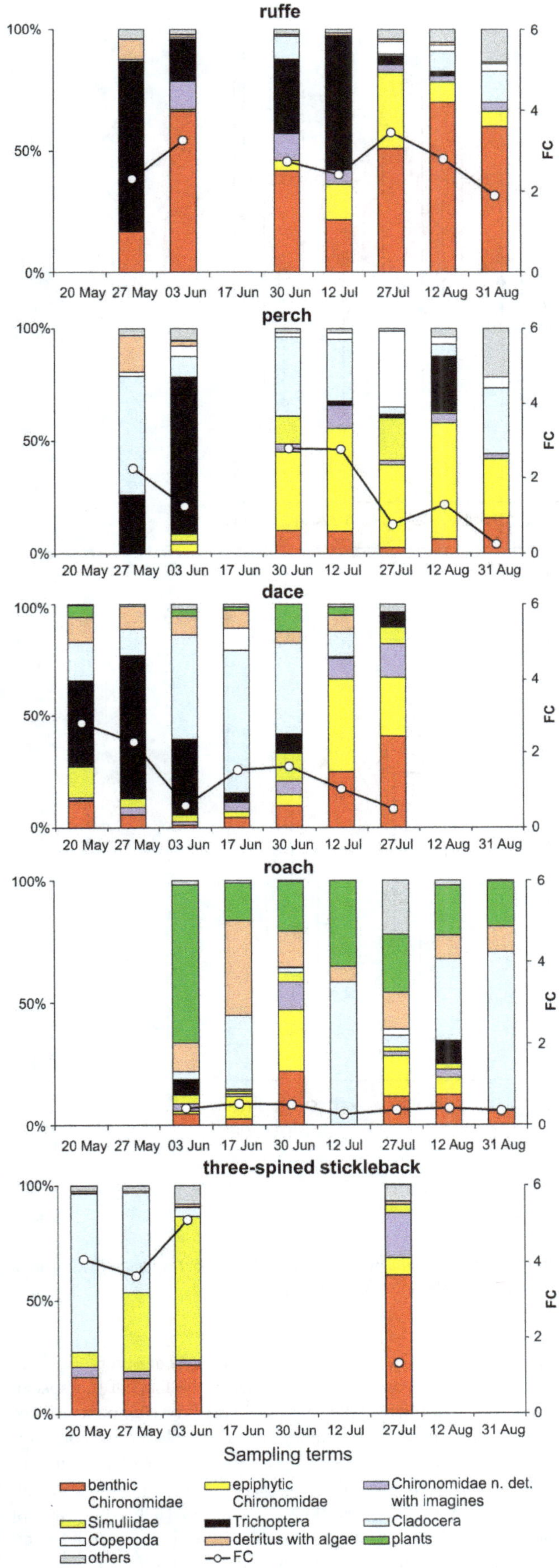

Figure 3. Fish diet composition. Food items and gut fullness coefficient (FC) of each fish species over the study period.

vertebrates showed quite opposite trends, mainly due to perch and roach, and to a lesser degree, to ruffe. This process of fish decline concerns, for example, dace, a rheophilic species (i.e. riverine specialist), which was present sporadically, and even absent in some years [3,24,25].

Dace, which exploits open water with fast water currents, usually suffer from human-induced changes in aquatic environment and is thus considered a good bioindicator [41–43]. The over-representation of dace among dense leaves and stems of *Potamogeton* recorded in the impacted stretch of the Warta River was rather unexpected. Dace showed a very high plasticity to food resources connected with SAM, feeding on larger, easily catchable benthic organisms, epiphytic fauna and/or zooplankton as well as imagines from water surface (mainly Chironomidae) which died after mating and/or rested on the surface above its pupal exuviae after eclosion. However, dace reached the highest value of FC when consuming large *Hydropsyche* larvae and at that time their niche overlapped that of ruffe. In June the diet of dace comprised also Cladocera, and the FC of dace was reduced. The presence of dace in SAM may testify to the greater attractiveness of this temporary habitat than the sandy mid-channel of the alluvial Warta River, where only tiny organisms, such as some Oligochaeta and Chironomidae, occasionally occur. Also, the potential migration of dace towards the depositional, SAM-less zone (see Material and methods), would not bring many benefits to the fish because the mud covering that zone is frequently flooded, or, to a high extent, exposed (to air) due to pulse water releases from the reservoir. Therefore, at the depositional zone benthic fauna was remarkably impoverished as compared with the natural river section (upstream of the reservoir); virtually no insects (except some families of Diptera), Hirudinea and Oligochaeta, were collected there [3,27,28,44]. Summing up, dace food spectrum in the very biologically productive SAM habitat was similar to those in other ecosystems [45–47] in which dace may also display daily

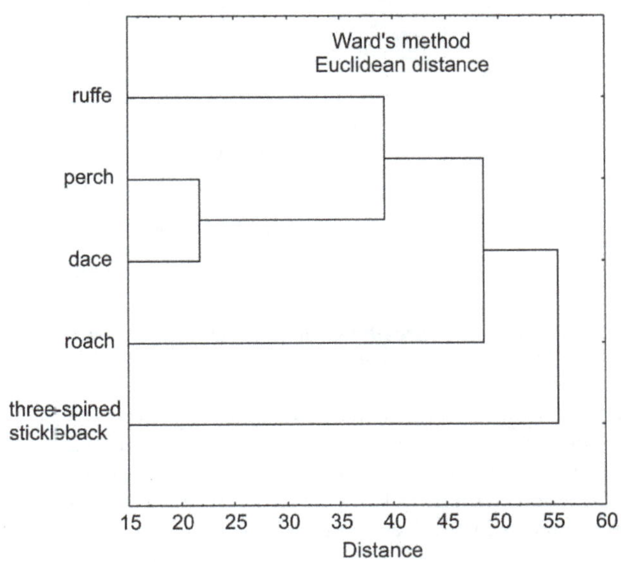

Figure 4. Similarity of fish species in terms of diet. Dendrogram resulting from the cluster analysis performed on gut contents of each species over the whole investigated period.

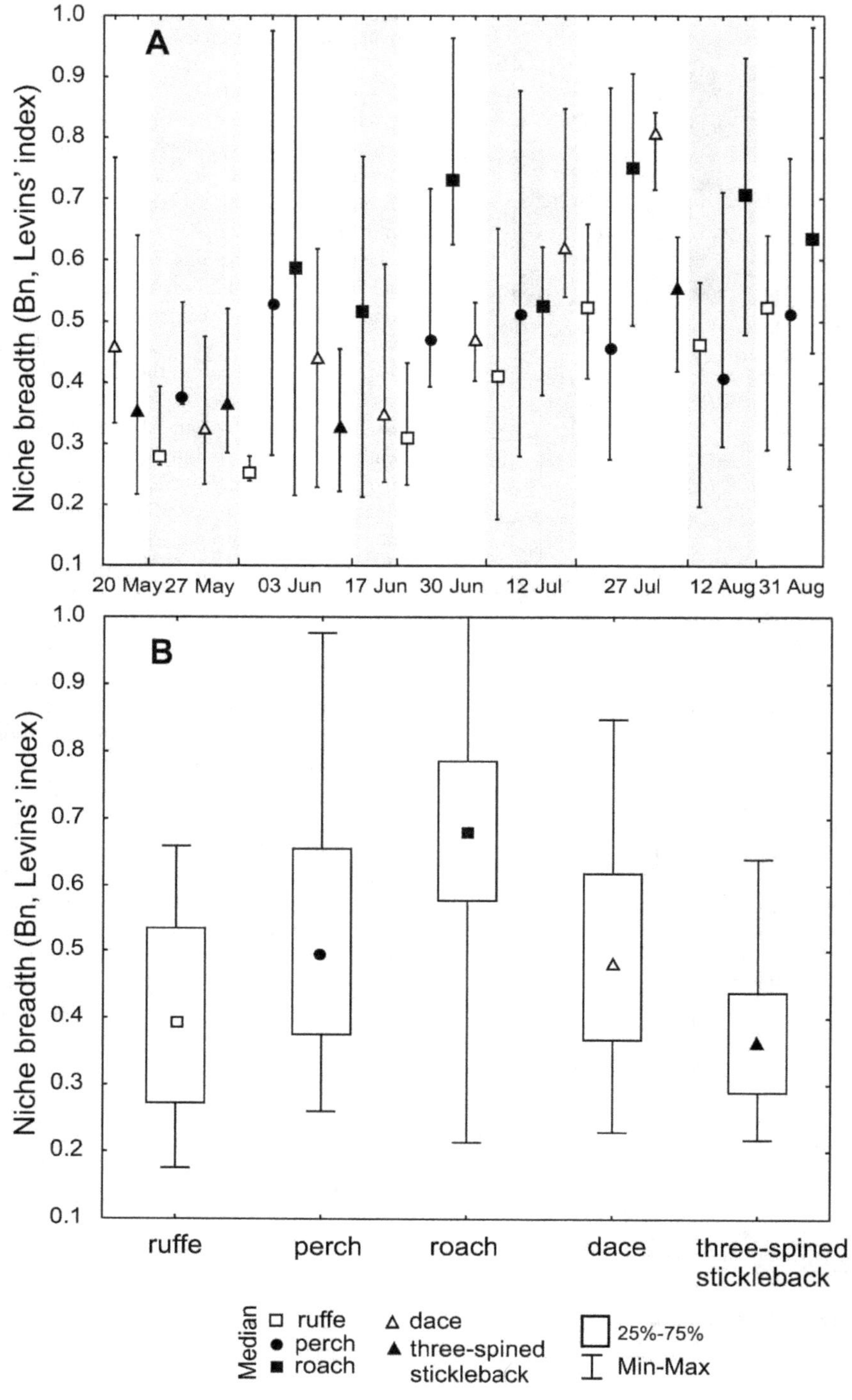

Figure 5. Food niche breadth of fishes. A. Intraseasonal variation in the niche breadth (medians of Levins' index, B_n) of each species. B. Median of the niche breadth for each species over the whole studied period. Vertical bars represent the interquartile range.

migrations to and from feeding places [48]. It is worth noting that this species also shows ontogenetic shifts in its food spectrum [49].

Three-spined stickleback was the second species for which overrepresentation in SAM as compared with its abundance in the whole tailwater reach was observed [50], but only at the beginning of the studied period. According to Bańbura [50], three-spined stickleback feed mainly on Copepoda, Cladocera, larvae of Chironomidae, and seasonally Mollusca, Oligochaeta and fish eggs, but none of these items exceeded 25% of the gut contents. This finding is not in accordance with the present observations. In the macrophyte beds of the Warta River, the food of this species varied intraseasonally; the extraordinary development of the epiphytic fauna caused a foraging shift from Cladocera (constituting at the beginning of the study period about 70% of gut contents, and consisting mainly of large sized species of *Daphnia*, of reservoir origin, [51]) to epiphytic fauna, especially to the largest (oldest) larvae of the dominant dipterans, both simuliids and chironomids (the majority of gut contents in June). Low niche

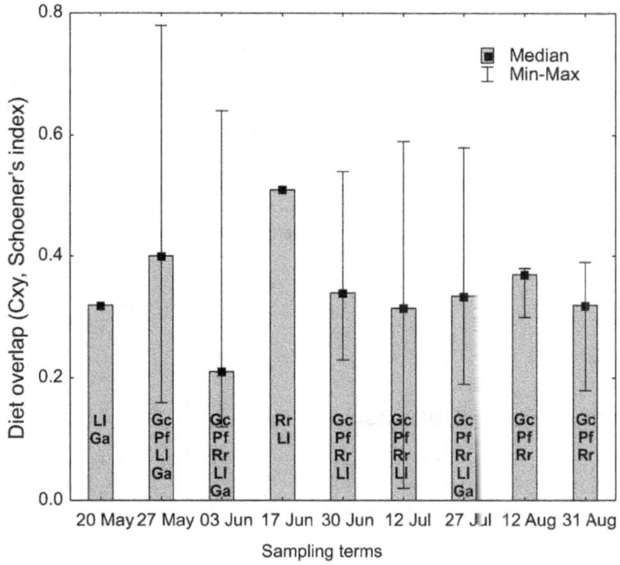

Figure 6. Interspecific diet overlaps. Interseasonal variation in the diet overlap (medians of the Schoener index, C_{xy}) between perch (Pf), ruffe (Gc), roach (Rr), dace (Ll) and three-spined stickleback (Ga); the above abbreviations in parentheses come from scientific names of fish species. Other explanations as in Fig. 5.

overlap between three-spined stickleback and other species was the effect of consuming epiphytic simuliids as the main prey and other prey types, such as fish eggs (the highest values of FC occurred when the species fed on these elements), rather untypical food items for other fish. This finding is confirmed by a dendrogram resulting from the cluster analysis.

The choice of older (larger) dipteran individuals by stickleback, as stated in our earlier paper [22], is consistent with the optimal foraging theory [52] - organisms forage in such a way as to maximize their net energy intake per unit time.

Ruffe, as a typical benthivorous fish, and partially three-spined stickleback and dace, play an important role in the internal nutrient cycling; firstly, during the searching for food (through bioturbation), secondly, during the translocation of nutrients from the bottom to the water column realized via their digesting and egestion. Ruffe, a small but aggressive fish native to Europe and Asia, may be classified rather among specialists [18,53–56] than generalists [57]. In lakes, ruffe may efficiently forage in deeper and darker bed patches due to its very sensitive lateral line system and the light-reflecting *tapetum lucidum* in its eye [58,59]. In the Warta River, this vertical gradient of food selection by ruffe was confirmed by Dukowska et al. [18], while its horizontal movement for searching food is rather unprofitable, similar to dace [3,27,28]. Overlaps between ruffe diet and those of other species were at the same level (from 0.21 to 0.34) regardless of ruffe's preference for benthic chironomids and *Hydropsyche*.

According to some studies, ruffe do not undergo ontogenetic dietary shifts, and remain the bottom feeders throughout the life cycle [57].

In rivers, high diversity and abundance values of fish are usually strongly associated with a high degree of trophic specialization (low amplitude of individual trophic niches) and a small degree of overlap between the diets of species constituting an assemblage [60]. But in the impacted stretch of the Warta River fish diversity has been low from the beginning of the functioning of the Jeziorsko Reservoir, although the abundance of several species was very high [24,25]. Each year, when the amount of water released from the reservoir increases, a mass escapement of fish of eurytopic species, predominantly juvenile stages, gets intensified. This mainly concerns the species that have attained reproductive success in the reservoir in a given year (including mostly perch and roach, but also ruffe) and may lead to an increase in the abundance of these species (two or three orders of magnitude higher than in the pre-impoundment period or in the upstream river stretch) [3,24,61].

Perch, a potential competitor for ruffe [56,62], is included among generalists. It shows an ontogenetic shift in its diet during its life history, from zooplankton (at the onset of exogenous feeding) to macroinvertebrates, and from macroinvertebrates to fish [23,63–67]. However, the adults of this species may also be classified as trophic generalists switching frequently between piscivorous, zooplanktivorous, and benthivorous feeding style depending on the food resources in the environment. In the Warta River, in spite of this mode of foraging in areas drastically overcrowded by perch [61], the species starved also at the end of the present study period, despite the increased transport of zooplankton from the reservoir [18,51]. This is in accordance with assumptions of the theory of the ideal free distribution stating that an increased number of individuals in a given patch of resources reduces its quality, through either increased scramble competition or increased interference competition (including aggressive behavior) [68,69].

In the Warta River, diet overlap between perch and ruffe was rather low (the Schoener index, range 0.21–0.34) as perch preferred to eat epiphytic chironomids, simuliids and *Daphnia*, while ruffe chose large sized benthic chironomids and trichopterans (if they were present) and occasionally zooplankton [18]. It is worth stressing that the identification of prey, mainly Chironomidae, of these two fish species, to genus (mainly) or species level helped to determine the food resource partition between these two closely related species, because these fishes generally consumed different chironomid taxa [18].

In the Warta River, the second numerically most abundant species connected with SAM was roach. The interaction between perch and roach has been studied by many ecologists, especially in lentic ecosystems [67,70,71]. Both young roach, which fed mainly on detritus, chironomids and zooplankton, as well as older individuals, which consumed mostly detritus, filamentous algae, vascular plants, macroinvertebrates and molluscs, represented typically omnivorous feeding habitats, and are thus considered generalists [71–73]. Besides, roach may be classified into opportunists. If huge amounts of easily accessible food appear, roach use it immediately; for example, during chironomid emergences the alimentary tracts of roach are filled in with numerous pupae of these insects [74]. For each chironomid pupa being in a water column is a very dangerous experience (as the pupa may then end up as the prey of macroinvertebrates and/or fish), however, at that time zooplankton, mainly *Daphnia*, is released from fish predation [75].

In the present material, an insufficient amount of food available for roach (starvation?) is indicated by the low values of its FC. Its niche breadth was the largest one of those of all the five species during the whole studied period. The niche overlap between this species and other fishes was low, thus we may suppose that rather an intraspecific than interspecific competition decided the fate of small roach in this overcrowded environment. Even if certain individuals of this eurytopic species die because of competitive interactions, they will soon be replaced by juveniles migrating massively from the reservoir [25,61,76]. It is worth mentioning that the consumption of such food categories as algae and detritus may have resulted in a slow growth rate [73]. A large spectrum of food types consumed by roach, larger than that of perch, was recorded by other ecologists [67,70].

Conclusions

In the SAM habitat the diet overlap was highest when the SAM patches, and the food resources associated with them, were most developed (twice during the investigated period). For the first time at the beginning of SAM development, when large-sized *Hydropsyche* were the main food category for ruffe, perch and dace, and for the second time throughout June and the first half of July, when benthic and/or epiphytic Chironomidae were the basic food items for these species. This finding is congruent with the niche overlap hypothesis saying that maximal tolerable niche overlap can be higher in less intensely competitive situations, i.e. in environments with lower demand/supply ratios [77].

One of the most important attributes of organisms to avoid direct overlap in the use of resources is diversification of body size of individuals of given species [60]. We put focus on three (time, space and resource) of the four niche axes of each of the five fish species living among the submersed macrophytes and we concluded that their diets only partly overlap, which allows them to coexist in this temporary, very rich habitat.

Acknowledgments

We are greatly indebted to L. Kucharski for the identification of macrophytes, to W. Jurasz for the identification of cladocerans, and to our colleagues, L. Marszał, G. Zięba and J. Lik for assistance in the field and/or laboratory work, as well as to Ł. Głowacki and R. Reddy for revising the English. We also thank the Department of Hydrography and Morphology of River Beds, the Institute of Meteorology and Water Management, Poland, for granting us a licence to use the Electronic Map of Hydrographic Partitions in Poland. The study was carried out in the Field Station at Pęczniew.

Author Contributions

Conceived and designed the experiments: MD MG. Performed the experiments: MD. Analyzed the data: MD. Wrote the paper: MD MG. Analyzed the food resources and gut contents of fish: MD MG. Prepared graphics: MD.

References

1. Ward JS, Stanford JA (1980) Tailwater biota: ecological response to environmental alternations. In:Proceedings of the symposium on surface water impoundments ASCE.
2. Petts GE (1984) Impounded rivers. Perspectives for ecological management. Chichester: John Wiley and Sons. 326 p.
3. Głowacki Ł, Grzybkowska M, Dukowska M, Penczak T (2011) Effects of damming a large lowland river on chironomids and fish assessed with (multiplicative partitioning of) true/Hill biodiversity measures. River Res Appl 27: 612–629.
4. Bednarek AT (2001) Undamming rivers: a reviews of the ecological impacts of dam removal. Environ Manage 27: 803–814.
5. Feld CK, Birk S, Bradley DC, Hering D, Kail J, et al. (2011) From natural to degraded rivers and back again: A test of restoration ecology theory and practice. Adv Ecol Res 44: 119–209.
6. Franklin P, Dunbar M, Whitehead P (2008) Flow controls on lowland river macrophytes: A review. Sci Total Environ 400: 369–378.
7. Dukowska M, Grzybkowska M, Sitkowska M, Zelazna-Wieczorek J, Szeląg-Wasielewska E (1999) Food resource partitioning between chironomid species associated with submerged vegetations in the Warta River below the dam reservoir, Poland. Acta Hydrobiol 41: 219–229.
8. Tokeshi M, Pinder LCV (1985) Microhabitats of stream invertebrates on two submersed macrophytes with contrasting leaf morphology. Holarctic Ecol 8: 313–319.
9. Pinder LCV (1992) Biology of epiphytic Chironomidae (Diptera: Nematocera) in chalk streams. Hydrobiologia 248: 39–51.
10. Grzybkowska M, Dukowska M, Takeda M, Majecki J, Kucharski L (2003) Seasonal dynamics of macroinvertebrates associated with submersed macrophytes in a lowland river downstream of the dam reservoir. Ecohydrol Hydrobiol 3: 399–408.
11. Chick JH, McIvor CC (1997) Habitat selection by three littoral zone fishes: effects of predation pressure, plant density and macrophyte type. Ecol Freshw Fish 6: 27–35.
12. Grenouillet G, Pont D (2001) Juvenile fishes in macrophyte beds: influence of food resources, habitat structure and body size. J Fish Biol 59: 939–959.
13. Li J, Huang P, Zhang R (2010) Modeling the refuge effect of submerged macrophytes in ecological dynamics of shallow lakes: A new model of fish functional response. Ecol Modell 221: 2076–2085.
14. Rozas LP, Odum WE (1988) Occupation of submerged aquatic vegetation by fishes: testing the roles of food and refuge. Oecologia 77: 101–106.
15. Manatunge J, Asaedaa T, Priyadarshana T (2000) The influence of structural complexity on fish–zooplankton interactions: a study using artificial submerged macrophytes. Environ Biol Fishes 58: 425–438.
16. Kleeberg A, Köchler J, Sukhodolova T, Sukhodolov A (2010) Effects of aquatic macrophytes on organic matter deposition, resuspension and phosphorus entrainment in a lowland river. Freshw Biol 55: 326–345.
17. Kohler J, Hachoł J, Hilt S (2010) Regulation of submersed macrophyte biomass in a temperate lowland river: Interactions between shading by bank vegetation, epiphyton and water turbidity. Aquat Bot 92: 129–136.
18. Dukowska M, Grzybkowska M, Kruk A, Szczerkowska-Majchrzak E (2013) Food niche partitioning between perch and ruffe: combined use of a self-organising map and the IndVal index for analysing fish diet. Ecol Modell 265: 221–229.
19. Chesson P (2000) Mechanisms of maintenance of species diversity. Annu Rev Ecol Syst 31: 343–366.
20. Schulze T, Dörner H, Baade U, Hölker F (2012) Dietary niche partitioning in a piscivorous fish guild in response to stocking of an additional competitor – The role of diet specialization. Limnologica 42: 56–64.
21. Dukowska M, Grzybkowska M, Folcholc I, Tszydel M, Szczerkowska E (2005) Predation of *Hydra* sp. on epiphytic fauna and zooplankton in a disturbed lowland river. Teka Commision of Protection and Formation of Natural Environment 2: 48–57.
22. Dukowska M, Grzybkowska M, Marszał L, Zięba G (2009) The food preferences of three-spined stickleback, *Gasterosteus aculeatus* L., downstream of a dam reservoir. Oceanol Hydrobiol Stud 38: 39–50.
23. Marszał L, Grzybkowska M, Penczak T, Galicka W (1996) Diet and feeding of dominant fish populations in the impounded Warta River, Poland. Polish Arch Hydrobiol 43: 185–202.
24. Penczak T, Głowacki Ł, Galicka W, Koszaliński H (1998) A long-term study (1985–1995) of fish populations in the impounded Warta River, Poland. Hydrobiologia 368: 157–173.
25. Penczak T, Głowacki Ł, Kruk A, Galicka W (2012) Implementation of a self-organizing map for investigation of impoundment impact on fish assemblages in a large, lowland river: Long-term study. Ecol Modell 227: 64–71.
26. EMPHP (Electronic Map of Hydrographic Partitions in Poland) (2007) Instituite of Meteorology and Water Management, Poland. Available: http://www.imgw.gov.pl. Accessed 10 January 2013.
27. Grzybkowska M, Dukowska M (2002) Communities of Chironomidae (Diptera) above and below a reservoir on a lowland river: long-term study. Annal Zool 52: 235–247.
28. Grzybkowska M, Hejduk J, Zieliński P (1990) Seasonal dynamics and production of Chironomidae in a large lowland river upstream and downstream from a new reservoir in Central Poland. Arch Hydrobiol 119: 439–455.
29. Petersen RC, Cummins KW, Ward GM (1989) Microbial and animal processing of detritus in a woodland stream. Ecol Monogr 59: 21–39.
30. Dumont HJ, Van de Velde I, Dumont S (1975) The dry weight estimate of biomass in a selection of Cladocera, Copepoda and Rotifera from the plankton, periphyton and benthos of continental waters. Oecologia 19: 75–97.
31. Opuszyński K (1983) The basics of fish biology. Warszawa: PWRiL. 590 p (in Polish).
32. Krebs CJ (1999) Ecological methodology. USA: Addison-Wesley Educational Publishers Inc. CA. 620 p.
33. Schoener TW (1970) Non-synchronous spatial overlap of lizards in patchy habitats. Ecology 51: 408–418.
34. Wallace RK (1981) An assessment of diet-overlap indexes. Trans Am Fish Soc 110: 72–76.
35. Zar JH (1984) Biostatistical analysis. Englewood Cliffs, New Jersey: Prentice-Hall Inc. 717 p.

36. StatSoft Inc. (2011) STATISTICA (data analysis software system), version 10. Avaiable: http://www.statsoft.com. Accessed 2014 March 3.
37. Ibáñez C, Caiola N, Rovira A, Real M (2012) Monitoring the effects of floods on submerged macrophytes in a large river. Sci Total Environ 440: 132–139.
38. De Nie HW (1987) The decrease in aquatic vegetation in Europe and its consequences for fish populations. EIFAC/CECPI Occasional paper 19: 52 p.
39. Vanderstukken M, Mazzeo N, Van Colen W, Declerck SAJ, Muylaert K (2011) Biological control of phytoplankton by the subtropical submerged macrophytes *Egeria densa* and *Potamogeton illinoensis*: a mesocosm study. Freshw Biol 56: 1837–1849.
40. Gross EM (2003) Allelopathy of aquatic autotrophs. Crit Rev Plant Sci 22: 313–339.
41. Penczak T, Kruk A (2000) Threatened obligatory riverine fishes in human-modified Polish rivers. Ecol Freshw Fish 9: 109–117.
42. Raat AJP (2001) Ecological rehabilitation of the Dutch part of the River Rhine with special attention to the fish. River Res Appl 17: 131–144.
43. Kruk A (2007) Role of habitat degradation in determining fish distribution and abundance along the lowland Warta River, Poland. J Appl Ichthyol 23: 9–18.
44. Grzybkowska M (1991) Development and habitat selection of chironomid communities at long- and short-term water discharge fluctuation. Regul Riv 6: 257–264.
45. Tadajewska M (2000) Dace *Leuciscus leuciscus* (Linnaeus, 1758). In: Brylińska M, editor. Freshwater fishes of Poland.Warszawa: PWN.pp. 311–314 (in Polish).
46. Kucharczyk D, Mamcarz A, Kujawa R, Targońska K (2008) Dace *Leuciscus leuciscus* (Linnaeus, 1758) - monography Olsztyn: Mercurius78 p (in Polish).
47. Vlach P, Švátora M, Dušek J (2013) The food niche overlap of five fish species in the Úpoř brook (Central Bohemia). Knowl Manag Aquat Ecosyst. Available: http://dx.doi.org/10.1051/kmae/2013070. Accessed: 3 March 2014.
48. Clough S, Ladle M (1997) Diel migration and site fidelity in a stream-dwelling cyprinid *Leuciscus leuciscus*. J Fish Biol 50: 1117–1119.
49. Nunn AD, Harvey JP, Cowx IG (2007) The food and feeding relationships of larval and 0+ year juvenile fishes in lowland rivers and connected waterbodies. I. Ontogenetic shifts and interspecific diet similarity. J Fish Biol 70: 726–742.
50. Bańbura J (2000) Three-spined stickleback. In: Brylińska M, editor. Freshwater fishes of Poland.Warszawa: PWN.pp. 439–443 (in Polish).
51. Grzybkowska M, Temech A, Najwer I (1996) Seston, (particles>400 μm) of the Warta River downstream from the new reservoir of Jeziorsko. Acta Univ Lodz, Folia limnol 6: 47–61.
52. MacArthur RH, Pianka ER (1966) On optimal use of a patchy environment. Am Nat 100: 603–609.
53. Gunderson JL, Klepinger MR, Bonte CR, Marsden JE (1998) Overview of the international symposium on Eurasian ruffe (*Gymnocephalus cernuus*) biology, impacts and control. J Great Lakes Res 24: 165–169.
54. Tarvainen M, Ventelä A, Helminen H, Sarvala J (2005) Nutrient release and resuspension generated by ruffe (*Gymnocephalus cernuus*) and chironomids. Freshw Biol 50: 447–458.
55. Schleuter D, Eckmann R (2006) Competition between perch *Perca fluviatilis* and ruffe *Gymnocephalus cernuus*: the advantage of turning night into day. Freshw Biol 51: 287–297.
56. Schleuter D, Eckmann R (2008) Generalist versus specialist: the performances of perch and ruffe in lake of low productivity. Ecol of Freshw Fishes 17: 86–99.
57. Rösh R, Kangur A, Kangur K, Krämer A, Ráb P, et al. (1996) Ruffe (*Gymnocephalus cernuus*). Acta Zool Litu 19: 18–24.
58. Ogle DH, Selgeby JH, Newman RM, Henry MG (1995) Diet and feeding periodicity of ruffe in the St. Louis River Estuary, Lake Superior. Trans Am Fish Soc 124: 356–369.
59. Fullerton AH, Lamberti GA (2006) A comparison of habitat use and habitat-specific feeding efficiency by Eurasian ruffe (*Gymnocephalus cernuus*) and yellow perch (*Perca flavescens*). Ecol Freshw Fish 15: 1–9.
60. Barili E, Agostinho AA, Gomes LC, Latin JD (2011) The coexistence of fish species in streams: relationships between assemblage attributes and trophic and environmental variables. Environ Biol Fishes 92: 41–52.
61. Penczak T, Kruk A (2005) Patternizing of impoundment impact (1985–2002) on fish assemblages in a lowland river using the Kohonen algorithm. J Appl Ichthyol 21: 169–177.
62. Bergman E (1988) Foraging abilities and niche breadths of two percids, *Perca fluviatilis* and *Gymnocephalus cernua*, under different environmental conditions. J Animal Ecol 57: 443–453.
63. Kornijów R (1997) The impact of predation by perch on the size-structure of Chironomus larvae - the role of vertical distribution of the prey in the bottom sediments, and habitat complexity. Hydrobiologia 342/343: 207–213.
64. Dieterich A, Baumgärtner D, Eckmann R (2004) Competition for food between Eurasian perch *Perca fluviatilis* and ruffe *Gymnocephalus cernuus* over different substrate types. Ecol Freshw Fish 13: 236–244.
65. Kezsu E, Specziár A (2006) Ontogenetic diet profiles and size-dependent diet partitioning of ruffe *Gymnocephalus cernuus*, perch *Perca fluviatilis* and pumpkinseed *Lepomis gibbosus* in Lake Balaton. Ecol Freshw Fish 15: 339–349.
66. Eorcherding J, Magnhagen C (2008) Food abundance affects both morphology and behaviour of juvenile perch. Ecol Freshw Fish 17: 207–218.
67. Nurminen L, Pekcan-Hekim Z, Horppila J (2010) Feeding efficiency of planktivorous perch *Perca fluviatilis* and roach *Rutilus rutilus* in varying turbidity: an individual-based approach. J Fish Biol 76: 1848–1855.
68. Kennedy M, Gray RD (1993) Can ecological theory predict the distribution of foraging animals? A critical analysis of experiments on the ideal free distribution. Oikos 68: 158–166.
69. Danchin E, Giraldeau LA, Cézilly F (2008) Behavioural ecology. Oxford: Oxford University Press. 912 p.
70. Persson L (1987) Effects of habitat and season on competitive interactions between roach (*Rutilus rutilus*) and perch (*Perca fluviatilis*). Oecologia 73: 170–177.
71. Kornijów R, Vakkilainen K, Horppila J, Luokkanen E, Kairesalo T (2005) Impacts of a submerged plant (*Elodea canadensis*) on interactions between roach (*Rutilus rutilus*) and its invertebrate prey communities in a lake littoral zone. Freshw Biol 50: 262–273.
72. Grzybkowska M (1988) Food of roach in the Widawka River. Acta Univ Lodz, Folia limnol 3: 85–100 (in Polish with English summary).
73. Horppila J, Nurminen L (2009) Food niche segregation between two herbivorous cyprinid species in a turbid lake. J Fish Biol 75: 1230–1243.
74. Grzybkowska M, Zalewski M (1983) The food of roach, bream and white bream in the Sulejów Dam Reservoir. In:Proceedings of the Conference of the Polish Hydrobiological Society. Lublin, pp 71–72 (in Polish).
75. Makino W, Kato H, Takamura N, Mizutani H, Katano N, et al. (2001) Did chironomid emergence release *Daphnia* from fish predation and lead to *Daphnia*-driven clear-water phase in Lake Towada, Japan? Hydrobiologia 442: 309–317.
76. Kruk A, Penczak T (2003) Impoundment impact on populations of facultative riverine fish. Ann Limnol 39: 197–210.
77. Pianka ER (1974) Niche overlap and diffuse competition. Proc Nat Acad Sci 71: 2141–2145.

16

Attribution and Expression of Incentive Salience Are Differentially Signaled by Ultrasonic Vocalizations in Rats

Juan C. Brenes[1,2,3]*, Rainer K. W. Schwarting[3]

1 Institute for Psychological Research, University of Costa Rica, Rodrigo Facio Campus, San Pedro, Costa Rica, 2 Neuroscience Research Center, University of Costa Rica, Rodrigo Facio Campus, San Pedro, Costa Rica, 3 Behavioral Neuroscience, Experimental and Biological Psychology, Philipps-University of Marburg, Marburg, Germany

Abstract

During Pavlovian incentive learning, the affective properties of rewards are thought to be transferred to their predicting cues. However, how rewards are represented emotionally in animals is widely unknown. This study sought to determine whether 50-kHz ultrasonic vocalizations (USVs) in rats may signal such a state of incentive motivation to natural, nutritional rewards. To this end, rats learned to anticipate food rewards and, across experiments, the current physiological state (deprived vs. sated), the type of learning mechanism recruited (Pavlovian vs. instrumental), the hedonic properties of UCS (low vs. high palatable food), and the availability of food reward (continued vs. discontinued) were manipulated. Overall, we found that reward-cues elicited 50-kHz calls as they were signaling a putative affective state indicative of incentive motivation in the rat. Attribution and expression of incentive salience, however, seemed not to be an unified process, and could be teased apart in two different ways: 1) under high motivational state (i.e., hunger), the attribution of incentive salience to cues occurred without being expressed at the USVs level, if reward expectations were higher than the outcome; 2) in all experiments when food rewards were devalued by satiation, reward cues were still able to elicit USVs and conditioned anticipatory activity although reward seeking and consumption were drastically weakened. Our results suggest that rats are capable of representing rewards emotionally beyond apparent, immediate physiological demands. These findings may have translational potential in uncovering mechanisms underlying aberrant and persistent motivation as observed in drug addiction, gambling, and eating disorders.

Editor: Ralph E Mistlberger, Simon Fraser University, Canada

Funding: This work was supported by the grant Schw 559/10-1 from the Deutsche Forschungsgemeinschaft. JCB was funded by the Deutscher Akademischer Austauschdienst (DAAD, Germany), and the University of Costa Rica. The funders had no role in study design, data collection and analysis, decision to publish, or preparation of the manuscript.

Competing Interests: The authors have declared that no competing interests exist.

* Email: brenesaenz@gmail.com

Introduction

Having affective representations in terms of pleasures and desires is a fundamental part of our subjective experience. Rewards and reward-related stimuli can make us feel good, and remind us how good they were in the past, but also how good they would be if experienced again. Being exposed to reward-related cues may also set a state of readiness for seeking and consuming that reward, even though we have not experienced it for a while or when physiological needs for it have been fulfilled [1–4]. In humans, such mechanisms play a critical role in drug addiction and relapse, overeating in obesity, and binge disorders [5–7]. The incentive valence of such reward-related stimuli (like places, odors, sounds, and time periods) is mainly determined by the affective experience resulting from preceding intake of that reward [8,9]. Following Pavlovian learning, sensory reward properties and associated cues are transformed into attractive and desired incentives [4,10–13]. This motivational component of reward is normally referred to as incentive salience [5,10]. In classical and modern incentive motivation theories, either activation of a "central emotive state", "expectations about rewards", or "subjective wanting" have been proposed as critical factors in the process of attributing incentive salience to reward cues [9–19]. In non-human animals, especially rodents, incentive motivation has been extensively investigated using traditional behavioral parameters, like nose-poking, lever-pressing, and approach behavior to cues and rewards in Pavlovian, instrumental, and Pavlovian-to-instrumental transfer paradigms [5,9,20]. The study of the emotional or affective conditioned responses underlying incentive motivation, however, has received less attention, first, because the study of emotions was disregarded in behavioristic tradition (for review see [10]) and second, due to the lack of direct and more precise measures of such states in animals.

Currently, there is an increasing interest in studying rodent ultrasonic vocalizations (USVs) in basic and clinically-oriented research, since USVs seem to provide a unique avenue to study the putative affective state of an animal which might not be accessible by conventional behavioral approaches. Rat USVs are complex affective and communicative signals expressed in different social and non-social situations, which vary according to age and context [21,22]. Out of these, high-frequency calls (i.e., 50-kHz calls) are normally emitted in naturalistic rewarding situations such as mating, and rough-and-tumble play, or triggered by non-naturalistic stimuli such as electrical stimulation of the mesolimbic dopamine pathways, or by psychostimulant drugs like amphetamine and cocaine [23–28]. For instance, individual differences in incentive salience attribution to food cues predicted conditioned place preference for cocaine and 50-kHz calls induced by cocaine related cues [29]. Whether 50-kHz calls may be indicative of incentive salience attributed to food cues, however, is still unclear: previous studies showed mixed results and were not conclusive due to the lack of proper controls groups and concomitant behavioral confirmations of incentive learning [23,30–32].

Encouraged by the translational potential of modeling subjective putative affective states in animals we decided to perform a series of studies to explore further the hypothesis that 50-kHz calls can come to signal a state of incentive motivation in the rat, which may constitute an emotional reward representation triggered by conditioned stimuli (CS) predicting reward or by some perceptual features of the food itself (unconditioned stimulus, UCS). One of the simplest conceivable tests to achieve this aim was training rats to anticipate their daily feeding taking place under certain predictable environmental cues. Within or across experiments the conditioning task was systematically modified so that the current physiological state of the subject (deprived vs. sated), the type of learning mechanism recruited (Pavlovian vs. instrumental), the hedonic properties of UCS (low vs. high palatable food), and the availability of the food reward (continued vs. discontinued) were manipulated.

General Methods

Ethics statement

All experimental procedures were approved by the appropriate governmental agency (Regierungspräsidium, Giessen, Germany) and complied with the EU directive 86/609/EEC. Every effort was made to minimize the number of animals used and their suffering.

Subjects

Adult male Wistar rats (Harlan-Winkelmann, Netherlands) served as subjects. They were housed 4–5 per polycarbonate cage (595×380×200 mm) in a climate-controlled room with a 12:12 h light–dark schedule (light on at 07:00 h). Food (Altromin, Lage, Germany) and water (0.0004% HCL-solution) were freely available unless otherwise specified. In all experiments, animal order of testing was counterbalanced within and across days and experiments to the fullest extent possible.

Screening cage test

Since rats show substantial and rather stable inter-individual variability in 50-kHz calls [33], we applied a screening test in which rats are tested for their levels of spontaneous USVs before being assigned in a counterbalanced order to further tests or treatments [27,33]. Briefly, at the beginning of each experiment all animals' cages were removed from the housing-rack and placed on a desk in the same room. Afterwards, a given rat was individually placed into a clean polycarbonate cage (425×266×185 mm) with fresh bedding (Tapvei) and then transported to an adjacent ultrasonic lab, where a recording session immediately started. The cage was placed on a desk under a microphone positioned at 35 cm above the center of cage floor. It was illuminated by red light (about 7 lx inside the cage) and visually separated from the data acquisition area by a curtain. The cage test was conducted on two consecutive days (5 min each). Testing took place from 8:00 to 17:00 h in a counterbalanced order between days and subjects. Based on the average number of spontaneous 50-kHz calls on both days, animals were equally assigned either to the control or the reward group.

Appetitive cage test

All test settings and the general procedure were the same as described in the screening cage test. Briefly, a given rat was put into a clean cage with bedding, which was then placed on a desk under the microphone, where the recording session immediately started. Two loudspeakers (Avemaster 60 PC stereo system, Germany) connected to a personal computer were placed on either side of the cage. As the conditioned stimulus (CS), a 3-kHz tone (49.2 dB inside the cage) was used. The unconditioned stimulus (UCS) was either normal rat chow (about 20 g) or sweetened condensed milk (10% concentrated milk diluted 1:3 in tap water, Milbona, Germany). For the reward groups, the CS predicted either the start of each daily feeding session (1.5 h access to food per day) or a 30 min-drinking time (milk). Throughout the whole experiment, reward intake took place in the same testing cage used for a given rat. During the first 120 s, animals were left undisturbed ("context" phase), then the CS was presented over another 120 s, subsequently followed by the UCS (food or milk). The overlapping CS-UCS period lasted 30 s once reward intake started. When the tone ended, the animal was allowed to continue consuming the reward for another 60 s before being transported back (in the same testing cage) to the adjacent animal room. A matched control rat was tested simultaneously in a test cage, where it received the same pairing schedule as the matched reward rat did, except that food or milk were never delivered there. Afterwards, the pair of control and reward animals was brought back to the animal room and placed on a rack, with controls on odd and reward rats on even rows, so that both group cages were never side by side. Each control rat remained in its own testing cage while the matched reward rat completed either the 1.5 h-feeding session or 30-min drinking time. At least 3 h after all controls rats had been brought back into their own group cages, namely once the night cycle entered, their 1.5 h-daily feeding session began. In the milk experiments (3 and 4), all animals were first habituated to the sweetened condensed milk for a week. During this period, controls rats had milk in the evening together with their daily food, whereas reward rats had milk in the light period, coinciding exactly with the daily time in which they would be further tested.

Runway maze

The apparatus was a single U-shaped runway maze constructed of black acrylic, which consisted of two arm alleys (50 cm L×20 cm W×24 cm H) connected by a 20 cm L corridor. The start box (40 cm L) was equipped with a guillotine door that was manually lifted from afar using a pulley cable. The maze was placed on a desk under a microphone held at 45 cm above the center of maze floor. At the distal wall of the goal box, a door was positioned, through which the rat could enter a cage. A second microphone was affixed at 35 cm above the center of the cage floor. The maze was thoroughly cleaned between trials and subjects with a 0.1% acetic acid solution. The testing area was illuminated by red light (about 10 lx inside the maze) and surrounded by curtains.

Behavioral analysis

Behavior was recorded with a video camera positioned at a longitudinal side of the cage. In Experiment 2, an additional camera recorded behavioral activity in the runway maze. Locomotion (i.e., the number of cage-halves crossed with three paws or the number of 20-cm segments crossed in the runway maze), rearing frequency (i.e., the number of upright postures sustained with hind–paws on the floor), digging (moving cage bedding with forepaws and snout, in seconds), eating or drinking time (seconds), and latency to consume the reward (i.e., time difference between the presentation of food or milk and the first eating or drinking bout, in seconds) were manually counted from videotapes using the EthoLog 2.25 software (University of São Paulo, Institute of Psychology SP, Brazil). Fluid intake (experiments 3 and 4) was determined by weighing bottles before and after testing.

Ultrasonic recording and analysis

As previously reported [27], USVs were monitored with an UltraSoundGate Condenser Microphone (CM16; Avisoft Bioacoustics, Berlin, Germany) and recorded with Avisoft Recorder 2.7 software (sampling rate: 214,285 Hz; format: 16 bit). High resolution spectrograms (frequency resolution: 0.488 kHz, time resolution: 0.512 ms) were obtained after fast Fourier transformation (512 FFT-length, 100% frame, Hamming window, 75% time window overlap), by using the Avisoft SASLabPro 4.38 software. Experienced observers manually counted USVs off-line from the spectrograms. All USVs emitted over 33 kHz were considered as 50-kHz calls. If two call elements were at least 0.048 s apart, two independent calls were counted. USVs occurring during the tasks were expressed as the number of calls emitted per time (calls/min), except otherwise specified. In the cage tests, the proportion of calls emitted during the tone presentation was expressed as: [(call number during tone/total call number) ×100]. The analysis of 50-kHz calls subtypes (e.g., flat, step-calls, trills) provided no relevant information as groups showed rather similar distributions of such USVs subtypes (data not shown). Therefore they were not included in the analyses and only total call number is presented. Since 22-kHz calls were only rarely and non-systematically observed, they were also omitted from the study.

Statistical analysis

Results were expressed as means ± SEM. The main effect of groups (G, control vs. reward), training days (D), and their interaction (DxG) was assessed by means of independent mixed ANOVA analyses. In one of the analyses, the repeated-measures factor was the food deprivation days, and in the other, the food ad libitum days. When only one group provided data (i.e., latency to eat and time spent eating in Experiments 1, 2, and 5), a repeated-measures ANOVA within the reward group was computed. All multiple comparisons among days were adjusted with the Bonferroni *post hoc* test. In all repeated-measures analyses that did not meet the sphericity assumption, the Greenhouse-Geisser correction was used. When appropriate, *t*-tests for related samples were used to compare feeding phases within groups. Statistical significance was defined as $p<.05$.

Results

Experiment 1

Introduction. The hypothesis that 50-kHz calls can come to signal a state of incentive motivation to food reward was investigated by training deprived rats to anticipate their daily feeding. In this experiment the CS signaled the start of each feeding session (1.5 h access to food per day), which began in the ultrasonic lab (~2 min in the testing cage) and ended in the animal room (see general materials and methods for details). A reward-unpaired rat (i.e., controls) was tested simultaneously in an adjacent room, where it received the same pairing schedule as the matched reward rat, except that a hopper of chow pellets was never placed upon the cage grid.

Methods. Thirty experimentally naïve rats weighing 277–351 g on arrival were used. One week before testing, animals were habituated to the experimental conditions and were handled during four days (5 min each). Afterwards, two consecutive screening cage tests were conducted (see screening cage test). Subsequently, animals were counterbalanced into two groups and put on a 22.5-h food deprivation (FD) schedule by being given free access to their maintenance diet for 1.5 h per day, starting one week before the appetitive cage test. During this period, rats were handled and weighed every other day. From day 1 to 7, animals were food deprived (FD); thereafter (days 8–10), they obtained food ad libitum (FAL) in their own home cages.

Results. *FD phase*: Reward rats (Fig. 1; days 1–7) showed typical motivational behavior, i.e. approach and food consumption. The latencies to approach the reward decreased over days (D: $F_{3,57}=9.57$, $p=.0001$). Locomotor activity was lower in reward rats than in controls (G: $F_{1,28}=9.24$, $p=.005$), whereas rearing activity did not differ between groups (Figure S1). Total call number increased over days (D: $F_{3,84}=12.79$, $p=.0001$), but contrary to our expectations this effect was observed in both groups (G: $p>.05$) (Figure 1C). The relative number of calls emitted during tone presentation (Figure 1D) did yield a higher percentage of tone-related calls in reward rats (G: $F_{1,28}=17.08$, $p=.0001$), which increased over days (D: $F_{3,57}=9.84$, $p=.0001$), indicating that the reward animals did learn the associations. *FAL phase:* After testing on day 7, animals received food in their home cages in order to devalue the food reward. If the previous lack of group differences seen on total call number was unrelated to incentive learning, no changes in USVs would be expected, but if part of the USVs in reward rats was emitted in anticipation of food, then satiation should decrease them. Surprisingly, we found that total call number increased in reward animals once they were sated (FD vs. FAL: $t_{19}=-13.10$, $p=.0001$), differing now from controls on all FAL days (G: $F_{1,28}=13.09$, $p=.001$). For instance, call rate in the reward group on day 8 exceeded both, their own levels of day 7 (160%), and controls levels (86%) on the same day (Figure 1C). After 48 h of FAL (i.e. on day 9), total 50-kHz calls reached a maximum, that is, an elevation of ~310% and ~166% over FD and control levels, respectively. In contrast, the proportion of calls emitted during tone presentations dropped, especially in the reward group, but was still significantly higher in reward rats (G: $F_{1,28}=10.51$, $p=.003$). Rearing behavior (Figure S1B), which occurred mostly at the cage side where the food reward was delivered (details not shown), increased in reward rats (FD vs. FAL: $t_{19}=-4.89$, $p=.0001$) and remained consistently high until the end of the FAL phase (G: $F_{1,28}=11.04$, $p=.002$). Remarkably, the increases in appetitive 50-kHz calls and rearing occurred even though approach and consummatory behaviors were completely abolished during all FAL days (Figure 1A and B). Thus, the devalued feeding conditions dramatically increased both total call number and tone-induced USVs even after 72 h of experiencing the reward in a low motivational state.

Discussion. These data suggest that attribution of incentive salience to reward predictive cues (i.e., cage context and tone CS) may have occurred while animals were deprived, and surprisingly cues were able to trigger conditioned motivational reactions to reward, i.e. USVs, even though it was fully devalued. Since the conditioned response was learned under FD, expression but not acquisition of such a response is what seemed to be suppressed during this phase. Perhaps, approach/consummatory responses taking place in the same testing environment may have overlapped with the preparatory/emotional elements of the UCS producing a sort of inhibition in the expression of the latter [34]. For example, species-specific foraging behavior such as digging/snout-down locomotion, which was also observed here (Table S1, supporting information) is known to increase during FD even when animals

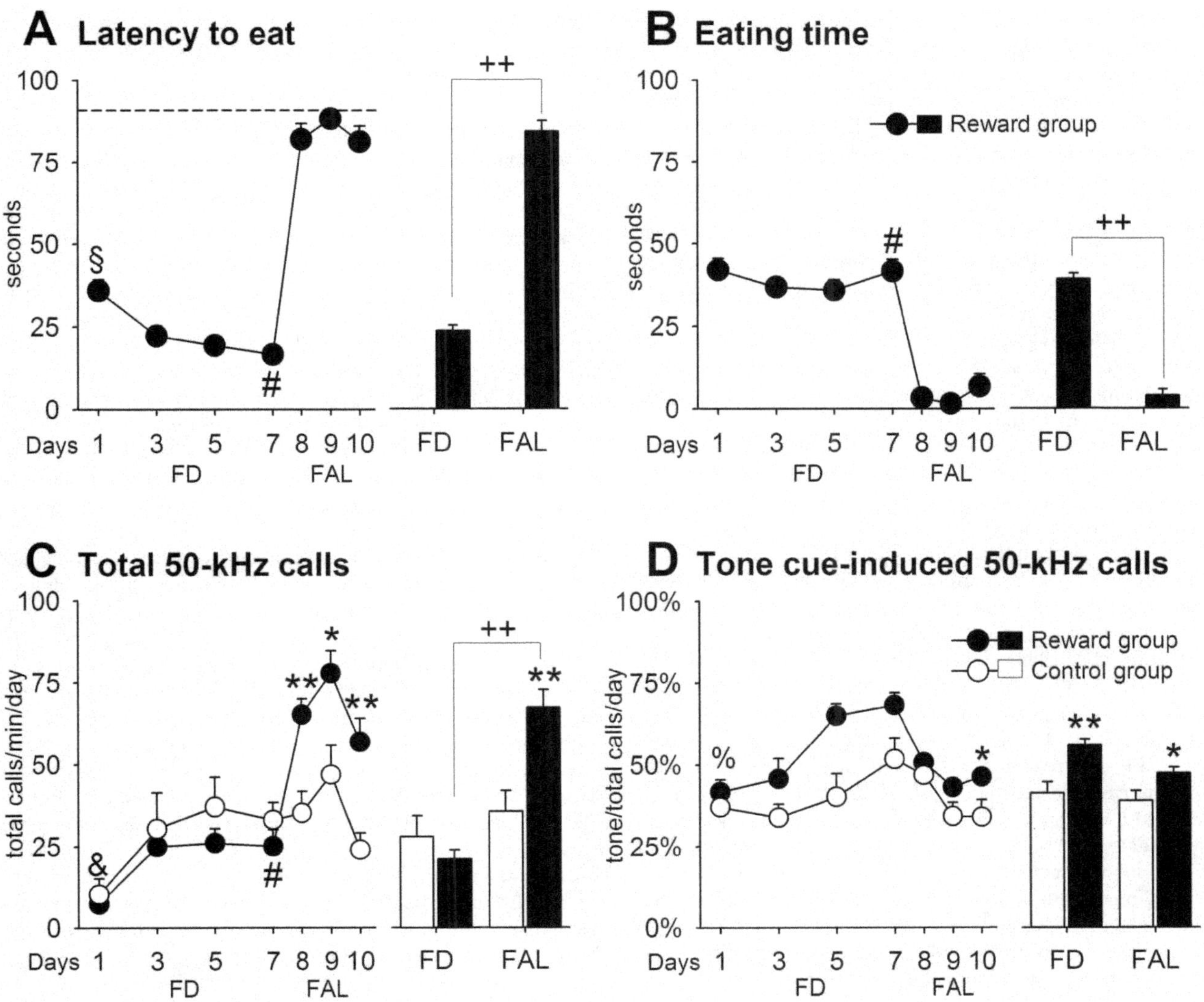

Figure 1. Experiment 1. Animals learned to associate incentive Pavlovian cues with access to daily feeding as reward. A. Latency to eat. B. Eating time. C. Total 50-kHz calls. D. Tone cue-induced 50-kHz calls. The dashed line indicates that a maximal latency time was set at 90 s. Control vs. reward: * $p<.05$, ** $p<.01$. FD vs. FAL: ++ $p<.01$. Day 1 differed from days 5 and 7 in reward rats: § $p<.05$. Day 7 differed from days 8 to 10 in reward rats: # all $p<.05$. Day 1 differed from days 3 to 7 in both groups: & $p<.05$. Data are expressed as mean+SEM (control = 10, reward = 20).

never obtained food by these means [35,36]. Since these and other approach/consummatory behaviors were reduced drastically when tested under FAL conditions, we consider the idea of competition between different behavioral systems.

Experiment 2

Introduction. Here, the procedure was modified so that USVs associated with anticipatory and consummatory acts could be measured in different testing compartments. A testing cage with bedding was also used here, but instead of training animals to passively wait for food reward to be delivered (i.e., Pavlovian schedule), they now learned to run down a runway maze connected to the cage, so that they could voluntarily enter it and access their daily food ration available there (i.e., instrumental component). With these modifications, animals motivation to attain the reward and cue-induced anticipatory 50-kHz calls in the runway could be assessed independently from consummatory responses in the goal cage. As anticipating and earning a reward appear to be distinct processes [8] we sought to elucidate whether the USV effects observed in experiment 1 rely upon the type of associative process. The cage was the same as in Experiment 1, so that each animal had its own cage for testing throughout the whole experiment.

Methods. The same 30 rats used in Experiment 1 served as subjects, weighing 361–440 g at the beginning of this experiment, which took place 27 days apart from the first experiment. Exactly as there, all animals were put on a 22.5-h schedule of FD with free access to their maintenance diet (1.5 h per day) either immediately after testing (for reward animals in their own testing cages) or at least 3 h later (for controls once they were returned to their group cages). After 3 handling days, habituation to the runway was begun. This consisted of taking the rats from their home cages and placing them in pairs into the start box of the maze (with the door opened) for about 15 min during three consecutive days. In parallel, we performed reinstatement of tone/food pairing by repeating the cage test procedure of Experiment 1. During seven days, starting from the second day of the runway habituation, animals were given a maze habituation session followed by a cage test procedure. On the next two days, both procedures were combined, that is, single animals were placed into the maze with the cage attached to it (with food for reward rats). When they entered the cage, a 3-kHz tone was played as in Experiment 1. During habituation, animals were weighed and handled every other day. Afterwards, reward animals were trained to run through the runway maze to access food in the cage attached to the end of the runway goal arm. Rats received daily training sessions for 10 consecutive days conducted as follows: A given rat was confined to the start box for 120 s, and during the last 60 s a 3-kHz tone was played, which ended with opening of the door. Afterwards, rats were free to locomote between runway and cage during approximately 4 min. Control rats followed the same procedure but food was never given in the cage. As in Experiment 1, animals were food deprived during days 1–7; thereafter (days 8–10) they received FAL in their own home cages. USVs were recorded during the entire testing period, since animals used to shuttle between runway and cage.

Results. *FD phase:* As shown in Figure 2, the latencies to eat declined (D: $F_{3,57} = 8.43$, $p = .0001$) and eating times increased over days in the reward group (D: $F_{3,57} = 5.03$, $p = .004$). In the runway maze, locomotion (D: $F_{3,84} = 26.79$, $p = .0001$) and rearing (D: $F_{3,84} = 90.17$, $p = .0001$) but not USV (D: $p > .05$) decreased over days (Figure S2A, S2B, and 2C, respectively). For all these variables, no group differences were observed (G: $p > .05$). In the cage, all animals emitted more 50-kHz calls per time than in the maze (Figure 2D). There, USVs diminished over days (D: $F_{3,84} = 9.67$, $p = .0001$) without differing between groups (G: $p > .05$). Cage locomotion (G: $F_{1,28} = 44.93$, $p = .0001$) and rearing (G: $F_{1,28} = 18.89$, $p = .0001$) were higher in controls (Figure S2C and S2D), perhaps since reward rats were now engaged in eating while controls still explored the cage. *FAL phase:* As in experiment 1, rats received FAL after testing on day 7. Again, the latencies to eat increased (FD vs. FAL: $t_{19} = -29.64$, $p = .0001$) and eating times decreased in the reward group (FD vs. FAL: $t_{19} = 10.31$, $p = .0001$). In contrast, and consistent with experiment 1, reward cues associated to the runway maze now elicited enhanced 50-kHz calls (Figure 2C). For instance, total call number in reward rats was now ~210% higher compared with their own USVs levels while FD (FD vs. FAL: $t_{19} = -13.10$, $p = .0001$), and ~195% higher than that in controls on all FAL days (G: $F_{1,28} = 7.07$, $p = .01$). In the cage (Figure 2D), 50-kHz calls increased in both groups (D: $F_{3,84} = 4.72$, $p = .004$), but did not differ from each other (G: $p > .05$). There were no group differences in locomotion or rearing (G: $p > .05$) (Figure S2).

Discussion. This experiment replicated the results from Experiment 1 in which no differences in total call number were observed under FD, but increased USVs occurred in reward animals once they became sated. The suppressive effect of FD probably did not depend on the type of learning recruited, the behavioral competition between approach/consummatory and anticipatory affective responses, or the interference of an opposite behavior such as digging since the maze had no bedding. Since animals were free to shuttle between maze and cage and most reward animals revisited the maze between eating bouts (details not shown), maze cues were not just temporally predicting further access to reward, but also became imbued with incentive salience after animals re-experienced the UCS, facilitating CS representations to be re-updated within and across training days. As a consequence, runway maze cues, but not cage cues, triggered appetitive 50-kHz calls suggesting that USVs were specifically sensitive to the type of learning mechanism recruited. Again, attribution of incentive salience to food cues seemed to take place during the FD period, whereas the expression of such an appetitive response occurred once animals became sated, that is, when the reward was devalued and when no other appetitive behaviors were emitted. Finally, the analysis of USVs in the cage revealed that satiation on its own increased 50-kHz calls irrespective of being food rewarded or not.

Experiment 3

Introduction. As just shown, the current physiological state of the rat produces a biphasic expression of 50-kHz calls in reward rats, which according to Experiment 2 is not dependent on the interference between preparatory and consummatory responses [16] or the competition between species-specific responses activated by the UCS (e.g., foraging inhibiting calling, for review see [37]). To simplify data collection and analysis we went back to the test settings of Experiment 1. Now, we asked whether increasing the incentive properties of the reward would enhance motivation for UCS during the FD period. To this end, a high palatable reward (i.e., sweetened condensed milk) was used. Since the reward delivered in the testing cage was different from normal rat chow, access to reward became independent from the daily feeding session. Thus, we expected that it could still be valuable when testing animals under satiation.

Methods. Twenty-four experimentally naïve rats weighing 231–256 g on arrival were used. Habituation to the animal facilities, handling, the screening cage test, and FD schedule were conducted as in Experiment 1, but now, the CS signaled access to a 30 min-drinking period: ~2 min in the cage and the remaining time in the animal room. The reward group had access to sweet condensed milk, whereas the control group had access to tap water. One week before testing, rats were habituated to sweetened condensed milk. During this period, all rats were handled and weighed every other day. Testing was performed with the former FD/FAL schedule: FD from day 1 to 7, and FAL thereafter (days 8–10).

Results. *FD phase:* The latencies to drink (Figure 3) diminished slightly once training began, with reward rats being ~6 times faster than controls, which were given a bottle with tap water (G: $F_{1,22} = 85.05$, $p = .0001$; DxG: $F_{3,66} = 16.34$, $p = .002$). The times spent drinking (G: $F_{1,22} = 538.80$, $p = .0001$; DxG: $F_{3,66} = 15.78$, $p = .0001$) and daily milk consumption (G: $F_{1,22} = 582.71$, $p = .0001$; DxG: $F_{3,66} = 4.19$, $p = .009$) were higher in the reward group where they increased also over days. Total call number augmented over days in all animals (D: $F_{3,66} = 12.05$, $p = .0001$), especially after the third day (Figure 3D), but did not differ significantly between groups (G: $p > .05$). In contrast, the percentage of tone-induced 50-kHz calls was higher in the reward group (G: $F_{1,22} = 19.05$, $p = .0001$) (Figure 3E). *FAL phase:* When tested without deprivation, there was a transitory increase in the latency to drink and a transitory reduction in the time spent drinking which fully recovered on the following FAL days. Despite such small variations when feeding conditions changed, reward rats still differed from controls on latencies to drink (G: $F_{1,22} = 76.23$, $p = .0001$) and times spent drinking ($F_{1,22} = 76.23$, $p = .0001$). Milk intake declined drastically (FD vs. FAL: $t_{11} = -11.41$, $p = .0001$), almost reaching control levels on the first FAL day, but was higher than controls again thereafter. On the following FAL days, milk intake partially recovered between about 25% to 43% of the maximal intake achieved under FD (G: $F_{1,22} = 17.08$, $p = .0001$; DxG: $F_{3,66} = 10.03$, $p = .0001$). In addition, locomotion (FD vs. FAL: $t_{11} = -8.45$, $p = .0001$) and rearing (FD vs. FAL: $t_{11} = -9.01$, $p = .0001$) increased in the reward group and exceeded those of controls (locomotion, G, $F_{1,22} = 758$, $p = .01$; rearing, G: $F_{1,22} = 18.06$, $p = .0001$; Figure S3A and S3B). Similar to Experiments 2 and 3, call rate was potentiated by shifting the feeding conditions, an effect which now occurred in both groups (D: $F_{3,66} = 3.14$, $p = .03$). Interestingly, the attenuation

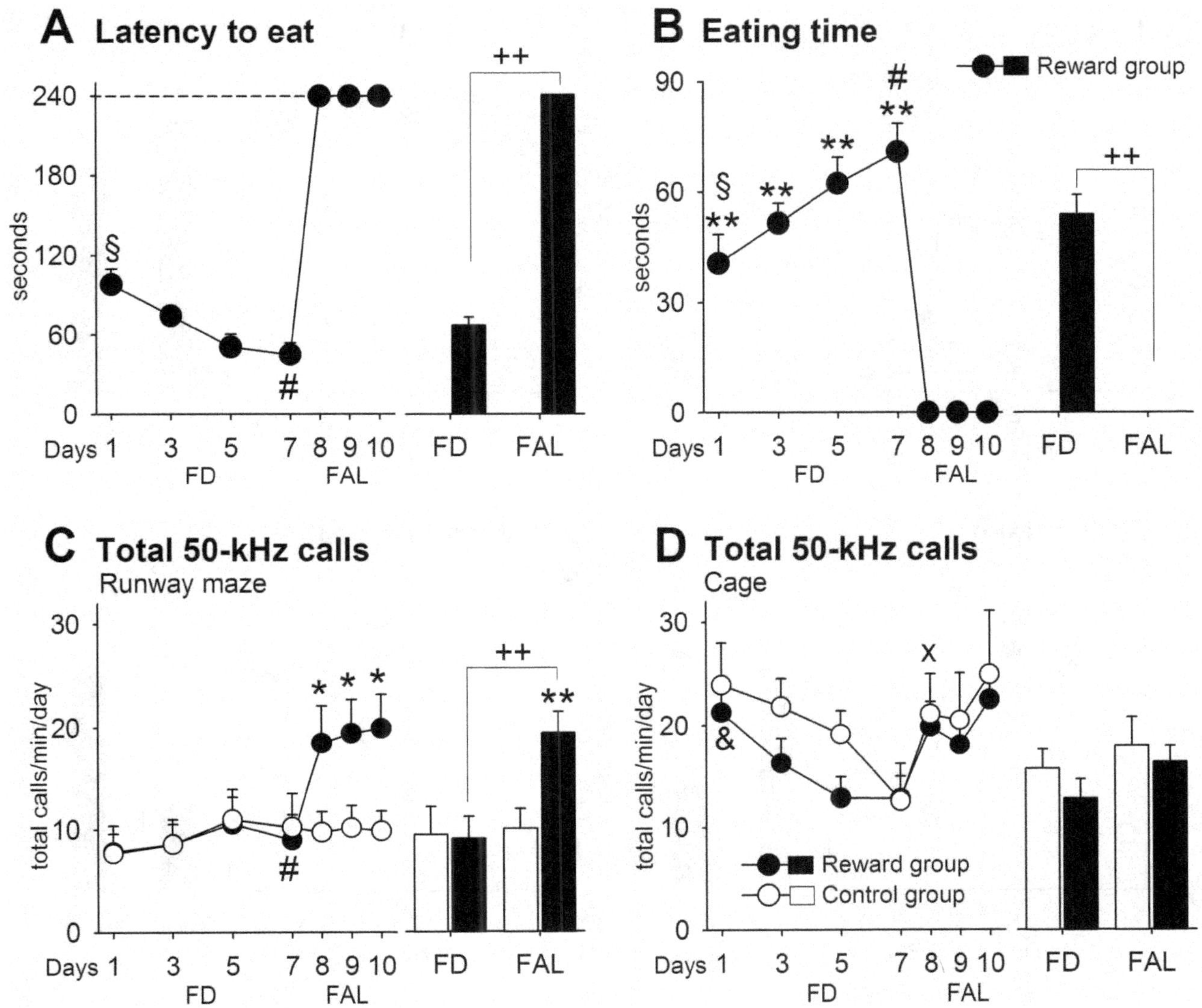

Figure 2. Experiment 2. Animals learned to access their daily feeding in a cage by running through a runway maze attached to it. A. Latency to eat. B. Eating time. C. Total 50-kHz calls in the runway maze. D. Total 50-kHz calls in the cage. The dashed line indicates that a maximal latency time was set at 240 s. Control vs. reward: * $p<.05$, ** $p<.01$. FD vs. FAL: ++ $p<.01$. Day 1 differed from days 5 and 7 in reward rats: § $p<.05$. % Day 1 differed from days 3 to 7 in reward rats: § $p<.05$. Days 1 and 3 differed from day 7 in both groups: & $p<.05$. Day 7 differed from days 8 to 10 in reward rats: # all $p<.05$. Day 7 differed from days 8 and 10 in both groups: x all $p<.05$. Data are expressed as mean+SEM (control = 10, reward = 20).

of approach and consummatory behaviors observed when shifting feeding conditions was not paralleled by a reduction in total call number and percentage of cue-induced calls. Instead, total call number (Figure 3D) was now significantly higher in the reward group (G: $F_{1,22} = 6.60$, $p = .02$), and tone cue-induced calls were also higher (G: $F_{1,22} = 5.18$, $p = .03$) but returned towards control levels over days (Figure 3E).

Discussion. Relative to previous experiments, USVs appeared slightly increased at the end of the FD period, although no overall effect on total call number was detected. However, the percentage of tone-induced calling increased during FD indicating that conditioning strengthened over days. Once again, reward devaluation decreased neither total call number nor tone-induced calling, as it had initially been expected. Instead, total call number increased while cue-induced USVs remained slightly high during FAL days. Regarding reward palatability, the higher incentive properties of the UCS (i.e., milk) plus the likely invigorating effect of the CS seemed to maintain latencies to drink and times spent drinking in the cage while the UCS was degraded in agreement with previous reports [1,3,4]. However, the amount of milk intake, most of which was consumed in the animal room without the influence of the CS, appeared to be drastically reduced by satiety.

Experiment 4

Introduction. So far, the increased percentage of 50-kHz calls induced by the tone cue indicated that attribution of incentive salience to reward-related stimuli had successfully taken place during FD, even thought it was not clearly translated into an overall elevation of 50-kHz calls. To account for such an inhibition in USVs utterance, we assume that the ability of food CS cues to elicit appetitive 50-kHz calls was possibly suppressed by FD, an effect that occurred independently from learning acquisition. So far, the three preceding experiments showed that restoring FAL feeding conditions after FD increased spontaneous USVs in controls and potentiated total call number and food cues-induced appetitive 50-kHz calls in reward rats. This may suggest that FD

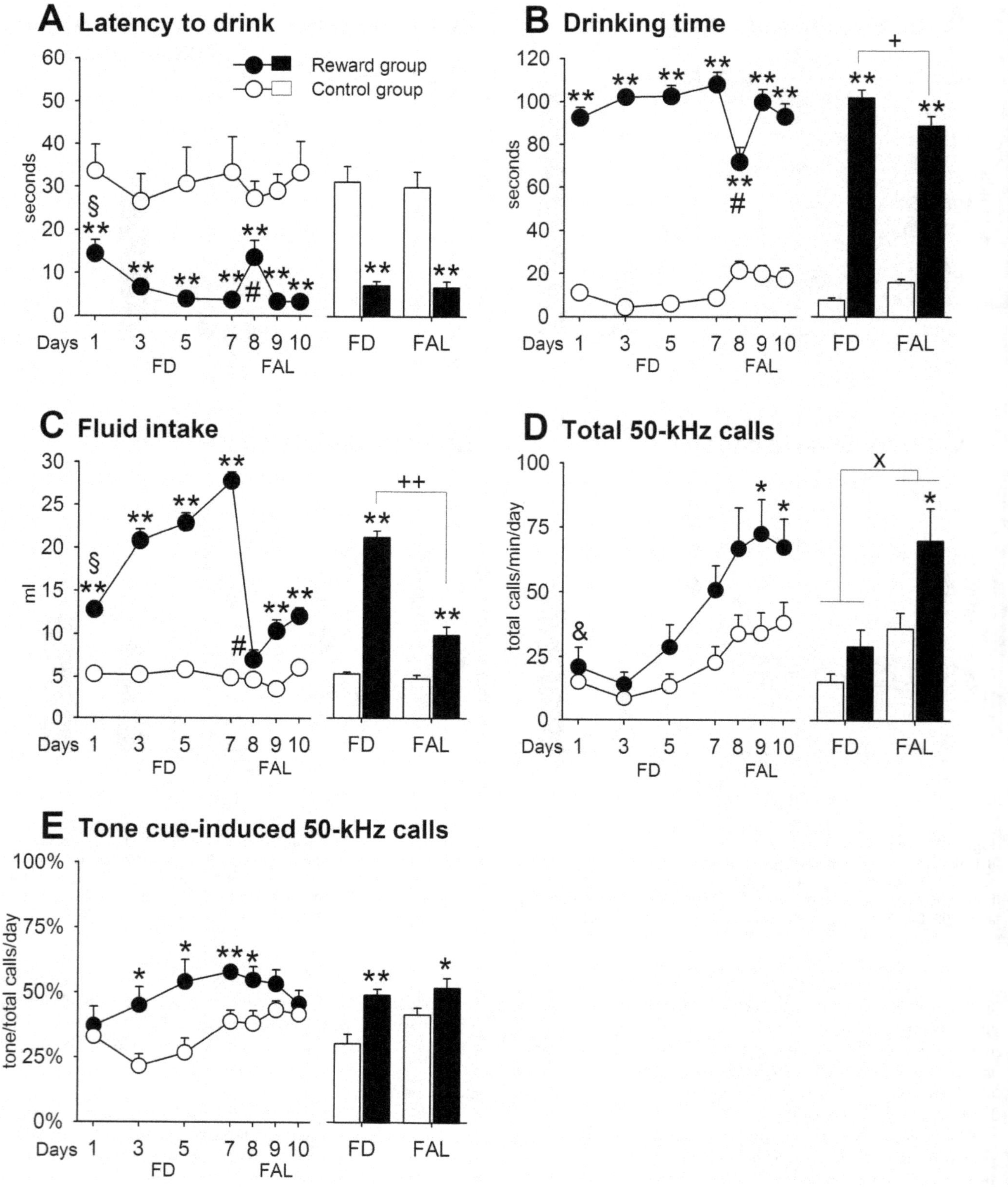

Figure 3. Experiment 3. Animals learned to associate incentive Pavlovian cues with access to sweetened condensed milk as reward. A. Latency to drink. B. Drinking time. C. Fluid intake. D. Total 50-kHz calls. E. Tone cue-induced 50-kHz calls. Control vs. reward: * $p<.05$, ** $p<.01$. FD vs. FAL: + $p<.05$, ++ $p<.01$. FD vs. FAL in both groups: x all $p<.05$. Day 1 differed from days 3 to 7 in reward rats: § $p<.05$. Day 1 to 5 differed from day 7 in both groups: & $p<.05$. Day 8 differed from days 7, 9, and 10 in reward rats: # all $p<.05$. Data are expressed as mean+SEM (control = 12, reward = 12).

itself was able to suppress USVs particularly at the time when animals were expecting the food reward. Having access to food after a long FD period recruits not only positive but also negative reinforcement mechanisms, and may be described as a transition from distress to pleasure [38]. FD can induce an aversive state so that animals will work to prevent starvation by either prolonging the period of food availability [39] or escaping from a CS signaling the omission of an expected food reward [40]. This evidence raised the question of whether the same palatable reward (i.e., milk), now acquired in the absence of FD, would be sufficient to increase appetitive 50-kHz calls.

Methods. Twenty experimentally naïve rats weighing 259–279 g on arrival were used. The experimental procedure was generally the same as in Experiment 3, with sweetened condensed milk also used as reward. However, contrary to all previous experiments, the acquisition phase (days 1–7) of UCS-CS pairing occurred first in the FAL phase and was followed by the FD phase (days 8–10).

Results. *FAL phase:* As expected, reward rats showed shorter latencies to drink (G: $F_{1,18} = 1252.46$, $p = .0001$) and more time spent drinking (G: $F_{1,18} = 172.56$, $p = .0001$) than controls which consumed almost none of the tap water (Figure 4A and B). As soon as reward animals had learned that milk was available, latencies and drinking times did not change over the FAL days (D: $p > .05$). However, the amount of milk (Figure 4C) consumed augmented with repeated testing (G: $F_{1,18} = 8.02$, $p = .01$; DxG: $F_{3,54} = 4.05$, $p = .01$). Total call number increased over days (D: $F_{3,54} = 24.86$, $p = .0001$), with no significant differences between groups (G: $p > .05$) (Figure 4D). Likewise, no differences were observed for the percentage of tone-induced calling (Figure 4E). Also, exploratory activity appeared unaffected by both, repeated testing and reward experience (Figure S4A and S4B). *FD phase:* Latencies to drink (G: $F_{1,18} = 147.51$, $p = .0001$) and times spent drinking (G: $F_{1,18} = 2039.35$, $p = .0001$) remained higher in the reward group compared to controls (Figure 4A–B). The more noticeable effect of FD occurred on the amount of milk consumed, which scaled up between 34% to 78% over preceding FAL levels (FD vs. FAL: $t_9 = -11.47$, $p = .0001$; Figure 4C), whereas water intake remained unaffected (G: $F_{1,18} = 190.58$, $p = .0001$). Contrary to approach and consummatory behaviors, call rate dropped drastically on the first FD day in both groups (Figure 4D) (D: $F_{3,54} = 16.58$, $p = .0001$). On the following FD days, total call number progressively returned to FAL levels only in the reward rats (DxG: $F_{3,54} = 3.74$, $p = .03$). Similarly, the percentage of tone-induced USVs was significantly higher in the reward group (G: $F_{1,18} = 11.82$, $p = .003$) (Figure 4E). Locomotion (FD vs. FAL: $t_9 = 3.31$, $p = .009$) and rearing behavior (FD vs. FAL: $t_9 = 5.96$, $p = .0001$) were reduced in controls (Figure S4), whereas in reward rats only locomotor activity was reduced by FD (FD vs. FAL: $t_9 = 2.96$, $p = .02$).

Discussion. This experiment shows first, that a highly palatable food reward was not sufficient to increase either total call number or tone cue-induced calling on its own and, second, that FD was able to suppress calling in both groups. Since the reward did not have a high hedonic value during the acquisition phase (i.e., when tested under FAL conditions), total call number and cue-induced 50-kHz calls recovered and differed from control levels only when the hedonic representation of that reward was updated while in the subsequent state of being hungry. This is consistent with studies showing that the instrumental response guided by previous reward expectations changes only when the new hedonic value of the incentive is experienced [8,9]. In this as well as in previous experiments, the motivational state of being FD seems to be required for reward cues to be imbued with incentive salience, even though it suppressed overall USVs utterance.

Experiment 5

Introduction. The likely aversive state provoked by long FD may have accounted for some suppressive effects in calling in our previous experiments. In experiment 3, however, total call number tended to increase while FD, an effect that, according to Experiment 4, may not solely be attributed to palatability. Another factor might be critical: By replacing rat chow with milk as a reward we also inevitably altered the predictive association between access to reward in the cage and daily feeding session. If expectations about reward were controlled by the very first access to food or milk (2 min) –and not by the whole period of eating (1.5 h) or drinking (30 min)–, it is very likely that animals learned to anticipate the short access to reward instead of the long one. Thus, when animals encountered the reward, a negative discrepancy between the reward expected and the one actually obtained may have been experienced, an effect probably energized by FD. We hypothesized, therefore, that providing continued access to reward in the testing environment would prevent such negative discrepancy to occur, 'releasing' the expression of reward-related appetitive USVs when FD. To test this idea, we adapted the procedure of Experiment 1 in which the higher suppression in calling was observed.

Methods. Twenty experimentally naïve rats weighing 240–265 g on arrival served as subjects. Habituation to the animal facilities, handling, and the screening cage test were conducted largely as in Experiments 1 and 2: Food pellets (normal rat chow) served as reward, but contrary to there, both access to reward and the completion of the daily feeding session took place exclusively in the testing room. Indeed, during habituation to FD, reward rats had access to the daily food ration only in the testing room, so that the fact of being fed after a 22.5-h FD period was specially linked to this environment. During testing, rats were FD from days 1 to 7. Controls never accessed their daily food ration either in the cage or in the experimental room where testing took place.

Results. Animals approached the food and started eating without any noticeable change from the beginning to the end of testing (D: $p > .05$) (Figure 5A and B). Contrary to our previous food experiments, reward cues did now increase total call number over FD days (DxG: $F_{3,54} = 8.19$, $p = .0001$) (Figure 5C), and calls were approximately 120% higher than that in controls (G: $F_{1,18} = 7.54$, $p = .01$), which showed rather stable call rates over days. Likewise, the percentage of tone-induced calling was significantly higher in reward rats than in controls (G: $F_{1,18} = 17.90$, $p = .001$) (Figure 5D). Unlike locomotion (Figure S5A), rearing behavior in reward rats showed a progressive increase mirroring the one observed for USVs (G: $F_{1,18} = 11.07$, $p = .004$; DxG: $F_{3,54} = 9.81$, $p = .0001$), yet to a lesser extent (Figure S5B).

Discussion. This experiment shows that providing continuous access to reward in the testing environment enables attribution and expression of incentive salience during the FD period, and contrary to previous experiments, this effect was now noted both in terms of total call number and the percentage of cue-induced 50-kHz calls.

General Discussion

Following Pavlovian incentive learning, a CS for reward comes to produce expectations and potentiates motivation about the UCS. Here, we sought to determine whether rat 50-kHz USVs may signal such a state of incentive motivation to a natural,

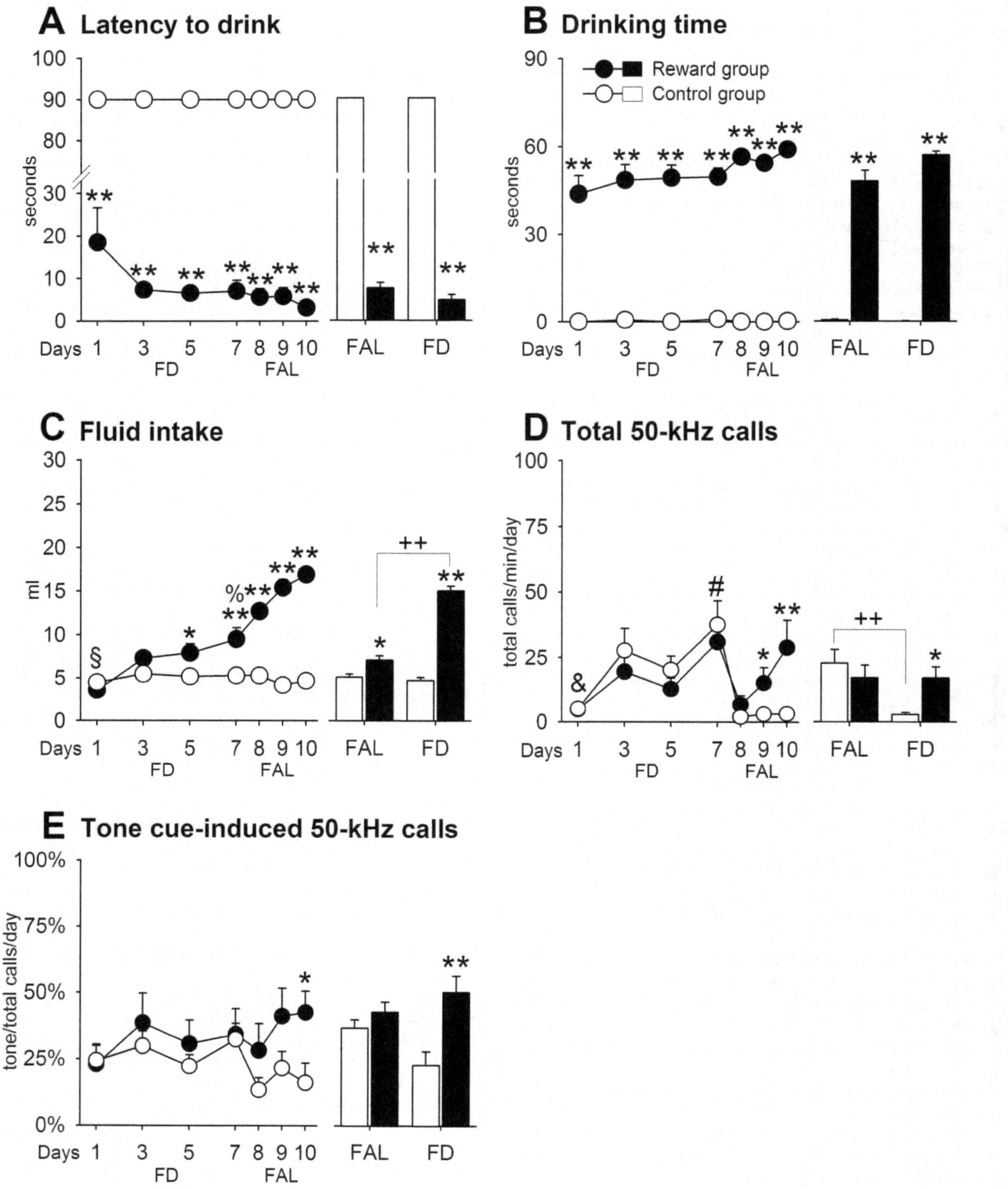

Figure 4. Experiment 4. Animals learned to associate incentive Pavlovian cues with access to sweetened condensed milk as reward. A. Latency to drink. B. Drinking time. C. Fluid intake. D. Total 50-kHz calls. E. Tone cue-induced 50-kHz calls. Control vs. reward: * $p<.05$, ** $p<.01$. FAL vs. FD: ++ $p<.01$. Day 1 differed from days 5 and 7 in reward rats: § $p<.05$. Day 1 differed from days 3 to 7, and day 5 differed from day 7 in both groups: & $p<.05$. Day 7 differed from days 8 to 10: % $p<.05$. Day 7 differed from all FD days in controls, and from day 8 in reward rats: # all $p<.05$. Data are expressed as mean+SEM (control = 10, reward = 10).

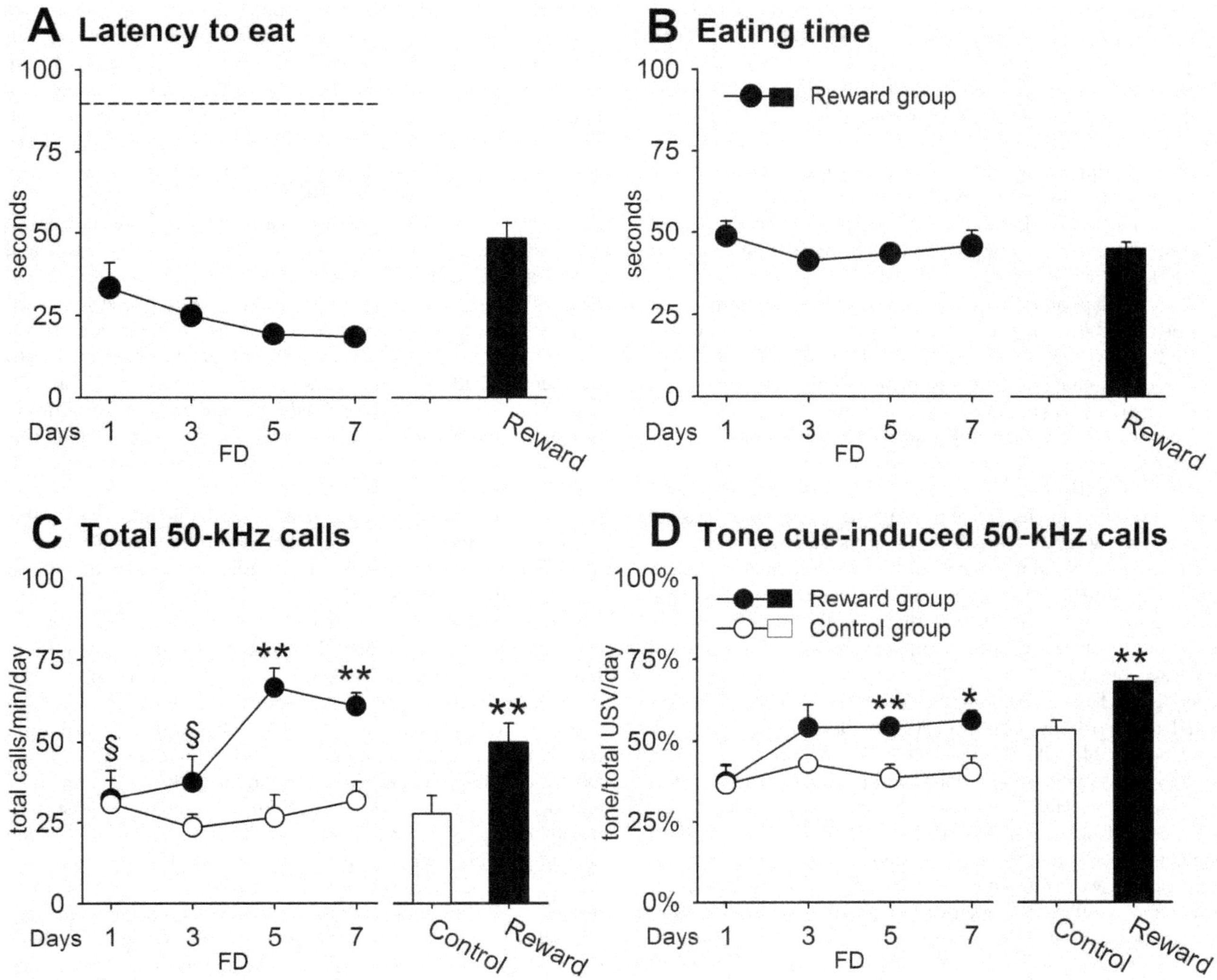

Figure 5. Experiment 5. Animals learned to associate incentive Pavlovian cues with access to daily feeding as reward. A. Latency to eat. B. Eating time. C. Total 50-kHz calls. D. Tone cue-induced 50-kHz calls. The dashed line indicated that a maximal latency time was set at 90 s. Control vs. reward: * $p<.05$, ** $p<.01$. Days 1 and 3 differed from days 5 and 7 in reward rats: § $p<.05$. Data are expressed as mean+SEM (control = 10, reward = 10).

nutritional reward. In general, we found that reward-cues become effective to elicit 50-kHz calls. Under certain conditions, however, utterance of 50-kHz calls can be either suppressed during a highly motivational state, or more strikingly, can be elicited when food rewards were devalued by satiation. In both cases, changes in calling occurred independently from motivation to approach and consume the reward. Interestingly, this phasic character of USVs was consistently seen across independent experiments.

We acknowledge that the question of whether 50-kHz calls can be elicited by food rewards has already been addressed. The pioneer study [23] showed an increase in anticipatory 50-kHz calls in FD rats (i.e., before daily feeding) at the end of a 6-days period of training. In a sucrose self-administration paradigm conducted with non-FD rats, 50-kHz calls increased over time when comparing different time points throughout a testing period of 4–5 weeks [30]. Others described differences in 50-kHz calls between adolescent and adult rats when offered chocolate chips in a one-trial test [32], and one study yielded differences in calling following positive and negative reward contrasts with different probabilities to obtain sucrose reinforcement [31]. In all these studies, however, it was unclear whether call rate in food-paired rats was different from spontaneous calling mainly because no control rats were included [23,30–32]. It has repeatedly been observed that rats call at moderate rates simply by the fact of placing them in certain testing environments [27,33,41]. For example, in the only two studies showing positive results [23,30] calling increased over days in a similar way as it did in our control rats in Experiments 1 and 4, in which no groups differences were found until feeding conditions were changed. Also, previous studies did not test whether increases in 50-kHz calls were accompanied by changes in other relevant learning or motivational parameters because no concomitant behavioral measures were described [23,30,32]. In general, we went beyond those studies showing that USVs in reward rats as compared to matched controls were differentially sensitive to the current physiological state of the subject (FD vs. FAL), the type of learning mechanism recruited (more Pavlovian vs. more instrumental), the hedonic properties of the UCS (low vs. high palatable food), its availability (continued vs. discontinued), and the relation between 50-kHz calls and other behavioral dimensions indicative of incentive learning and conditioning.

Our results also make us believe that FD on its own induced a putative negative state that affected USVs likelihood. This assumption is also supported by our previous findings in which FD consistently suppressed spontaneous calling over four consecutive days [33]. Since FD is aversive enough to strongly motivate escape and avoidance responses [38–40], it is not surprising that FD exerted a suppressive effect on 50-kHz calls utterance similar to those produced by other aversive stimuli [21,22,25]. Still the question remains, how FD particularly suppressed the expression of the emotional conditioned response during acquisition while being FD. In all experiments in which reward intake was discontinued (Experiments 1–4), animals seemed to learn about the association between testing and the 2-min access to reward permitted while they remained in the testing room. Figure 6 depicts a model that summarizes our assumptions in terms of a suppression-release hypothesis, in which we propose that FD played a critical role in the suppression of cue-induced calling by increasing the negative contrast between reward expectation and outcome. As training progressed, the 2-min access to food became gradually insufficient for experiencing the positive effects of consuming the food and therefore the expectation of being fed and becoming sated did not match each other. For example, in the rat chow experiment access to the reward in the cage predicted the 1.5-h feeding session, which was the only feeding opportunity animals had. In the milk experiment, conversely, access to reward in the cage predicted only a 30-min drinking time, which was independent of feeding. Although the duration of daily feeding was adjusted to keep body weight at 90% of baseline based on the caloric income of milk, animals still had two unrelated feeding opportunities as compared to only one in rat chow experiments. Thus, reward expectation should have been proportional to the magnitude and density of reward, being therefore greater when giving chow pellets than when giving milk. To better illustrate this point, calling was compared between Experiments 1 and 3: Figure 7 shows call rate as relative to control levels to normalize the fluctuations in calling due to the FD itself. As can be seen in FD rats receiving normal rat chow, the score for cue-induced calling is negative, namely, 25% lower than spontaneous calling in controls. Once sated, calling increased by 90% over control levels. In rats receiving milk reward, in contrast, the relative increase in cue-induced calling was about 90% over control levels while FD but also in the FAL phase. This indicates that suppression in cue-induced calling depended upon the predictive strength of the reward in relation to feeding: the larger the discrepancy between expectation and UCS outcome, the greater the suppression. Once sated, the magnitude of suppression released was inversed to the strength of suppression that preceded it. We acknowledge that both rewards differed in their incentive properties, but as shown in Experiment 4, palatability on its own is unlikely to account for all differences observed between experiments using chow pellets vs. milk. In addition, we plotted calling results of Experiments 1 and 5 to highlight the contribution of reward expectations on USVs suppression (Figure 7B). When providing continued access to reward while all other factors remained equal, reward expectation matched outcome and thus, suppression was no longer observed. Then, attribution and expression of cue-induced calling occurred simultaneously over FD days. Based on this assumption one might think, even counter-intuitively, that what FAL did was removing the negative expectation of the outcome given by the difference between being hungry and having access to an insufficient reward. Without the urge for food, the outcome matched the expectation of being rewarded. In other words, restoring the normal feeding conditions acted as a 'releasing' factor of the negative difference between reward expectation and outcome, which did not require updating and occurred afresh as soon as the current physiological state shifted (for an example of instant transformation of an aversive cue into a desired one see [42]). The suppression in the conditioned response cannot be explained in terms of conditioned inhibition, because the UCS was always presented and therefore no CS signaled its absence. A negative difference between reward expectations and the actual outcome has previously been described in terms of a frustration effect [40,43] (for review see [44]). Such a reward discrepancy or devaluation can induce a putative, negative affective state able to elicit escape responses [39,40], intra- and hetero-specific aggression [45], high corticosterone levels [46], and distress USVs. For example, 11-day-old rat pups that had learned to approach an anesthetized dam with dry suckling as a reward showed distress USVs when reward was denied [47]. In adult rats, reductions in 50-kHz calls or increases in distress USVs (i.e., 22-kHz calls) have also been reported following timeout, withdrawal, or devaluation of different rewards [26,31,48]. Here, it should be noted that distress calls were only rarely observed in our present experiments.

It is still surprising however, that the updating of hedonic value of the UCS under a state of satiation did not reduce the ability of the CS to induce appetitive 50-kHz calls across experiments. If animals had not experienced the reward during the FAL phase we can perhaps assume that rats were behaving based on previous expectations built up when the reward was still valued [8,9]. However, some animals in the rat chow experiments approached the food, sniffed it or gnawed it; something that may have been enough to re-update the new hedonic value of that reward, even though none actually ate a piece of food in the cage (it was freely available in home cages). In contrast, in the milk experiment (3) all animals re-experienced the reward during satiation. At least from day 8 to day 9, and from there to day 10, a re-update of the current hedonic value of the food reward should have happened. Nevertheless, it did not impede incentive motivation reactions to occur (i.e., 50-kHz calls and, to a lesser extent, rearing behavior). We acknowledge that the FAL period measured may not have been long enough for a back-to-baseline drop in USVs rate, however, it was apparently sufficient for consummatory behavior to be completely abolished (rat chow experiments) or drastically reduced (milk experiment). We have provided a putative explanation for this effect consistent with the suppression-release hypothesis developed here. According to the Konorskian opponent-process model [16] (e.g., see [9]), we propose that the release of a motivational system (i.e., appetitive) from inhibition by the opponent system (i.e., aversive state induced by negative reward expectations maximized by FD) produced a rebound appetitive excitation, which may have lasted longer and decayed slower for preparatory/emotional responses than for consummatory/sensorial ones [16,34]. The latter responses are normal unconditioned feeding behaviors that are expected to be rapidly suppressed or activated according to physiological demands. Cue-induced USVs and exploratory activity, in contrast, are acquired conditioned responses controlled more by environmental stimuli rather than by the current appetitive state. It seems quite reasonable that cues that had signaled food availability while in a state of need were still able to guide behavior despite physiological needs were transiently fulfilled, since requirements of food may change as a matter of hours and, therefore, places where it was consistently available should be well remembered. This differential expression of incentive motivation responses may explain why right after satiation 50-kHz calls appeared detached from food seeking and consumption. To our knowledge, there is no such evidence as the one presented here, and as recently reviewed elsewhere [5], persistent incentive motivation has only been described when the

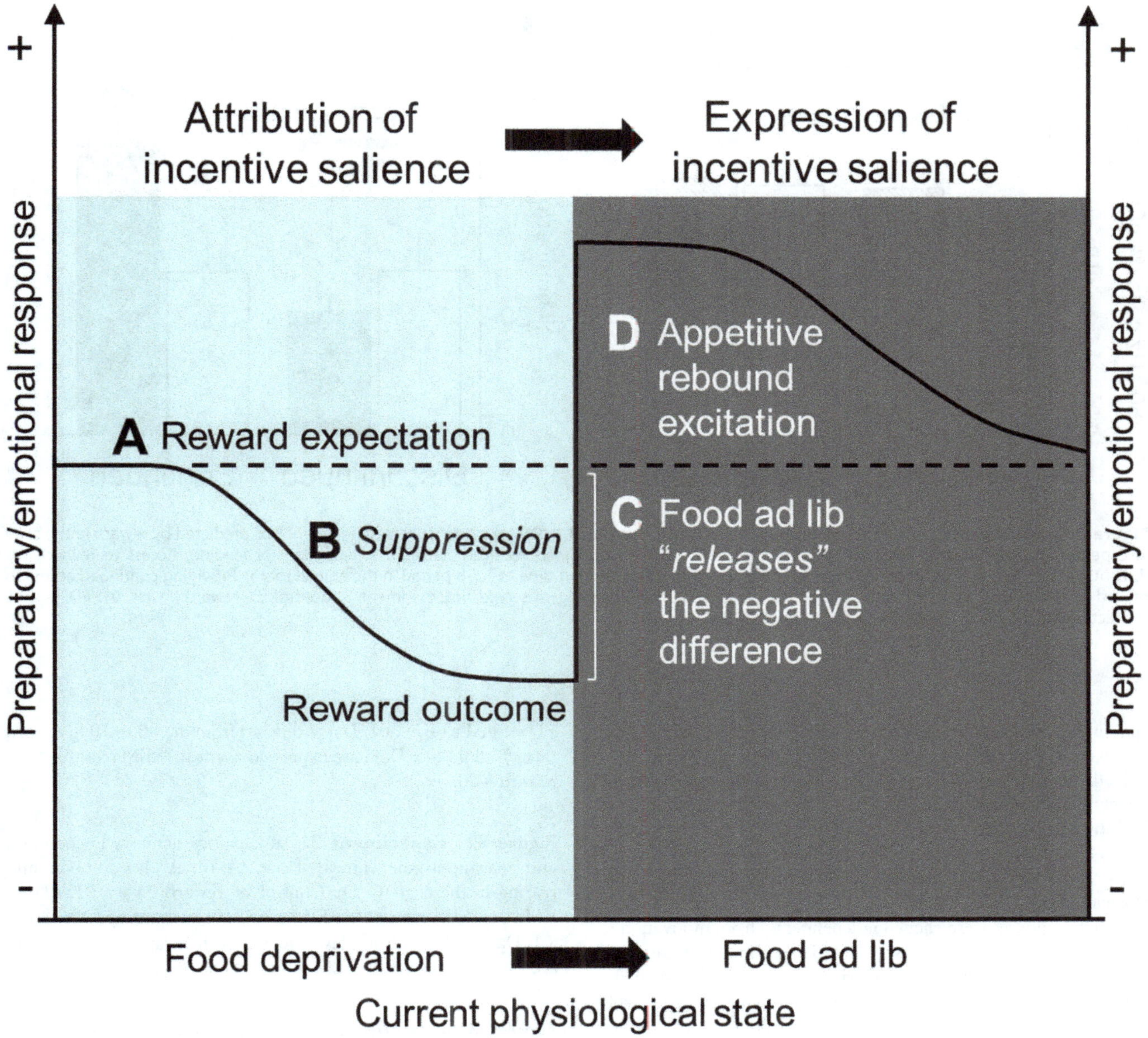

Figure 6. Suppression-release hypothesis. This hypothesis integrates statements modified from previous models [16,34]. A) If the strength (positive magnitude) of the actual UCS is less than the strength of the subject's expectation (maximized by food FD), the result will be suppression in the expression of the conditioned response. B) The larger the discrepancy between the strength of the expectation and the strength of the UCS outcome, the greater the suppression. C) If the strength of the actual UCS equals the strength of the subject's expectation, no suppression will be observed. Then, the magnitude of the suppression released would be proportionally inversed to the strength of the suppression that precedes it. Restoring the normal feeding conditions acts as a "releasing" factor of the negative difference between reward expectation and outcome, which does not require updating and which occurs afresh as soon as the current physiological state shifts. In the present experiments, the suppression in the expression of the conditioned response cannot be explained in terms of conditioned inhibition, because the UCS was always presented and therefore no CS- signaled its absence. D) The release of a motivational system (i.e., appetitive) from inhibition by the opponent system (i.e., aversive state induced by negative reward expectations) produces a rebound appetitive excitation that may last longer and decay slower for preparatory/emotional conditioned responses than for consummatory/sensorial ones.

UCS was devalued in the absence of the previous CS or following over-training, which was not our issue. Further experiments employing different conditioning paradigms with longer and more diverse testing schedules are required to elucidate the phenomena shown here, especially regarding USVs. However, it seems clear so far that independent of Pavlovian or instrumental task demands, reward palatability, reward accessibility and availability, devaluation of reward did not reduce cue-induced appetitive 50-kHz and rearing behavior, and more strikingly, shifting the current physiological state of the animals, and probably their subjective emotional state too, elicited appetitive 50-kHz calls by the pure incentive salience attributed to the environmental cues of the testing situation.

Conclusions

After Pavlovian incentive learning, reward-cues became able to elicit 50-kHz calls presumably signaling a state indicative of

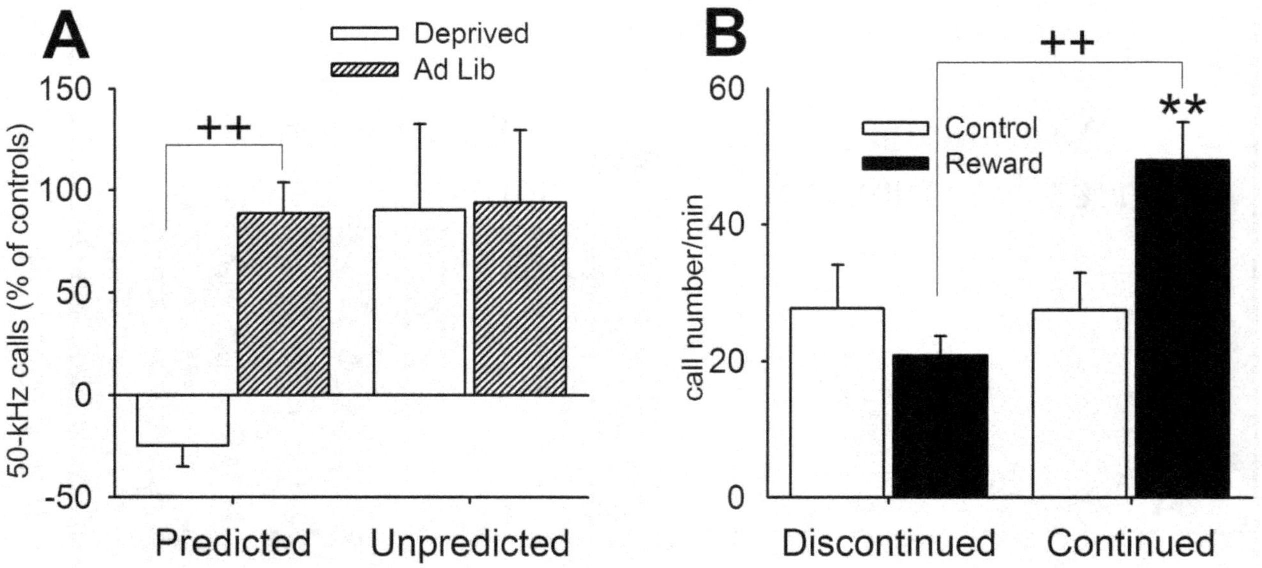

Figure 7. Comparisons between Experiments 1 and 3 (A) and 1 and 5 (B). Access to daily feeding (1.5-h) was predicted by reward in the cage in Experiment 1 (A, left) but not in Experiment 3 (A, right), in which animals received a reward independent of feeding. Access to reward was discontinued (B, left) in Experiment 1 (~2 min in the cage and the remaining time of 1.5-h period in the animal room). Providing continued access to reward in the testing cage (B, right) prevented the suppression in calling observed in Experiment 3. Control vs. reward: ** $p<.01$. FD vs. FAL interaction: ++ $p<.01$. Data are expressed as mean+SEM.

appetitive incentive motivation in the rat. Attribution and expression of incentive salience, however, do not seem to be a unified process, and were teased apart in two different ways: 1) under a high motivational state (i.e., hunger) the attribution of incentive salience to cues occurred without being expressed at the USVs level; and 2) under a low motivational state (i.e., food satiation), expression of appetitive USVs persisted despite physiological needs being fulfilled. In both cases, putative affective incentive responses were elicited independently from motivation to approach and consume the reward. While in a hungry state, short access to rewards may have led to a discrepancy between the reward expected and the one actually obtained that likely suppressed expression of USVs. When such a discrepancy between reward expectations and outcome was prevented by providing continued access to food, attribution and expression of incentive salience synchronized. Similarly, shifting feeding conditions from deprivation to satiation acted as a 'releasing' factor of the putative aversive state induced by both reward discrepancy and food deprivation. Such a release of a motivational system from inhibition led to a rebound appetitive excitation that lasted longer and decayed slower for preparatory/emotional responses than for consummatory/sensorial ones. The latter may explain why appetitive 50-kHz calls increased while sated but detached from reward seeking and consumption. Finally, the fact that rats seem to represent rewards emotionally (for review see, [21]) and beyond apparent, immediate physiological demands, provides an unparalleled translational tool to model motivational mechanisms underlying eating disorders, and may even be extendable to other forms of aberrant or persistent motivation such as in drug addiction, or gambling disorders.

Supporting Information

Figure S1 Experiment 1. Anticipatory activity. Locomotion (A) and rearing behavior (B). Control vs. reward: * $p<.05$, ** $p<.01$. FD vs. FAL: ++ $p<.01$. Day 7 differed from days 8 to 10 in reward rats: # all $p<.05$. Data are expressed as mean+SEM (control = 10, reward = 20).

Figure S2 Experiment 2. Anticipatory activity. Locomotion and rearing in the runway maze (A–B). A. Locomotion and rearing in the cage (C–D). Control vs. reward: ** $p<.01$. FD vs. FAL: + $p<.05$, ++ $p<.01$. FD vs. FAL in both groups: xx all $p<.01$. Day 1 differed from days 3 to 7 in both groups: § $p<.05$. Data are expressed as mean+SEM (control = 10, reward = 20).

Figure S3 Experiment 3. Anticipatory activity. Locomotion (A) and rearing behavior (B). Control vs. reward: ** $p<.01$. FD vs. FAL in both groups: xx all $p<.01$. Data are expressed as mean+SEM (control = 12, reward = 12).

Figure S4 Experiment 4. Anticipatory activity. Locomotion (A) and rearing behavior (B). Control vs. reward: * $p<.05$, ** $p<.01$. FD vs. FAL in both groups: xx all $p<.01$. FD vs. FAL: ++ $p<.01$. Day 7 differed from all FD days in controls, and from day 8 in reward rats: & all $p<.05$. Day 8 differed from day 10 in reward rats: # $p<.05$. Data are expressed as mean+SEM (control = 10, reward = 10).

Figure S5 Experiment 5. Anticipatory activity. Locomotion (A) and rearing behavior (B). Control vs. reward: ** $p<.01$. Day 1 differed from days 3 to 7 in reward rats: § $p<.05$. Data are expressed as mean+SEM (control = 10, reward = 10).

Acknowledgments

We thank Natalie Heyse for assistance with data collection and analysis.

Author Contributions

Conceived and designed the experiments: JCB RKWS. Performed the experiments: JCB. Analyzed the data: JCB. Contributed reagents/materials/analysis tools: RKWS. Wrote the paper: JCB RKWS.

References

1. Cornell CE, Rodin J, Weingarten H (1989) Stimulus-induced eating when satiated. Physiol Behav 45: 695–704.
2. Nair SG, Adams-Deutsch T, Epstein DH, Shaham Y (2009) The neuropharmacology of relapse to food seeking: methodology, main findings, and comparison with relapse to drug seeking. Prog Neurobiol 89: 18–45.
3. Petrovich GD, Ross CA, Gallagher M, Holland PC (2007) Learned contextual cue potentiates eating in rats. Physiol Behav 90: 362–367.
4. Weingarten HP (1983) Conditioned cues elicit feeding in sated rats: a role for learning. Science 220: 431–433.
5. Berridge KC (2012) From prediction error to incentive salience: mesolimbic computation of reward motivation. Eur J Neurosci 35: 1124–1143.
6. Schachter S (1968) Obesity and eating. Internal and external cues differentially affect eating behavior of obese and normal subjects. Science 161: 751–756.
7. Volkow ND, Wang GJ, Tomasi D, Baler RD (2013) The addictive dimensionality of obesity. Biol Psychiatry 73: 811–818.
8. Balleine BW (2005) Neural bases of food-seeking: Affect, arousal and reward in corticostriatolimbic circuits. Physiol Behav 86: 717–730.
9. Dickinson A, Balleine BW (2002) The role of learning in the operation of motivational systems. In: Gallistel CR, editor. Learning, motivation and emotion, volume 3 of Steven's Handbook of Experimental Psychology, Third edition. New York' John Wiley & Sons. pp. 497–533.
10. Berridge KC (2001) Reward learning: reinforcement, incentives, and expectations. In: Medin DL, editor. Psychology of Learning and Motivation, vol. 40. New York: Academic Press. pp. 223–278.
11. Bolles RC (1975) Theory of Motivation (2nd edition). New York: Harper & Row. Pp. 330–368.
12. Bindra D (1978) How adaptive behavior is produced: a perceptual-motivation alternative to response reinforcement. Behav Brain Sci 1: 41–91.
13. Toates FM (1986) Motivational Systems. Cambridge: Cambridge University Press. pp. 121–139.
14. Crespi LP (1942) Quantitative variation of incentive and performance in the white rat. Amer J Psychol 55: 467–517.
15. Hull C (1952) A Behavior System: An Introduction to Behavior Theory concerning the individual Organism. New Haven: Yale University Press. pp. 151–181.
16. Konorski J (1967) Integrative Activity of the Brain: An Interdisciplinary Approach. Chicago: University of Chicago Press. pp. 29–59.
17. Mowrer OH (1960) Learning Theory and Behavior. New York: John Wiley & Sons.
18. Rescorla RA, Solomon RL (1967) Two-process learning theory: relationships between Pavlovian conditioning and instrumental training. Psychol Rev 74: 151–182.
19. Panksepp J (1992) A critical role for "affective neuroscience" in resolving what is basic about basic emotions. Psychol Rev 99: 554–560.
20. Flagel SB, Akil H, Robinson TE (2009) Individual differences in the attribution of incentive salience to reward-related cues: implications for addiction. Neuropharmacology 56: 139–148.
21. Knutson B, Burgdorf J, Panksepp J (2002) Ultrasonic vocalizations as indices of affective states in rats. Psych Bull 128: 961–977.
22. Wöhr M, Schwarting RKW (2013) Affective communication in rodents: ultrasonic vocalizations as a tool for research on emotion and motivation. Cell Tissue Res 354: 81–97.
23. Burgdorf J, Knutson B, Panksepp J (2000) Anticipation of rewarding electrical brain stimulation evokes ultrasonic vocalization in rats. Behav Neurosci 114: 320–327.
24. Burgdorf J, Knutson B, Panksepp J, Ikemoto S (2001) Nucleus accumbens amphetamine microinjections unconditionally elicit 50 kHz ultrasonic vocalizations in rats. Behav Neurosci 115: 940–944.
25. Burgdorf J, Kroes RA, Moskal JR, Pfaus JG, Brudzynski SM, et al. (2008) Ultrasonic vocalizations of rats (*Rattus norvegicus*) during mating, play, and aggression: behavioral concomitants, relationship to reward, and self-administration of playback. J Comp Psychol 122: 357–367.
26. Burgdorf J, Wood PL, Kroes R, Moskal JR, Panksepp J (2007) Neurobiology of 50-kHz ultrasonic vocalizations in rats: Electrode mapping, lesion, and pharmacological studies. Behav Brain Res 182: 274–283.
27. Natusch C, Schwarting RKW (2010) Using bedding in a test environment critically affects 50-kHz ultrasonic vocalizations in laboratory rats. Pharmacol Biochem Behav 96: 251–259.
28. Williams SN, Undieh AS (2010) Brain-derived neurotrophic factor signaling modulates cocaine induction of reward-associated ultrasonic vocalization in rats. J Pharmacol Exp Ther 332: 463–468.
29. Meyer PJ, Ma ST, Robinson TE (2012) A cocaine cue is more preferred and evokes more frequency-modulated 50-kHz ultrasonic vocalizations in rats prone to attribute incentive salience to a food cue Psychopharmacology 219: 999–1009.
30. Browning JR, Browning DA, Maxwell AO, Dong Y, Jansen HT, et al. (2011) Positive affective vocalizations during cocaine and sucrose self-administration: a model for spontaneous drug desire in rats. Neuropharmacology 61: 268–275.
31. Coffey KR, Barker DJ, Ma S, Root DH, Martinez L, et al. (2013) Effects of varying reinforcement probability on pavlovian approach behavior and ultrasonic vocalizations in rats. Behav Brain Res 237: 256–262.
32. Willey AR, Spear LP (2013) The effects of pre-test social deprivation on a natural reward incentive test and concomitant 50 kHz ultrasonic vocalization production in adolescent and adult male Sprague-Dawley rats. Behav Brain Res 245: 107–112.
33. Schwarting RKW, Jegan N, Wöhr M (2007) Situational factors, conditions and individual variables which can determine ultrasonic vocalizations in male adult Wistar rats. Behav Brain Res 182: 208–222.
34. Brandon SE, Vogel EH, Wagner AR (2003) Stimulus representation in SOP: I. Theoretical rationalization and some implications. Behav Processes 62: 5–25.
35. Pecoraro NC, Timberlake WD, Tinsley M (1999) Incentive downshifts evoke search repertoires in rats. J Exp Psychol Anim Behav Process 25: 153–167.
36. Wong PT A (1979) Behavioral field approach to general activity: Sex differences and food deprivation in the rat. Anim Learn Behav 7: 111–118.
37. Timberlake W (2001) Motivational modes in behavior systems. In: Mowrer RR, Klein SB editors. Handbook of Contemporary Learning Theories. Hillsdale: Erlbaum Associates. pp. 155–209.
38. Baron A, Galizio M (2005) Positive and negative reinforcement: Should the distinction be preserved? Behav Anal 28: 85–98.
39. D'Andrea T (1971) Avoidance of timeout from response-independent reinforcement. J Exp Anal Behav 15: 319–325.
40. Daly HB (1974) Reinforcing properties of escape from frustration aroused in various learning situations. In: GH Bower, editor. The Psychology of Learning and Motivation Vol. 8. New York: Academic Press. pp. 187–231.
41. Wöhr M, Houx B, Schwarting RKW, Spruijt B (2008) Effects of experience and context on 50-kHz vocalizations in rats. Physiol Behav 93:766–776.
42. Robinson MJF, Berridge KC (2013) Instant transformation of learned repulsion into motivational "wanting". Curr Biol 23: 282–289.
43. Amsel A (1958) The role of frustrative nonreward in noncontinuous reward situations. Psycho Bull 55: 102–119.
44. Papini MR, Dudley TR (1997) Consequences of surprising reward omissions. Rev Gen Psychol 1: 175–197.
45. Azrin NH, Hutchinson RR, Hake DF (1966) Extinction-induced aggression J Exp Anal Behav 9: 191–204.
46. Flaherty CF, Becker HC, Pohorecky L (1985) Correlation of corticosterone elevation and negative contrast varies as a function of postshift day. Anim Learn Behav 13: 309–314.
47. Amsel A, Radek CC, Graham M, Letz R (1977) Ultrasound emission in infant rats as an indicant of arousal during appetitive learning and extinction. Science 197: 786–788.
48. Covington HE III, Miczek KA (2003) Vocalizations during withdrawal from opiates and cocaine: possible expressions of affective distress. Eur J Pharmacol 467: 1–13.

17

High-Resolution Mapping of a Genetic Locus Regulating Preferential Carbohydrate Intake, Total Kilocalories, and Food Volume on Mouse Chromosome 17

Rodrigo Gularte-Mérida[1¤], Lisa M. DiCarlo[2], Ginger Robertson[2], Jacob Simon[2], William D. Johnson[4], Claudia Kappen[3], Juan F. Medrano[1], Brenda K. Richards[2*]

1 Department of Animal Science, University of California Davis, Davis, California, United States of America, **2** Genetics of Eating Behavior Laboratory, Pennington Biomedical Research Center, Louisiana State University System, Baton Rouge, Louisiana, United States of America, **3** Department of Developmental Biology, Pennington Biomedical Research Center, Louisiana State University System, Baton Rouge, Louisiana, United States of America, **4** Biostatistics Department, Pennington Biomedical Research Center, Louisiana State University System, Baton Rouge, Louisiana, United States of America

Abstract

The specific genes regulating the quantitative variation in macronutrient preference and food intake are virtually unknown. We fine mapped a previously identified mouse chromosome 17 region harboring quantitative trait loci (QTL) with large effects on preferential macronutrient intake-carbohydrate (*Mnic1*), total kilcalories (*Kcal2*), and total food volume (*Tfv1*) using interval-specific strains. These loci were isolated in the [C57BL/6J.CAST/EiJ-17.1-*(D17Mit19-D17Mit50)*; B6.CAST-17.1] strain, possessing a ~40.1 Mb region of CAST DNA on the B6 genome. In a macronutrient selection paradigm, the B6.CAST-17.1 subcongenic mice eat 30% more calories from the carbohydrate-rich diet, ~10% more total calories, and ~9% more total food volume per body weight. In the current study, a cross between carbohydrate-preferring B6.CAST-17.1 and fat-preferring, inbred B6 mice was used to generate a subcongenic-derived F_2 mapping population; genotypes were determined using a high-density, custom SNP panel. Genetic linkage analysis substantially reduced the 95% confidence interval for *Mnic1* (encompassing *Kcal2* and *Tfv1*) from 40.1 to 29.5 Mb and more precisely established its boundaries. Notably, no genetic linkage for self-selected fat intake was detected, underscoring the carbohydrate-specific effect of this locus. A second key finding was the separation of two energy balance QTLs: *Mnic1/Kcal2/Tfv1* for food intake and a newly discovered locus regulating short term body weight gain. The *Mnic1/Kcal2/Tfv1* QTL was further de-limited to 19.0 Mb, based on the absence of nutrient intake phenotypes in subcongenic HQ17IIa mice. Analyses of available sequence data and gene ontologies, along with comprehensive expression profiling in the hypothalamus of non-recombinant, *cast/cast* and *b6/b6* F_2 controls, focused our attention on candidates within the QTL interval. *Zfp811*, *Zfp870*, and *Btnl6* showed differential expression and also contain stop codons, but have no known biology related to food intake regulation. The genes *Decr2*, *Ppard* and *Agapt1* are more appealing candidates because of their involvement in lipid metabolism and down-regulation in carbohydrate-preferring animals.

Editor: Tongming Yin, Nanjing Forestry University, China

Funding: This research was funded through National Institutes of Health grant DK-53113 to B.K.R. The Genomics Core Facility (GCF) was supported, in part, by Center of Biomedical Research Excellence (COBRE) (NIH 8 P20 GM103528) and Nutrition Obesity Research Center (NORC), (NIH 2P30DK072476) center grants from the National Institutes of Health. W.D.J. was funded by 1 U54 GM104940 from the National Institute of General Medical Sciences of the National Institutes of Health which funds the Louisiana Clinical and Translational Science Center. The funders had no role in study design, data collection and analysis, decision to publish, or preparation of the manuscript.

Competing Interests: The authors have declared that no competing interests exist.

* Email: richarbk@pbrc.edu

¤ Current address: Unit of Animal Genomics, GIGA-Research, Université de Liège, Liège, Belgium

Introduction

Genes influencing the quantitative variation in caloric and macronutrient-specific intakes, which can predispose individuals to obesity and obesity-related diseases, are virtually unknown [1,2]. Whole-genome linkage analysis is the most commonly used approach for discovering the genetic contribution to eating behavior [3]. In humans, genome-wide linkage analyses have identified several regions of significant linkage for macronutrient intake [4–7], e.g., for energy and macronutrient intakes on human chromosome 3q27.3 [6] which corresponds to the region between 22,776,516 and 22,776,729 bp on mouse chromosome (MMU) 16 (GRCh37/hg19 assembly, UCSC). To our knowledge, none of the quantitative trait loci (QTL) found in humans correspond to those identified in mice, with the exception of a locus for total energy on human chromosome 20q13.13 [7] that overlaps *Kcal3*, a body weight-dependent QTL for kilocalorie intake on MMU2 [8]. Mice are excellent models for genetic mapping because interval-specific strains can be bred to isolate and test loci associated with specific traits. Another key advantage of using laboratory animals for studies of eating behavior instead of humans [9] is the ability to provide a controlled environment, including manipulation of the diet and accurate measurement of food consumption.

Despite its importance in energy balance and thus the obesity equation, very few studies have identified QTL for energy intake in mammals. In mice, Allan *et al.* [10] found eight loci influencing energy consumption on five chromosomes by recording chow intake at weekly intervals. Mathes *et al.* [11] detected a QTL on MMU12 for chow intake during exercise that was determined by the C57BL/6J-derived allele. We and others have shown that mice, similar to people, exhibit a wide range in the amounts of carbohydrate and fat eaten when selecting among food choices [12–19], providing evidence for naturally occurring variation. We previously investigated the genetic basis for total energy and macronutrient-specific intakes in F_2 progeny derived from an intercross of carbohydrate-preferring CAST/EiJ (CAST) and fat-preferring C57BL/6J (B6) mouse inbred strains [14]. We identified six significant and two suggestive QTL for self-selected macronutrient intake (fat-rich *vs.* carbohydrate-rich diets), as well as three significant loci for total kilocalorie intake [8], providing strong evidence for multiple genetic determinants of food intake. In particular, highly significant QTL for macronutrient intake-carbohydrate (*Mnic1)* and total kilocalorie intake (*Kcal2*) were uncovered on proximal MMU17. *Mnic1* was consistent with the parental strain phenotype, i.e., CAST alleles at *Mnic1* increased the preferential intake of carbohydrate over fat, independent of body weight.

The *Mnic1* and *Kcal2* QTLs were successfully captured in both congenic and subcongenic strains, eventually narrowing the interval to a 40.1 Mb region [20–22]. The subcongenic strain B6.CAST-*D17Mit19-D17Mit50* (referred to here as B6.CAST-17.1) possesses CAST genetic material between 4.8 and 45.4 Mb of MMU17 on an otherwise B6 genome. Congenic strains, by design, eliminate genetic variation outside the locus of interest, and thus can establish whether the locus of interest acts independently to exert its phenotypic effects. In a diet choice paradigm, the B6.CAST-17.1 subcongenic mice ate 30% more carbohydrate-rich diet and 10% more total calories per gram body weight, yet consumed similar amounts of the fat-rich diet when compared to B6 littermates [20], demonstrating that the MMU17 subcongenic interval retained and confirmed the effects of *Mnic1* and *Kcal2*. In accordance with the higher volume/weight and lower calorie density of carbohydrate relative to fat, the B6.CAST-17.1 strain also consumed a larger food volume, consistent with a QTL for total food volume (*Tfv1*) that we identified in the same genomic region [23].

To shorten the responsible interval and thereby reduce the number of candidate genes, we have now performed single nucleotide polymorphism- (SNP-) based fine mapping of the *Mnic1/Kcal2/Tfv1* QTL using an interval-specific congenic F_2 mapping population. To further de-limit the causative interval, we also evaluated the macronutrient diet selection and kcal/g intake phenotypes of an existing subcongenic strain (C57BL/6J$^{hg/hg}$.CAST-(*rs49640908–rs47909630*). In addition to the fine mapping strategies, we analyzed bioinformatics data, including available sequence, and generated gene expression data from a trait-relevant tissue–hypothalamus–to highlight potential candidate genes. Genes uncovered using both approaches have been proposed as likely causative genes underlying a QTL [24].

Materials and Methods

Mouse lines and breeding strategy

The development of the B6.CAST-17.0 speed congenic and B6.CAST-17.1 subcongenic strains has been described previously [20–22]. The MMU17 subcongenic interval was previously defined as a 40.6 Mb CAST minimal donor region extending from *D17Mit19* to *D17Mit50* [20]. In the current study, this region was more precisely defined as a 42.5 Mb interval bounded by SNP markers *rs49640908* (proximal) and *rs48762654* (distal) (Figure 1). For mapping purposes, a congenic-by-recipient F_2 population was generated by mating a single B6.CAST-17.1 congenic male to multiple C57BL/6J (stock #000664) females purchased from The Jackson Laboratory (Bar Harbor, ME). The resulting F_1 mice were intercrossed and in this manner, a large cohort of B6.CAST-17.1 congenic F_2 was generated. To further map the causative interval on proximal chromosome 17, we also phenotyped subcongenic (n = 14) and wildtype (n = 14) mice from the C57BL/6J$^{hg/hg}$.CAST(*rs49640908–rs47909630*) line (referred to as HQ17IIa). This HQ17IIa subcongenic mouse strain, developed in the laboratory of Dr. Juan F. Medrano at the University of California, Davis, is homozygous for CAST/EiJ (CAST) alleles from 3.19 to 26.08 Mb on MMU 17 on a *high growth* background (Figure 1). *High growth* mice (C57BL/6J$^{hg/hg}$) show an increased body weight without obesity due to the high growth (*hg*) deletion which eliminates expression of the *Socs2* (suppressor of cytokine signaling 2), a negative regulator of growth hormone signaling [25].

All animals were bred and reared in polycarbonate cages on sterilized corncob bedding, and maintained under controlled conditions of temperature (21±2°C), humidity (30–70%), and lighting (14 h light:10 h dark). Mice were fed standard chow diet (LabDiet 5001; 28% protein, 12% fat, and 60% carbohydrate kcal/g) and tap water ad libitum. Pups were weaned at 24–26 days of age and housed with siblings in same-sex groups of 1–4. Only progeny from litters containing 4–10 pups were used for breeding and experiments, and the average litter size was 7.48 pups. All animal husbandry protocols were in accordance with the guidelines of the American Association for Accreditation of Laboratory Animal Care (AAALAC). All experimental protocols conducted in this study were approved by the Pennington Biomedical Research Center Institutional Animal Care and Use Committee.

Experimental design

The general experimental approach used to fine map the MMU 17 QTL involved phenotyping and genotyping male F_2 mice possessing at least one recombination within the subcongenic region (n = 168), as well as their non-recombinant F_2 littermates, i.e., *cast/cast* (n = 44), *b6/b6* (n = 47), and *cast/b6* (n = 60), for a total of 319 congenic F_2. These numbers were based on power calculations which determined that ~170 animals with at least one recombination within the subcongenic region were needed to detect a significant difference in carbohydrate/protein (C/P; see below) kcal at 80% power. A variety of body weight, body composition, food intake, and organ weight phenotypes were assessed in five experimental cohorts of randomly selected, age contemporary male F_2 mice. Standardized phenotyping methods have been previously described in detail [8]. Briefly, 10–16 week old F_2 mice were first weighed and then housed individually in a hanging, stainless steel mouse cage with wire mesh floor, containing a polyvinylchloride tube for nesting. To minimize heat loss via convection in these cages, animals were maintained at an ambient temperature of 26–27°C. Before being presented with a

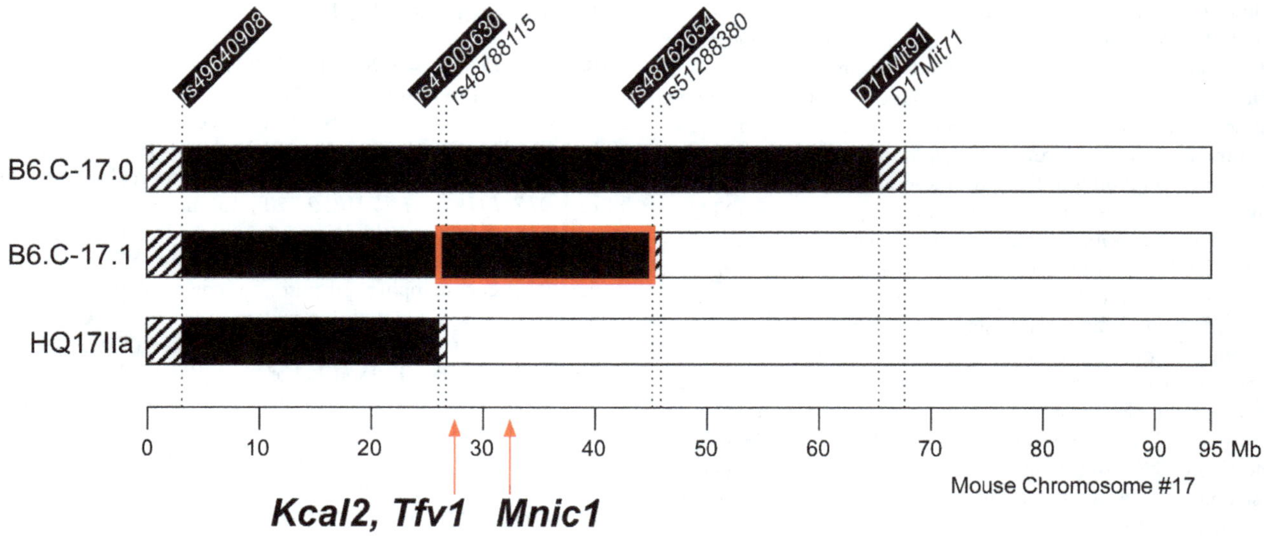

Figure 1. The critical *Mnic1/Kcal1/Tfv1* QTL region on mouse chromosome 17 was reduced to 19.0 Mb. Legend: Congenic and subcongenic strains with CAST/EiJ alleles introgressed on the wild type C57BL/6J (B6) or mutant C57BL/6J-$^{hg/hg}$ genome are illustrated. Solid bars indicate CAST donor regions, open bars indicate B6 genotype, and hatched bars designate intervals of undetermined genotype, as defined by SNP or Mit markers (top). The fine-mapped interval encompassing carbohydrate-specific macronutrient intake (*Mnic1*; peak at 32.49 Mb), total kilocalories (*Kcal1*; peak at 27.19 Mb) and total food volume (*Tfv1*; peak at 27.10) is specified by the bar outlined in red.

choice between macronutrient diets, animals were allowed a minimum of 7 d to adapt to the special housing conditions, as evidenced by a return to baseline body weight. When not tested in the macronutrient diet selection protocol, mice were housed in polycarbonate cages and fed standard chow *ad libitum* (LabDiet No. 5001, Richmond, IN).

Measurement of phenotypes

Body weights and body composition were measured twice: immediately before and after the 10 d diet selection study. Nuclear magnetic resonance (NMR) with a Bruker Mice Minispec MQ10 series NMR analyzer (Bruker Optics, Inc., Billerica, MA) was used to provide estimates of body fat, lean body tissue, and fluid in awake animals. This instrument was calibrated daily according to the manufacturer's instructions. Intakes of fat/protein, carbohydrate/protein, and total calories were determined in singly-housed, adult male mice, using a macronutrient diet protocol. Specifically, for 10 days mice were provided a choice between fat/protein (F/P) and carbohydrate/protein (C/P) diet mixtures, equivalent for protein (22% of energy) and with the balance of calories contributed by either fat or carbohydrate (78%). Both diets contained casein (protein), minerals and vitamins. The C/P diet was composed of corn starch and powdered sucrose, whereas the F/P diet contained vegetable shortening from one of two sources, according to availability. The experimental diet composition and complete details of the phenotyping procedures have been described previously [8]. Briefly, each diet was presented in a custom two oz. glass jar with stainless steel lid (Unifab, Kalamazoo, MI); food intake and all spillage were measured daily to the nearest 0.1 g. Following the 10 d diet self-selection protocol, animals were returned to a standard chow diet for at least two weeks. Two days before euthanasia, animals were again provided access to the macronutrient selection diets. The mice were fasted for 4 h prior to euthanasia, which consisted of an overdose of isoflurane gas inhalation followed by decapitation. Bilateral epididymal (EPI) fat pads and whole liver were dissected and wet weights were determined. The hypothalamus was carefully lifted from the ventral surface of the brain based on visual localization, e.g., relative to the optic chiasm and pituitary. Spleens were collected for DNA isolation.

Genotyping and SNP selection

Genomic DNA was isolated from spleens using phenol/chloroform extraction and suspended in TE buffer (10 mM Tris, pH 7.5, 1 mM EDTA) at a final concentration of 50 ng/µl, as determined by Quant-iT PicoGreen (Invitrogen). To perform QTL analysis, a custom SNP panel was designed based on the Perlegen SNP dataset available at the Mouse Phenome database (http://phenome.jax.org/). We identified a total of 384 polymorphic markers between CAST/EiJ and C57BL/6J, located from 3.18 to 47.1 Mb on MMU 17. SNP were selected at uniform intervals, giving preference to those located within coding regions and previous QTL locations (Table S1), resulting in an average spacing of 0.114±0.066 Mb across the interval. This SNP panel containing 301 markers (Table S1) was used to genotype 319 mice from the B6.CAST-17.1 F_2 intercross, and additional controls, using the Illumina GoldenGate assay and VeraCode technology on the BeadXpress platform. Genotype calls were carried out using Illumina Genome Studio software. The genotype call rate averaged 98.7% for the DNA samples and 47 control samples showed complete genotype concordance.

Fine-mapping of QTL for body composition, macronutrient diet selection and total food intake (kcal, g)

Measurements of daily consumption of fat/protein (F/P) kcal, carbohydrate/protein (C/P) kcal, total kcal and total gram intake were expressed as 10 d sums as previously described [8]. Gain in body weight and body composition components (lean mass, fat mass, fluid mass) was defined as the difference between the ending (e.g., BW2) and starting values (e.g., BW1) over the 10 d of macronutrient diet selection. Gain was also determined for the difference between end-of-study body weight (BW3) and earlier weights (BW1, BW2). Phenotypic differences among F_2 non-recombinant controls, possessing *cast/cast*, *b6/cast*, and *b6/b6* genotypes across the subcongenic segment, were estimated using a mixed effects, general linear statistical model (*Proc MIXED, SAS v9.3*) to perform a repeated measures analysis of variance (covariance) while accounting for the effects of fat source, initial age, baseline body weight and baseline lean mass. These covariates were considered to be the most biologically and experimentally relevant, e.g., lean body mass is metabolically active and contributes significantly to energy expenditure [26]. Significance of specific discrepancies among genotypes was tested using orthogonal contrasts on the three genotypes (*b6/b6, b6/cast, cast/cast*). Relevant outcomes were summarized in either tables or graphs as covariate-adjusted (least squares) mean ± standard error of mean (SEM). Pearson correlation coefficients among dependent variables were determined and are reported for four categories of phenotypes, including food intake, body composition, body weight, and tissue end weights.

Statistical genetic analyses

Linkage analysis was carried out using both interval mapping and single marker analysis. Interval mapping was performed using the scanone function with the Halley-Knott regression method and imputation of pseudomarkers at 0.01 Mb from the R/qtl package of R: Language and Environment [27,28]. Fat source, initial age (age1), baseline body weight (BW 1), and initial lean body mass (NMR Lean 1) were included as additive covariates as described above. To define the genome-wide LOD score threshold required as significant or suggestive for each specific trait, genome-wide significance levels were estimated by using 1,000 permutations with the n.perm argument in scanone [29]. Ninety-five percent confidence intervals (CI) were determined by the bayesint function in R/qtl. To estimate the QTL effect, genotypes were coded as 1, 2, and 3 for b6/b6, b6/cast and cast/cast, respectively. The genotype coefficient was considered as the estimate of the additive effect of the cast allele. Single marker analysis was carried out at each individual SNP using a general linear model (glm function) that included fat source, initial age, baseline body weight and initial lean body mass as covariates. These results were similar to those from interval mapping, and therefore are not presented.

The results of single QTL analysis suggested the presence of multiple QTL segregating in the congenic strain, thus we tested for the presence of multiple QTL using the *stepwiseqtl* function in R/qtl [30]. To increase the power to detect multiple QTL a combined cross analysis was performed by combining the genotype and phenotype results from two separate mapping populations [31]: C57BL/6J×B6.CAST-17.1 subcongenic (n = 319 F_2) in the current study, and our previous C57BL/6J×CAST/EiJ strain intercross (n = 502 F_2) [8]. The results of this combined cross analysis provided insufficient evidence to support the hypothesis of multiple QTL in the region.

Experimental design for gene expression analyses

Global gene expression profiles in the hypothalamus were compared between non-recombinant subcongenic-derived F_2 mice, possessing a genotype of *cast/cast* (n = 12) or *b6/b6* (n = 12) across the Chr 17 subcongenic segment and *b6/b6* across the rest of the genome. RNA was isolated from individual mice of each genotype that were selected for study. Specifically, twelve mice of each genotype that displayed the most divergent phenotypic values for self-selected carbohydrate and total kcal intake were chosen for gene expression analysis, i.e., *cast/cast* mice with the highest and *b6/b6* mice with the lowest kcal intake from carbohydrate, or the 25% tails of the distribution. Tissues were harvested ~48 h after re-initiation of the carbohydrate/protein *vs.* fat/protein diets, following an extended wash-out period on chow diet after completion of the 10 d macronutrient selection test (see Methods above). The hypothalamus was selected for study based on its key role in the behavioral and metabolic control of food intake [32].

Gene expression profiling

Total RNA from the hypothalamus was extracted and purified using an AllPrep RNA/Protein kit (Qiagen, Valencia, CA) and re-suspended in Nanopure water. RNA quality was assessed by electrophoresis using an Agilent 2100 Bioanalyzer (Total RNA Nano; Agilent) and all samples showed an RIN number (RNA integrity number) of ≥7.0. Gene expression profiling was performed by serial analysis of gene expression followed by high-throughput sequencing (SAGE-Seq) using the 5500XL SOLiD system (Life Technologies). Briefly, SAGE libraries containing 27-bp, 3′ tags for all transcripts within a sample were constructed using a SOLiD SAGE kit (Life Technologies), at the PBRC Genomics Core Facility. Each library was then labeled with a unique barcode sequence and high-throughput sequencing was performed using SOLiD technology (Life Technologies). Sequence mapping was performed using a modified version of the SOLiD SAGE Analysis Software v1.10 (Life Technologies) and defined analysis parameters. Sequenced reads were aligned using the mouse transcriptome RefSeq mRNA database and genome build GRCm38/mm10. Tag hits, i.e., successfully aligned reads, were normalized according to DESeq by estimating the size factor for each sample and dividing the sample counts by the corresponding size factor. Differential expression analysis was performed using the DESeq R/Bioconductor package [33]. Genes with significantly altered expression in the *cast/cast* congenic F_2 samples compared to that of *b6/b6* congenic F_2 were stringently defined by a fold change of ≥1.5 and a P value of ≤0.01. Two-way hierarchical clustering, by means of Ward's minimum variance criterion method, was applied to normalized and standardized expression data using the tools in JMP Genomics, Version 10 (SAS Institute Inc., Cary, NC). The SAGE-Seq analyses reported here have been deposited to GEO (http://ncbi.nlm.nih.gov/geo/; accession number GSE60756).

Gene annotation

Biological process annotation was performed using the WEB-based Gene SeT AnaLysis Toolkit (WebGestalt; http://bioinfo.vanderbilt.edu/webgestalt/) which draws on a number of centrally and publicly curated databases including Gene Ontology (GO) and KEGG (Kyoto Encyclopedia of Genes and Genomes) [34]. The results of this analysis are illustrated in Figure S3. For the enrichment calculations in WebGestalt (Figure S4), we executed a Gene Ontology analysis against a background of all mouse RefSeq genes, using the default settings for classification stringency. The significance of gene enrichment was based on P-values generated by the hypergeometric test, adjusted for multiple testing. Gene annotation categories were considered to be significantly overrepresented if the associated P value was less than 0.05.

Results

Phenotypes in non-recombinant subcongenic-derived-F_2 mice

Macronutrient and total calorie intakes, body weight, and body composition were measured in non-recombinant subcongenic-derived F_2 mice (see Table 1). The mean kcal intake selected from carbohydrate/protein (C/P) diet was ~25% higher in *cast/cast* F_2 compared to *b6/b6* F_2 mice, thus confirming and extending previous observations [20,21]. Based on least squares means, over-dominance, i.e., the mean of the *b6/cast* hybrid population as being less or more than the average value of the two parental strains [35], was observed for eight phenotypes (Table 1). Both the *cast/cast* F_2 and *b6/cast* F_2 mice consumed more total kcal from carbohydrate and less from fat compared to *b6/b6* F_2 littermates ($P<0.005$), indicating a dominant effect of the *cast* allele. The cumulative intake of total kilocalories for 10 d was also higher in non-recombinant *cast/cast* compared to *b6/b6* ($P<0.005$) F_2 mice. A dominant effect of the *cast* allele on cumulative total food volume ($P<0.05$) was observed, which may reflect higher consumption of the less-energy-dense carbohydrate/protein diet (3.61 kcal/g), than the fat/protein diet (5.96 kcal/g), as indicated by the strong positive correlation between C/P kcal and food volume ($r = 0.87$, $P<0.0001$; Table S4). In non-recombinant F_2 mice, short-term weight gain was positively associated with total calorie intake ($r = 0.51$, $P<0.0001$) and, to some extent, fat calories ($r = 0.22$, $P<0.01$), but not carbohydrate ($r = 0.12$, P = NS) (Table S5).

The 10 d time-course of genotype effects on C/P versus F/P intake in non-recombinant subcongenic F_2 animals is illustrated in Figure 2. Relative to the *b6/b6* genotype, both *cast/cast* ($P<0.005$, Tukey-Kramer) and *b6/cast* ($P<0.001$) F_2 mice consumed more C/P kcal (Figure 2A), with the exception of *day 1* when *b6/cast*> *b6/b6* F_2 mice = *cast/cast* F_2 [genotype by day: F (18, 1187) = 2.16, $P<0.003$]. By contrast, the *b6/b6* F_2 ate more F/P kcal over 10 d, when compared to *cast/cast* F_2 ($P<0.008$) but not *b6/cast* F_2 ($P = 0.10$) (Figure 2B). Based on both total calorie and g consumption, the animals displayed a pronounced hyperphagic response to the novel diets at the beginning of the study, which gradually subsided over time [e.g., total kcal, day: F (9, 938) = 21.10, $P<0.0001$], independent of genotype [genotype × day: F (18, 938) = 0.94, $P = 0.53$]. Relative to the *b6/b6* genotype, non-recombinant F_2 with the *cast/cast* ($P<0.005$) and *b6/cast* ($P<0.0001$) genotype consumed more total g over 10 d.

Both body weight and body fat content of the non-recombinant, littermate F_2 control mice were similar among genotypes at baseline (Table 1). After 10 d of macronutrient diet selection, all three genotypes gained similar amounts of body weight (~5–6%) and body fat (28–32%). By the end of the entire study period (BW3), both the *cast/cast* F_2 and *b6/cast* F_2 mice had gained a small (~9%) but significantly greater amount of weight compared to *b6/b6* F_2 littermates ($P<0.005$; Table 1). There were no genotype effects on epididymal fat pad or liver weights.

High resolution mapping of *Mnic1*, *Kcal2* and *Tfv1* QTL

A subcongenic-derived intercross was constructed to reduce the QTL influencing preferential carbohydrate intake, total calories and food volume to a smaller region containing fewer genes. Compared with a whole-genome scan, this approach to linkage analysis provides a substantial increase in statistical power to detect and resolve QTL due to the elimination of background genetic noise. As a result, we narrowed and more precisely localized the QTL for macronutrient intake-carbohydrate (*Mnic1*) (*rs46437881*, 32.49 Mb; LOD = 5.77) (Table 2). In addition, the peak position of co-localized QTL for total kilocalorie intake (*Kcal2*) and total food volume (*Tfv1*) was localized to 27.19 Mb

Table 1. Phenotypic data for food intake, body weight, body composition and organ weights in non-recombinant B6.CAST-17.1-derived F_2 mice.

	B/B (n = 47)	B/C (n = 60)	C/C (n = 44)
10d sum C/P kcal[a, b]	52.9±2.6[§]	67.6±2.5**	70.5±2.9
10d sum F/P kcal[a, b]	55.9±2.5*	47.6±2.3*	43.6±2.7
10d sum Total kcal[a]	108.8±1.5**	115.2±1.4	114.1±1.7
10d sum Total g[a, b]	24.0±0.5§	26.7±0.4*	26.9±0.5
Baseline BW 1 (g)	23.7±0.1	23.8±0.1	23.9±0.1
BW 2 after 10 d diet (g)	25.0±0.1	25.2±0.1	25.4±0.2
BW3 - dissection (g)[a, b]	25.7±0.1**	26.2±0.1*	26.3±0.1
BW gain (2 minus 1)	1.2±0.1	1.4±0.1	1.6±0.2
NMR fat 1	1.85±.05	1.81±0.05	1.97±0.06
NMR fat 2	2.58±0.12	2.70±0.11	2.88±0.13
NMR fat gain	0.73±0.10	0.89±0.10	0.92±0.11
NMR lean 1[b]	18.30±0.06	18.19±0.06*	18.02±0.07
NMR lean 2[b]	18.56±0.10	18.58±0.09*	18.86±0.11
NMR lean gain[b]	0.25±0.11	0.39±0.11**	0.84±0.12
NMR fluid 1	0.68±0.02	0.66±0.02	0.66±0.02
NMR fluid 2[a]	0.76±0.02**	0.66±0.02	0.69±0.02
NMR fluid gain[a]	0.08±0.02*	0.00±0.02	0.03±0.03
EPI fat pad weight (g)	0.350±0.013	0.380±0.012	0.375±0.014
Liver weight (g)	1.405±0.027	1.467±0.025	1.462±0.029

Values indicate least squares means ± SE.

[a]Difference between B/B and C/C; probability value indexed in B/B column.

[b]Difference between the B/C population and the average of its two parental strains combined, adjusted for fat source, initial age, baseline body weight, and baseline lean mass; probability value indexed in B/C column.

*$P<0.05$; **$P<0.005$; [§]$P<0.0001$. Carbohydrate/protein (C/P) and fat/protein (F/P) diets were presented simultaneously for 10 days. BW, body weight; NMR, nuclear magnetic resonance; EPI, epididymal.

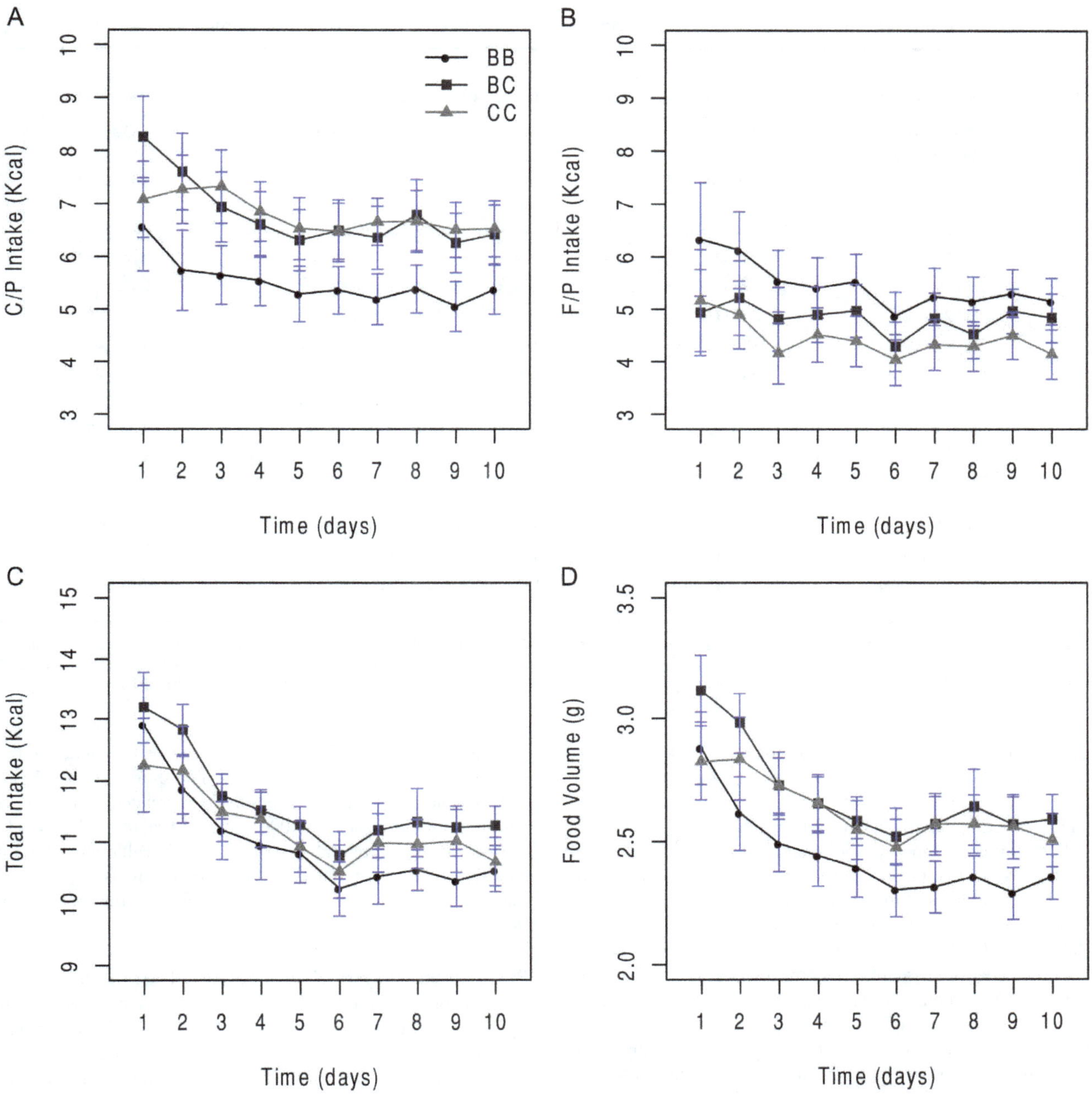

Figure 2. Non-recombinant B6.CAST-17.1 F_2 mice exhibit increased intake of carbohydrate kcal, total kcal and total food volume. Legend: Daily consumption of (A) carbohydrate/protein kcal (C/P) versus (B) fat/protein kcal (F/P), total kcal (C) and total food volume (D) in non-recombinant B6.CAST-17.1 F_2 mice. Values are mean ± SE. Relative to *b6/b6* F_2, both *cast/cast* ($P<0.005$, Tukey-Kramer) and *b6/cast* ($P<0.001$) F_2 mice consumed more C/P kcal (A), with the exception of *day 1* when *b6/cast*>*b6/b6* F_2 mice = *cast/cast* F_2 [genotype by day: F (18, 1187) = 2.16, $P<0.003$]. By contrast, the *b6/b6* F_2 ate more F/P kcal when compared to *cast/cast* F_2 ($P<0.008$) but not *b6/cast* F_2 ($P=0.10$) (B), during the 10 d study. With respect to total kcal, all genotypes displayed a pronounced hyperphagic response to the diets at the beginning of the study, which subsided gradually over time [day: F (9, 938) = 21.10, $P<0.0001$], independent of genotype [genotype × day: F (18, 938) = 0.94, $P=0.53$]. Relative to *b6/b6* F_2, both *cast/cast* ($P<0.005$) and *b6/cast* ($P<0.0001$) F_2 mice consumed more total g over 10 d.

(*rs33797547*), with highly significant LOD scores of 5.86 and 8.05, respectively (Table 2; Figure 3). No significant linkage for F/P kcal intake was detected (LOD = 1.92) in this subcongenic interval. These results clearly replicated, yet with far greater mapping resolution, the Chr 17 QTL identified in the original F_2 intercross [8]. Specifically, the peak locus for *Kcal2* and *Tfv1* (*rs33797547*), was fine mapped to ~27.1 Mb (*rs33797547*). Positioned ~5.30 Mb distal to this locus, is the peak for *Mnic1* (*rs46437881*), suggesting that a minimum of two loci are responsible, for both the amount of food consumed in a diet choice paradigm and the macronutrient composition of that food. Sub-peaks within the CI suggest the possibility of more than one genetic element that is contributing to the major phenotypic effects of these QTL [36]. An examination of The Jackson Laboratory QTL database (www.informatics.jax.org) revealed a total of 37 documented mouse QTL within the 15.55–45.12 Mb CI for *Mnic1*, as determined by linkage analysis. Only two of these QTL are obesity-related, i.e., *Obrq13* [37] and *Wta4* [38], and none

Table 2. QTLs for nutrient intake, body weight, and body composition in B6.CAST-17.1-derived F_2 mice.

QTL name	*Phenotype*	*Peak (Mb) (Marker)*	*LOD*	*95% CI (Mb) (Markers)*	*Effect of CAST allele*
Tfv1	10d sum Total food volume (g)	27.19 (*rs33797547*)	8.05	16.41–34.18 (*rs33750505–rs46967024*)	+1.30±0.25***
Kcal2	10d sum Total (Kcal)	27.19 (*rs33797547*)	5.86	16.41–42.12 (*rs33750505–rs33341718*)	+3.61±0.81***
Mnic1	10d sum C/P (Kcal)	32.49 (*rs46437881*)	5.77	15.55–45.12 (*rs48970296–rs46074101*)	+6.87±1.40***
----	NMR fat gain (g)	21.74 (*rs48587745*)	3.46	10.49–41.83 (*rs33750661–rs47337390*)	+0.17±0.05**
----	BW 2 (g)	11.06 (*rs33738432*)	3.45	3.19–31.84 (*rs49640908–rs45936635*)	+0.31±0.08***
----	NMR 2 fat (g)	16.53 (*rs33747676*)	3.18	3.19–37.64 (*rs49640908–rs33721754*)	+0.21±0.06***
----	EPI Weight (g)	21.31 (*rs51776929*)	3.08	5.44–38.20 (*rs48030175–rs33809121*)	+0.022±0.006***
----	NMR 2 lean (g)	31.44 (*rs51849267*)	2.48	9.14–45.50 (*rs46011679–rs49209168*)	+0.19±0.05**
----	BW 3 (g)	45.12 (*rs46074101*)	2.07	6.73–45.73 (*rs33695293–rs48762654*)	+0.27±0.08***
----	10d sum F/P (Kcal)	3.86 (*rs33651689*)	1.92	3.19–45.73 (*rs49640908–rs48762654*)	−2.44±1.26[§]
----	NMR 2 free fluid (g)	5.89 (*rs47725817*)	1.60	3.19–45.73 (*rs49640908–rs48762654*)	−0.01±0.01
----	Liver Weight (g)	8.17 (*rs48213049*)	1.23	3.19–45.73 (*rs49640908–rs48762654*)	−0.02±0.01
----	NMR 1 fat (g)	33.79 (*rs33219958*)	1.14	3.19–45.73 (*rs49640908–rs48762654*)	0.02±0.03
----	NMR 1 free fluid (g)	45.73 (*rs48762654*)	0.97	11.53–45.73 (*rs33653408–rs48762654*)	−0.01±0.01

Genome coordinates are based on the Genome Reference Consortium Mouse Build 38 (GRCm38). Mb = megabase. LOD = logarithm (base 10) of odds. Significant linkage ($P<0.01$ and $P<0.05$) was defined as LOD>2.98 and LOD>2.14 respectively, based on 1,000 permutations. "----", un-named. CI = confidence interval. C/P = carbohydrate/protein; BW = body weight. NMR = nuclear magnetic resonance. F/P = fat/protein. EPI = epididymal fat. ***$P\leq0.0001$; **$P\leq0.001$; *$P\leq0.01$; [§]$P\leq0.05$.

pertain to macronutrient preference, energy intake, or food consumption, with the exception of *Mnic1*, *Kcal2*, and *Tfv1* [8,23].

The intersecting pattern of QTLs determining the consumption of carbohydrate, total energy, and total food volume in this model was reflected by the inter-correlations among phenotypes. For example, the measures of total food consumed by recombinant F_2 in both calories and g, showed a strong positive correlation ($r = 0.85$, $P<0.0001$; Table S2; Table S3). The lack of a perfect correlation between these two phenotypes can be attributed to variation in energy densities per weight (g) that exists between the two diet formulations. With respect to macronutrient-specific intake, the total volume of food consumed in g was strongly and positively correlated with carbohydrate/protein g intake ($r = 0.86$, $P<0.0001$), but inversely correlated with fat/protein g intake ($r = -0.36$, $P<0.0001$), as illustrated in Figure 4.

Identification of QTL for body weight and body composition

Following 10 d of macronutrient diet selection, two novel QTL not detected in our original F_2 mapping study [8] were identified for BW2 (*rs33738432*, 11.06 Mb; LOD = 3.45) and body fat gain (*rs48587745*, 21.74 Mb; LOD = 3.46) (Table 2; Figure 5). It should be noted that the BW2 QTL is essentially the same as body weight gain over the 10 d period because BW1 was included as an additive covariate in the statistical model. A QTL influencing short-term body weight gain is located near marker *rs33738432*, with a CI between 3.19 and 31.84 Mb that partially overlaps the CI for a body fat gain QTL. A suggestive QTL for NMR2 lean mass also was identified (*rs51849267*, 31.44 Mb; LOD = 2.48). A significant QTL for epididymal fat pad weight was located at 21.31 Mb (*rs51776929*; LOD = 3.08), which replicated a previously identified *cast*-linked locus [39]. The effect of the CAST allele for each of these QTL was to increase body weight and body fat, relative to the B6 allele (Table 2). The short-term weight gain in recombinant F_2 mice was positively correlated with total kcal consumption ($r = 0.51$, $P<0.0001$) and fat kcal ($r = 0.22$, $P>0.01$), but not carbohydrate kcal ($r = 0.12$, P = NS) (Table S3). Thus total energy-, rather than macronutrient-specific intake, may be the major contributor to short-term weight gain in this subcongenic-derived F_2 population.

Phenotypic analysis of subcongenic HQ17IIa mice

To refine the critical segment containing the *Mnic/Kcal2/Tfv1* QTLs, we evaluated the macronutrient selection phenotypes of an existing HQ17IIa subcongenic strain, harboring a 22.8 Mb segment of CAST genomic DNA on proximal MMU17 that is smaller than the B6.CAST-17.1 CAST donor segment (Figure 1). The time-course of the genotype effect on carbohydrate *vs.* fat intake in HQ17IIa mice over the 10 d period is shown in Figure S1. Compared to wild type (WT) controls, the HQ17IIa strain (C/C) selected/consumed similar, cumulative amounts of carbohydrate/protein kcal (73±7 C/C vs. 77±9 WT), fat/protein kcal (71±8 C/C vs. 65±8 WT), total kilocalories (127±2 CC vs. 129±3 WT), or total grams of food (27.8 C/C±0.7 vs. 29.1±1.2 WT) over the 10 d period. In addition, there were no strain differences in baseline body weight (35.5±0.5 g C/C vs. 36.8±0.7 g WT; $P = 0.14$) or percent lean mass (77±0.4% C/C vs. 76±0.6% WT; $P = 0.16$) (Table S6), therefore adjusting the animals' food intake values for body size or metabolically active lean mass was deemed unnecessary. The phenotypes of HQ17IIa animals were determined in two experiments, including both a pilot study (unpublished) and a replicate study of 14 subcongenic and 14 controls (Figure S1). The results demonstrated clearly that HQ17IIa mice, compared to the appropriate B6 background controls, failed to exhibit the food intake phenotypes in question

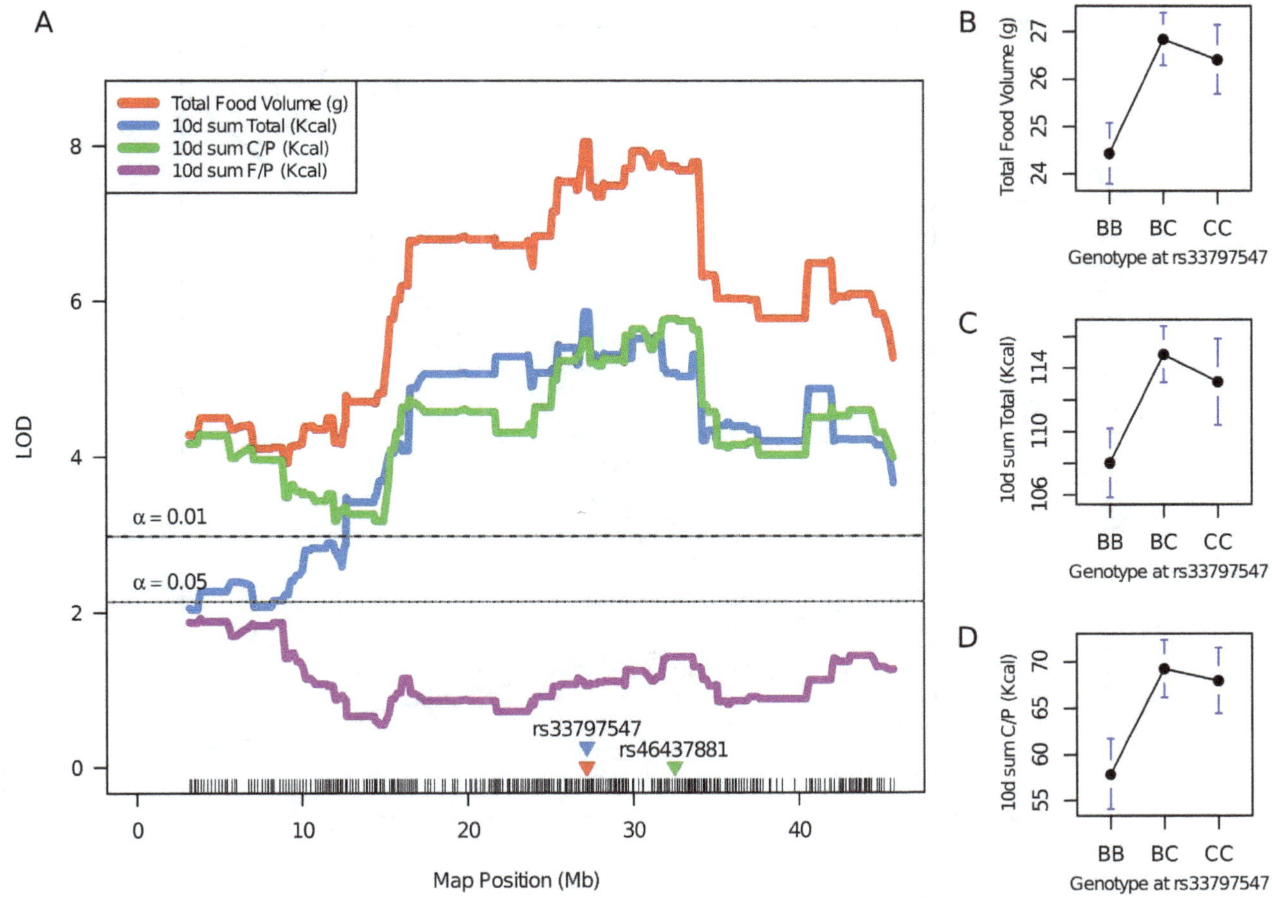

Figure 3. Preferential carbohydrate and total food intake is controlled by *Mnic1* and *Kcal/Tfv1* loci, respectively. Legend: Interval plot of proximal Chr 17 illustrates fine-mapped QTL for carbohydrate intake (*Mnic1*), total calorie intake (*Kcal2*) and total food volume consumed (*Tfv1*) in B6.CAST-17.1 subcongenic F_2 mice (left) and uncorrected phenotypic means for the peak marker of each QTL (right). Significance threshold values established for $\alpha = 0.01$ and $\alpha = 0.05$ were LOD scores of 2.98 and 2.14, respectively, as determined by 1,000 permutation tests. On the interval map, locations of markers nearest the peak LOD scores are shown on the x-axis, e.g., *rs33797547*. On the right, genotype effect plots at marker *rs33797547* show the CAST (CC) allele is associated with a higher intake of g, total kcal, and carbohydrate/protein kcal compared to the B6 (BB) allele, and the F1 (BC) responses for all three phenotypes resembled those of the CC, indicating dominance of the CAST allele. Values are mean ± SEM. See Table 2 for a list of all QTLs.

(preferential carbohydrate intake, increased total calorie/g intake), making it extremely likely that the causal genetic variant is located distal to the 26.08 Mb breakpoint in the mutant. Based on this result, the responsible region therefore can be reduced to a 19.044035 Mb interval located between 26.081867 and 45.125902 Mb (Figure 1), containing approximately 599 RefSeq genes.

Analysis of sequence variation between strains

Using a combination of high-resolution fine-mapping and phenotypic analyses of subcongenic mouse strain HQ17IIa, we determined that the critical QTL spans the interval between 26.08 and 45.12 Mb (Figure 1). Based on the assumption that causative polymorphisms must be contained within the QTL region, we compiled a list of coding variants between CAST and B6 within these boundaries using data from the Wellcome Trust Sanger Institute Mouse Genome Project and the Mouse Phenome Database (http://phenome.jax.org/SNP). Thus we calculated, within the QTL boundaries, a total of 296 nonsynonymous coding SNPs in 71 genes. These genetic variants included nucleotide changes that result in the gain or loss of 3 stop codons, as well as 27 deletions and 19 insertions, e.g., some as long as 30 nucleotides; 5 inversions; 1 frame-shift variant, and 2 copy number variants.

To look for variation that could predict altered protein function, missense mutations in the QTL intervals were evaluated by *in silico* analysis using the SIFT program [40]. SIFT predicts deleterious and tolerated substitutions for nonsynonymous coding (Cn) SNP based on the evolutionary conservation of amino acids within protein families. The results of this analysis predicted with high confidence that 14 of the 296 Cn SNP identified within the reduced QTL boundaries would have a possible detrimental effect. Although this program generates approximations, it can identify missense mutations that have potential functional significance and thus may warrant further investigation.

Differential gene expression in *cast/cast* and *b6/b6* subcongenic-derived F_2 mice

Gene expression analysis, independent of sequence-based analysis, can be helpful in identifying genes that are affecting a trait [24]. To highlight potentially relevant genes in the critical interval, a SAGE-seq experiment was performed to analyze gene expression in the hypothalamus of non-recombinant F_2 progeny possessing *cast/cast* vs. *b6/b6* alleles across the subcongenic segment, and *b6/b6* alleles in the rest of the genome. Expression

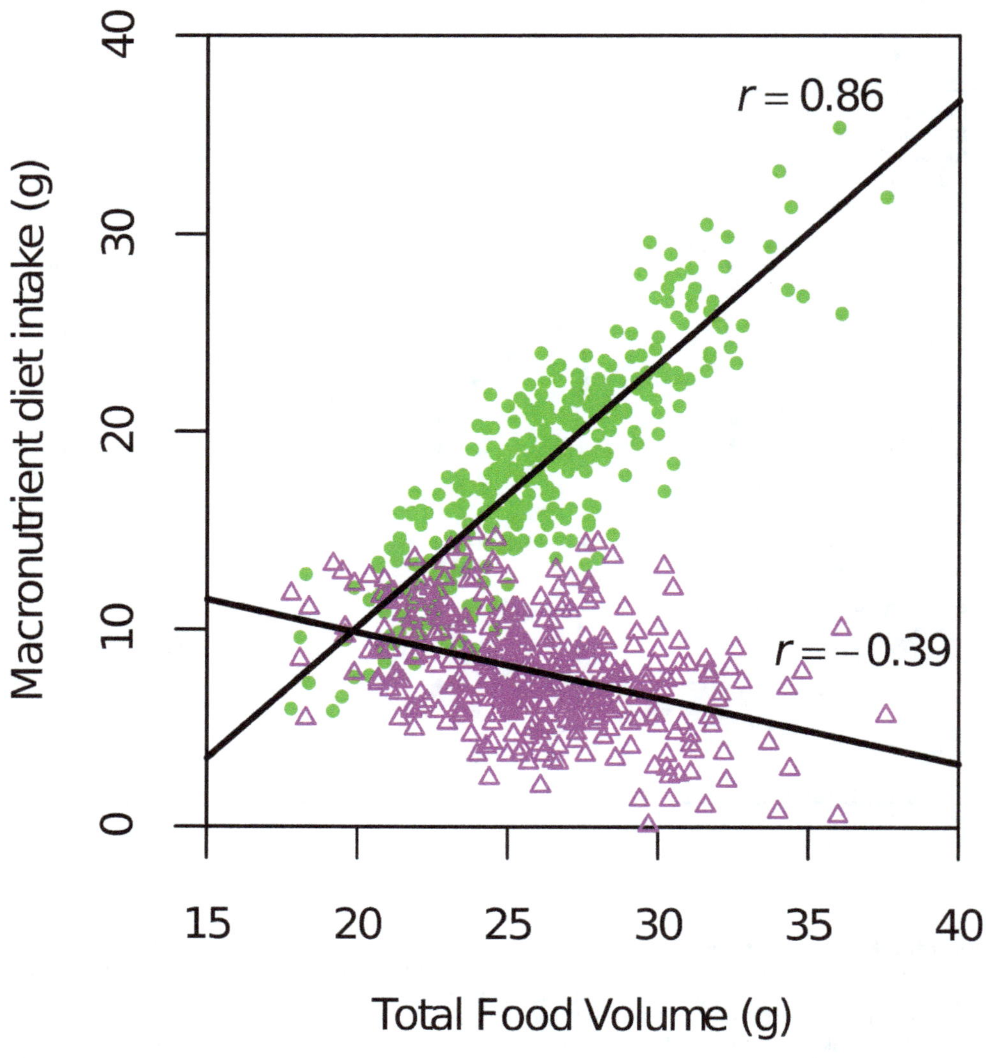

Figure 4. Preferential carbohydrate intake was positively correlated with total food volume in recombinant subcongenic-derived F_2 mice. Legend: The macronutrient diet selection phenotype of preferential carbohydrate- versus fat-specific intake, unique to this genetic model, is illustrated. The total volume of food consumed in g was strongly and positively correlated with carbohydrate/protein (C/P) intake ($r = 0.86$, $P < 0.0001$), but inversely correlated with fat/protein (F/P) intake ($r = -0.39$, $P < .0001$) in this macronutrient diet choice paradigm.

of these genes is regulated in *cis*, suggesting that local sequence variation within the QTL region accounts for the observed expression differences. The hypothalamus was chosen for analysis because it is an integration site for acute and long-term metabolic signals and is the tissue most likely to influence behavioral feeding and macronutrient-specific appetites [32]. Results from the SAGE-Seq analysis indicated that 55 genes or 9% of RefSeq genes in the 19.0 Mb interval were differentially expressed (DE) in the hypothalamus of littermate, non-recombinant subcongenic F_2 mice (Table 3), selected from the 25% tails of the phenotype distribution for self-selected 10 d carbohydrate intake (see Methods). Gene expression was significantly increased (*cast/cast* genotype relative to *b6/b6*) in 13 genes and decreased in 42 genes (Table 3) in animals fed the macronutrient selection diet. Of the total 55 DE genes, *Glo1*, *Pla2g7* and *Pde9a* were validated previously in chow-fed B6.CAST-17.1-*(D17Mit19-D17Mit50)* subcongenic mice [20]. Because the differential expression of these three genes, by genotype, was independent of diet, they are unlikely to be causal for the phenotypic effects of *Mnic1/Kcal2/Tfv1* on macronutrient-specific intake.

Hierarchical clustering analyses of significant genes are illustrated in Figure 6, which revealed five main clusters of differentially regulated genes that were evident when the magnitude and direction of changes were considered. Genes whose expression changed significantly (*adjP*<0.01) in animals with the *cast/cast* genotype (higher carbohydrate consumption), relative to *b6/b6* (higher fat consumption), cluster together as increased (red) or decreased (blue) cells. Additional clusters with smaller magnitude of differences in gene expression level (less intense red or blue color), by genotype, are also shown.

WebGestalt was used to organize the differentially expressed genes into Gene Ontology (GO) Slim categories (Figure S3). Nearly 50% of these DE genes were classified as metabolism genes (Table S3), of which seven were associated with lipids and/or fatty acids (*Decr2*, *Ppard*, *Agpat1*, *Tnxb*, *Neu1*, *Pla2g7*, *Cyp39a1*; all down-regulated), and two with carbohydrate metabolism (*Glo1*, *Neu1*; up-regulated). We then used WebGestalt to visualize significantly enriched GO categories according to biological process, molecular function, and cellular component (Figure S4). The most significantly enriched GO category under biological

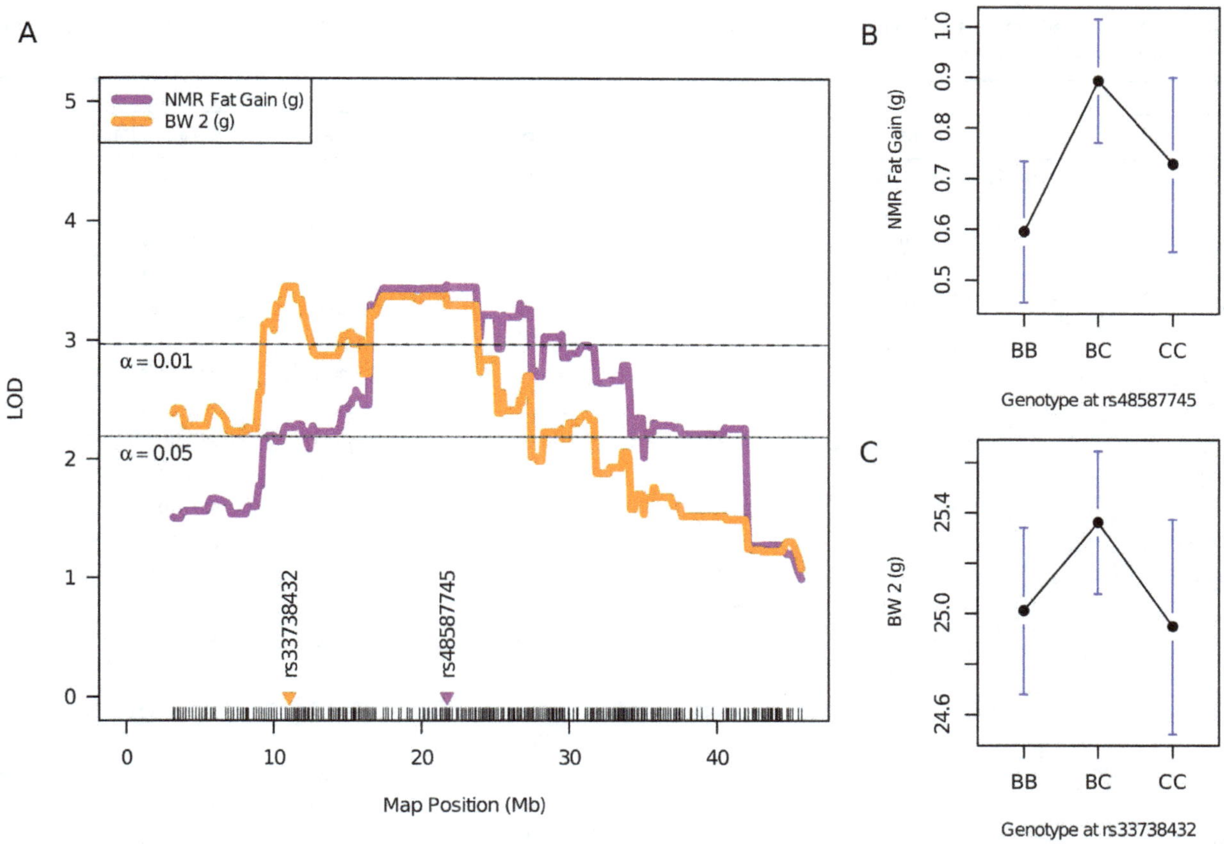

Figure 5. Short-term body fat and weight gain is controlled by a proximal chromosome 17 locus. Legend: Interval map of proximal chromosome 17 illustrates fine-mapped QTL for body fat gain and body weight gain after 10 d of macronutrient diet selection, in B6.CAST-17.1 subcongenic-derived F_2 mice (left), and includes uncorrected phenotypic means for the peak marker of each QTL (right). The significant LOD threshold values for α = 0.01 and α = 0.05 were 2.97 and 2.19, respectively, as determined by 1,000 permutation tests. The locations of markers nearest the peak LOD scores are shown on the x-axis, e.g., *rs48587745*.

process was antigen processing and presentation (7 genes, *adjP*< 0.0001; Figure S4). Approximately 36% of the 55 differentially expressed genes have molecular functions related to metal ion binding (*adjP* = 0.0001). These include several transcription factors, e.g., *Ring1*, and members of the cytochrome P450 family. Long-chain fatty acid binding, represented by *Ppard* and *Cyp4f14*, was also noted (*adjP* = 0.004).

Identification of potentially relevant candidate genes

To focus attention on candidate genes within the fine mapped *Mnic1/Kcal2/Tfv1* QTL interval, we employed both bio-informatic and genomic methods. We analyzed available mouse sequence data via http://phenome.jax.org/SNP, that was based on the following sources: GRCm38 coordinates, dbSNP 138 annotation, and Sanger data updates (28 Aug 2013). We identified 296 protein coding differences contained within the fine mapped interval. Next, using SIFT analysis, we determined *in silico* that 14 of these protein coding changes between strains are likely to be detrimental by impairing protein function. Strain-specific polymorphisms could also affect expression level, which can be valuable in identifying candidate genes [41]. To further understand the molecular mechanisms underlying *Mnic1/Kcal2/Tfv1*, hypothalamic gene expression was evaluated between homozygous *cast/cast* subcongenic and *b6/b6* wild-type F_2 littermates using SAGE seq. We identified 55 differentially expressed positional candidates located within the critical 19.0 Mb region (Table 3) and among these, only two genes showed evidence of both altered mRNA abundance and a coding nonsynonymous SNP predicted as damaging: *Zfp811* and *Morc2b* (microrchidia 2B), including a stop gain codon in *Zfp811*. Available sequence data for *Zfp870*, while not differentially expressed in hypothalamus, shows seven nonsynonymous SNPs between B6 and CAST, two of which are calculated as damaging and one that predicts the gain of a premature stop codon. *Btnl6* (butyrophilin-like 6) has two potentially deleterious SNPs that are predicted to result in the loss of a stop codon. The four candidate genes described above are located from ~32.80 to 34.50 Mb, in close proximity to the *Mnic1* peak for preferential carbohydrate intake. However, nothing is known thus far about a functional role of these candidate genes in any food intake phenotypes.

To further search for possible candidates, we used the MGI ontologies database version 5.15 (www.informatics.jax.org) to examine available annotation for genes located in the minimal QTL region. Using the query terms food intake or energy intake, this search found only six biologically relevant genes: *Glp1r*, *Clps*, *Itpr3*, *Mut*, *Rcan2* and *Cdkn1a*. Based on our previous investigations, *Glp1r* remains a viable candidate gene for *Mnic1/Kcal2/Tfv1*, while evidence for *Clps* and *Itpr3* is lacking (see below and Discussion). Using bioinformatic resources, we found no evidence for an amino acid change or altered gene expression to support *Mut*, and *Rcan2* as candidates, but SIFT analysis predicted a deleterious SNP in *Cdkn1a* between the CAST and

Table 3. Differentially expressed genes in the hypothalamus of homozygous *cast/cast* vs. *b6/b6* subcongenic-derived F_2 mice, located within the fine mapped QTL interval of 26.08–45.12 Mb.

Gene Symbol	Mean BB	Mean CC	Fold change	*P* value	Location (Mb)
Decr2	183.6	84.4	−2.174	0.0097	26.081211
Kifc5b	24.3	4.3	−5.682	≤0.0001	26.917091
Phf1	305.9	14.5	−21.075	≤0.0001	26.933127
Lemd2	36.6	13.2	−2.782	0.0001	27.189601
Gm10505	16.7	0.4	−47.588	≤0.0001	27.342460
Nudt3	906.9	417.9	−2.170	0.0057	27.579382
Uhrf1bp1	89.2	46.7	−1.911	0.0016	27.856490
Ppard	25.3	7.5	−3.352	0.0001	28.232754
Brpf3	732.6	49.8	−14.700	≤0.0001	28.801090
4930539E08Rik	106.1	368.2	3.470	≤0.0001	28.896397
Mtch1	3760.5	2032.3	−1.850	0.0009	29.332072
Tbc1d22b	29.7	12.0	−2.479	0.0015	29.549788
Gm6402	13.2	68.7	5.219	≤0.0001	30.394825
Glo1	1232.3	2575.0	2.090	≤0.0001	30.592866
Umodl1	14.7	1.1	−13.062	≤0.0001	30.954683
Rsph1	42.1	248.3	5.894	≤0.0001	31.255019
Pde9a	287.9	164.1	−1.754	0.0023	31.386234
Cbs	112.5	50.3	−2.236	0.0031	31.612623
Hsf2bp	16.6	59.6	3.584	≤0.0001	31.944769
Cyp4f16	52.9	4.5	−11.747	≤0.0001	32.536558
Zfp811	357.3	212.2	−1.684	0.0015	32.797406
Cyp4f14	44.6	3.0	−14.938	≤0.0001	32.905071
Zfp472	66.2	26.4	−2.511	≤0.0001	32.965814
Zfp763	80.9	23.9	−3.377	≤0.0001	33.016863
Morc2b	6.6	16.6	2.532	0.0048	33.135588
Zfp955a	638.3	256.4	−2.489	≤0.0001	33.241519
BC051226	32.1	10.8	−2.976	≤0.0001	33.908182
Zbtb22	262.4	15.6	−16.833	≤0.0001	33.915904
Wdr46	270.3	11.3	−24.002	≤0.0001	33.940660
Vps52	237.0	366.9	1.548	0.0099	33.955812
H2-K2	63.9	3.5	−18.311	≤0.0001	33.974786
AA388235	54.9	0.2	−348.820	≤0.0001	33.981492
H2-K1	129.8	57.6	−2.255	0.0030	33.996017
Ring1	1652.2	2534.3	1.534	0.0059	34.020792
Rxrb	969.4	208.9	−4.641	≤0.0001	34.031812
H2-DMa	47.4	107.1	2.258	0.0020	34.135182
Psmb9	11.8	29.0	2.463	0.0008	34.181988
Psmb8	66.4	8.8	−7.523	≤0.0001	34.197721
H2-Aa	125.9	1.2	−105.436	≤0.0001	34.282744
H2-Eb2	10.1	22.0	2.169	0.0093	34.325665
Agpat1	342.3	196.9	−1.739	0.0008	34.604262
Tnxb	147.2	48.2	−3.055	0.0002	34.670535
Neu1	310.1	151.3	−2.049	≤0.0001	34.931253
1110038B12Rik	179.2	5.6	−32.090	≤0.0001	34.950238
H2-Q1	677.6	390.8	−1.734	0.0014	35.320405
H2-Q4	26.9	1.3	−20.938	≤0.0001	35.379617
Ddr1	541.3	22.8	−23.761	≤0.0001	35.681567
Abcf1	1238.6	174.7	−7.089	≤0.0001	35.956819
A930015D03Rik	13.0	63.5	4.890	≤0.0001	35.994453

Table 3. Cont.

Gene Symbol	Mean BB	Mean CC	Fold change	*P* value	Location (Mb)
Rpp21	127.1	5.7	−22.294	≤0.0001	36.255645
Znrd1	448.4	5.3	−84.073	≤0.0001	36.954358
E130008D07Rik	34.4	2.6	−13.293	≤0.0001	43.146041
Pla2g7	773.3	6.2	−125.196	≤0.0001	43.568098
Cyp39a1	23.0	10.2	−2.252	0.0038	43.667425
Enpp4	323.1	534.0	1.653	0.0034	44.096308

Positive fold change indicates increased expression, negative value indicates decreased expression in homozygous *cast/cast* (CC) subcongenic-derived F_2 mice (n = 12) relative to *b6/b6* (BB) subcongenic-derived F_2 (n = 12). Genes were selected based on a significance value of $P<0.01$ and an expression change of ≥1.5-fold, based on sequence tag counts.

B6 strains. Our SAGE-Seq results showed clearly that *Cdkn1* is expressed in the hypothalamus, but was not differential between strains. We are unaware of any evidence for a physiological role of *Cdkn1a* in food intake regulation. A literature search uncovered one report suggesting that *Cdkn1a,* a cyclin-dependent kinase inhibitor, may have a role in the obesity-inducing effects of high-fat diet feeding beyond one generation [42]. However this study examined the effects of *Cdkn1a* activation to promote lipid accumulation, and did not explore its association with food intake or selection.

Candidate gene analysis of *Itpr3*

Based on its physical location and possible physiological relevance to ingestive behavior phenotypes, we carried out candidate gene analyses of *Itpr3*. *Itpr3,* encoding inositol 1,4,5-triphosphate receptor, type 3, is a component of the taste transduction cascade and is located under the LOD peak for *Kcal2* at ~27.1 Mb. Specifically, the intracellular calcium channel ITPR3 releases calcium from the endoplasmic reticulum in response to signals from small molecules and proteins including nucleotides, kinases, and phosphatases, as well as non-enzyme proteins [43,44]. The ITPR3 is widely expressed in tissues including taste buds, olfactory epithelium, brain, epidermis, intestine, kidney, pancreatic islets and stomach [45,46]. It has been suggested that *Itpr3* may play a role in macronutrient diet choice [47]. We therefore investigated the possibility that *Itpr3* contributes to the effects of *Mnic1/Kcal2*. We examined the expression of *Itpr3* in the hypothalamus of B6.CAST-17.1 subcongenic compared to wild-type mice using quantitative PCR, but found no difference in expression level. Next, using allele-specific PCR, we verified a non-synonymous coding SNP in *Itpr3* that changes G to T at 27,098,333 base pair (bp) of chromosome 17 and produces a alanine-to-serine missense mutation at position 821 (A821S). The amino acid change resulting from this polymorphism was classified as 'tolerated' by SIFT [40]. Next, we hypothesized that altered taste perception of the experimental diets might contribute to carbohydrate preference in our selection paradigm. Thus we examined the taste preferences of B6.CAST-17.1 subcongenic mice for sucrose using 48-h two-bottle tests. The result was that B6.CAST-17.1 displayed normal behavioral responses to sucrose compared to wild type controls (Figure S2). Although the strain difference in ITPR3 protein sequence could possibly affect protein function, it did not severely impair sensitivity for sweet stimuli in our genetic model, as has been reported in ITPR3 knockout mice [46] Therefore the phenotype of preferential carbohydrate intake does not appear to be driven by a preference for sweet taste, and must depend on some other mechanism. Nonetheless, the location of *Itpr3* coincides closely with the peak map position for *Kcal2/Tfv1* (Table 2), allowing the possibility that *Itpr3* contributes to total calorie intake and/or food volume, but this has not been determined.

Discussion

In this study, we have clearly confirmed and refined the locations of QTL regulating self-selected macronutrient intake-carbohydrate (*Mnic1*), as well as the consumption of total kilocalories (*Kcal2*) and total food volume (*Tfv1*). These food intake QTL were originally identified through genome-wide mapping [8,23] and now have been reproduced in a subcongenic-derived F_2 mapping population. The absence of genetic linkage for self-selected fat intake in the results underscores the carbohydrate-specific effect of this mouse chromosome 17 locus on macronutrient selection. The fine mapped *Mnic1/Kcal2/Tfv2* QTL was then further de-limited by evaluating macronutrient diet selection phenotypes in an interval-specific subcongenic strain. Consequently, we are now able to infer that a 19.04 Mb interval between 26.08 and 45.12 Mb harbors the responsible sequence variation regulating these food intake traits.

To our knowledge, no other genetic loci for macronutrient preference have been reported in laboratory rodents until recently. Specifically, a number of food consumption QTL in animals selecting their intake from separate macronutrient (protein, carbohydrate and fat) sources were mapped in a LOU/C×Fischer 344 F_2 rat population [48]. Two QTL influencing the percentage of carbohydrate consumed were identified on rat chromosomes 10 (*Foco17*) and 20 (*Foco23*). These rat QTL regions share synteny blocks with the fine mapped mouse *Mnic1* region for preferential carbohydrate intake described in the current study (www.rgd.mcw.edu), providing further support for its authenticity.

Our study also revealed two partially overlapping QTL, affecting short term gains in both body fat (NMR fat gain) and body weight (BW 2) (Figure 5) (Table 2), positioned between the centromere and lower boundary of the 95% CI for *Mnic1* (preferential carbohydrate intake QTL). The body weight/fat gain QTL peaks are situated ~10–20 Mb away from the food intake QTL (Figures 3 & 5). The separation of these energy balance loci, *Mnic1/Kcal2/Tfv1* for food intake and the newly discovered locus regulating short term body weight/fat gain, suggests the possibility of different quantitative trait genes for two energy balance traits, i.e., intake and storage. This region co-localizes with at least four other obesity-related QTLs, previously mapped to this region in other strains [49–51], including the *Obrq13* locus where the A/J-

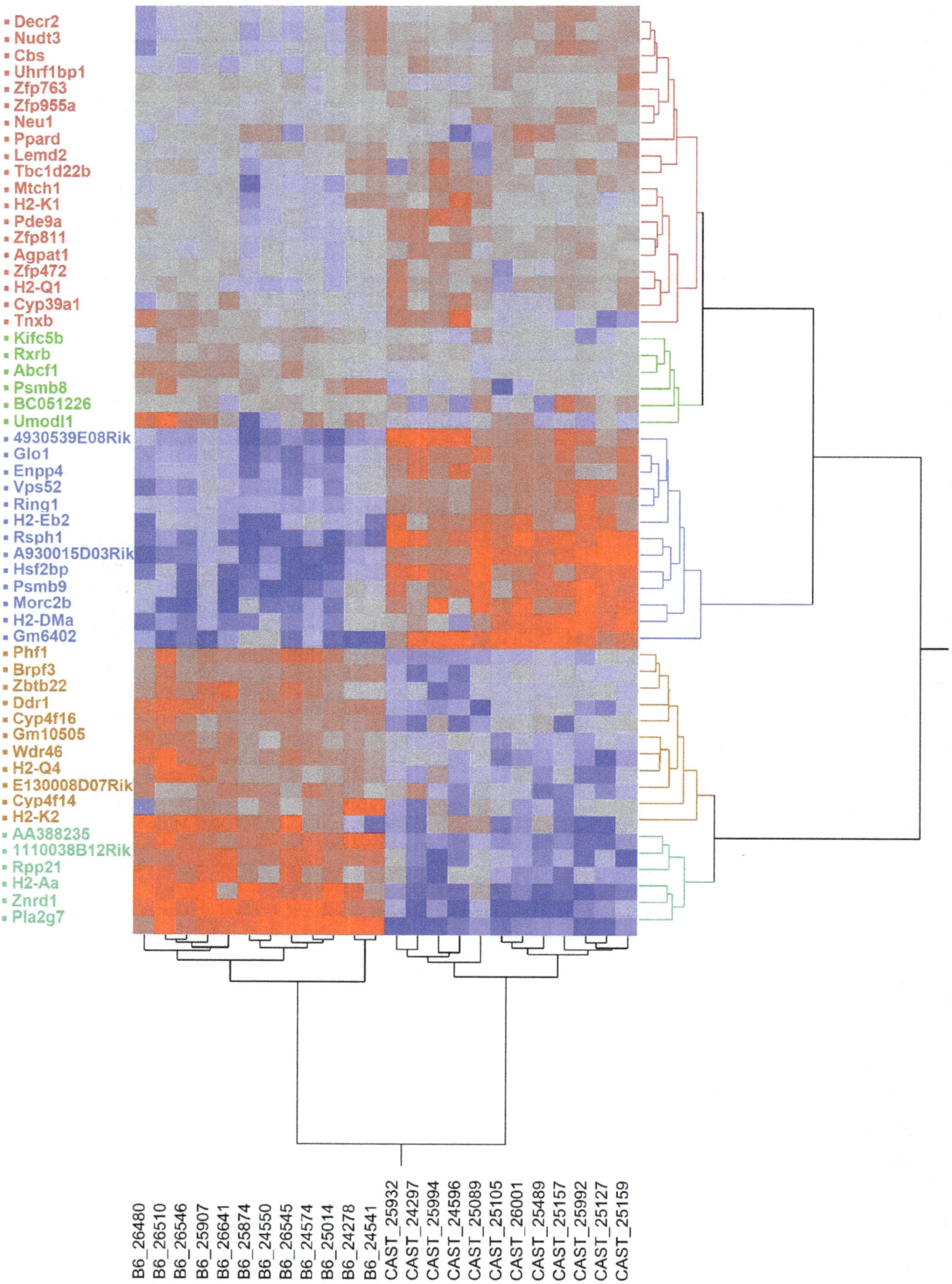

Figure 6. Hierarchical clustering of differential gene expression in the hypothalamus of non-recombinant B6.CAST-17.1-derived F_2 mice. Legend: Gene expression was measured in hypothalamus on day 2 of macronutrient selection diet using tag-based transcriptome sequencing (n = 12 individual libraries per genotype). Animals used in this experiment were either *cast/cast* (carbohydrate-preferring) or *b6/b6* (fat-preferring) within the subcongenic segment, and *b6/b6* across the rest of the genome. Genes were filtered based on ≥1.5-fold change and *P* value≤0.01 using

the DESeq method. The resulting 55 differentially expressed genes are displayed on the vertical axis; individual animals are clustered by genotype on the horizontal axis. Genes whose expression changed significantly in animals with the *cast/cast* genotype (higher carbohydrate consumption), relative to *b6/b6* (higher fat consumption), cluster together as increased (red) or decreased (blue) cells, with gray representing no change. Brighter shades of red and blue reflect higher degrees of up- and down-regulation.

derived allele protects against the diet-induced obesity that characterizes B6 males when fed a high-fat diet [37]. In the current study, the QTL for body fat gain after 10 d of macronutrient diet selection coincides with a locus for retroperitoneal fat pad weight identified previously in a C57BL/6J×CAST/Ei intercross [39]. The effect of the *cast* allele on body fat gain, although modest, was highly significant ($P<0.001$; Table 2) and occurred over a very short period of time. This finding is remarkable because the CAST strain has been characterized for obesity-resistant phenotypes [52,53] in studies employing a single, obesity-inducing diet of moderate fat content, while the *b6* allele usually confers obesity in mapping crosses [37,51].

Among the genes that exhibited differential mRNA expression between *cast/cast* and *b6/b6* in the hypothalamus, three showed ontologies with possible relevance to eating behavior phenotypes. Specifically, *Decr2*, *Ppard*, and *Agpat1* are associated with fatty acid oxidation or lipid metabolism and were down-regulated in *cast/cast* subcongenic F_2 compared to *b6/b6*. *Ppard* (peroxisome proliferator-activated receptor, delta), also known as *Nr1c2*, is a lipid-activated transcription factor that forms an obligate heterodimer with the retinoid × receptor to induce fatty acid transport and oxidation [54]. In our SAGE-Seq experiment (Table 3), *Ppard* and its binding partner *Rxrb* (retinoid × receptor beta) showed 3-fold and nearly 5-fold down-regulation, respectively, in the hypothalamus of carbohydrate- compared to fat-preferring mice. *Ppard* is the most highly expressed PPAR isoform in the CNS, where it is enriched in medio-basal hypothalamus [55], an area involved in energy homeostasis. Evidence for a role of *Ppard* in feeding behavior is limited, e.g., mice with neuron-specific deletion of *Ppard* showed a blunted feeding response to fasting [56]. There are no reports of an association of *Decr2* or *Agpat1* with food intake regulation. Nevertheless, *Decr2* encodes 2,4-dienoyl CoA reductase, an enzyme which catalyzes a reaction considered to be the rate-limiting step in the beta-oxidation of polyunsaturated fatty acids [57]. It is intriguing that expression of a QTL region gene with a key metabolic function in lipid metabolism is significantly decreased in the hypothalamus of carbohydrate-preferring mice. More studies will be needed to address whether the decreased expression of any of these lipid-related genes is a cause or consequence of macronutrient diet selection behavior.

Three positional candidates previously investigated by our group (*Clps*, *Glo1*, and *Glp1r*) reside within the critical interval. Pancreatic colipase (*Clps*) at 28.5 Mb, encodes a cofactor involved in fat digestion; however, sequencing uncovered only two silent nucleotide polymorphisms [8] and no expression differences were observed in the current study. *Glo1* (glyoxalase I), located at 30.59 Mb, is involved in the detoxification of methylglyoxal, a highly reactive dicarbonyl compound formed as a by-product of glycolysis, which can be toxic to the genome and proteome [58]. A mechanistic link between *Glo1* and food preferences has not been established. The strain difference in hypothalamic *Glo1* expression, observed in the current study, replicates previous observations of an up-regulation of *Glo1* in B6.CAST-17 carbohydrate-preferring congenic mice compared to fat-preferring wild type mice [21,22]. These observations initially led us to hypothesize that high carbohydrate consumption produces a higher flux of MG, leading to increased *Glo1* expression. However, our studies have consistently demonstrated a several-fold higher *Glo1* mRNA and enzyme activity in B6.CAST-17 congenic and subcongenic mice, whether animals were fed standard rodent chow, high- or low-carbohydrate diets, or macronutrient selection diets [20–22]. Together, these findings provide convincing evidence for intrinsic strain variation in *Glo1* expression, independent of the level of carbohydrate intake, and when combined with the lack of evidence for a functional SNP [21], weaken support for *Glo1* as a candidate for *Mnic1*. *Glp1r*, located nearby at ~30.90 Mb under a sharp LOD curve inflection (Figure 3), remains a strong candidate for *Mnic1* (preferential carbohydrate intake) based on its physiological roles in glucose homeostasis and gastric emptying. We demonstrated previously that *Glp1r* is differentially expressed in both the pancreas and stomach (yet in opposite direction), but not in hypothalamus of B6.CAST-17 congenic mice compared to B6 [21]. Furthermore, *Glp1r* expression in the stomach of F1 heterozygous mice showed allelic imbalance, i.e., a significant deviation from the theoretical 50:50 allelic ratio [23], suggesting that a stomach-specific, *cis*-acting regulatory element may underlie the strain difference in gastric *Glp1r* expression. Sequencing of *Glp1r* identified a non-synonymous coding SNP (C416Y) between strains which could have functional implications in the downstream regulation of protein activity [21]. These collective results, along with the close proximity of *Glp1r* near the refined *Mnic1* peak (32.49 Mb), support its further investigation and the consideration of a possible gastrointestinal mechanism.

We combined high-density SNP-mapping and subcongenic strain analyses to reduce the critical QTL interval for preferential carbohydrate and total food intake to a 19.0 Mb region on proximal Chr 17. We also obtained evidence that suggests the existence of separate QTLs determining food intake and short term body weight/fat gain and raises the prospect of distinct molecular genetic mechanisms for these energy balance phenotypes. To approach the question of which gene or genes within the fine-mapped 19.0 Mb interval could be causal, we examined available sequence data and gene ontologies, and performed comprehensive gene expression profiling in the hypothalamus of *cast/cast* and *b6/b6* non-recombinant F_2 controls. From these analyses, genes such as *Zfp811*, *Zfp870*, and *Btnl6* were shown to be differentially expressed and also to contain stop codons, although they have no known biology related to food intake regulation. In particular, *Decr2*, *Ppard* and *Agpat1* drew our attention as appealing candidates because of their involvement in lipid metabolism and down-regulation in carbohydrate-preferring animals. Additional studies, e.g., genetic modifications targeting priority candidates to determine their phenotypic effects, are required to uncover their potential contributions to the effects of *Mnic1/Kcal2/Tfv1*.

Supporting Information

Figure S1 Title: HQ17IIa mice, compared to WT controls, did not exhibit increased intake of carbohydrate kcal, total kcal and total food volume. Legend: Daily consumption of (A) carbohydrate/protein kcal (C/P) versus (B) fat/protein kcal (F/P), total kcal (C) and total food volume (D) in

HQ17IIa (CC) and wild type (WT) mice. Values are mean ± SE. The HQ17IIa subcongenic mouse strain is homozygous for CAST/EiJ (CAST) alleles from 3.19 to 26.08 Mb on MMU 17 (Figure 1). These results show clearly that HQ17IIa mice, compared to the appropriate B6 background controls, failed to exhibit the food intake phenotypes in question, making it extremely likely that the causal genetic variant is located distal to the 26.08 Mb breakpoint in the mutant.

Figure S2 Mean taste preference ratios of B6.CAST-17.1 WT and subcongenic mice using 48-hour two-bottle (tastant vs. distilled water) preference tests. Legend: Behavioral responses to sucrose (15, 30, and 60 mM) in B6.CAST-17.1 WT and subcongenic mice. The values are means ± SE (n = 7 per strain group). #$P<0.05$, *$P<0.001$ vs. a preference ratio of 0.50, using the one-sample *t*-test.

Figure S3 Biological process categories. Legend: WEB-based Gene SeT AnaLysis Toolkit (WebGestalt; http://bioinfo.vanderbilt.edu/webgestalt/) was used to organize the differentially expressed genes into Gene Ontology (GO) biological process categories. Nearly 50% of all 55 DE genes were classified as metabolism genes, of which seven were associated with lipids and/or fatty acids (*Decr2*, *Ppard*, *Agpat1*, *Tnxb*, *Neu1*, *Pla2g7*, *Cyp39a1*; all down-regulated), and two with carbohydrate metabolism (*Glo1*, *Neu1*; up-regulated).

Figure S4 Enriched gene ontology categories. Legend: WebGestalt was also used to visualize significantly enriched GO categories according to biological process, molecular function, and cellular component. For biological process, the most significantly enriched GO category was antigen processing and presentation (7 genes, *adjP*<0.0001). Approximately 36% of the 55 differentially expressed genes have molecular functions related to metal ion binding (*adjP* = 0.0001), including several transcription factors, e.g., *Ring1*, and members of the cytochrome P450 family. Long-chain fatty acid binding, represented by *Ppard* and *Cyp4f14*, was also noted (*adjP* = 0.004).

Table S1 SNP markers and their physical and genetic positions. Legend: SNP markers and their chromosomal positions according to http://genome.ucsc.edu. Mm9 sequence was obtained from the Build 37 assembly by NCBI and the Mouse Genome Sequencing Consortium. Excluded, markers not used in the analysis.

Table S2 Correlation matrix for nutrient intake phenotypes and baseline, pre-diet selection characteristics in the recombinant congenic F_2 population. Legend: Carbohydrate/protein (C/P), fat/protein (F/P), total kilocalories (kcal) and total food volume (g) consumed; body weight (BW 1), body fat (NMR1 fat), and body lean mass (NMR1 lean) when diet selection began. $^{a}P<0.05$; $^{b}P<0.01$; $^{c}P<0.001$, $^{d}P<0.0001$.

Table S3 Correlation matrix for nutrient intake phenotypes and post-diet selection characteristics in the recombinant congenic F_2 population. Legend: Carbohydrate/protein (C/P), fat/protein (F/P), total kilocalories (kcal) and total food volume (g) consumed; body weight (BW 2), body weight gain from BW 1 to BW 2; body fat (NMR2 fat) and body lean mass (NMR2 lean) after 10 d macronutrient diet selection; fat mass gain (Fat gain 12) and lean mass gain (lean gain12) over 10 d diet selection. $^{a}P<0.05$; $^{b}P<0.01$; $^{c}P<0.001$, $^{d}P<0.0001$.

Table S4 Correlation matrix for nutrient intake phenotypes and baseline, pre-diet selection characteristics in the non-recombinant congenic F_2 population. Legend: Carbohydrate/protein (C/P), fat/protein (F/P), total kilocalories (kcal) and total food volume (g) consumed; body weight (BW 1), body fat (NMR1 fat), and body lean mass (NMR1 lean) when diet selection began. $^{a}P<0.05$; $^{b}P<0.01$; $^{c}P<0.001$, $^{d}P<0.0001$.

Table S5 Correlation matrix for nutrient intake phenotypes and post-diet selection characteristics in the non-recombinant congenic F_2 population. Legend: Carbohydrate/protein (C/P), fat/protein (F/P), total kilocalories (kcal) and total food volume (g) consumed; body weight (BW 2), body weight gain from BW 1 to BW 2; body fat (NMR2 fat) and body lean mass (NMR2 lean) after 10 d macronutrient diet selection; fat mass gain (Fat gain 12) and lean mass gain (lean gain12) over 10 d diet selection. $^{a}P<0.05$; $^{b}P<0.01$; $^{c}P<0.001$, $^{d}P<0.0001$.

Table S6 Body weight and composition data for HQ17IIa sub-congenic mice. Legend: Values (mean ± SE) were obtained immediately before and then after the 10 d period of macronutrient diet selection.

Acknowledgments

We thank Aamir Zuberi for helpful discussions during the early stages of this project and Tuomo Rankinen, of the Human Genomics Laboratory at the Pennington Center, for performing the Illumina SNP genotyping. We also thank Michael Salbaum, Director of the Genomics Core Facility (GCF) at Pennington Biomedical for advice on the SAGE experiment, along with Susan Newman and Richard Carmouche for analytical and technical assistance, respectively.

Author Contributions

Conceived and designed the experiments: BKR JFM. Performed the experiments: BKR LMD GR JS. Analyzed the data: RGM BKR WDJ JS. Contributed reagents/materials/analysis tools: JFM. Contributed to the writing of the manuscript: BKR RGM CK.

References

1. Grimm ER, Steinle NI (2011) Genetics of eating behavior: established and emerging concepts. Nutr Rev 69: 52–60.
2. Reed DR, Bachmanov AA, Beauchamp GK, Tordoff MG, Price RA (1997) Heritable variation in food preferences and their contribution to obesity. Behav Genet 27: 373–387.
3. Rankinen T, Bouchard C (2006) Genetics of food intake and eating behavior phenotypes in humans. Annu Rev Nutr 26: 413–434.
4. Cai G, Cole SA, Bastarrachea RA, Maccluer JW, Blangero J, et al. (2004) Quantitative trait locus determining dietary macronutrient intakes is located on human chromosome 2p22. Am J Clin Nutr 80: 1410–1414.
5. Cai G, Cole SA, Butte N, Bacino C, Diego V, et al. (2006) A quantitative trait locus on chromosome 18q for physical activity and dietary intake in Hispanic children. Obesity (Silver Spring) 14: 1596–1604.
6. Choquette AC, Lemieux S, Tremblay A, Chagnon YC, Bouchard C, et al. (2008) Evidence of a quantitative trait locus for energy and macronutrient intakes on chromosome 3q27.3: the Quebec Family Study. Am J Clin Nutr 88: 1142–1148.
7. Collaku A, Rankinen T, Rice T, Leon AS, Rao DC, et al. (2004) A genome-wide linkage scan for dietary energy and nutrient intakes: the Health, Risk Factors, Exercise Training, and Genetics (HERITAGE) Family Study. Am J Clin Nutr 79: 881–886.

8. Smith Richards BK, Belton BN, Poole AC, Mancuso JJ, Churchill GA, et al. (2002) QTL analysis of self-selected macronutrient diet intake: fat, carbohydrate, and total kilocalories. Physiol Genomics 11: 205–217.
9. Schoeller DA, Thomas D, Archer E, Heymsfield SB, Blair SN, et al. (2013) Self-report-based estimates of energy intake offer an inadequate basis for scientific conclusions. Am J Clin Nutr 97: 1413–1415.
10. Allan MF, Eisen EJ, Pomp D (2005) Genomic Mapping of Direct and Correlated Responses to Long-Term Selection for Rapid Growth Rate in Mice.
11. Mathes WF, Aylor DL, Miller DR, Churchill GA, Chesler EJ, et al. (2011) Architecture of energy balance traits in emerging lines of the Collaborative Cross. Am J Physiol Endocrinol Metab 300: E1124–1134.
12. Smith Richards BK, Belton BN, York B, Volaufova J (2004) Mice bearing Acads mutation display altered postingestive but not 5-s orosensory response to dietary fat. Am J Physiol Regul Integr Comp Physiol 286: R311–319.
13. Smith BK, West DB, York DA (1997) Carbohydrate versus fat intake: differing patterns of macronutrient selection in two inbred mouse strains. Am J Physiol 272: R357–362.
14. Smith BK, Andrews PK, West DB (2000) Macronutrient diet selection in thirteen mouse strains. Am J Physiol Regul Integr Comp Physiol 278: R797–805.
15. Smith BK, Andrews PK, York DA, West DB (1999) Divergence in proportional fat intake in AKR/J and SWR/J mice endures across diet paradigms. Am J Physiol 277: R776–785.
16. Mayer J, Dickie MM, Bates MW, Vitale JJ (1951) Free selection of nutrients by hereditarily obese mice. Science 113: 745–746.
17. South T, Huang XF (2006) Phenotypic variations between a fat-preferring strain and a macronutrient non-preferring strain of mouse. Diabetes Obes Metab 8: 302–310.
18. Koegler FH, Schaffhauser RO, Mynatt RL, York DA, Bray GA (1999) Macronutrient diet intake of the lethal yellow agouti (Ay/a) mouse. Physiol Behav 67: 809–812.
19. Alexander J, Chang GQ, Dourmashkin JT, Leibowitz SF (2006) Distinct phenotypes of obesity-prone AKR/J, DBA2J and C57BL/6J mice compared to control strains. Int J Obes (Lond) 30: 50–59.
20. Kumar KG, DiCarlo LM, Volaufova J, Zuberi AR, Richards BK (2010) Increased physical activity cosegregates with higher intake of carbohydrate and total calories in a subcongenic mouse strain. Mamm Genome 21: 52–63.
21. Kumar KG, Poole AC, York B, Volaufova J, Zuberi A, et al. (2007) Quantitative trait loci for carbohydrate and total energy intake on mouse chromosome 17: congenic strain confirmation and candidate gene analyses (Glo1, Glp1r). Am J Physiol Regul Integr Comp Physiol 292: R207–216.
22. Kumar KG, Smith Richards BK (2008) Transcriptional profiling of chromosome 17 quantitative trait Loci for carbohydrate and total calorie intake in a mouse congenic strain reveals candidate genes and pathways. J Nutrigenet Nutrigenomics 1: 155–171.
23. Kumar KG, Byerley LO, Volaufova J, Drucker DJ, Churchill GA, et al. (2008) Genetic variation in Glp1r expression influences the rate of gastric emptying in mice. Am J Physiol Regul Integr Comp Physiol 294: R362–371.
24. Arbilly M, Pisante A, Devor M, Darvasi A (2006) An integrative approach for the identification of quantitative trait loci. Anim Genet 37 Suppl 1: 7–9.
25. Horvat S, Medrano JF (2001) Lack of Socs2 expression causes the high-growth phenotype in mice. Genomics 72: 209–212.
26. Butler AA, Kozak LP (2010) A recurring problem with the analysis of energy expenditure in genetic models expressing lean and obese phenotypes. Diabetes 59: 323–329.
27. Broman KW, Wu H, Sen S, Churchill GA (2003) R/qtl: QTL mapping in experimental crosses. Bioinformatics 19: 889–890.
28. R Core Team (2013) R: A language and environment for statistical computing. R-devel-r62600 ed. Vienna, Austria.
29. Churchill GA, Doerge RW (1994) Empirical threshold values for quantitative trait mapping. Genetics 138: 963–971.
30. Manichaikul A, Moon JY, Sen S, Yandell BS, Broman KW (2009) A model selection approach for the identification of quantitative trait loci in experimental crosses, allowing epistasis. Genetics 181: 1077–1086.
31. Cox A, Sheehan SM, Klöting I, Paigen B, Korstanje R (2010) Combining QTL data for HDL cholesterol levels from two different species leads to smaller confidence intervals. Heredity 105: 426–432.
32. Berthoud HR, Munzberg H, Richards BK, Morrison CD (2012) Neural and metabolic regulation of macronutrient intake and selection. Proc Nutr Soc 71: 390–400.
33. Anders S, Huber W (2010) Differential expression analysis for sequence count data. Genome Biol 11: R106.
34. Wang J, Duncan D, Shi Z, Zhang B (2013) WEB-based GEne SeT AnaLysis Toolkit (WebGestalt): update 2013. Nucleic Acids Res 41: W77–83.
35. Mather R, Jinks J (1977) Introduction to Biometrical Genetics. New York: Cornell University Press.
36. Flint J (2011) Mapping quantitative traits and strategies to find quantitative trait genes. Methods 53: 163–174.
37. Millward CA, Burrage LC, Shao H, Sinasac DS, Kawasoe JH, et al. (2009) Genetic factors for resistance to diet-induced obesity and associated metabolic traits on mouse chromosome 17. Mamm Genome 20: 71–82.
38. Cheverud JM, Vaughn TT, Pletscher LS, Peripato AC, Adams ES, et al. (2001) Genetic architecture of adiposity in the cross of LG/J and SM/J inbred mice. Mamm Genome 12: 3–12.
39. Smith Richards BK, Belton BN, Poole AC, Mancuso JJ, Churchill GA, et al. (2002) QTL analysis of self-selected macronutrient diet intake: fat, carbohydrate, and total kilocalories. Physiological Genomics 11: 205–217.
40. Sim NL, Kumar P, Hu J, Henikoff S, Schneider G, et al. (2012) SIFT web server: predicting effects of amino acid substitutions on proteins. Nucleic Acids Res 40: W452–457.
41. Smith JD (2008) Quantitative Trait Locus Mapping to Identify Genes for Complex Traits in Mice. In: Walker JM, Rapley R, editors. Molecular Biomethods Handbook. 2nd ed. Totowa, NJ: Humana Press.
42. Takasaki M, Honma T, Yanaka M, Sato K, Shinohara N, et al. (2012) Continuous intake of a high-fat diet beyond one generation promotes lipid accumulation in liver and white adipose tissue of female mice. J Nutr Biochem 23: 640–645.
43. Patterson RL, Boehning D, Snyder SH (2004) Inositol 1,4,5-trisphosphate receptors as signal integrators. Annu Rev Biochem 73: 437–465.
44. Nakashima K, Ninomiya Y (1999) Transduction for sweet taste of saccharin may involve both inositol 1,4,5-trisphosphate and cAMP pathways in the fungiform taste buds in C57BL mice. Cell Physiol Biochem 9: 90–98.
45. Hegg CC, Jia C, Chick WS, Restrepo D, Hansen A (2010) Microvillous cells expressing IP3 receptor type 3 in the olfactory epithelium of mice. Eur J Neurosci 32: 1632–1645.
46. Hisatsune C, Yasumatsu K, Takahashi-Iwanaga H, Ogawa N, Kuroda Y, et al. (2007) Abnormal taste perception in mice lacking the type 3 inositol 1,4,5-trisphosphate receptor. J Biol Chem 282: 37225–37231.
47. Tordoff MG, Jaji SA, Marks JM, Ellis HT (2012) Macronutrient choice of BTBR.NZW mice congenic for a 21-gene region of chromosome 17. Physiol Behav 106: 556–561.
48. Marissal-Arvy N, Diane A, Moisan MP, Larue-Achagiotis C, Tridon C, et al. (2013) QTLs influencing carbohydrate and fat choice in a LOU/CxFischer 344 F2 rat population. Obesity (Silver Spring).
49. Stylianou IM, Korstanje R, Li R, Sheehan S, Paigen B, et al. (2006) Quantitative trait locus analysis for obesity reveals multiple networks of interacting loci. Mamm Genome 17: 22–36.
50. Taylor BA, Phillips SJ (1997) Obesity QTLs on mouse chromosomes 2 and 17. Genomics 43: 249–257.
51. Ishimori N, Li R, Kelmenson PM, Korstanje R, Walsh KA, et al. (2004) Quantitative trait loci that determine plasma lipids and obesity in C57BL/6J and 129S1/SvImJ inbred mice. J Lipid Res 45: 1624–1632.
52. Mehrabian M, Wen PZ, Fisler J, Davis RC, Lusis AJ (1998) Genetic loci controlling body fat, lipoprotein metabolism, and insulin levels in a multifactorial mouse model. J Clin Invest 101: 2485–2496.
53. York B, Lei K, West DB (1996) Sensitivity to dietary obesity linked to a locus on chromosome 15 in a CAST/Ei x C57BL/6J F2 intercross. Mamm Genome 7: 677–681.
54. Kleiner S, Nguyen-Tran V, Bare O, Huang X, Spiegelman B, et al. (2009) PPAR{delta} agonism activates fatty acid oxidation via PGC-1{alpha} but does not increase mitochondrial gene expression and function. J Biol Chem 284: 18624–18633.
55. Moreno S, Farioli-Vecchioli S, Ceru MP (2004) Immunolocalization of peroxisome proliferator-activated receptors and retinoid X receptors in the adult rat CNS. Neuroscience 123: 131–145.
56. Kocalis HE, Turney MK, Printz RL, Laryea GN, Muglia LJ, et al. (2012) Neuron-specific deletion of peroxisome proliferator-activated receptor delta (PPARdelta) in mice leads to increased susceptibility to diet-induced obesity. PLoS One 7: e42981.
57. Wanders RJ, Waterham HR (2006) Biochemistry of mammalian peroxisomes revisited. Annu Rev Biochem 75: 295–332.
58. Thornalley PJ (2003) Glyoxalase I–structure, function and a critical role in the enzymatic defence against glycation. Biochem Soc Trans 31: 1343–1348.

18

Shifting the Circadian Rhythm of Feeding in Mice Induces Gastrointestinal, Metabolic and Immune Alterations Which Are Influenced by Ghrelin and the Core Clock Gene Bmal1

Jorien Laermans, Charlotte Broers, Kelly Beckers, Laurien Vancleef, Sandra Steensels, Theo Thijs, Jan Tack, Inge Depoortere*

Gut Peptide Research Lab, Translational Research Center for Gastrointestinal Disorders, KU Leuven - University of Leuven, Leuven, Belgium

Abstract

Background: In our 24-hour society, an increasing number of people are required to be awake and active at night. As a result, the circadian rhythm of feeding is seriously compromised. To mimic this, we subjected mice to restricted feeding (RF), a paradigm in which food availability is limited to short and unusual times of day. RF induces a food-anticipatory increase in the levels of the hunger hormone ghrelin. We aimed to investigate whether ghrelin triggers the changes in body weight and gastric emptying that occur during RF. Moreover, the effect of genetic deletion of the core clock gene Bmal1 on these physiological adaptations was studied.

Methods: Wild-type, ghrelin receptor knockout and Bmal1 knockout mice were fed *ad libitum* or put on RF with a normal or high-fat diet (HFD). Plasma ghrelin levels were measured by radioimmunoassay. Gastric contractility was studied *in vitro* in muscle strips and *in vivo* (^{13}C breath test). Cytokine mRNA expression was quantified and infiltration of immune cells was assessed histologically.

Results: The food-anticipatory increase in plasma ghrelin levels induced by RF with normal chow was abolished in HFD-fed mice. During RF, body weight restoration was facilitated by ghrelin and Bmal1. RF altered cytokine mRNA expression levels and triggered contractility changes resulting in an accelerated gastric emptying, independent from ghrelin signaling. During RF with a HFD, Bmal1 enhanced neutrophil recruitment to the stomach, increased gastric IL-1α expression and promoted gastric contractility changes.

Conclusions: This is the first study demonstrating that ghrelin and Bmal1 regulate the extent of body weight restoration during RF, whereas Bmal1 controls the type of inflammatory infiltrate and contractility changes in the stomach. Disrupting the circadian rhythm of feeding induces a variety of diet-dependent metabolic, immune and gastrointestinal alterations, which may explain the higher prevalence of obesity and immune-related gastrointestinal disorders among shift workers.

Editor: Ralph E. Mistlberger, Simon Fraser University, Canada

Funding: Jorien Laermans is supported by the Research Foundation Flanders (FWO) as an aspirant (11A8414N) (http://www.fwo.be/). Sandra Steensels is holder of a PhD grant of the Agency for Innovation by Science and Technology (IWT) (http://www.iwt.be/). This work is supported by a Methusalem grant from the University of Leuven for research on "The Brain-Gut Axis in Health and Disease: from Mucosal Integrity to Cortical Processing." The funders had no role in study design, data collection and analysis, decision to publish, or preparation of the manuscript.

Competing Interests: The authors have declared that no competing interests exist.

* Email: inge.depoortere@med.kuleuven.be

Introduction

Not only the amount or type of food we ingest, but also the timing of food consumption seems to play a crucial role in the development of obesity and associated metabolic disorders [1]. In our 24-hour society, people are voluntarily shifting their normal activity patterns to unusual times of day, for instance by shift working or frequent time zone traveling. As a result, they are seriously compromising their circadian system, an evolutionary conserved timekeeping mechanism that generates daily behavioral rhythms that allow organisms to actively anticipate and adapt to predictable environmental changes, thereby increasing the likelihood of survival [2]. In mammals, this timing system is comprised, in a hierarchical way, of a hypothalamic master clock and peripheral oscillators in numerous body cells. At the molecular level, circadian rhythms depend on the concerted co-expression of a set of clock genes (Clock, Bmal1, Per1-3, Cry1-2) [2]. These genes participate in transcription-translation feedback loops, through which they not only regulate their own activity, but also that of downstream clock-controlled genes.

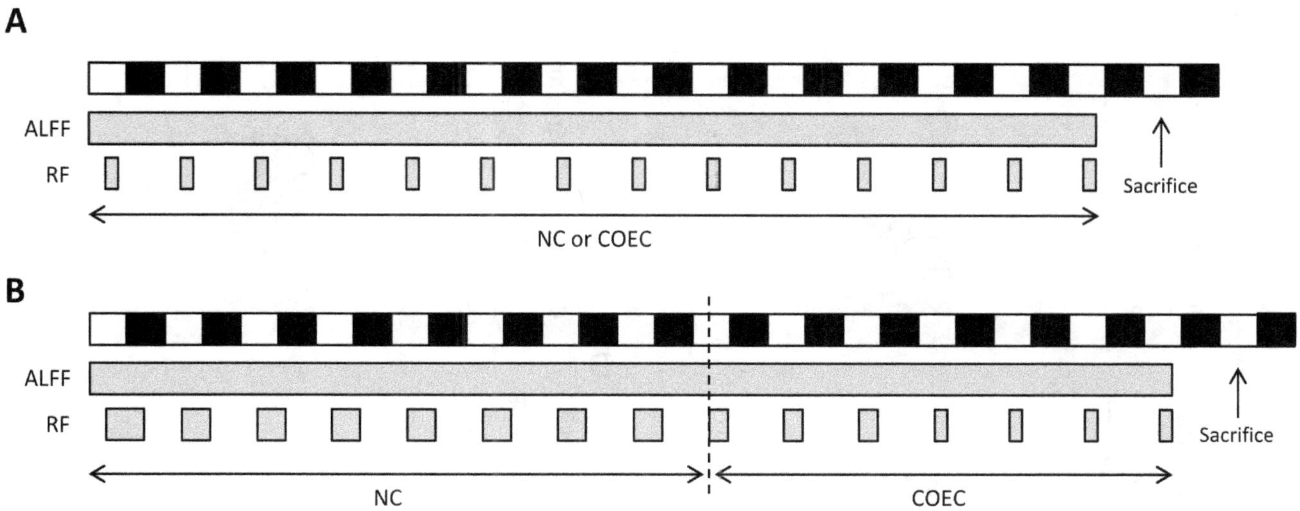

Figure 1. Restricted feeding protocols. (**A**) Scheme of the standard RF schedule in which food availability was limited to 4 hours a day (ZT 5–9) from day 1 until day 14. White and black bars represent times of lights on and off, respectively. Gray bars represent times of food availability of either normal chow (NC) or canola oil-enriched chow (COEC). (**B**) Scheme of the adapted RF schedule in which food availability was gradually decreased during the experiment. Both groups received NC for 8 days (RF group: 1 day 12 h food available (ZT 5–17) and 7 days 9 h food available (ZT 5–14)) and COEC during the remaining 7 days (RF group: 3 days 6 h food available (ZT 5–11) and 4 days 4 h food available (ZT 5–9)). Note that the time of onset of food availability is the same each day (ZT 5).

In order to maintain a near 24 h-rhythm, circadian clocks need to be entrained to daily environmental cues. Under normal circumstances, the master clock is synchronized by the light/dark-cycle and will further entrain the peripheral clocks. However, during restricted feeding (RF), when food availability is limited to short and abnormal times of the day, the phase of peripheral clock gene expression becomes uncoupled from the master clock and shifts in order to realign with mealtime [3]. The entrainment of these peripheral clocks by feeding cues is still present in mice given lesions in the master clock [4], suggesting that the circadian function of feeding depends on separate food-entrainable oscillators (FEOs). The FEOs predict food availability and ensure that the organism retains a positive energy balance, even if food is available at unusual times. The anatomical location of these FEOs remains elusive despite extensive research. Recently, LeSauter *et al.* found that the expression of ghrelin and of the clock genes PER1 and PER2 within the ghrelin-secreting cells of the stomach was rhythmic and entrained by food availability [5]. Hence, they proposed that these ghrelin-secreting cells might serve as one of the FEOs, producing a timed ghrelin output signal that acts widely at both brain and peripheral sites.

Ghrelin is a 28-amino acid peptide mainly secreted by the stomach [6]. The octanoylation of ghrelin at Ser^3 by ghrelin O-acyltransferase (GOAT) is crucial to its biological activity. Besides being the only circulating hormone that stimulates food intake, ghrelin increases body weight by preventing fat utilization, accelerates gastric emptying and initiates hunger contractions in the fasted state [7]. Plasma ghrelin levels fluctuate diurnally, with a nocturnal elevation in humans [8]. In addition, levels surge during fasting and decrease postprandially to dictate the timing of meals [9,10]. Studies in animals subjected to RF have highlighted this tight relationship between ghrelin and timing of feeding. Indeed, a preprandial rise in plasma ghrelin levels is observed in anticipation of a scheduled meal in rodents [11,12]. Nevertheless, although controversial, the majority of the studies in ghrelin receptor knockout (GHSR-KO) and ghrelin knockout mice reveal that ghrelin and its receptor are not necessary for food-anticipatory behavior [13].

This study aimed to examine whether ghrelin might serve as an output signal of the FEO that triggers physiological adaptations to alterations in the circadian rhythm of feeding induced by RF. Here we showed for the first time that RF not only results in changes in food intake, body weight and gastric emptying, but also induces alterations in gastric proinflammatory cytokine expression and myeloperoxidase (MPO) activity. Studies in wild-type (WT) and GHSR-KO mice revealed that ghrelin was merely involved in the restoration of body weight loss during RF. Next, we investigated whether the core clock gene Bmal1 might serve as the key driver behind the adaptations by studying the effects of RF in Bmal1 knockout (Bmal1-KO) mice, which is the only single clock gene knockout in which the mouse loses all rhythmic behavioral activity [14]. We found that Bmal1 not only determines the extent of body weight restoration during RF, but also defines the type of infiltrating immune cells and influences the changes in contractility prior to food availability during RF with a high-fat diet.

Materials and Methods

Ethics Statement

All mouse experiments were approved by the Ethical committee for Animal Experiments of the KU Leuven (project number P106/2011). All efforts were made to minimize animal suffering. After being anesthetized using a mixture of ketamine and xylazine, mice were sacrificed by decapitation.

Animals

Breeding couples of mice heterozygous for GHSR and Bmal1 were kindly provided by Janssen Pharmaceutica (Beerse, Belgium) [15] and R. Lijnen (KU Leuven, Leuven, Belgium) [16], respectively. All KO mice and their WT littermates were bred in the animal facility of the KU Leuven and genotyped by polymerase chain reaction (PCR) analysis performed on total

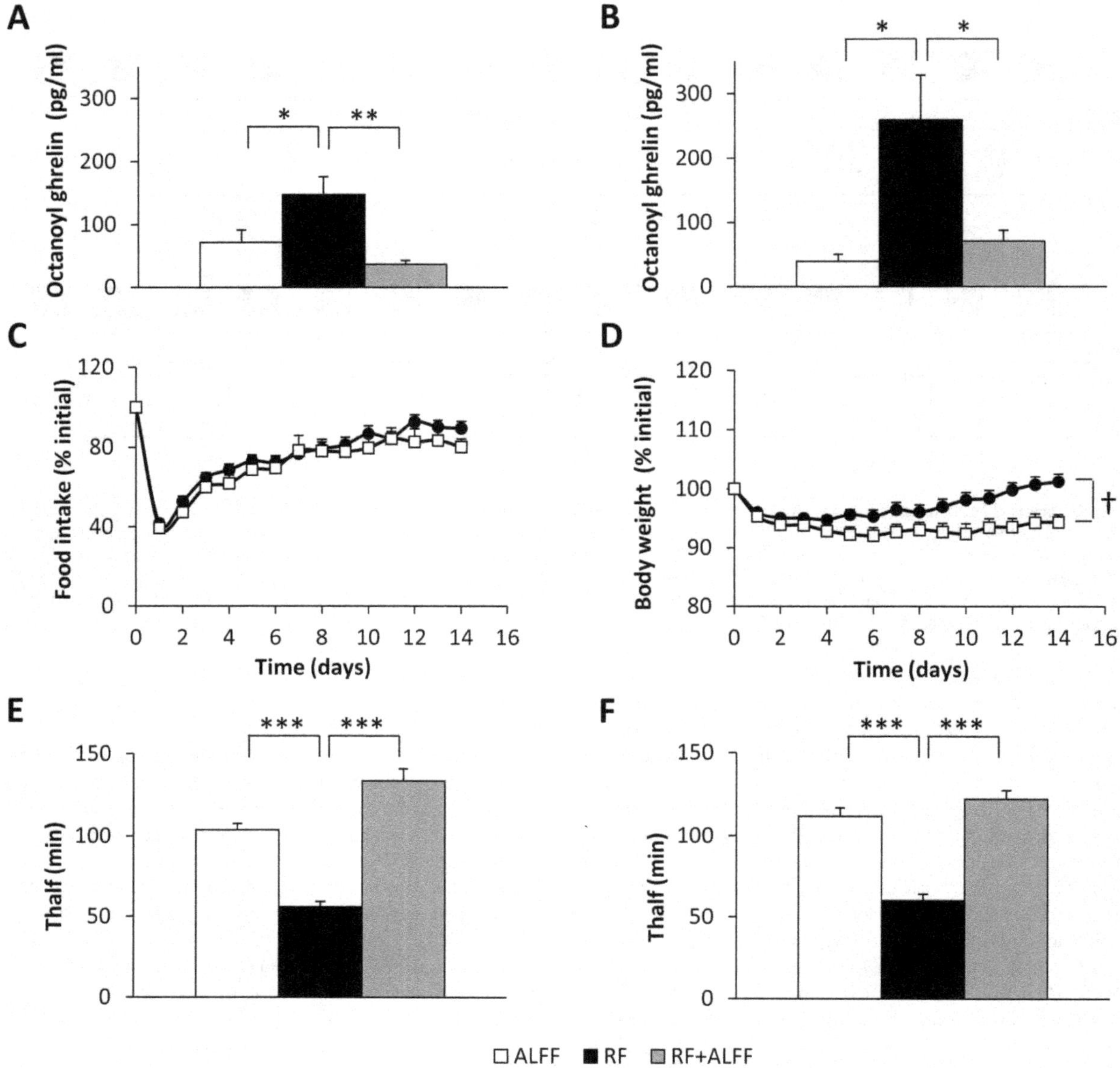

Figure 2. Role of ghrelin in the RF-induced changes in food intake, body weight and gastric emptying. (**A–B**) Plasma octanoyl ghrelin levels in WT (n = 6/group) (**A**) or GHSR-KO mice (n = 2–5/group) (**B**) under ALFF, RF or RF+ALFF conditions. (**C–D**) Food intake and body weight of WT (●)(n = 21) or GHSR-KO (□)(n = 17) mice on RF. (**E–F**) Gastric emptying in WT (n = 12) (**E**) or GHSR-KO mice (n = 10) (**F**) under ALFF, RF or RF+ALFF conditions. **P*<0.05,***P*<0.01,****P*<0.001 vs. RF; † *P*<0.05 WT vs. GHSR-KO.

genomic DNA from the tail. Mice were housed (20–22°C) under a 12-h/12-h light/dark-cycle (lights on at 7 AM) and had *ad libitum* access to food and drinking water, unless stated otherwise.

Diets

During RF experiments, mice were fed normal chow (Ssniff R/M-H, Ssniff Spezialdiäten GmbH, Soest, Germany; 9% kcal from fat) or canola oil-enriched chow (COEC) (powdered normal chow mixed with canola oil, 4:1 wt/wt; 47% kcal from fat). When using COEC, mice were allowed to habituate to the newly introduced diet before starting the actual experiment.

Experimental design

Standard RF schedule. Mice were randomly assigned to either of two groups, subjected to different feeding regimes during two weeks. The RF group only had access to food for 4 hours between *zeitgeber* time (ZT) 5 and 9 (where ZT 0 is lights-on by convention), while the other group received food *ad libitum* (Figure 1*A*). In parallel with the RF group, food was removed from the *ad libitum* group at ZT 9 the day before being sacrificed. Hence, this group was termed *ad libitum* fed fasted (ALFF). A third group of mice, hereinafter referred to as the RF+ALFF group, was first subjected to two weeks of RF and then refed *ad libitum* during a period of four weeks. All mice were sacrificed at ZT 4.5.

Adapted RF schedule with gradually decreased food availability. WT and Bmal1-KO mice were either fed *ad libitum* or subjected to a RF schedule in which food availability was gradually decreased and chow was enriched with canola oil to increase the caloric content of the meal [17] (Figure 1*B*). Because of a low tolerance rate of the *ad libitum*-fed Bmal1-KO mice towards the amount of fat in the COEC, resulting in 80% mortality, both ALFF and RF mice received normal chow during

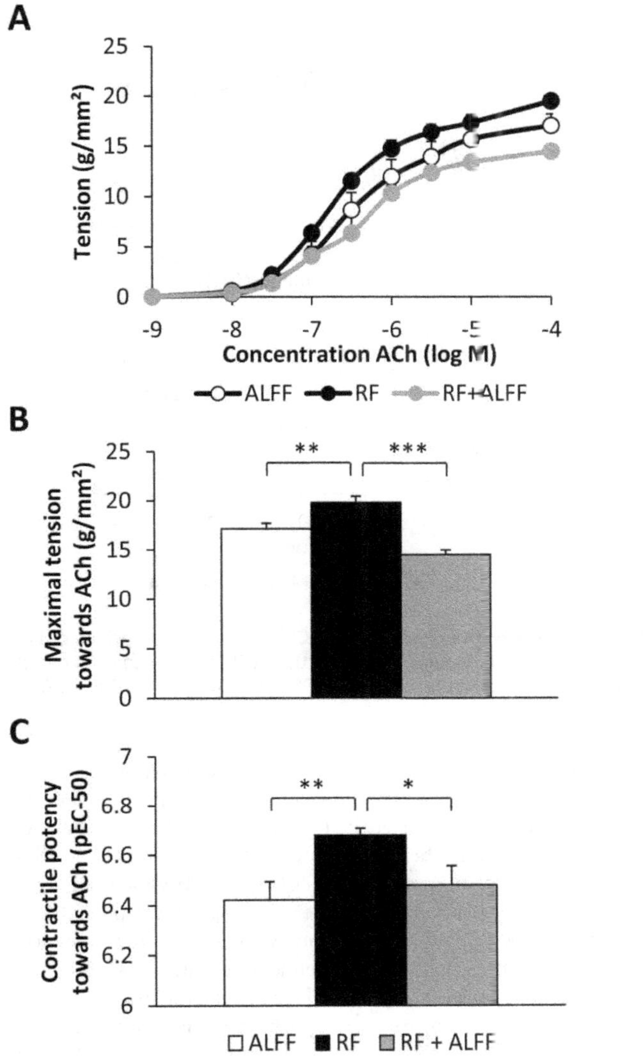

Figure 3. RF with normal chow induces hypercontractility towards ACh in gastric smooth muscle strips. (**A**) Concentration-response curve towards ACh in fundic smooth muscle strips of normal chow-fed WT mice under different feeding conditions. (**B**) Maximal tension and (**C**) contractile potency (pEC-50 value) derived from the concentration-response curves. (ALFF and RF: N = 4 mice, n = 2–3 strips/mouse; RF+ALFF: N = 3 mice, n = 1–3 strips/mouse). * $P < 0.05$, ** $P < 0.01$, *** $P < 0.001$ vs. RF.

the first 8 days and COEC during the next 7 days. All mice were sacrificed at ZT 4.5 after a 19.5 h fast.

Ghrelin radioimmunoassay

Blood samples (1 mg/mL EDTA and 4 mM AEBSF) were centrifuged and acidified (10% HCl). After extraction on Sep-Pak C18 column, radioimmunoassay was performed as previously described [18].

Gastric emptying. Gastric emptying was measured using the ^{13}C octanoic acid breath test, as described previously [15,19]. T_{half} is the time point at which 50% of the total amount of $^{13}CO_2$ was exhaled.

In vitro contractility studies

Mucosal-free fundic smooth muscle strips were suspended along their circular axis in a Krebs-filled tissue bath. Concentration-response curves to acetylcholine (ACh) (10^{-9} to 10^{-4} mol/L) were established isometrically. The maximal tension (g/mm^2) and concentration necessary to induce 50% of the maximal contraction (EC-50) were calculated. Neural responses were elicited by electrical field stimulation (EFS) (pulse duration 1 ms, train duration 10 s, amplitude 6 V) at increasing frequencies (0.5–16 Hz) [20]. On-relaxations were expressed relative to the response induced by 10^{-5} mol/L nitroglycerin. The area under the curve (AUC) of the off-contractions was expressed as g/mm^2.

Quantitative real-time PCR

Total RNA was isolated from stomach using the Qiagen RNeasy Mini Kit (Qiagen, Hilden, Germany) and reverse transcribed to cDNA using SuperScript II Reverse Transcriptase (Invitrogen, Carlsbad, CA, USA). Quantitative real-time PCR was performed as previously described [15]. Primer sequences were as follows: GAPDH: forward CCCCAATgTgTCCgTCgTg, reverse gCCTgCTTCACCACCTTCT; IL-1β: forward gACCTTCCAg-gATGAggACA, reverse TCCATTgAggTggAgAgCTT; IL-6: forward CCATAgCTACCTggAgTACATg, reverse TggAA-ATTggggTAggAAggAC; IL-1α: forward gAgAgCCgggTgACAg-TATC, reverse ACTTCTgCCTgACgAgCTTC; ghrelin: forward CCAgAggACAgAggACAAgC, reverse ACATCgAAgggAgCAT-TgAA; GOAT: forward ACCCgggCCAggTACCT, reverse ACCCATggCAgCAAAAgC.

MPO activity assay

Fundic MPO activity was determined using the O-dianisidine-H_2O_2 method. In brief, tissue samples were homogenized in 50 mM phosphate buffer containing 14 mM hexadecyltrimethyl ammonium bromide (HTAB; pH 6.0). After two freeze-thaw cycles, samples were centrifuged. After adding the supernatant to an O-dianisidine buffer (50 mM phosphate buffer, 0.52 mM O-dianisidine and 0.15 mM H_2O_2), changes in absorbance were measured at 460 nm. Results were expressed as units of MPO per mg tissue, where 1 unit of MPO was defined as the amount of enzyme degrading 1 µmol H_2O_2 per minute at 25°C.

H&E and peroxidase staining

Frozen fundic sections (6 µm) were stained with hematoxylin and eosin. The number of polymorphonuclear (PMN) cells was determined by counting 10 randomly chosen representative high-power fields (40x). The number of peroxidase-positive cells was quantified in sections stained with Hanker Yates reagent (Sigma-Aldrich, St. Louis, MO, USA).

Statistical analysis

Results are presented as means ± SEM. Data were analyzed using Statistica 11 (StatSoft Inc., Tulsa, OK, USA). Data obtained at different time points in the same mice were analyzed using repeated measures ANOVA. For the EFS-induced responses, post hoc Bonferroni testing was used to detect overall differences between feeding conditions followed by planned comparison testing. Differences between the COEC-fed ALFF and RF groups were detected with an unpaired Student's t-test. All other data were analyzed using a one- or two-way ANOVA, followed by post hoc Bonferroni testing. Significance was accepted at the 5% level.

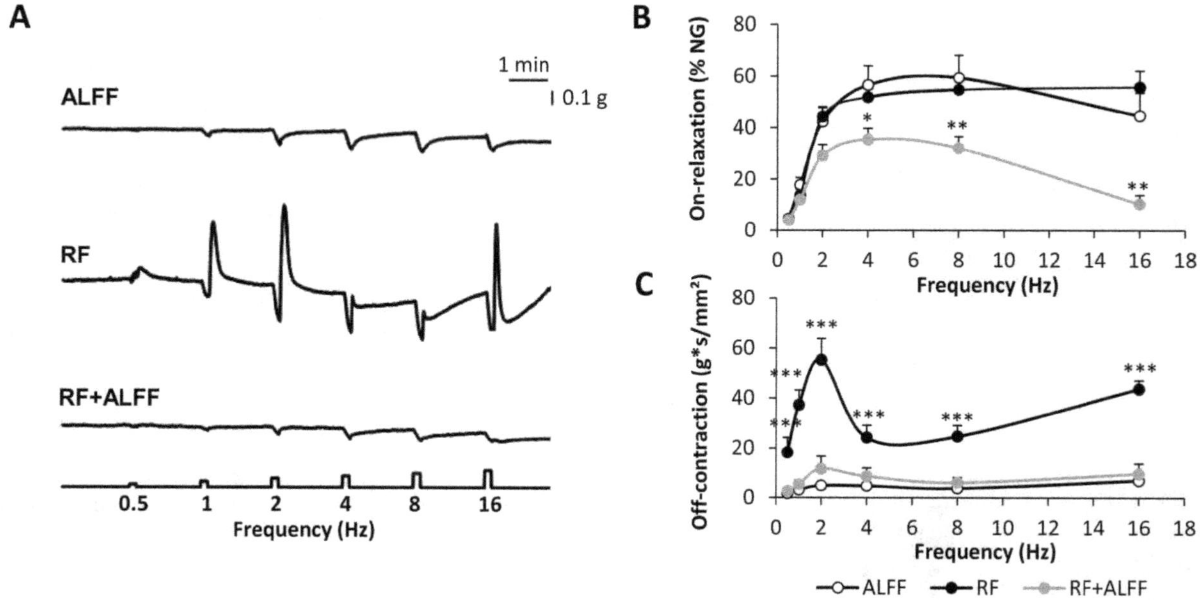

Figure 4. RF with normal chow causes neural hyperexcitability of gastric smooth muscle strips. (**A–C**) Representative tracings of EFS-induced neural responses (**A**) and graphs summarizing changes in on-relaxations (**B**) and post-stimulus off-contractions (**C**) of fundic smooth muscle strips of NC-fed WT mice under ALFF, RF or RF+ALFF conditions (N = 3–4 mice/group, n = 1–3 strips/mouse). *$P<0.05$, **$P<0.01$, ***$P<0.001$ vs. ALFF.

Results

1. Role of ghrelin in the physiological adaptations induced by RF

RF increases plasma ghrelin levels. Two weeks of RF increased ($P<0.05$) plasma concentrations of octanoyl (Figure 2*A*) and total ghrelin (RF: 2337±204 vs. ALFF: 1333±243 pg/ml; $P<0.01$) in WT mice. GHSR-KO mice even displayed a 5.3 fold higher rise in octanoyl ghrelin levels (Figure 2*B*). A similar effect was observed on total ghrelin levels (data not shown). In both genotypes, refeeding the mice *ad libitum* for four weeks after two weeks of RF (RF+ALFF) normalized plasma ghrelin levels.

RF induces body weight loss. The role of ghrelin signaling in the RF-induced changes in food intake and body weight was studied in WT and GHSR-KO mice. In both genotypes, food intake and body weight dropped to a similar extent at the beginning of the RF schedule (Figure 2 *C–D*). While food intake recovered in both genotypes by the end of the 2-week RF schedule, body weight of GHSR-KO mice remained 9% lower ($P<0.05$) compared to WT mice.

RF accelerates gastric emptying. Since ghrelin displays gastroprokinetic properties, gastric emptying rate during RF was assessed. RF accelerated ($P<0,001$) gastric emptying in both WT and GHSR-KO mice to a similar extent, suggesting that this effect is not mediated via the increase in ghrelin levels (Figure 2 *E–F*). Refeeding the mice *ad libitum* (RF+ALFF) normalized gastric emptying in both genotypes.

To identify the mechanisms involved in the acceleration of gastric emptying, *in vitro* contractility studies were performed with fundic smooth muscle strips of WT mice. Figure 3A depicts the concentration-response curves towards ACh for the three feeding conditions. RF resulted in a fully reversible increase in maximal tension ($P<0.01$) and contractile potency (pEC_{50}) ($P<0.001$) towards ACh (Figure 3 *B–C*). This coincided with a significant increase in the cross-sectional area of the smooth muscle strips (RF: 0.088±0.002 mm^2 vs. ALFF: 0.073±0.002 mm^2; $P<0.01$). RF also affected neural responses of the smooth muscle strips elicited by EFS at increasing frequencies of stimulation (Figure 4). There was a significant effect of feeding condition*frequency ($P<0.001$) on the relaxations elicited during the period of stimulation (on-relaxations) and the post-stimulus off-contractions. The EFS-induced on-relaxations did not differ between ALFF and RF mice, but were less pronounced in mice refed *ad libitum* ($P<0.05$ vs. ALFF) (Figure 4*B*). Off-contractions were significantly enhanced ($P<0.001$) in a frequency-dependent manner by RF and normalized again in the RF+ALFF group (Figure 4*C*).

RF alters proinflammatory cytokine expression and MPO activity. Since ghrelin has been shown to exert anti-inflammatory effects, cytokine expression was quantified in the stomach of WT and GHSR-KO mice. Two-way ANOVA analysis revealed that RF increased IL-1β and IL-6 mRNA expression in the stomach, regardless of the genotype (feeding condition*genotype not significant) (Figure 5 *A–B*). On the contrary, IL-1α mRNA expression was downregulated during RF in WT, but not in GHSR-KO mice (feeding condition*genotype $P<0.05$) (Figure 5*C*). In addition, RF increased MPO activity in both genotypes (feeding condition*genotype not significant) (Figure 5*D*). In both WT and GHSR-KO mice, MPO activity was normalized in the RF+ALFF group (data not shown).

2. Role of the core clock gene Bmal1 in the physiological adaptations induced by RF

Since our study in WT and GHSR-KO mice demonstrated that the role of ghrelin in the physiological adaptations to RF was limited to the restoration of body weight loss, our focus shifted to the circadian system itself. As expected, RF mice displayed a 6-fold increase in Per2 and an 8-fold decrease in Bmal1 mRNA expression levels in the stomach (data not shown), indicating a phase-shift in clock gene expression. Subsequently, we aimed to determine the role of the core clock gene Bmal1 in the RF-induced physiological adaptations.

When subjected to RF with normal chow, Bmal1-KO mice failed to adapt to the RF schedule and died within 4 days, due to a

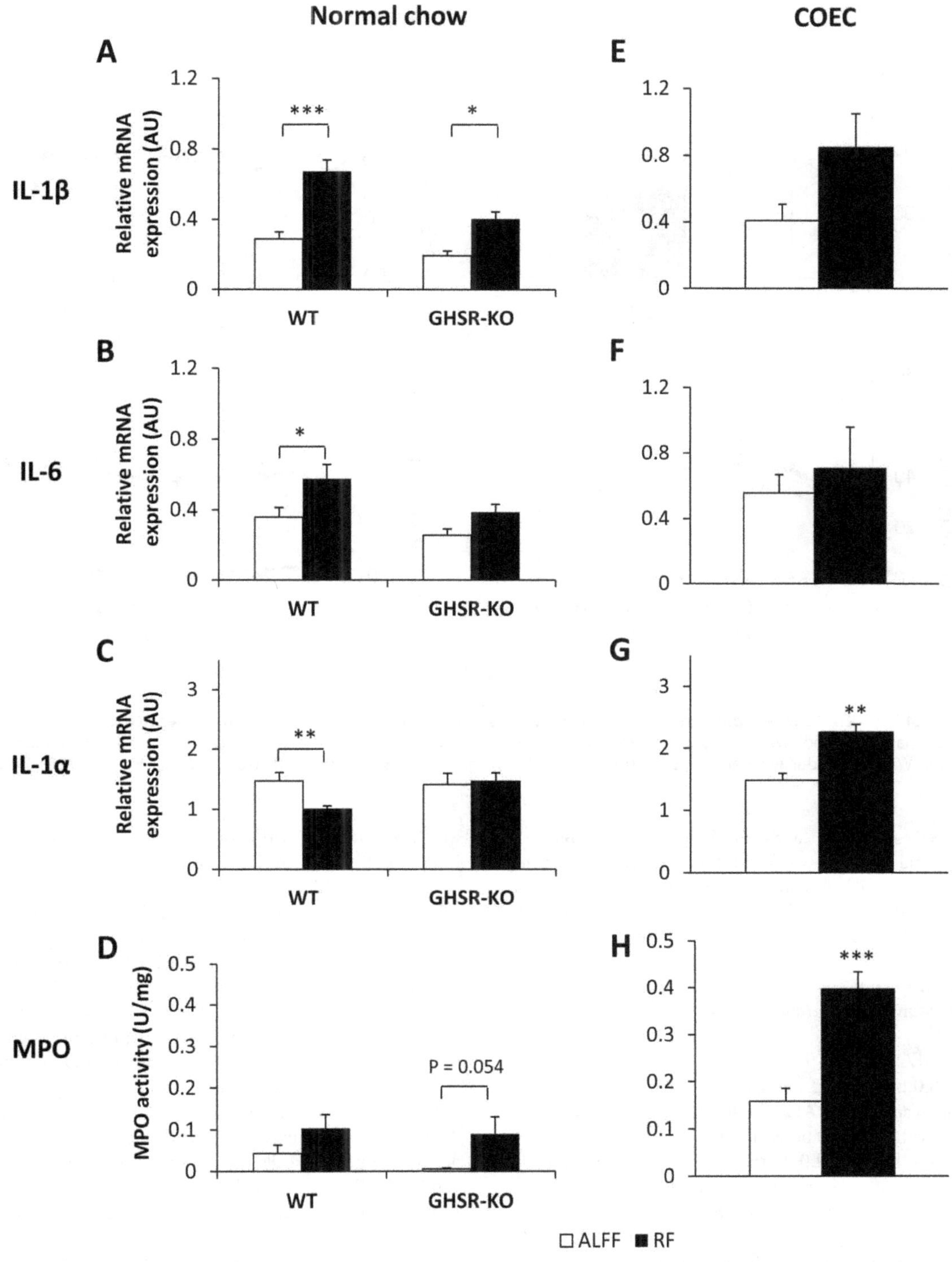

Figure 5. RF with normal chow or COEC alters gastric cytokine mRNA expression and MPO activity levels. Gastric mRNA expression of the proinflammatory cytokines IL-1β (**A, E**), IL-6 (**B, F**) and IL-1α (**C, G**) and MPO activity (**D, H**) of normal chow-fed WT (n = 7–16/group) or GHSR-KO (n = 6–9/group) mice (**A–D**) or COEC-fed WT mice (n = 5–6/group) (**E–H**) under different feeding conditions. *$P<0.05$, **$P<0.01$, ***$P<0.001$ vs. ALFF. (AU = arbitrary units).

persisting decrease in food intake and body weight (data not shown). Therefore, several adjustments had to be made to the RF schedule according to a previous study [17]. In the final scheme (Figure 1*B*), food availability was decreased gradually and during the last 7 days, chow was enriched with canola oil to increase the caloric content of the meal.

However, since a high-fat diet itself is capable of perturbing circadian rhythms at the molecular and behavioral level [21] and stimulating low-grade inflammation [22], we first investigated the impact of the COEC on the physiological adaptations during the standard RF schedule (Figure 1*A*) in WT mice, before imposing the adapted RF schedule onto Bmal1-KO mice.

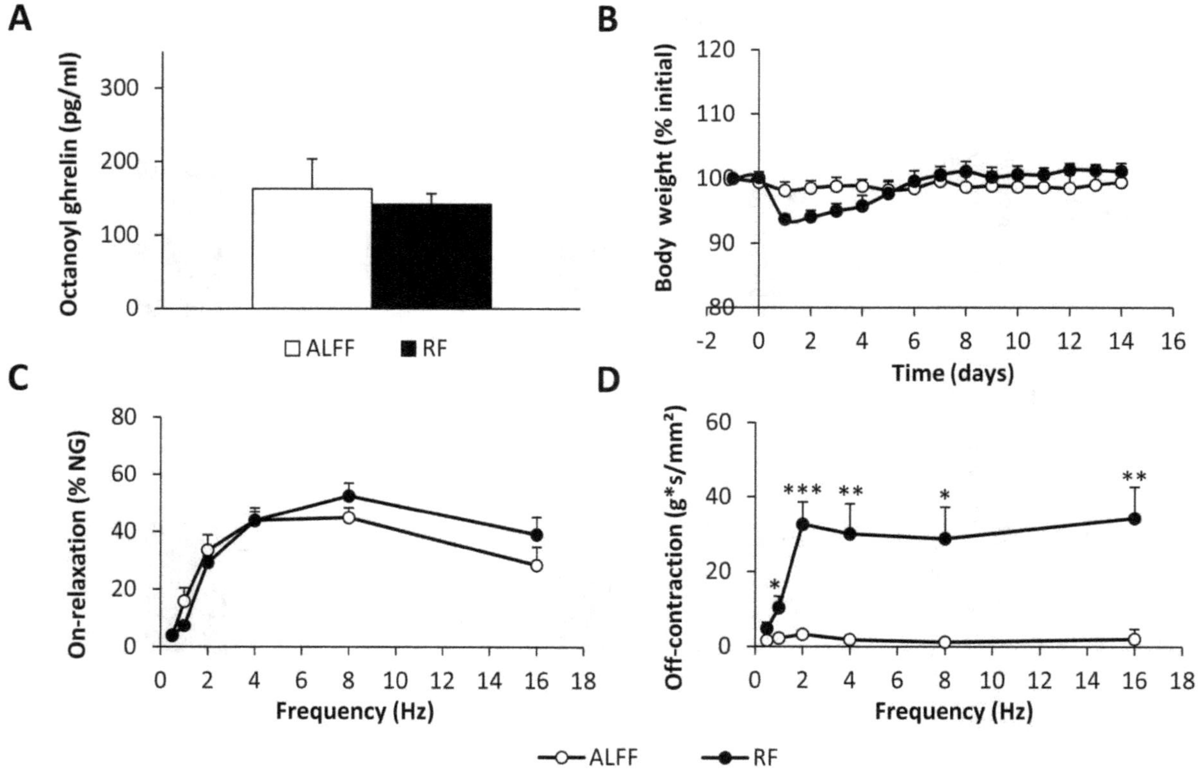

Figure 6. Effect of RF with COEC on plasma octanoyl ghrelin levels, body weight and gastric *in vitro* contractility. (**A**) Plasma octanoyl ghrelin levels, (**B**) changes in body weight and (**C–D**) EFS-induced on-relaxations (**C**) and post-stimulus off-contractions (**D**) of fundic smooth muscle strips of COEC-fed WT mice under ALFF and RF conditions (N = 5–7 mice/group, n = 8–10 strips). *$P<0.05$, ** $P<0.01$, ***$P<0.001$ RF vs. ALFF.

Standard RF schedule with COEC in WT mice. In contrast to normal chow, 2 weeks of RF with COEC did not increase plasma octanoyl ghrelin levels (Figure 6*A*). In addition, under fasting conditions (ALFF), plasma octanoyl ghrelin was 127% higher ($P<0.01$) in COEC-fed mice compared to normal chow-fed mice.

COEC-fed mice were able to restore their body weight in less than one week's time, compared to two weeks with normal chow (Figure 6*B*).

RF with COEC tended ($P = 0.07$) to increase the maximal tension (RF: 18.0±0.7 vs. ALFF: 15.1±1.4 g/mm^2; $P = 0.07$) of the contractile response to ACh in fundic strips. However, in contrast to RF with normal chow, the pEC$_{50}$-value towards ACh was not increased (RF: 6.31±0.04 vs. ALFF: 6.24±0.08). RF also resulted in neuronal hyperexcitability of fundic strips, as reflected by a frequency-dependent increase in the post-stimulus off-contractions (feeding condition*frequency, $P<0.001$) (Figure 6*D*). Inhibitory on-responses were not affected (Figure 6*C*).

In contrast to normal chow, RF with COEC did not significantly ($P = 0.10$) alter IL-1β mRNA expression, but upregulated ($P<0.01$) IL-1α mRNA expression (Figure 5 *E,G*). IL-6 mRNA expression remained unaffected (Figure 5*F*). Moreover, MPO activity was markedly increased ($P<0.001$) after RF with COEC (Figure 5*H*).

Adapted RF schedule with COEC in WT and Bmal1-KO mice. WT mice on the adapted RF schedule, in which food availability was gradually decreased, did not display a drop in body weight, but immediately outweighed ($P<0.001$) their *ad libitum*-fed counterparts (Figure 7*A*). This coincided with an increase ($P<0.001$) in total fat pad mass, consisting of gonadal and perirenal retroperitoneal fat (Figure 7*C*). In contrast, body weight and total fat pad mass did not differ between ALFF and RF Bmal1-KO mice (Figure 7 *B–C*).

RF led to thickening of the fundic wall, which was more pronounced in the longitudinal muscle layer (Bmal1-KO vs. WT: 100% vs. 30% increase), submucosa (Bmal1-KO vs. WT: 66% vs. 21% increase) and mucosa (Bmal1-KO vs. WT: 49% vs. 23% increase) of Bmal1-KO mice compared to WT mice (Figure 8). The RF-induced increase in the number of inflammatory PMN cells (neutrophils and eosinophils) was more pronounced (genotype*feeding condition $P<0.001$) in Bmal1-KO compared to WT mice (Figure 8*I*). Under ALFF conditions, few peroxidase positive cells (eosinophils, neutrophils and monocytes) were present (Figure 8*J*). The increasing effect of RF on the number of peroxidase positive cells was more pronounced (genotype*feeding condition $P<0.001$) in Bmal1-KO mice. In addition, MPO activity, determined by infiltrating neutrophils and monocytes, was lower ($P<0.05$) in Bmal1-KO mice during ALFF conditions (Figure 8*K*). RF significantly increased MPO activity in WT, but not in Bmal1-KO mice (genotype*feeding condition $P<0.01$). IL-1β and IL-6 mRNA expression did not differ between WT and Bmal1-KO mice during ALFF or RF conditions (Figure 7 *D–E*). In contrast, IL-1α mRNA expression was significantly ($P<0.01$) higher in the stomach of ALFF Bmal1-KO mice (Figure 7*F*). RF significantly upregulated IL-1α mRNA expression in WT, but not in Bmal1-KO mice (genotype*feeding condition $P<0.01$). In summary, these results indicate that Bmal1 promotes infiltration of neutrophils and mRNA expression of IL-1α in the stomach during RF.

In both genotypes, RF increased ($P<0.05$) the maximal tension (WT: RF 17.1±0.9 vs. ALFF 14.0±1.0 g/mm^2, $P<0.05$; Bmal1-KO: RF 17.0±0.5 vs. ALFF 14.4±0.2 g/mm^2, $P<0.05$) towards

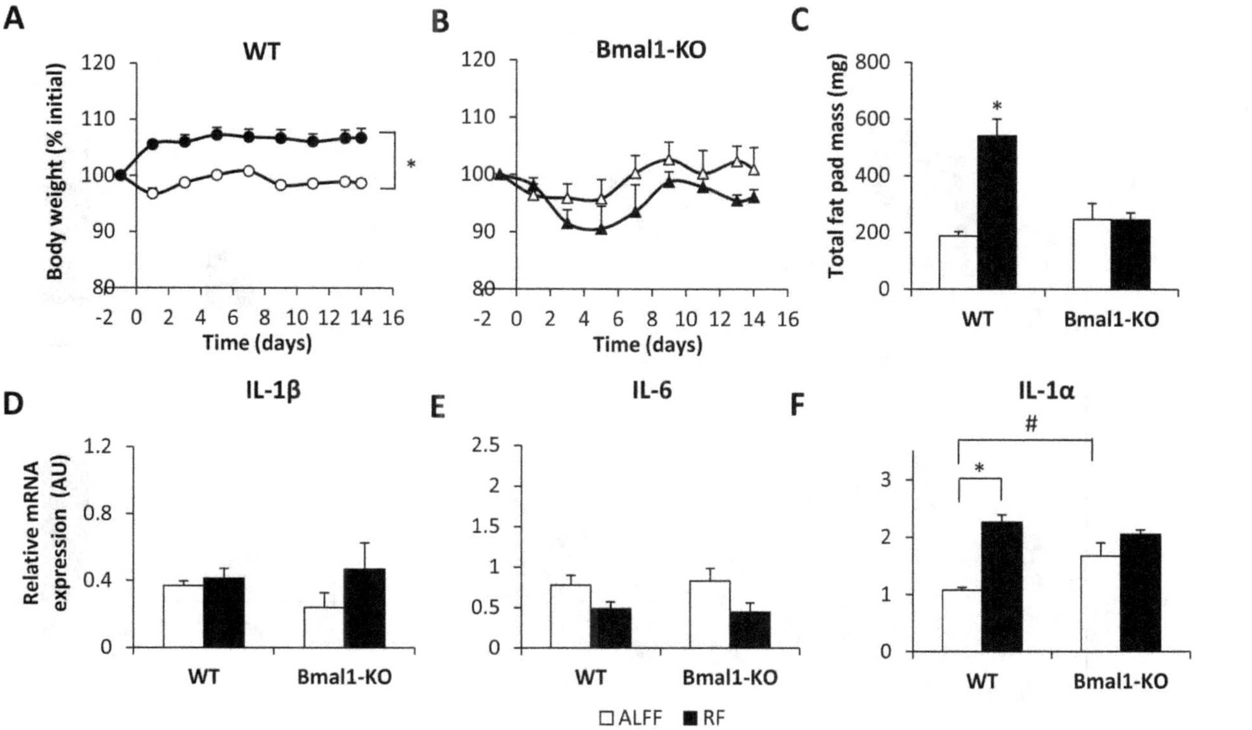

Figure 7. Bmal1 regulates body weight and upregulates gastric IL-1α mRNA expression during RF with COEC. (**A–B**) Changes in body weight of (**A**) COEC-fed WT (n = 11–21/group) or (**B**) Bmal1-KO mice (n = 7–11/group) under ALFF or RF conditions with gradually restricted food availability. (**C**) Total fat pad mass of COEC-fed WT (n = 7–12/group) and Bmal1-KO (n = 6/group) mice under ALFF or RF conditions with gradually restricted food availability. (**D–F**) Gastric mRNA expression of the proinflammatory cytokines IL-1β (**D**), IL-6 (**E**) and IL-1α (**F**) of COEC-fed WT (n = 9–19 mice/group) or Bmal1-KO mice (n = 6–7 mice/group) under ALFF or RF conditions with gradually restricted food availability. *$P<0.001$ ALFF vs. RF; # $P<0.01$ WT vs. Bmal1-KO.

ACh to a similar extent. The RF-induced increase in contractile potency (pEC_{50}) towards ACh in WT mice (RF: 6.42±0.05 vs. ALFF: 6.22±0.05; $P<0.05$) was abolished in Bmal1-KO mice (RF: 6.20±0.06 vs. ALFF: 6.12±0.04). Under ALFF conditions, EFS-induced on-relaxations were more pronounced in Bmal1-KO than in WT mice (genotype, $P<0.05$) (Figure 9*A*). In WT, but not in Bmal1-KO mice, RF enhanced the on-relaxations (feeding condition*frequency, $P<0.001$). Similarly, neural off-contractions were increased (feeding condition*frequency, $P<0.001$) after RF in WT mice (Figure 9*B*). This increase was less pronounced in Bmal1-KO mice (feeding condition*frequency $P<0.01$).

Discussion

Circadian clocks are widely accepted to act as the timekeeping system of nearly every living organism, ensuring that physiological processes are carried out at the right time of day or night. However, the concept that the gut is home to one of the food-entrainable oscillators that predicts the availability of food, especially when food becomes restricted, is rather new in the field. Our aim was to study the role of ghrelin and the core clock gene Bmal1 in the physiological adaptations to an altered circadian rhythm of feeding, induced by RF. We show that the food-anticipatory increase in ghrelin during RF depends on the type of nutrients ingested. Furthermore, we demonstrate that during RF, ghrelin and Bmal1 are involved in the restoration of body weight. We also provide the first evidence that RF alters cytokine mRNA expression levels in the stomach prior to food availability. A high-fat diet modulates this expression profile and results in a heightened proinflammatory state in the stomach right before food becomes available. Moreover, the type of inflammatory cells infiltrating the stomach is modulated by Bmal1, which specifically promoted the infiltration of neutrophils and upregulated IL-1α expression. RF also results in a thickening of the smooth muscle layers, which is counteracted by Bmal1. Our findings suggest that this thickening, whether or not in combination with the proinflammatory state, but not ghrelin signaling, leads to hyperexcitability of gastric smooth muscle, thereby promoting gastric emptying during RF. These findings are schematically represented in Figure 10.

We acknowledge that data collection and analysis of only a single time point is a limitation of this study. However, due to several practical reasons, obtaining data at additional time points was not feasible. Nevertheless, our data underpin a clear link between the circadian, metabolic, gastrointestinal and immune system and emphasize that not only "what" but also "when" you eat may determine whether you are prone to develop inflammation, gastrointestinal symptoms or obesity.

We showed that changes in plasma ghrelin levels during fasting (ALFF) were nutrient-dependent. Although it is well established that ghrelin levels are decreased during obesity, fasting levels in mice with *ad libitum* access to COEC for two weeks were twice as high as in mice fed normal chow. Similar observations were made in mice fed a high-fat diet for two weeks and in humans that were subjected to overfeeding during one week [23,24]. Since a high-fat diet can phase-shift and alter the amplitude of clock genes and clock-controlled humoral and central metabolic systems [21,25], we propose that the higher fasting plasma ghrelin levels originate from the clock altering capacities of the COEC.

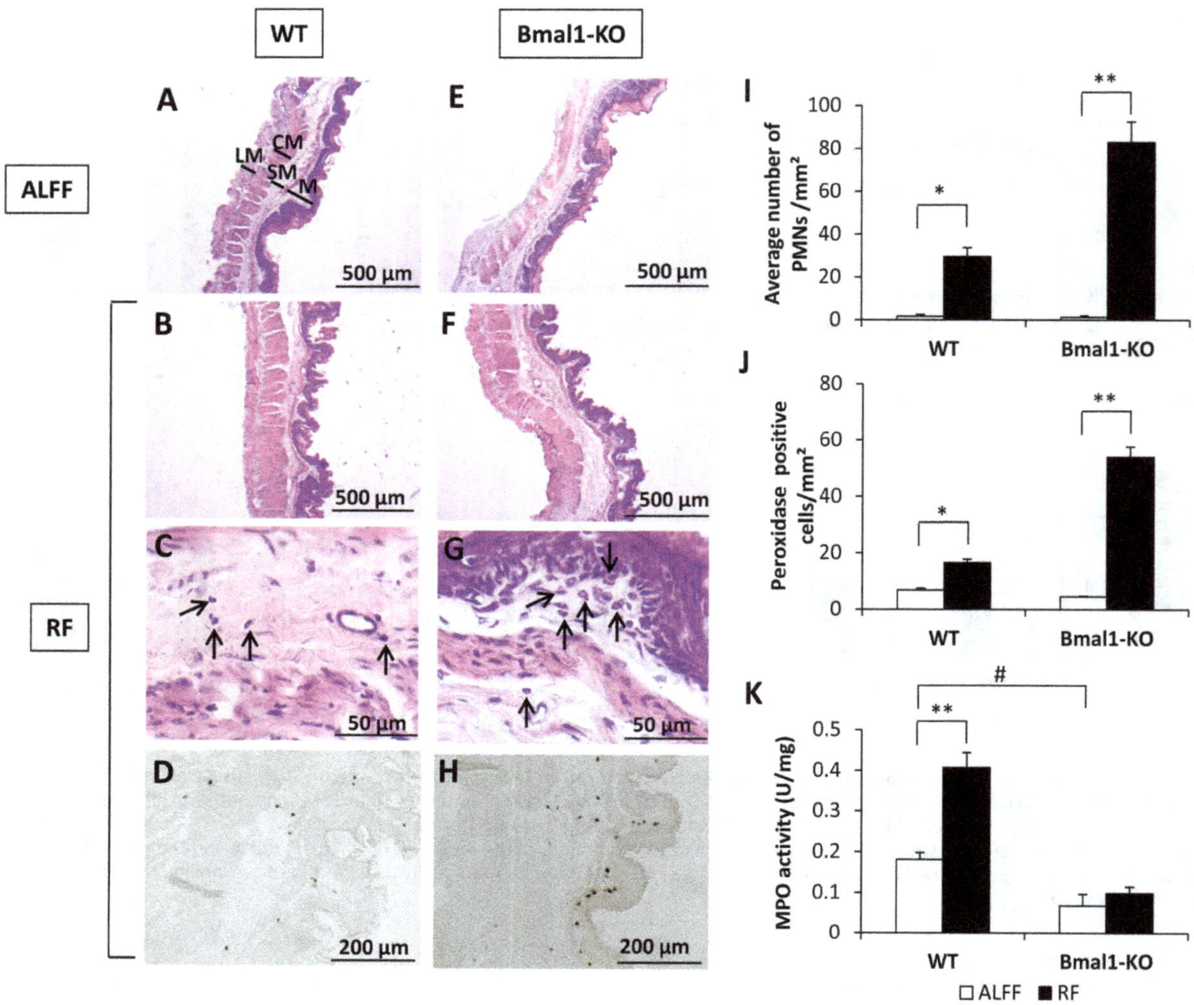

Figure 8. Bmal1 promotes infiltration of neutrophils in the stomach during RF with COEC. Representative H&E stained fundic sections of COEC-fed WT or Bmal1-KO mice under ALFF (**A,E**) or RF (**B,F**) conditions with gradually restricted food availability. (**C,G**) Higher magnifications of RF sections with arrows pointing towards PMNs. Representative peroxidase-stained fundic sections of WT (**D**) and Bmal1-KO (**H**) mice under RF conditions. Average number of PMNs per mm^2 (**I**) and peroxidase positive cells per mm^2 (**J**) in the fundus of WT (n = 4–5/group) or Bmal1-KO mice (n = 4/group) under ALFF or RF conditions. (**K**) MPO activity levels of WT (n = 9–20/group) or Bmal1-KO mice (n = 6–7/group) under ALFF or RF conditions. **P*<0.01, ***P*<0.001 ALFF vs. RF; # *P*<0.05 WT vs. Bmal1-KO. (LM = longitudinal muscle layer, CM = circular muscle layer, SM = submucosa, M = mucosa).

Similar to previous studies [11,12], we showed that RF with normal chow increased plasma octanoyl ghrelin levels of mice 30 minutes before food anticipation, an effect that can be reversed by refeeding *ad libitum*. Bodosi *et al.* previously demonstrated that this increase was the consequence of both a phase-shift and an increase in the amplitude of the circadian rhythm of ghrelin levels [12]. However, since ghrelin signaling may not be necessary for food-anticipatory activity, ghrelin might either be redundant with other (signals entraining) FEOs or act downstream of or in parallel with other FEOs that drive this activity [13]. Use of the COEC abolished the RF-induced increase in octanoyl ghrelin levels. We speculate that the high-fat feeding resulted in a lack of phase-shift or difference in amplitude between the diurnal rhythms of the plasma ghrelin levels of the ALFF and RF groups. However, this remains to be investigated further.

Our studies in GHSR-KO mice showed that ghrelin signaling was important to restore body weight loss during RF with normal chow. Ghrelin does not only affect body weight through its orexigenic effect, but also by preventing the utilization of fat [26]. Martínez-Merlos *et al.* demonstrated that RF induced epididymal and perirenal retroperitoneal fat loss in rats [27]. Since we did not observe any changes in food intake between WT and GHSR-KO mice, we speculate that the increased ghrelin levels during RF were not able to stimulate adipogenesis in GHSR-KO due to the absence of a functional ghrelin receptor.

Mice subjected to RF with COEC during 4 hours for 2 weeks restored their body weight much faster than normal chow-fed mice. When the availability of the COEC during RF was gradually decreased, mice were protected from entering a negative energy balance, allowing them to quickly outweigh their *ad libitum* fed counterparts. Arble *et al.* showed that mice fed a high-fat diet only during the light-phase, similar to our study, gained significantly more weight than mice fed solely during the dark-phase [28]. Similarly, Mistlberger *et al.* demonstrated that weight gain in a genetic model of obesity was reduced by preventing food intake in the light-phase, without reducing total daily caloric intake [29]. These results again stress the importance of the timing of food intake. Indeed, people that consume most of their food during

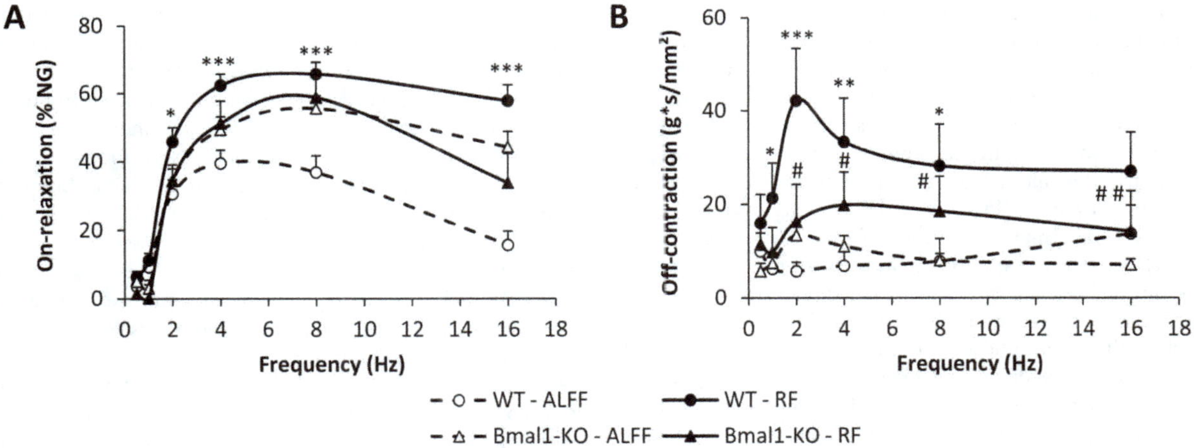

Figure 9. Bmal1 is involved in the contractility changes induced by RF with COEC. (**A**) On-relaxations and (**B**) off-contractions of COEC-fed WT or Bmal1-KO mice under ALFF and RF conditions with gradually restricted food availability. (ALFF: N = 8–14 mice/genotype, n = 16–17 strips; RF: N = 4–8 mice/genotype, n = 6–12 strips). *$P<0.05$, **$P<0.01$, ***$P<0.001$ WT vs. ALFF; # $P<0.05$, ## $P<0.001$ Bmal1-KO vs. ALFF.

their normal sleep period – such as shift workers, breakfast skippers and individuals suffering from night eating syndrome – suffer from obesity and related metabolic diseases more frequently [30,31,32]. However, in contrast to the findings in short-term studies like ours, weight gain resulting from high-fat feeding in mice can be prevented by restricting food availability to the dark-phase or even the light-phase during a long-term period of 18 weeks [33,34].

Similar to timing of food intake, deleting circadian clock genes in mice can drastically affect body weight and composition [16,35,36,37]. Here, we show that the increase in body weight during RF with COEC was regulated by Bmal1, since Bmal1-KO mice were protected from the increase in body weight and fat pad mass. This again highlights the crucial role of Bmal1 in the control of adipogenesis and lipid metabolism [38,39].

Ghrelin is an important gastroprokinetic agent and accelerates gastric emptying in humans and rodents [7]. Ariga *et al.* hypothesized that the RF-induced increase in ghrelin might be responsible for the acceleration in gastric emptying in rats [40]. We showed that RF reversibly accelerated gastric emptying in both WT and GHSR-KO mice, indicating that this acceleration is independent from ghrelin signaling. Our *in vitro* contractility studies in fundic smooth muscle strips demonstrated that RF with normal chow resulted in fully reversible neural hyperexcitability and hypercontractility to ACh. Thus, RF promotes numerous metabolic and physiological adaptations to optimize biochemical handling of a sudden increase in nutrients. In addition, our results show that Bmal1 is involved in the RF-induced increase in contractile potency towards ACh and the neural hyperexcitability.

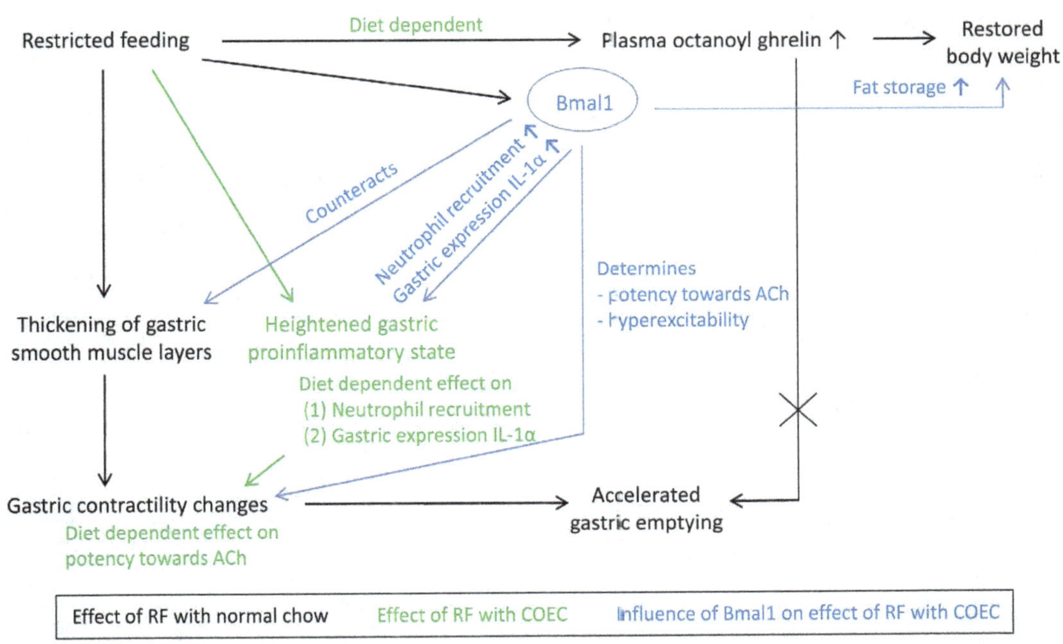

Figure 10. Schematic overview of the role of ghrelin and the clock gene Bmal1 in the physiological adaptations induced by RF with different diets, half an hour prior to food availability.

Circadian regulation has been described for levels of circulating proinflammatory cytokines, different populations of leukocytes, but also for NK cell function and phagocytic activity by macrophages and neutrophils [41]. The current study indicates for the first time that RF probably shifts the rhythm of cytokine mRNA expression and infiltrating immune cells in the stomach, as evidenced by the altered gastric proinflammatory cytokine expression profiles and MPO activity levels. This is strengthened by the study of Sherman *et al.* which showed that long-term (4 months) RF altered mRNA expression levels of proinflammatory cytokines in the liver, jejunum and white adipose tissue [42].

In addition, we show that it is likely that RF with a high-fat diet further shifts this rhythm, leading to increased MPO activity and IL-1α mRNA expression at the expense of IL-1β, which was upregulated by RF with normal chow. Our histological studies confirm that RF with a high-fat diet induces a heightened proinflammatory state in the stomach half an hour before food availability, characterized by infiltrating immune cells. This adds to the finding of Luna-Moreno *et al.* that RF was capable of inducing local immune responses in the liver [43].

Furthermore, Bmal1 seems to upregulate IL-1α expression in the stomach during RF with COEC. In addition, we showed that the type of inflammatory infiltrate is altered in the absence of Bmal1. Indeed, the results of the PMN cell and peroxidase positive cell countings in combination with the MPO activity assay showed that Bmal1 is involved in the recruitment of neutrophils, but not of eosinophils, to the stomach during RF. Since the circadian and immune systems are closely intertwined [41], it is not surprising that genetic circadian disruption can modulate innate immunity. Indeed, Bmal1-KO mice suffer from progressive corneal inflammation [44]. Also, myeloid cell-specific Bmal1 deletion induces expression of monocyte-attracting chemokines and disrupts rhythmic trafficking of proinflammatory Ly6C^{hi} monocytes, leading to predisposition to inflammation-associated pathologies [45]. In addition, recent evidence has emerged for a role of clock genes in natural killer cell and neutrophil function after activation of innate immune responses [46,47].

Our histological studies indicate a thickening of the fundic smooth muscle layers during RF which may contribute to the hypercontractility of the stomach and the accelerated gastric emptying, in order to adequately process the large amounts of food ingested during the period of food availability. Bmal1 seems to play a pivotal role in this process, since the thickening of the fundic longitudinal muscle layer during RF was more pronounced in Bmal1-KO mice than in WT mice. Nevertheless, we cannot exclude that the expressed cytokines are also contributing to this hypercontractility and neural hyperexcitability. Several studies provide a causal relationship between the presence of cytokines in the gastrointestinal tract and alterations of intestinal transit and smooth muscle contractility. The proinflammatory cytokine IL-1β has been shown to enhance fundic smooth muscle contractility and to induce hyperexcitability of neurons of the myenteric plexus [48,49]. On the contrary, TNF-α inhibited contraction of ileal smooth muscle tissue of mice [50]. Similarly, IFNγ decreased carbachol-induced longitudinal smooth muscle contraction [51]. To our knowledge, there have been no studies reporting the influence of IL-1α on smooth muscle contractility. The upregulation of this cytokine might offer an explanation for the hypercontractility observed during RF with COEC.

In conclusion, our findings provide a clear link between the circadian, gastrointestinal, immune and metabolic system. This interconnection may provide a rationale why disruption of biological rhythms in shift workers or frequent time zone travelers not only results in obesity and its associated comorbidities, but also in immune-related gastrointestinal pathologies such as gastric ulcers and irritable bowel syndrome, which is often associated with low-grade inflammation [52].

Acknowledgments

The authors thank Linda Nys and Anneleen Geuzens for their skillful technical assistance.

Author Contributions

Conceived and designed the experiments: JT ID. Performed the experiments: JL CB KB LV SS TT. Analyzed the data: JL CB KB TT ID. Wrote the paper: JL ID.

References

1. Froy O (2010) Metabolism and circadian rhythms–implications for obesity. Endocr Rev 31: 1–24.
2. Reppert SM, Weaver DR (2002) Coordination of circadian timing in mammals. Nature 418: 935–941.
3. Mendoza J (2007) Circadian clocks: setting time by food. J Neuroendocrinol 19: 127–137.
4. Hara R, Wan K, Wakamatsu H, Aida R, Moriya T, et al. (2001) Restricted feeding entrains liver clock without participation of the suprachiasmatic nucleus. Genes Cells 6: 269–278.
5. LeSauter J, Hoque N, Weintraub M, Pfaff DW, Silver R (2009) Stomach ghrelin-secreting cells as food-entrainable circadian clocks. Proc Natl Acad Sci U S A 106: 13582–13587.
6. Kojima M, Hosoda H, Date Y, Nakazato M, Matsuo H, et al. (1999) Ghrelin is a growth-hormone-releasing acylated peptide from stomach. Nature 402: 656–660.
7. Avau B, Carbone F, Tack J, Depoortere I (2013) Ghrelin signaling in the gut, its physiological properties, and therapeutic potential. Neurogastroenterol Motil 25: 720–732.
8. Spiegel K, Tasali E, Leproult R, Scherberg N, Van Cauter E (2011) Twenty-four-hour profiles of acylated and total ghrelin: relationship with glucose levels and impact of time of day and sleep. J Clin Endocrinol Metab 96: 486–493.
9. Cummings DE, Frayo RS, Marmonier C, Aubert R, Chapelot D (2004) Plasma ghrelin levels and hunger scores in humans initiating meals voluntarily without time- and food-related cues. Am J Physiol Endocrinol Metab 287: E297–304.
10. Cummings DE, Purnell JQ, Frayo RS, Schmidova K, Wisse BE, et al. (2001) A preprandial rise in plasma ghrelin levels suggests a role in meal initiation in humans. Diabetes 50: 1714–1719.
11. Blum ID, Patterson Z, Khazall R, Lamont EW, Sleeman MW, et al. (2009) Reduced anticipatory locomotor responses to scheduled meals in ghrelin receptor deficient mice. Neuroscience 164: 351–359.
12. Bodosi B, Gardi J, Hajdu I, Szentirmai E, Obal F, Jr., et al. (2004) Rhythms of ghrelin, leptin, and sleep in rats: effects of the normal diurnal cycle, restricted feeding, and sleep deprivation. Am J Physiol Regul Integr Comp Physiol 287: R1071–1079.
13. Patton DF, Mistlberger RE (2013) Circadian adaptations to meal timing: neuroendocrine mechanisms. Front Neurosci 7: 185.
14. Bunger MK, Wilsbacher LD, Moran SM, Clendenin C, Radcliffe LA, et al. (2000) Mop3 is an essential component of the master circadian pacemaker in mammals. Cell 103: 1009–1017.
15. Verhulst PJ, De Smet B, Saels I, Thijs T, Ver Donck L, et al. (2008) Role of ghrelin in the relationship between hyperphagia and accelerated gastric emptying in diabetic mice. Gastroenterology 135: 1267–1276.
16. Hemmeryckx B, Himmelreich U, Hoylaerts MF, Lijnen HR (2011) Impact of clock gene Bmal1 deficiency on nutritionally induced obesity in mice. Obesity (Silver Spring) 19: 659–661.
17. Storch KF, Weitz CJ (2009) Daily rhythms of food-anticipatory behavioral activity do not require the known circadian clock. Proc Natl Acad Sci U S A 106: 6808–6813.
18. Janssen S, Laermans J, Verhulst PJ, Thijs T, Tack J, et al. (2011) Bitter taste receptors and alpha-gustducin regulate the secretion of ghrelin with functional effects on food intake and gastric emptying. Proc Natl Acad Sci U S A 108: 2094–2099.
19. Kitazawa T, De Smet B, Verbeke K, Depoortere I, Peeters TL (2005) Gastric motor effects of peptide and non-peptide ghrelin agonists in mice in vivo and in vitro. Gut 54: 1078–1084.

20. De Smet B, Thijs T, Peeters TL, Depoortere I (2007) Effect of peripheral obestatin on gastric emptying and intestinal contractility in rodents. Neurogastroenterol Motil 19: 211–217.
21. Kohsaka A, Laposky AD, Ramsey KM, Estrada C, Joshu C, et al. (2007) High-fat diet disrupts behavioral and molecular circadian rhythms in mice. Cell Metab 6: 414–421.
22. Calder PC, Ahluwalia N, Brouns F, Buetler T, Clement K, et al. (2011) Dietary factors and low-grade inflammation in relation to overweight and obesity. Br J Nutr 106 Suppl 3: S5–78.
23. Delhanty PJ, Huisman M, Baldeon-Rojas LY, van den Berge I, Grefhorst A, et al. (2013) Des-acyl ghrelin analogs prevent high-fat-diet-induced dysregulation of glucose homeostasis. FASEB J 27: 1690–1700.
24. Wadden D, Cahill F, Amini P, Randell E, Vasdev S, et al. (2012) Serum acylated ghrelin concentrations in response to short-term overfeeding in normal weight, overweight, and obese men. PLoS One 7: e45748.
25. Barnea M, Madar Z, Froy O (2009) High-fat diet delays and fasting advances the circadian expression of adiponectin signaling components in mouse liver. Endocrinology 150: 161–168.
26. Tschop M, Smiley DL, Heiman ML (2000) Ghrelin induces adiposity in rodents. Nature 407: 908–913.
27. Martinez-Merlos MT, Angeles-Castellanos M, Diaz-Munoz M, Aguilar-Roblero R, Mendoza J, et al. (2004) Dissociation between adipose tissue signals, behavior and the food-entrained oscillator. J Endocrinol 181: 53–63.
28. Arble DM, Bass J, Laposky AD, Vitaterna MH, Turek FW (2009) Circadian timing of food intake contributes to weight gain. Obesity (Silver Spring) 17: 2100–2102.
29. Mistlberger RE, Lukman H, Nadeau BG (1998) Circadian rhythms in the Zucker obese rat: assessment and intervention. Appetite 30: 255–267.
30. Giovannini M, Verduci E, Scaglioni S, Salvatici E, Bonza M, et al. (2008) Breakfast: a good habit, not a repetitive custom. J Int Med Res 36: 613–624.
31. Knutsson A (2003) Health disorders of shift workers. Occup Med (Lond) 53: 103–108.
32. Stunkard AJ, Allison KC, Lundgren JD, O'Reardon JP (2009) A biobehavioural model of the night eating syndrome. Obes Rev 10 Suppl 2: 69–77.
33. Hatori M, Vollmers C, Zarrinpar A, DiTacchio L, Bushong EA, et al. (2012) Time-restricted feeding without reducing caloric intake prevents metabolic diseases in mice fed a high-fat diet. Cell Metab 15: 848–860.
34. Sherman H, Genzer Y, Cohen R, Chapnik N, Madar Z, et al. (2012) Timed high-fat diet resets circadian metabolism and prevents obesity. FASEB J 26: 3493–3502.
35. Hemmeryckx B, Hoylaerts MF, Lijnen HR (2012) Effect of premature aging on murine adipose tissue. Exp Gerontol 47: 256–262.
36. Lamia KA, Storch KF, Weitz CJ (2008) Physiological significance of a peripheral tissue circadian clock. Proc Natl Acad Sci U S A 105: 15172–15177.
37. Turek FW, Joshu C, Kohsaka A, Lin E, Ivanova G, et al. (2005) Obesity and metabolic syndrome in circadian Clock mutant mice. Science 308: 1043–1045.
38. Shimba S, Ishii N, Ohta Y, Ohno T, Watabe Y, et al. (2005) Brain and muscle Arnt-like protein-1 (BMAL1), a component of the molecular clock, regulates adipogenesis. Proc Natl Acad Sci U S A 102: 12071–12076.
39. Shimba S, Ogawa T, Hitosugi S, Ichihashi Y, Nakadaira Y, et al. (2011) Deficient of a clock gene, brain and muscle Arnt-like protein-1 (BMAL1), induces dyslipidemia and ectopic fat formation. PLoS One 6: e25231.
40. Ariga H, Imai K, Chen C, Mantyh C, Pappas TN, et al. (2008) Fixed feeding potentiates interdigestive gastric motor activity in rats: importance of eating habits for maintaining interdigestive MMC. Am J Physiol Gastrointest Liver Physiol 294: G655–659.
41. Scheiermann C, Kunisaki Y, Frenette PS (2013) Circadian control of the immune system. Nat Rev Immunol 13: 190–198.
42. Sherman H, Frumin I, Gutman R, Chapnik N, Lorentz A, et al. (2010) Long-term restricted feeding alters circadian expression and reduces the level of inflammatory and disease markers. J Cell Mol Med 15: 2745–2759.
43. Luna-Moreno D, Aguilar-Roblero R, Diaz-Munoz M (2009) Restricted feeding entrains rhythms of inflammation-related factors without promoting an acute-phase response. Chronobiol Int 26: 1409–1429.
44. Kondratov RV, Kondratova AA, Gorbacheva VY, Vykhovanets OV, Antoch MP (2006) Early aging and age-related pathologies in mice deficient in BMAL1, the core componentof the circadian clock. Genes Dev 20: 1868–1873.
45. Nguyen KD, Fentress SJ, Qiu Y, Yun K, Cox JS, et al. (2013) Circadian gene Bmal1 regulates diurnal oscillations of Ly6C(hi) inflammatory monocytes. Science 341: 1483–1488.
46. Liu J, Malkani G, Shi X, Meyer M, Cunningham-Runddles S, et al. (2006) The circadian clock Period 2 gene regulates gamma interferon production of NK cells in host response to lipopolysaccharide-induced endotoxic shock. Infect Immun 74: 4750–4756.
47. Murphy BA (2008) Equine neutrophils respond to PGE2 by activating expression of core circadian clock genes. The Open Veterinary Science Journal 2: p. 96–103.
48. Kindt S, Vanden Berghe P, Boesmans W, Roosen L, Tack J (2010) Prolonged IL-1beta exposure alters neurotransmitter and electrically induced Ca(2+) responses in the myenteric plexus. Neurogastroenterol Motil 22: 321–e385.
49. Moreels TG, De Man JG, Bogers JJ, De Winter BY, Vrolix G, et al. (2001) Effect of Schistosoma mansoni-induced granulomatous inflammation on murine gastrointestinal motility. Am J Physiol Gastrointest Liver Physiol 280: G1030–1042.
50. Ohama T, Hori M, Momotani E, Iwakura Y, Guo F, et al. (2007) Intestinal inflammation downregulates smooth muscle CPI-17 through induction of TNF-alpha and causes motility disorders. Am J Physiol Gastrointest Liver Physiol 292: G1429–1438.
51. Akiho H, Khan WI, Al-Kaabi A, Blennerhassett P, Deng Y, et al. (2007) Cytokine modulation of muscarinic receptors in the murine intestine. Am J Physiol Gastrointest Liver Physiol 293: G250–255.
52. Knutsson A, Boggild H (2010) Gastrointestinal disorders among shift workers. Scand J Work Environ Health 36: 85–95.

19

The Growing Price Gap between More and Less Healthy Foods: Analysis of a Novel Longitudinal UK Dataset

Nicholas R. V. Jones[1], Annalijn I. Conklin[1], Marc Suhrcke[1,2], Pablo Monsivais[1]*

1 UK Clinical Research Collaboration (UKCRC) Centre for Diet and Activity Research, Department of MRC Epidemiology, University of Cambridge School of Clinical Medicine, Addenbrooke's Treatment Centre, Cambridge Biomedical Campus, Cambridge, United Kingdom, **2** Faculty of Medicine and Health Sciences, University of East Anglia, Norwich, United Kingdom

Abstract

Objectives: The UK government has noted the public health importance of food prices and the affordability of a healthy diet. Yet, methods for tracking change over time have not been established. We aimed to investigate the prices of more and less healthy foods over time using existing government data on national food prices and nutrition content.

Methods: We linked economic data for 94 foods and beverages in the UK Consumer Price Index to food and nutrient data from the UK Department of Health's National Diet and Nutrition Survey, producing a novel dataset across the period 2002–2012. Each item was assigned to a food group and also categorised as either "more healthy" or "less healthy" using a nutrient profiling model developed by the Food Standards Agency. We tested statistical significance using a t-test and repeated measures ANOVA.

Results: The mean (standard deviation) 2012 price/1000 kcal was £2.50 (0.29) for less healthy items and £7.49 (1.27) for more healthy items. The ANOVA results confirmed that all prices had risen over the period 2002–2012, but more healthy items rose faster than less healthy ones in absolute terms:£0.17 compared to £0.07/1000 kcal per year on average for more and less healthy items, respectively ($p<0.001$).

Conclusions: Since 2002, more healthy foods and beverages have been consistently more expensive than less healthy ones, with a growing gap between them. This trend is likely to make healthier diets less affordable over time, which may have implications for individual food security and population health, and it may exacerbate social inequalities in health. The novel data linkage employed here could be used as the basis for routine food price monitoring to inform public health policy.

Editor: Harry Zhang, Old Dominion University, United States of America

Funding: The present study was undertaken by the Centre for Diet and Activity Research (CEDAR), a UKCRC Public Health Research Centre of Excellence. The authors gratefully acknowledge the funding from the British Heart Foundation, Cancer Research UK, Economic and Social Research Council, Medical Research Council, the National Institute for Health Research, and the Wellcome Trust, under the auspices of the UK Clinical Research Collaboration. AIC was fully supported by the Gates Cambridge Trust. The funding sources had no role in the design and conduct of the study or in the collection, management, analysis, and interpretation of the data.

Competing Interests: The authors have declared that no competing interests exist.

* Email: pm491@medschl.cam.ac.uk

Introduction

The association between foods, nutrients and diets and certain health outcomes is well established, [1] with the World Health Organization identifying energy-dense, nutrient-poor foods that are high in fat, sugar and salt as contributing to excess risk of chronic disease. [2] Accordingly, dietary recommendations, including those from the UK Department of Health (DH), discourage the consumption of such foods and emphasise vegetables and fruits, whole grains, low fat dairy foods and lean sources of protein. [3] However, on average the UK population consumes an excess of saturated fat and non-milk extrinsic sugars, and fails to consume enough oily fish or fruit and vegetables, falling short of government recommendations. [4] These patterns have a marked effect on public health: the 2010 Global Burden of Disease Study found that unhealthy diets accounted for 14.3% of the UK's disease burden (measured in disability-adjusted life years). [5] The burden on the healthcare system is also considerable with diet-related ill health estimated to be responsible for £5.8 billion of National Health Service expenditure annually, more than either smoking, alcohol consumption or physical inactivity (based upon data from 2006–7). [6].

One factor that might limit the uptake of healthier diets is the cost of healthier foods, which has not been recognised by the majority of UK public health policy outside of the context of national food security. [7,8] The notion that healthier foods are more expensive and that this expense contributes to the consumption of unhealthy diets is not new, and has a strong evidence base and conceptual framework to support it. [9] In a 2013 survey, price was rated by UK consumers as the most important factor influencing their choices of food products, with 39% stating it was the factor of greatest importance and 91% listing it in their top five criteria. [10] In contrast, just 9% of UK consumers considered a food's healthiness to be the most important factor and only 49% placed it in the top five. [10]

These findings suggest that cost considerations may override health concerns in consumer dietary choices.

Both researchers and policymakers have recognised that the price of healthy diets and foods ought to be monitored to inform public health nutrition policy but no monitoring system has hitherto been established in the UK. [8,11] Here we outline a method for examining the cost of foods in relation to nutrient content by linking existing UK government economic and nutrition surveillance data. Using the resulting dataset, we then examine changes in the price of food between 2002 and 2012, by Eatwell food group and by category of healthfulness as determined by a widely used nutrient profiling score. Our approach to linking such existing data could provide the basis for routine monitoring of the affordability of healthy foods and diets, thereby allowing for a better understanding of how price differs between more or less healthy foods.

Methods

Ethics Statement

NDNS was conducted according to the guidelines laid down in the Declaration of Helsinki and all procedures involving human subjects were approved by the Oxfordshire A Research Ethics Committee. Written informed consent was obtained from all participants [12].

Methods summary

We obtained food price and nutrition data from two separate and publicly available sources and linked the two together to create a novel dataset. We then converted prices to a price-per-unit-of-energy value and classified food items according to their nutritional content and by food group. Finally, we compared the mean prices of these categories in 2012 and examined the change in price since 2002.

Food price data

We selected the foods and beverages in our sample from the list of goods and services used to calculate the Consumer Price Index (CPI), a tool used to measure inflation in the UK based upon a basket of goods for which prices are measured across the nation each quarter. [13] In 2012, this basket included 157 foods and beverages which did not include an element of service, for example, a hot meal in a pub. We excluded such items because the cost of the service could not be separated from the cost of the food. However, to ensure that a meaningful comparison was being made over time, we restricted the contents of the basket analysed to include only those goods that remained in the basket during our study period between 2002 and 2012. Research in the USA has indicated that market baskets that change over time can contribute to apparent differences in the rate of change in the price of food groups. [14] We further excluded an additional four items in the basket as they contained no nutrients meaningful to the research questions (Instant Coffee, Filter Coffee, Tea Bags, Bottled Mineral Water), leaving a final list of 94 foods and beverages for comparison across 10 years.

We took the median price for each good in a given quarter and produced a mean value for the year, using data taken from the Office for National Statistics. [15] These data were per-unit prices, with no separate field for unit weight. To establish the price per 100 g, we used information on the purchased weight where it was included in the food name (e.g. "Grapes per kg"), or inferred the purchased mass using information on similar items available for purchase on an online supermarket aggregator, *mySupermarket*. [16] We chose items from the site when the price was closest to the 2012 price taken from the CPI data. For items with variable weights, e.g. peaches, we assigned the weight recorded for that type of item in the USDA National Nutrient Database for Standard Reference. [17] Using this combined method we established a price per 100 g for all 94 items in our list.

Nutrition data

We obtained nutrition data from survey years 1–3 of the rolling programme of the nationally-representative National Diet and Nutrition Survey (NDNS), which was available from the Economic and Social Data Service. [18] Foods consumed by 1,491 adult survey respondents have their nutrient content reported in detail, with the content of 60 nutrients and 27 disaggregated foods (e.g. mass of dried fruit) per portion and total portion mass reported. We removed non-nutrient information from the Food Level Dietary Data file, removed duplicate entries, and converted the values to a 100 g scale, thus creating a database of 3790 unique foods and beverages.

Linkage process

We used a qualitative process to determine the most appropriate NDNS items for each of the 94 items from the CPI list. Where multiple NDNS items were deemed a suitable match for a CPI item we calculated mean nutrition data, weighted by the frequency of consumption for each NDNS item. We adopted this approach to account for the fact that some CPI items were only described in very broad terms and could cover a range of different foods (e.g. "frozen ready meal, cooked – serves 1"), and also to account for the range of different methods of preparation (for instance, a potato could be boiled, baked or fried) which were associated with NDNS food items and would alter the nutrient content. The most NDNS items matched to any one item was 14 and the least was 1, with a median of 2 NDNS items match for a given CPI item.

Once matches had been made, the nutrition data needed to be adjusted to account for the fact that the NDNS data concern foods as consumed and the CPI data foods as purchased. The incongruence in the data occurs because there are either losses or gains associated with preparation and cooking of many of the listed foods. To remedy this we adjusted the CPI food price data so that they expressed price in terms of price per 100 g edible portion, using edible portion figures from the *United States Department of Agriculture's Handbook 102* where necessary. [19].

Following this adjustment, we converted prices per 100 g into price per 1000 kcal using the data on energy content provided by the NDNS. We produced a dataset with detailed nutrient content per 100 g and 11 years of data on price per 1000 kcal which would allow us to analyse price changes over time in relation to nutrient content.

Food group-based classification of foods

We classified food items in our new dataset according to five distinct food groups, defined by the Eatwell Plate—a tool for nutrition communication developed by the DH to define a healthy diet. [3] The five groups analysed were: (i) bread, rice potatoes and pasta; (ii) fruit and vegetables; (iii) milk and dairy foods; (iv) meat, fish, eggs, beans and other sources of protein; and (v) food and drinks high in fat and/or sugar. We assigned foods to food groups using a reference table in the Livewell Report which matched NDNS food categories to Eatwell food groups. [20] When NDNS items corresponding to a CPI item included more than one food group, we applied only one food group based on the item most frequently consumed according to the NDNS survey data.

Nutrient-based classification of foods

Food items were also classified as "more healthy" or "less healthy" based upon nutrient profiling, a technique which accounts for a food or drink's overall nutritional characteristics. We used the WXYfm model detailed in the DH's Nutritional Profiling Technical Guide, hereafter referred to as the "FSA score" due to its historical usage by the Food Standards Agency (FSA), because this score provides a categorical distinction between more and less healthy foods. [21] This model assigns an overall numeric score according to per 100 g levels of: energy, saturated fat, total sugar, sodium, fibre, protein, and fruit, vegetable and nut content. This particular model was originally developed to highlight foods which should not be advertised to children and consequently gives a definition of less healthy foods, allowing for objective classification of the items in our sample. [21] When used to classify foods this score has been shown to have good agreement with the subjective opinions of nutrition professionals. [22].

Statistical analyses

Descriptive statistics were used to characterise the mean economic cost and change in cost over time, according to food group and FSA score healthfulness categories. The distributions of the nutrient profile score for each Eatwell food group were tested with ANOVA using the data for 2012. The difference in price in 2012 between the categories "less healthy" and "more healthy" was tested using a t-test and between the Eatwell groups with ANOVA. Repeated measures ANOVA were used to determine whether (a) there was a statistically significant change in price over the period 2002–2012 for all foods and (b) the prices changed differently between Eatwell food group and FSA categories over this period.

Analyses were conducted using Stata (version SE 12.1). [23] Figures were produced using *R* (version 2.15.1 for *Windows*) and the *ggplot2* package. [24,25].

Sensitivity Analyses

We conducted two sensitivity analyses: we analysed the difference in price between more and less healthy foods with fruit and vegetables removed from the healthy foods category, to test whether any price difference was due only to this group. We also tested for the possibility of bias caused by excluding items which did not appear in all years, by looking at the difference in price between more and less healthy foods when all items in 2012 were included, not just those which appeared in the CPI basket across the entire 2002–12 period.

Results

Table 1 shows the 2012 mean price and changes in price for 2002–2012, 2002–2007 and 2007–2012, in both absolute and relative terms, for all foods and by Eatwell and FSA score categories. Between 2002 and 2012 the mean price of all foods in our sample rose 35%, from £3.87/1000 kcal to £5.21/1000 kcal. This increase was not constant, with the prices rising at a greater rate after 2007 than before, with the absolute change for the period 2002–07 being £0.27/1000 kcal compared to £1.07/1000 kcal for the period 2007–12. This increase in the rate of change after 2007 applied to all food groups and nutrient composition categories.

Price differences by Eatwell food group

The mean prices per 1000 kcal for each of the Eatwell food groups for the period 2002–2012 are shown in **Figure 1**. The

Table 1. 2012 mean, absolute and relative changes in price for all foods, by Eatwell group and by FSA score category.

		All foods	*Bread, rice, potatoes, pasta*	*Fruit and vegetables*	*Milk and dairy foods*	*Meat, fish, eggs, beans, other sources of protein*	*Food & drinks high in fat and/or sugar*	*More healthy*	*Less healthy*
2012 mean price (£/1000 kcal)		5.21	1.26	9.13	4.75	4.93	3.11	7.49	2.50
Relative change in price (%)	2002–12	35	12	23	29	54	49	33	41
	2002–07	7	-9	4	9	11	11	7	8
	2007–12	26	22	18	18	39	33	24	31
Absolute change in price (£/1000 kcal)	2002–12	1.34	0.13	1.73	1.07	1.73	1.02	1.84	0.73
	2002–07	0.27	−0.10	0.32	0.34	0.34	0.24	0.37	0.14
	2007–12	1.07	0.23	1.41	0.73	1.39	0.78	1.47	0.59

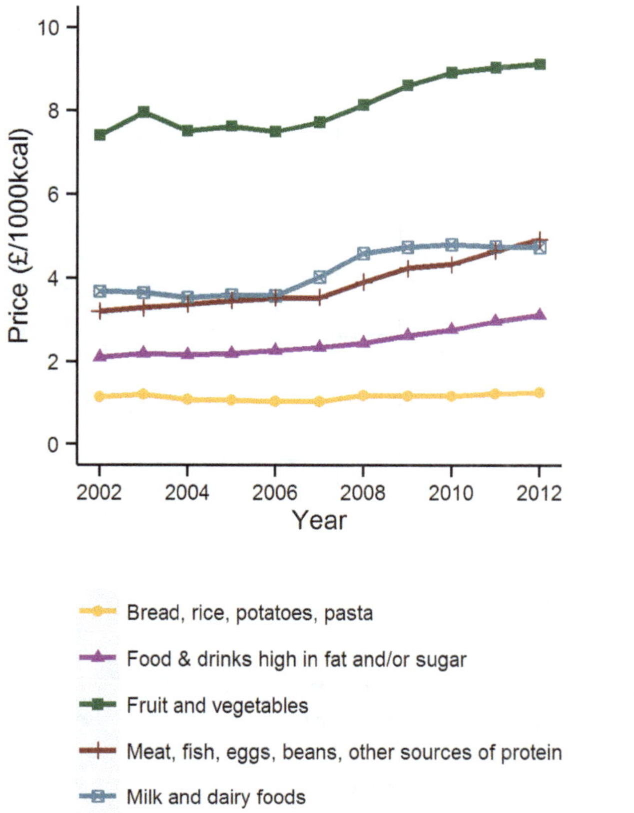

Figure 1. Mean price of foods by Eatwell food group, 2002–2012. Mean price (£/1000 kcal) by Eatwell food group of foods and beverages remaining in the UK Consumer Price Index basket across the entirety of the period 2002–2012 (n = 94).

figure shows that there is a clear hierarchy of prices across the period in which fruit and vegetables are always the most expensive foods and starchy carbohydrates the least expensive. All food groups saw price increases over the observation period, except for starchy foods, whose average price remained broadly constant throughout. The difference between groups was significant across all years ($p<0.001$).

Comparison of food groups' nutrient composition

Figure 2 shows the distribution of nutritional value for each Eatwell group according to the FSA score. We found that only the fruits and vegetables group showed a distinct, healthier nutrient profile, while all other groups contained food items overlapping the Ofcom categories of more and less healthy (for visual clarity, this plot excludes the sample's six beverages sample because the score uses different cut-offs for foods and beverages. All other analyses include all 94 foods and beverages). When tested with an ANOVA, there was a significant difference between FSA scores by groups ($p<0.001$) but this was not the case when the "Fruit and Vegetables" category was removed ($p = 0.267$). This result indicates that with the exception of this category, a food's Eatwell group cannot be used to determine whether a food is more or less healthy. This plot excludes the six beverages in the sample because the score uses a separate cut-off for foods and beverages. The beverages are included for all other analyses.

Price differences by nutrient profile category

We found an absolute difference in price between the nutrient profile categories in 2012, with more healthy foods approximately three times more expensive than less healthy foods ($p<0.001$). The mean price was £2.50 (standard deviation = 0.29) for less healthy items and £7.49 (1.27) for more healthy items. The mean prices per 1000 kcal for foods categorised as less healthy and foods categorised as more healthy for the period 2002–2012 are shown in **Figure 3**. Across the study period, we found that there was a consistent difference in price between these groups ($p<0.001$) and that there was a difference in the change over time by group ($p = 0.008$).

Sensitivity Analyses

When we included all foods and beverages in the CPI in 2012 rather than only those which has been included in the CPI basket since 2002, the difference in mean price between more and less healthy foods was £6.57/1000 kcal and £2.96/1000 kcal respectively ($p<0.001$). We also tested for a difference between more and less healthy foods over time when fruit and vegetables were removed from the analysis, finding that the difference between groups remained ($p<0.001$) and that they showed different time trends ($p = 0.004$), with the price of more healthy foods rising by £1.95/1000 kcal over the period in comparison to £0.73/1000 kcal for less healthy foods. With fruit and vegetables excluded, the mean price for more healthy foods in 2012 was £5.78/1000 kcal whereas the mean price of less healthy foods did not change.

Discussion

Our results show that the price of more healthy foods was consistently greater than that of less healthy foods over the period 2002–2012, and that the absolute price gap between healthy and less healthy foods has grown over this period. This finding strengthens the case for monitoring the affordability of healthy foods and diets in order to inform potential economic policy responses.

This study is the first to use UK data to examine price trends by the nutrient composition of foods. Our results tally with the general trend of increasing food prices observed in similar high income nations, as reported in a review, [26] where studies have found that in recent years healthy foods had increased more in price than foods which were less healthy, [27–30] and that healthier versions of particular foods were more expensive. [31,32] Another recent review has again found that within given food groups, the healthier option was typically more expensive for meats/protein, snacks/sweets, grains, and fats/oils, whilst healthier dairy foods were found to be less expensive. [33].

The broadly consistent observation of disparities in food prices across countries is likely to have multiple causes. In the UK it may be the case that food prices are heavily influenced by certain features of the Common Agricultural Policy (CAP) which intervenes in food markets to subsidise the production of certain goods, including grains, dairy products, oils and sugar. [34] Such subsidies have the potential to affect public health by influencing the availability and price of foods, with modelling studies showing that the CAP's presence may reduce the quantity of fruit and vegetables consumed and increase cardiovascular mortality through encouraging the consumption of saturated fats. [35,36] If public health policy is required to address the issue of the higher price of more healthy foods, it is likely to be necessary to engage with supply-side issues such as CAP reform to achieve long-term change.

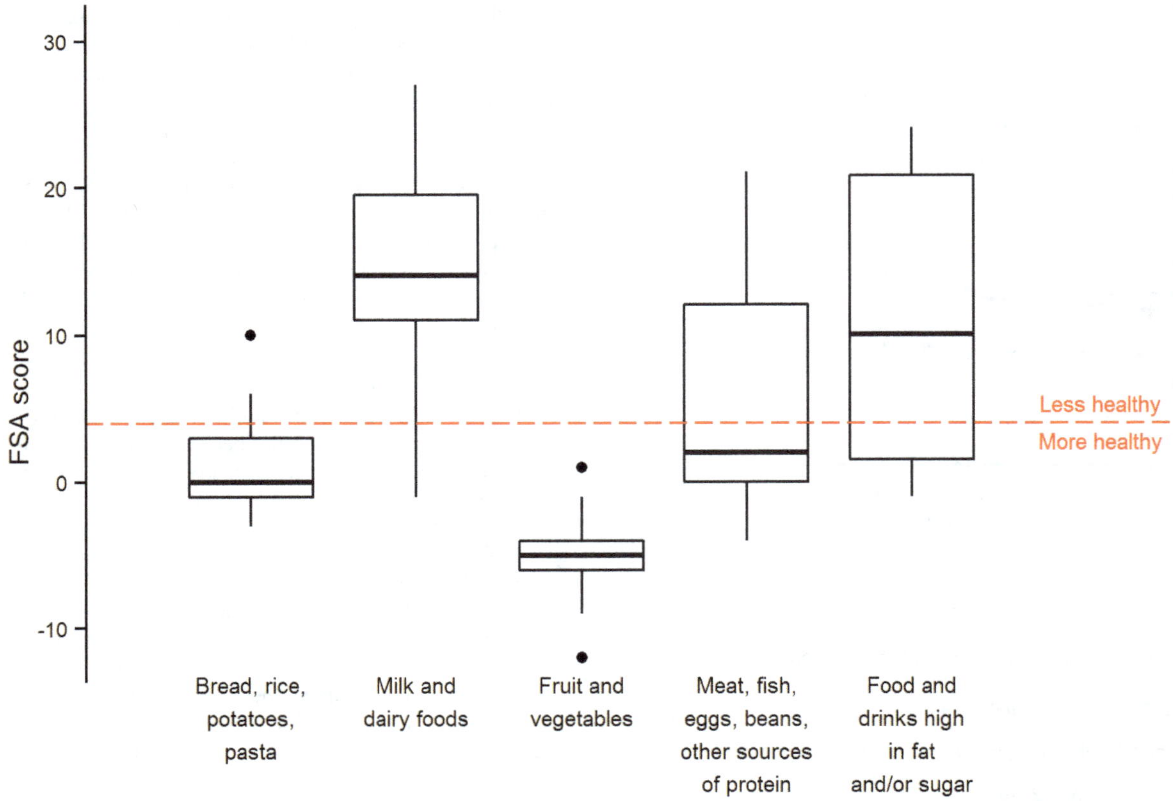

Figure 2. Box plots of nutrient density by Eatwell food group. Box plots of nutrient density as defined by the Food Standards Agency nutrient profiling score for foods (and not beverages) remaining in the UK Consumer Price Index basket across the entirety of the period 2002–2012 (n = 88), by Eatwell food group.

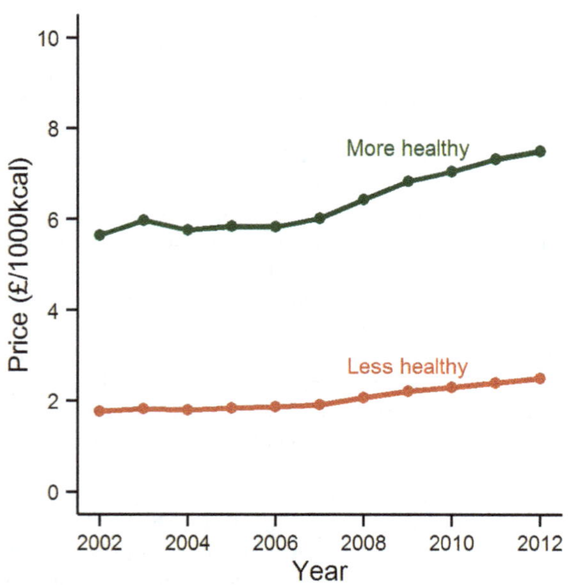

Figure 3. Mean price of foods by Food Standards Agency nutrient profiling score category, 2002–2012. Mean price (£/ 1000 kcal) by Food Standards Agency nutrient profiling score category of foods and beverages remaining in the UK Consumer Price Index basket across the entirety of the period 2002-2012 (n = 94).

In recent years the issue of food poverty has been of increasing concern in the UK and the rising use of food banks has been recognised as an issue of public health importance. [37,38] Our results suggest that we should consider not only the issue of people being able to afford to eat enough food to avoid hunger but also being able to eat enough food which is healthy. The standard definition of food security is that people should have physical and economic access to "sufficient, nutritionally adequate and safe food", [39,40] meaning that if economic constraints are gradually forcing people to replace more healthy foods with less healthy ones, they are becoming increasingly exposed to the risk of food insecurity. Analyses of UK food spending data by the Institute for Fiscal Studies has shown that, in recent years, all SES groups have changed their purchasing habits to both spend less on food and purchase calories which are both cheaper and less healthy, for example purchasing less fruit but more grains, cheese and prepared dishes. [41] Our findings help to explain this observation by uncovering the magnitude of the price difference between more and less healthy foods, which is a factor that drives increasing food insecurity and could contribute to a deterioration in population health.

In addition to our main finding we also observed that, with the exception of "fruit and vegetables", the Eatwell food groups were not distinct in terms of the FSA scores of their constituent foods. This finding is consistent with earlier work in the US showing that food groups have limited value in classifying healthy and less healthy foods. [42] If monitoring of food prices is to start in the UK, we would echo these authors in arguing for the development of a monitoring tool that merges nutritional profiling techniques with current guidance for eating a balanced diet rather than relying on monitoring prices by food group alone.

Methodological considerations and limitations

A key weakness to acknowledge is that the number of foods and beverages included in this study is small and only reflects those foods included in the CPI rather than a full range of available foods. Nevertheless, the items included for analysis should reflect those most commonly purchased by UK consumers, given the CPI's role as a measure of consumer inflation. Our study also does not account for variation in price by region or outlet, which is likely to affect the absolute and relative difference in price between food types in given instances. Another potential weakness is the use of price per unit energy rather than price per unit mass or any other price denominator, given that one of the factors determining a food's health categorisation is its energy content, an issue which has been raised by others. [33,43] We analysed price per unit of energy in line with the approach used by international organisations to assess food poverty. [44,45] Moreover, price per unit energy is more consistent with dietary guidance than price per unit weight and with observed household purchasing behaviour which shows that energy consumption is broadly consistent in the UK, even across differing SES groups. [46,47].

The main strength of our study is that we demonstrate the utility of existing government datasets on the prices and nutrition content of foods purchased and consumed in the UK, addressing the recent call by the International Network for Food and Obesity/ Non-communicable Diseases Research, Monitoring and Action Support (INFORMAS) for a cost-effective and simple tool for monitoring the price of healthy foods. [11] The study also provides information on recent price trends pertinent to the health of the UK population, using an objective and nutritionally relevant tool to categorise the foods and beverages examined.

Unanswered questions and future research

In conjunction with other work in the area of food prices, food poverty and food security, our findings highlight the need for the routine monitoring of food prices in relation to the food's nutrient composition. For greater relevance these prices should also be considered in the context of income and other unavoidable expenditure, such a rent or utilities, making it possible to consider the affordability of a healthy diet. Future research in this area ought to build on our findings and examine the cost of observed diets in relation to their quality, since the quality and cost of the overall diet is not simply a function of the price of certain healthy foods being more expensive. Future research should also seek to go beyond a descriptive analysis of the price trends by themselves and try to assess the cause of the observed link between the price and healthiness of foods, and also to examine the link between food purchases, actual consumption and health outcomes.

Conclusions

We have demonstrated a novel linkage of existing economic and nutrition surveillance data to assess trends in the prices of foods in relation to their nutritional value. The growing gap in the price of more healthy and less healthy foods revealed by our analysis leads us to suggest that ongoing monitoring of food prices for public health is warranted. The data linkage we describe could underpin such food price monitoring and provide evidence to inform policy responses to the problem of rising food prices.

Author Contributions

Conceived and designed the experiments: NRVJ AIC MS PM. Analyzed the data: NRVJ. Wrote the paper: NRVJ AIC MS PM.

References

1. Mozaffarian D, Appel LJ, Van Horn L (2011) Components of a cardioprotective diet: new insights. Circulation 123: 2870–2891.
2. World Health Organization (2004) Global Strategy on Diet, Physical Activity and Health. Geneva.
3. National Health Service. The Eatwell Plate. Available: http://www.nhs.uk/Livewell/Goodfood/Pages/eatwell-plate.aspx. Accessed 2013 Jun 30.
4. Department of Health (2012) National Diet and Nutrition Survey: headline results from Years 1, 2 and 3. London.
5. Murray CJL, Richards MA, Newton JN, Fenton KA, Anderson HR, et al. (2013) UK health performance: findings of the Global Burden of Disease Study 2010. Lancet 381: 997–1020.
6. Scarborough P, Bhatnagar P, Wickramasinghe KK, Allender S, Foster C, et al. (2011) The economic burden of ill health due to diet, physical inactivity, smoking, alcohol and obesity in the UK: an update to 2006-07 NHS costs. J Public Health 33: 527–535.
7. Dowler E (2008) Symposium on "Intervention policies for deprived households" Policy initiatives to address low-income households' nutritional needs in the UK. The Proceedings of the Nutrition Society. Vol. 67.pp. 289–300.
8. Department for Environment Food and Rural Affairs (2010) UK Food Security Assessment: Detailed Analysis UK Food Security Assessment. London.
9. Drewnowski A, Specter S (2004) Poverty and obesity: the role of energy density and energy costs. Am J Clin Nutr 79: 6–16. Available: http://ajcn.nutrition.org/content/79/1/6.long. Accessed 2013 Aug 30.
10. Department for Environment Food and Rural Affairs (2013) Food Statistics Pocketbook 2013. London.
11. Lee A, Mhurchu CN, Sacks G, Swinburn B, Snowdon W, et al. (2013) Monitoring the price and affordability of foods and diets globally. 14: 82–95.
12. Department of Health (2011) National Diet and Nutrition Survey Years 1–3 2008/09–2010/11: User Guide.
13. Office for National Statistics (2012) Consumer Price Indices Technical Manual. London.
14. Kuchler F, Stewart H (2008) Price Trends are Similar for Fruits, Vegetables, and Snack Foods. Washington D.C.
15. Office for National Statistics (2013) Office for National Statistics: Data. Available: http://www.ons.gov.uk/ons/datasets-and-tables/index.html. Accessed 2013 Dec 16.
16. MySupermarket (2013) mySupermarket.co.uk. Available: http://www.mysupermarket.co.uk/. Accessed 2013 Dec 1.
17. United States Department of Agriculture. USDA National Nutrient Database for Standard Reference. Available: http://ndb.nal.usda.gov/. Accessed 2013 Jun 27.
18. UK Data Service. National Diet and Nutrition Survey, 2008–2011. Available: http://discover.ukdataservice.ac.uk/catalogue/?sn=6533&type=Data catalogue. Accessed 2013 Jun 30.
19. United States Department of Agriculture (1975) Agriculture Handbook 102: Food Yields. Washington D.C.
20. Macdiarmid JI, Kyle J, Horgan G, Loe J, Fyfe C, et al. (2011) Livewell: a balance of healthy and sustainable food choices. London.
21. Rayner M, Scarborough P, British Heart Foundation (2009) The UK Ofcom Nutrient Profiling Model. Oxford.
22. Scarborough P, Boxer A, Rayner M, Stockley L (2007) Testing nutrient profile models using data from a survey of nutrition professionals. Public Health Nutr 10: 337–345.
23. StataCorp (2011) Stata Statistical Software: Release 12.
24. R_Development_Core_Team (2008) R: A language and environment for statistical computing.
25. Wickham H (2009) ggplot2: elegant graphics for data analysis.
26. Lee JH, Ralston RA, Truby H (2011) Influence of food cost on diet quality and risk factors for chronic disease: A systematic review. Nutr Diet 68: 248–261.
27. Burns C, Sacks G, Gold L (2008) Longitudinal study of Consumer Price Index (CPI) trends in core and non-core foods in Australia. Aust N Z J Public Health 32: 450–453.
28. Harrison M, Lee A, Findlay M, Nicholls R, Leonard D, et al. (2010) The increasing cost of healthy food. Aust N Z J Public Health 34: 179–186.
29. Monsivais P, Drewnowski A (2007) The rising cost of low-energy-density foods. J Am Diet Assoc 107: 2071–2076.
30. Williams P, Hull A, Kontos M (2009) Trends in affordability of the Illawarra Healthy Food Basket 2000-2007. Nutr Diet 66: 27–32.
31. Andreyeva T, Blumenthal DM, Schwartz MB, Long MW, Brownell KD (2008) Availability and prices of foods across stores and neighborhoods: the case of New Haven, Connecticut. Health Aff 27: 1381–1388.

32. Ni Mhurchu C, Ogra S (2007) The price of healthy eating: cost and nutrient value of selected regular and healthier supermarket foods in New Zealand. N Z Med J 120: U2388.
33. Rao M, Afshin A, Singh G, Mozaffarian D (2013) Do healthier foods and diet patterns cost more than less healthy options? A systematic review and meta-analysis.
34. European Union (2007) Common organisation of agricultural markets. Available: http://europa.eu/legislation_summaries/agriculture/agricultural_products_markets/l67001_en.htm. Accessed 2013 Dec 4.
35. Veerman JL, Barendregt JJ, Mackenbach JP (2006) The European Common Agricultural Policy on fruits and vegetables: exploring potential health gain from reform. Eur J Public Health 16: 31–35.
36. Loyd-Williams F (2008) Estimating the cardiovascular mortality burden attributable to the European Common Agricultural Policy on dietary saturated fats. Bull World Health Organ 86: 535–541.
37. Dowd AO (2013) Half a million people using food banks in UK as food poverty grows. BMJ: 3578.
38. Taylor-Robinson D, Rougeaux E, Harrison D, Whitehead M, Barr B, et al. (2013) The rise of food poverty in the UK. BMJ: 7157.
39. FAO (1996) Rome Declaration on World Food Security. Available: http://www.fao.org/docrep/003/w3613e/w3613e00.HTM. Accessed 2013 Aug 10.
40. Pinstrup-Andersen P (2009) Food security: definition and measurement. Food Secur 1: 5–7.
41. Griffith R, Connell MO, Smith K (2012) Food purchases and nutrition over the recession. London.
42. Monsivais P, Mclain J, Drewnowski A (2010) The rising disparity in the price of healthful foods: 2004–2008. Food Policy 35: 514–520.
43. Carlson A, Frazão E (2012) Are Healthy Foods Really More Expensive? It Depends on How You Measure the Price. Washington D.C.
44. The World Bank. Measuring Poverty Lines. Available: http://info.worldbank.org/etools/docs/library/93518/Hung_0603/Hu_0603/Module3MeasuringPovertyLines.pdf. Accessed 2013 Nov 28.
45. Anríquez G, Karfakis P, Daidone S, Mane E (2010) Measuring dietary energy deficiency and the impact of food price variations at the household level. Rome.
46. Change4Life (2013) Healthy living tips and benefits for you and your kids. Available: http://www.nhs.uk/Change4Life/Pages/why-change-for-life.aspx. Accessed 2013 Aug 30.
47. Office for National Statistics (2012) Living Cost and Food Survey.

20

Taste and Physiological Responses to Glucosinolates: Seed Predator *versus* Seed Disperser

Michal Samuni-Blank[1,2]*, Ido Izhaki[2], Yoram Gerchman[3], M. Denise Dearing[4], William H. Karasov[5], Beny Trabelcy[2], Thea M. Edwards[6], Zeev Arad[1]

1 Department of Biology, Technion-Israel Institute of Technology, Haifa 3200003, Israel, **2** Department of Evolutionary and Environmental Biology, Faculty of Natural Sciences, University of Haifa, Haifa 3498838, Israel, **3** Department of Biology and Environment, Faculty of Natural Sciences, University of Haifa, Oranim, Tivon 3600672, Israel, **4** Department of Biology, University of Utah, Salt Lake City, UT 84103, United States of America, **5** Department of Forest and Wildlife Ecology, University of Wisconsin, Madison, WI 53706, United States of America, **6** Department of Biology, Sewanee: The University of the South, Sewanee, TN 37383, United States of America

Abstract

In contrast to most other plant tissues, fleshy fruits are meant to be eaten in order to facilitate seed dispersal. Although fleshy fruits attract consumers, they may also contain toxic secondary metabolites. However, studies that link the effect of fruit toxins with seed dispersal and predation are scarce. Glucosinolates (GLSs) are a family of bitter-tasting compounds. The fleshy fruit pulp of *Ochradenus baccatus* was previously found to harbor high concentrations of GLSs, whereas the myrosinase enzyme, which breaks down GLSs to produce foul tasting chemicals, was found only in the seeds. Here we show the differential behavioral and physiological responses of three rodent species to high dose (80%) *Ochradenus'* fruits diets. *Acomys russatus,* a predator of *Ochradenus'* seeds, was the least sensitive to the taste of the fruit and the only rodent to exhibit taste-related physiological adaptations to deal with the fruits' toxins. In contrast, *Acomys cahirinus*, an *Ochradenus* seed disperser, was more sensitive to a diet containing the hydrolyzed products of the GLSs. A third rodent (*Mus musculus*) was deterred from *Ochradenus* fruits consumption by the GLSs and their hydrolyzed products. We were able to alter *M. musculus* avoidance of whole fruit consumption by soaking *Ochradenus* fruits in a water solution containing 1% adenosine monophosphate, which blocks the bitter taste receptor in mice. The observed differential responses of these three rodent species may be due to evolutionary pressures that have enhanced or reduced their sensitivity to the taste of GLSs.

Editor: Maik Behrens, German Institute of Human Nutrition Potsdam-Rehbruecke, Germany

Funding: Support for this study was available through grants from the U.S.-Israel Bi-National Science Foundation Grant (#2006043), Israel Science Foundation (#189/08) and Middle East Regional Cooperation (#TA-MOU-08-M28-013). The funders had no role in study design, data collection and analysis, decision to publish, or preparation of the manuscript.

Competing Interests: The authors have declared that no competing interests exist.

* Email: michal.samuni@gmail.com

Introduction

Fleshy fruits are commonly used by plants to facilitate seed dispersal by animals. However, as there are also seed predators, the nature of plant-animal interactions is dependent on the consumers' fruit eating behavior. Generally, there are three ways to utilize fruits: a) Utilize only the pulp - the fleshy ripe pulp is used by plants as a reward for seed dispersing animals [1–3]; b) utilize only the seeds - seeds are a valuable food source for many animal species [4], being of higher nutritional quality compared to ripe fruit pulp [5]; or c) utilize the pulp and the seeds - while seed dispersers utilize only the pulp, seed predators may utilize both the pulp and the seeds [6,7].

Although fruits are intended to facilitate seed dispersal, the ripe fruits of many plants contain secondary metabolites in toxic concentrations [1,8–11]. Fruit toxins are a widespread phenomenon but the study of their function is a relatively new field in ecology and ecophysiology [12]. At least seven adaptive hypotheses have been proposed for the existence of toxins in fruit [10,13]. The majority of these hypotheses assume that toxins have an effect, either negative or positive, on fruit consumers. For example, the Gut Retention Time Hypothesis [10,13] assumes that fruit toxins alter gut passage rates of vertebrates, while the Directed Nutritional Benefits Hypothesis [10,13] assumes that fruit improves the health, longevity and performance of the consumer. Furthermore, several of the adaptive hypotheses assume that fruit toxins have different effects among different consumers. The Directed Deterrence Hypothesis states that fruit toxins in ripe fruit deter seed predators, but have no or little toxic effect on seed-dispersers [10,13–15]. However, few data are available for the evaluation of these hypotheses, considering that the effect of fruit toxins is tightly linked to seed dispersal and predation, and thus to plant fitness. In this paper, we are going to directly address the Directed Deterrence Hypothesis.

Like all examined plant species from the order Brassicales (which includes the Resedaceae family), *Ochradenus baccatus* contains Glucosinolates (GLSs) [16]. GLSs are a family of bitter-tasting compounds [17,18]. Bitter taste and toxicity are often coupled traits, enabling consumers to avoid toxicity [19,20]. However, different species may have different taste sensitivities [21]. The defensive properties of bitter, intact GLSs are further enhanced upon hydrolysis by the myrosinase enzyme, a mechanism known as the "mustard-oil bomb" [22]. The defensive properties of the mustard-oil bomb include growth depression, decreased food efficiency and lesions in the liver, pancreas and kidney [22–24]. In Brassicales, GLSs occur throughout the tissues of plant organs, whereas myrosinases are localized in scattered myrosin cells, which are free of GLSs [24–26]. Other *Ochradenus* plant organs are also protected by the mustard-oil bomb [16,27]. In the fruits of *Ochradenus* there is a unique compartmentalization, where GLSs are found only in the pulp and the myrosinase enzyme is found only in the seeds [16]. Thus, consumers that simultaneously eat the pulp and crush the seeds will have to face the hydrolyzed products of the GLSs [16].

Ochradenus plants co-occur with two of the three omnivorous rodent species used in this study (*Acomys russatus* and *A. cahirinus*) that differ in their interactions with the plant. *Acomys russatus* is a seed predator that eats *Ochradenus* fruit pulp and seeds; whereas *A. cahirinus* eats the fruit pulp but expels the seeds intact [6,16]. A third omnivorous rodent, the house mouse (*Mus musculus*), is less likely to naturally feed on *Ochradenus* fruits or seeds as it is absent from desert areas were the *Ochradenus* is found. Comparing taste sensitivities of different species of rodents, and especially sympatric species can be illuminating. For example, it is known that two out of three common mouse species that share their habitat with monarch butterflies, are sensitive to the bitter-toxic taste of the glycosides and alkaloids in the butterflies [21]. Moreover, in rodents, the T2R bitter taste receptors are found to be expressed not only in the tongue, but also in the gastrointestinal tract [28]. Rodents have also been shown to behaviorally regulate bitter-toxic food intake [29] and finally, in rodents, gut retention time may be extended in response to bitter taste and thus may also regulate bitter-toxic food intake [28].

We predicted that the two *Acomys* species would be less sensitive than *M. musculus* to the taste of GLSs and their hydrolyzed products, as *Acomys* encounter and consume *Ochradenus* fruits in their natural habitat [6,7,16]. In this study we used high dose (80% of the diet), short-term, feeding trials. We also predicted that within a few days, we should be able to observe the negative impact of a high dose of pulp or mashed fruit diets in all three rodents. As intact GLSs are generally non-toxic, we predicted that seed disposers, like *A. cahirinus*, should not be deterred by the taste of intact GLSs in the pulp, but would keep away from pulp and seed co-consumption to avoid the mustard-oil bomb physiological consequences. As different species may have different taste sensitivities [21], it is plausible that the seed predator, *A. russatus,* has a higher perception threshold (i.e., lower sensitivity) to the taste of GLSs and their hydrolyzed products. Thus, it should be able to overcome the taste and physiological effects of intact GLSs as well as GLS-myrosinase combination. A new introduced species, like *M. musculus,* should reject intact as well as hydrolyzed GLSs.

We used adenosine monophosphate (AMP), known to block bitter taste receptors in mice [30], and monitored the rodents' feeding behavior. We also used diets that contained intact GLSs and activated GLSs and monitored the rodents' body mass, food intake, digestibility and gut retention time (as bitter compounds can extend retention time). We measured estrogenic activity in *Ochradenus* fruit pulp and seeds as some phytoestrogens are known for their bitter taste [18]. In addition, estrogenicity in the fruits may affect rodent metabolism and weight gain [31].

Materials and Methods

Ethics Statement

The experimental protocols were approved by the University of Haifa Committee of Animal Experimentation (Permit number 096/08). No specific permissions were required for the collection of fruits, as they were not collected from protected areas. The plant, *Ochradenus baccatus*, is not an endangered or protected species.

Estrogenic Activity in Fruits

For measurement of phytoestrogen activity in *Ochradenus* fruit, pulp and seeds, we collected 200 ripe fruits in early March 2013 from five individual plants growing wild in Almog junction (31°48′N, 35°27′E). Fruits were kept at 4°C and pulp was manually separated from the seeds within one day of collection. Samples were dried for 24 h at 40°C and stored at −20°C (pulps) or room temperature (seeds). Combined pulps and combined seeds from each plant ($n = 5$ per organ type; 0.3–0.5 g dry tissue per sample) were ground using a mortar and pestle and double extracted in 55% ethanol. Samples were reconstituted in 55% ethanol to a final concentration that represented 2.7 g dry weight/ml for pulps and 3.0 g dry weight/ml for seeds (equivalent to 13.3 and 3.1 g fresh weight/ml for pulps and seeds, respectively). Dilution curves to measure estrogenic activity of pulp and seed extracts were compared to estradiol and soybean leaf extracts using transgenic *Saccharomyces cerevisiae* (baker's yeast) expressing human estrogen receptor β (ESR2) linked to a β-galactosidase reporter gene (lacZ) [32]. Dilution curves ranged from 0.3–82 mg fresh weight per well for pulps and 0.14–19.4 mg fresh weight per well for seeds. Estrogenicity was expressed as pg estradiol equivalents per mg fresh weight.

Study System

General information on the study system including a description of the plant, fruit collection, fruit concentration of GLSs in the pulp and myrosinase activity in the seeds and animal maintenance can be found in Samuni-Blank *et al.* [7,16].

Fruit Taste - Behavior

Animals (*Acomys cahirinus* $n = 8$; body mass = 55.0±4.4 g SE; *Acomys russatus* $n = 8$; body mass = 59.3±2.5 g SE; *Mus musculus* $n = 8$; body mass = 25.8±0.9 g SE) were placed in separate cages with 5 intact *Ochradenus* fruits ('natural') over-night. After 24 h the cage floor was examined for intact fruits or fruit parts (pulp or seeds). We counted the intact fruits and documented whether the mice ate only the pulp, only the seeds or both. Then, we gave the same individuals five fruits from the same batch that were soaked for ten minutes in distilled water containing 1% adenosine monophosphate (AMP), known to block bitter taste receptors in mice [30]. Remains of AMP-treated fruits were categorized after 24 h as mentioned above. Throughout the experiments, carrots, rodent chow and dog chow were provided *ad libitum*.

Fruit Taste - Physiology

To examine the effect of taste of a mashed fruit diet (fruit pulp and seeds mashed together, causing hydrolysis of GLSs) *versus* a pulp diet (no seeds, therefore containing intact GLSs), we performed feeding trials and monitored the effects of the different diets on body mass, dry matter (DM) food intake and DM digestibility. We used adult males of: *A. cahirinus* (body mass = 50.9±1.2 g SE; $n = 117$), *A. russatus* (body mass = 53.8±1.1 g SE; $n = 110$) and wild house mouse (*M. musculus*; body mass = 29.6±0.7 g SE; $n = 22$) from captive breeding colonies maintained at the Department of Biology and Environment at the University of Haifa, Oranim.

The rodents were fed for two days with one of three possible diets (treatments): pulp (containing intact GLSs), mash (containing hydrolyzed products of GLSs) and a control (rodent chow) diet (n = 6–8 individuals per treatment). In each case the diet

Table 1. Average number (± S.E.) of intact fruits (Natural) and AMP-treated fruits (AMP) fruits after 24 h by the seed predator, *A. russatus*, the seed disperser, *A. cahirinus* and a naïve rodent, *M. musculus* ($n=8$ for each species in each of the treatments).

	Fruit left	
	Natural	**AMP**
Predator$^{N.S}$	0.0±0.0	0.63±0.63
Disperser$^{N.S}$	1.25±0.62	0.75±0.31
M. musculus	3.8±0.72^{A}	0. 5±0.5^{B}

Different letters adjacent to means indicate significant difference (Wilcoxon Signed Ranks Test, $P>0.05$) among means. N.S., not significant.

treatments contained on a wet mass basis: 20% rodent chow (Koffolk serial no. 19510, Tel Aviv, Israel) combined with 80% pulp (pulp was manually separated from the seeds) or mash (pulp and seeds crushed together). The control diet contained 70% rodent chow combined with 30% tap water. The total calories available in the pulp, mash and control diet was analyzed by Parr microbomb calorimeter with a benzoic acid standard.

A body mass loss of 15% was defined as the limit of tolerance. During the experiment we took daily measurements of body mass and food intake. Excreta and food leftovers were collected every day from the plastic cage floor, weighed, dried (at 50°C for 24 h) and stored at room temperature. The dry matter (DM) digestibility of food consumed by an animal was calculated from its DM intake and fecal DM output as: DM digestibility = (DM intake – fecal DM output)/DM intake.

Gut Retention Time

To examine the effect of *Ochradenus* fruits on the *Acomys* gut retention time, we used captive adult males and females of *A. russatus* (body mass = 58.2±2.2 g SE; $n=25$) and *A. cahirinus* (body mass = 49.3±1.6 g SE; $n=25$). Animals were fed according to one of the four following treatments: 1) 'Control' - rodent chow (Koffolk serial no. 19510) homogenized with 70% tap water; 2) 'Pulp' – pulp, which contain the intact GLSs, manually separated from fruits. 3) 'Seeds' – seeds, which contain the myrosinase enzyme, manually separated from fruits and homogenized with 80% water. 4) 'Mash' - pulp and seeds mashed together, contain the hydrolyzed products of GLSs. Food treatment was orally administrated using 10 ml syringe into the animal mouth. All other food was denied from the animals an hour before and an hour after feeding. Orally administrated food was homogenized with 1% of inert blue plastic marker pieces that can pass through a 40 mesh screen. Fecal samples were collected every 15 min (coprophagy was not prevented), each sample was mashed in water and examined until the first markers appeared in the feces.

Statistical Analyses

To test for differences in consumption with or without AMP, that did not fulfill normality criteria (Kolmogorov-Simirnov test), we used the Wilcoxon Signed Ranks Test. All other variables tested fulfilled normality criteria. Therefore, to compare species and treatments we used two-way ANOVA and to test for differences within each species we performed a one-way ANOVA followed by Bonferroni multiple comparisons. In all cases, significance level was set at $P<0.05$. All data are reported as means ± standard error (SE). Statistical analyses were conducted using SPSS 19.0 (SPSS, USA).

Results

For phytoestrogen activity in pulp, we tested extracts that represented 2–510 mg fresh weight/ml (equivalent to 0.4–102 mg dry weight/ml). For phytoestrogen activity in seeds, we tested extracts that represented 1–120 mg fresh weight/ml (equivalent to 0.96–115 mg dry weight/ml). No phytoestrogenic activity was found in *Ochradenus* fruits (pulp or seeds).

Fruit Taste - Behavior

A clear and significant difference was apparent between the two *Acomys* species in the number of seeds left intact. The seed predator, *A. russatus,* left 0.13±0.13 and 0.25±0.25 intact seeds, while the seed disperser, *A. cahirinus,* left 16.14±3.42 and 15.75±2.91 intact seeds on the non-treated and AMP treated fruits respectively. For each of the two *Acomys* species, there were no significant differences ($P>0.05$) in the number of fruits eaten and seeds left intact in the natural fruits versus the AMP-treated fruits (Table 1).

For *M. musculus,* there was a significant difference between ingestion of natural and AMP treated fruits with *M. musculus* avoiding ingestion of natural fruits but consuming AMP treated fruits ($Z=2.26$, $n=8$, $P=0.024$; Table 1). For non-treated fruits, five of eight *M. musculus* individuals left the natural fruits intact, two individuals ate only the seeds and one ate one whole fruit (pulp and seeds) out of five offered. As a results there were no intact seeds left separated from the pulp in the cages (seeds were either all consumed or were left inside the whole fruit). For fruits soaked with AMP, only one individual left intact fruits. The other seven individuals ate both pulp and seeds leaving 5.25±1.41 intact seeds separated from the pulp. Altogether, significantly more AMP-treated pulp and AMP-treated seeds were consumed compared to the natural pulp and seeds ($Z=2.45$, $n=8$, $P=0.014$; $Z=2.24$, $n=8$, $P=0.025$; respectively).

Fruit Taste - Physiology

The total calories available in the pulp, mash and control diet were 4060±44, 4433±80 and 4154±35 cal/g, respectively.

The experiment for all *M. musculus* individuals on mash diet was terminated after one day, due to loss of 15% of body mass on mash diet.

Body mass. There were significant differences in body mass changes among species ($F_{2,54}=36.9$, $P<0.0001$) and among treatments ($F_{2,54}=33.2$, $P<0.0001$), as well as a significant treatment*species interaction ($F_{4,54}=8.3$, $P<0.0001$). *M. musculus* significantly lost body mass on both pulp and mashed diets after only 24 h, while in the two *Acomys,* body mass was maintained on the control and pulp diets (Fig. 1A). All individuals recovered and returned to their original body mass a few days after the experiment ended.

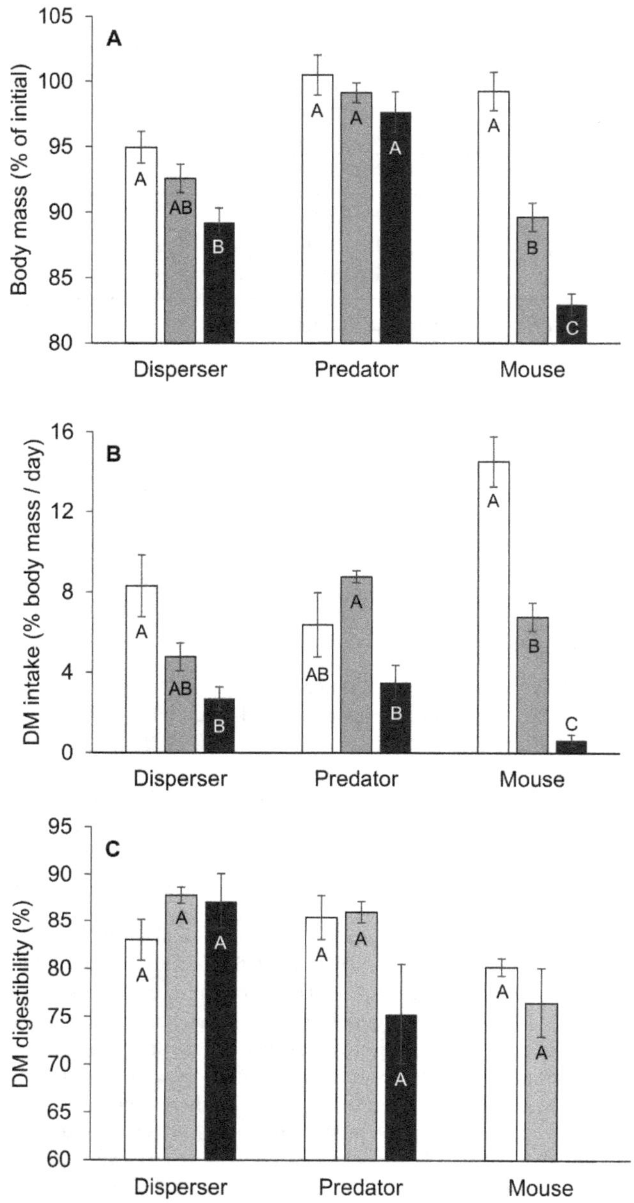

Figure 1. Feeding trials. Control (white bars), 80% *Ochradenus* pulp (gray bars) and 80% *Ochradenus* mash (black bars) diet of *A. cahirinus* (disperser) and *A. russatus* (predator) after two days and of *M. musculus* (mouse) after one day. $n = 6–8$ for each diet within each species. A. Body mass (% of initial). B. Dry matter intake (% body mass/day). C. Dry matter digestibility (%). Within each species, different letters at the top of the columns indicate significant differences (Bonferroni Multiple Comparison, $P<0.05$). Data are presented as means ± SE.

Food intake. A significant difference in the normalized DM intake (% body mass/day) was found among treatments ($F_{2,54} = 35.5$, $P<0.0001$) and there was no main effect of species on DM intake ($F_{2,54} = 2.7$, $P = 0.08$). However, there was a significant interaction between species and treatments ($F_{4,54} = 9.2$, $P<0.0001$); *Acomys russatus* maintained DM intake on the pulp diet, while the same diet depressed DM intake of *M. musculus* (Fig. 1B).

Digestibility. There was a significant difference in the DM digestibility among species ($F_{2,49} = 6.4$, $P<0.005$) and there were no significant differences in DM digestibility among treatments ($F_{2,49} = 1.6$, NS). There was a significant interaction between species and treatments ($F_{3,49} = 3.0$, $P<0.05$); the DM digestibility in *A. russatus,* but not in *A. cahirinus*, decreased on the mash diet (Fig. 1C).

Gut Retention Time

There were significant differences in gut retention time among treatments ($F_{3,40} = 3.4$, $P<0.05$) but no main effect of species ($F_{1,40} = 0.0$, NS). However, there was a significant treatment*species interaction ($F_{3,40} = 7.7$, $P<0.0001$); the mash treatment significantly increased the gut retention time in *A. russatus* but not in *A. cahirinus*. Average retention time for all groups, except for *A. russatus* mash treatment, was less than eight hours (Fig. 2).

Discussion

Previously [6,7,16], we revealed divergent behavioral and physiological strategies and adaptations in two coexisting species of desert rodents, *A. cahirinus* and *A. russatus,* dealing with fleshy fruit toxins. Here we demonstrate that these different strategies are probably mediated by taste.

The *Ochradenus* GLSs are likely to be an important factor limiting fruits consumption by rodents. GLSs and their hydrolyzed products are known for the deterrent quality of their bitter taste [18]. The bitter taste of the fruits that originate from GLSs in the pulp appears to be the cause of *M. musculus*' fruit avoidance, as we were able to alter *M. musculus* behavior by using AMP. Even though *M. musculus* was first exposed to the natural fruits and only later to the AMP treated fruits, there was no evidence of learning effect as it consumed significantly more AMP treated fruits. We cannot rule out neophobia as a possible explanation to the fact that 5 out of 8 *M. musculus* did not sample the untreated fruits, since we first gave the mice untreated fruits and only later the AMP treated fruits. However, over the years, we have observed numerous first-time encounters of rodents with *Ochradenus* fruits; some rodents hold the fruit in their mouth and spit it out intact. Thus, we believe that it is more likely that the mice avoided the fruits because of their taste and not because of neophobia.

From the results we conclude that the seed predator, *A. russatus,* has as a higher perception threshold (i.e., lower sensitivity) to the taste of GLSs and their hydrolyzed products; after two days in the feeding trial *A. russatus* was the only species that consistently ate the whole fruit and maintained body mass on 80% pulp and mash diets. Also, it was the only species to have higher DM food intake on the pulp diet compared to the control diet. The differences between species are consistent with our previous work, where we have shown that after four days in the feeding trial on 50% mash diet, *A. russatus* maintained ~90% of its initial body mass, while the seed disperser, *A. cahirinus,* maintained only ~80% of its initial body mass [7]. In addition, on the mash treatment, *A. russatus,* but not *A. cahirinus,* significantly extended its gut retention time and decreased its DM digestibility. These physiological responses may provide more time for the operation of detoxification enzymes in the gut and liver, decrease the concentrations and slow the rate of hydrolyzed products entering the systemic circulation [28]. We suggest that these differential responses of the two species to *Ochradenus* fruits have stemmed from interspecific competition.

Another observation that emerges from comparison to [7] is that *A. russatus* performs better on high-concentration, short-term diet (80% mashed fruit, two days) than on low-concentration, long-term mash diet (one day at 25% followed by three days at 50%). Likewise, compared to the pulp diet, DM intake of *A.*

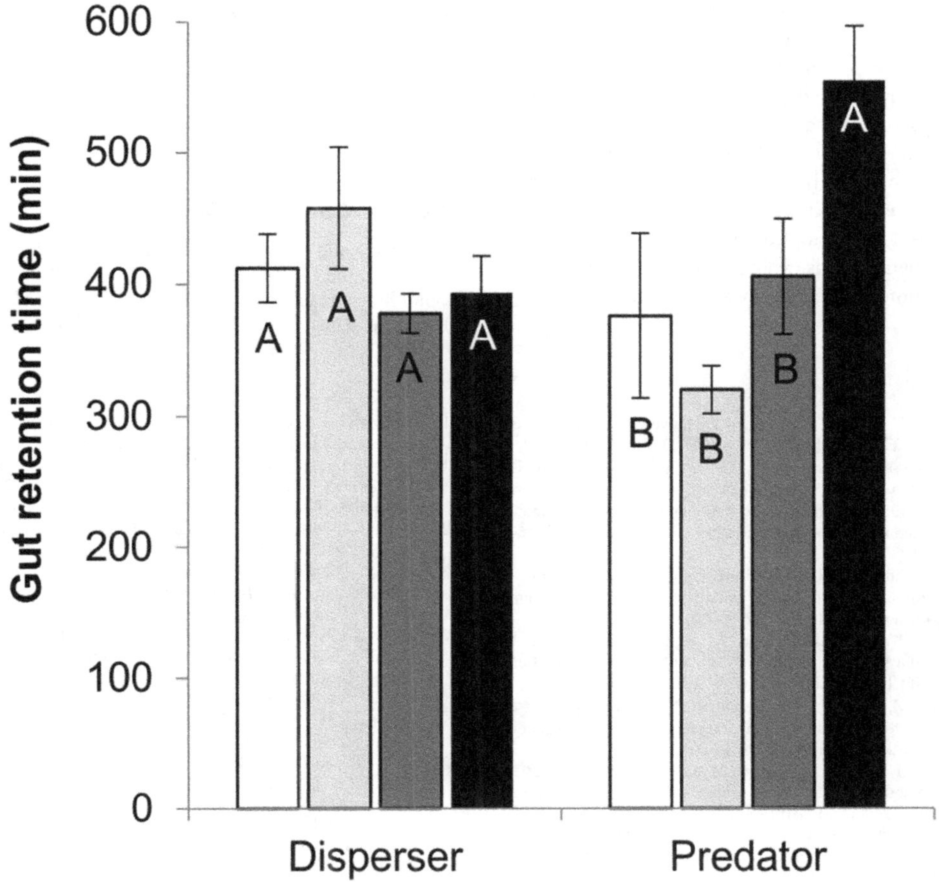

Figure 2. Gut retention time. Gut retention time in *Acomys cahirinus* (seed disperser) and *A. russatus* (seed predator; $n = 6–8$ for each group within each species) fed with a control diet (white bars), with *Ochradenus* pulp (light-gray bars), with *Ochradenus* seeds (dark-gray bars) or with mashed *Ochradenus* fruits (black bars). Within each species, different letters at the top of the columns indicate significant differences (Bonferroni Multiple Comparison, $P<0.05$). Data are presented as means ± SE.

russatus is lower by ~50% on a lower concentration of mash in our previous study [7], while the difference in this study was not significant. This could be evidence of adaptive physiological mechanisms such as detoxification enzymes that *A. russatus* can employ when toxicity levels increase. Another explanation is that post-ingestional effects are not as immediate as taste and thus are less pronounced in short term trials. A third hypothesis is that the high concentration of mash increases the likelihood of *A. russatus* using torpor to conserve energy [33].

Like the *Acomys, M. musculus* exhibited a higher tolerance level (in terms of defending body mass) when feeding on the pulp diet than on the mash diet, despite its avoidance of the GLSs. Although mash diet has the highest energetic value, after only one day on this diet, *M. musculus* lost ~15% of its initial body mass. Individuals of *M. musculus* preferred to face rapid and life threatening loss of body mass, rather than to feed on the mash diet. *Mus musculus* also significantly reduced DM food intake when feeding on the pulp diet. However, *M. musculus* consumed significantly more food on the pulp diet than on the mash diet, suggesting a preference of intact GLSs over their toxic hydrolyzed products.

This study, provides some evaluation to the existence of toxins in fruit adaptive hypotheses. In agreement with The Directed-Deterrence Hypothesis [13], *A. cahirinus* and *M. musculus* showed highest loss of mass while on mash diet. These findings also extend The Directed-Deterrence Hypothesis to the intraspecific level, in addition to the interspecific level, as they also performed better on seed dispersers' diet (pulp) than on seed predators' diet (mash). However, other findings of our work are in contradiction with The Directed-Deterrence Hypothesis, as they demonstrate the ability of *A. russatus* to consume the whole fruit of *Ochradenus* while exhibiting behavioral and physiological traits that allow it to avoid the negative effects of GLSs hydrolyzed products (see also [6,7]). Moreover, our previous study demonstrated the ability of another seed predator, *A. minous*, to circumvent the activation of the GSLs by making a hole in the pulp and consuming only the seeds [7]. Our results are ambiguous also with respect to The Gut Retention Time Hypothesis, which states that fruit secondary metabolites act to alter seed passage rates; *Ochradenus baccatus* fruit toxins did alter gut passage in *A. russatus,* but not in *A. cahirinus*. This study does not provide strong support for either of the hypotheses, probably due to the fact that the two species (*A. cahirinus* and *A. russatus*) are closely related. This fact, however, is what makes this study system particularly fascinating, as it allows to study the function of fruits' toxins in finer detail.

In the present study, we revealed the ability of *Ochradenus* plants to deter seed predators from co-consumption of pulp and seeds. Our results demonstrate that the mustard oil bomb mechanism in *Ochradenus* fruits shapes the behavioral responses of its consumers at an ecological timescale. This is also supported by our previous studies, which show, for example, that the evolutionary naïve *A. minous* was able to behaviorally avoid the GLSs-myrosinase combination in *Ochradenus* fruits. The bitter taste of the GLSs is a first line of defense against naïve rodents. The bitter taste of the hydrolyzed products of GLSs is a second barrier. Finally, seed predators that co-consume the pulp and seeds will encounter the toxic products of the GLSs. Nevertheless, the value of fleshy fruits cannot be overestimated in the desert ecosystem; thus, there is an evolutionary pressure on consumers to develop behavioral and physiological adaptations, in order to extract the greatest benefit. In this evolutionary arms race between the plant and its consumers, one will always lag behind.

Acknowledgments

We are grateful to the members of the Oranim College animal house staff, particularly to Nina Dainov for her help with animal maintenance and to Noa Sheena and Yonatan Lev-el for their help with the experiments. We would also like to thank the two anonymous reviewers for their thoughtful comments.

Author Contributions

Conceived and designed the experiments: MSB II MDD WHK ZA. Performed the experiments: MSB BT TME. Analyzed the data: MSB II. Contributed reagents/materials/analysis tools: MSB II YG TME ZA. Wrote the paper: MSB II YG MDD WHK TME ZA.

References

1. Izhaki I, Safriel UN (1989) Why are there so few exclusively frugivorous birds? experiments on fruit digestibility. Oikos 54: 23. doi:10.2307/3565893.
2. Herrera CM (1982) Defense of ripe fruit from pests: its significance in relation to plant-disperser interactions. Am Nat 120: 218–241.
3. Corlett RT, Lucas PW (1990) Alternative seed-handling strategies in primates: seed-spitting by long-tailed macaques (Macaca fascicularis). Oecologia 82: 166–171. doi:10.1007/BF00323531.
4. Kelt DA, Meserve PL, Gutiérrez JR (2004) Seed removal by small mammals, birds and ants in semi-arid Chile, and comparison with other systems. J Biogeogr 31: 931–942. doi:10.1111/j.1365-2699.2004.01045.x.
5. Norconk MA, Grafton BW, Conklin-Brittain NL (1998) Seed dispersal by neotropical seed predators. Am J Primatol 45: 103–126. doi:10.1002/(SICI)1098-2345(1998)45: 1<103::AID-AJP8>3.0.CO;2.-#.
6. Samuni-Blank M, Arad Z, Dearing MD, Gerchman Y, Karasov WH, et al. (2013) Friend or foe? Disparate plant–animal interactions of two congeneric rodents. Evol Ecol: 1–12. doi:10.1007/s10682-013-9655-x.
7. Samuni-Blank M, Izhaki I, Dearing D, Karasov W, Gerchman Y, et al. (2013) Physiological and behavioural effects of fruit toxins on seed-predating versus seed-dispersing congeneric rodents. J Exp Biol. doi:10.1242/jeb.089664.
8. Izhaki I (1992) A comparative analysis of the nutritional quality of mixed and exclusive fruit diets for yellow-vented bulbuls. The Condor 94: 912–923. doi:10.2307/1369288.
9. Barnea A, Harborne JB, Pannell C (1993) What parts of fleshy fruits contain secondary compounds toxic to birds and why? Biochem Syst Ecol 21: 421–429. doi:10.1016/0305-1978(93)90100-6.
10. Cipollini M (2000) Secondary metabolites of vertebrate-dispersed fruits: evidence for adaptive functions. Rev Chil Hist Nat 73: 421–440.
11. Izhaki I (2002) Emodin – a secondary metabolite with multiple ecological functions in higher plants. New Phytol 155: 205–217. doi:10.1046/j.1469-8137.2002.00459.x.
12. Stanley MC, Lill A (2001) Response of silvereyes (Zosterops lateralis) to dietary tannins: the paradox of secondary metabolites in ripe fruit. Aust J Zool 49: 633–640.
13. Cipollini ML, Levey DJ (1997) Secondary metabolites of fleshy vertebrate-dispersed fruits: adaptive hypotheses and implications for seed dispersal. Am Nat 150: 346–372. doi:10.1086/286069.
14. Janzen DH (1975) Ecology of plants in the tropics. Edward Arnold. 71.
15. Cipollini ML, Levey DJ (1997) Why are some fruits toxic? Glycoalkaloids in solanumand fruit choice by vertebrates. Ecology 78: 782–798.
16. Samuni-Blank M, Izhaki I, Dearing MD, Gerchman Y, Trabelcy B, et al. (2012) Intraspecific directed deterrence by the mustard oil bomb in a desert plant. Curr Biol CB 22: 1218–1220. doi:10.1016/j.cub.2012.04.051.
17. Tepper BJ, Koelliker Y, Zhao L, Ullrich NV, Lanzara C, et al. (2008) Variation in the Bitter-taste receptor gene TAS2R38, and adiposity in a genetically isolated population in southern Italy. Obesity 16: 2289–2295.
18. Drewnowski A, Gomez-Carneros C (2000) Bitter taste, phytonutrients, and the consumer: a review. Am J Clin Nutr 72: 1424–1435.
19. Chandrashekar J, Mueller KL, Hoon MA, Adler E, Feng L, et al. (2000) T2Rs function as bitter taste receptors. Cell 100: 703–711. doi:10.1016/S0092-8674(00)80706-0.
20. Burns KC (2012) Seed dispersal: The blind bomb maker. Curr Biol 22: R535–R537. doi:10.1016/j.cub.2012.05.014.
21. Glendinning JI (1990) Responses of three mouse species to deterrent chemicals in the monarch butterfly. II. Taste tests using intact monarchs. Chemoecology 1: 124–130. doi:10.1007/BF01241653.
22. Fenwick GR, Griffiths NM, Heaney RK (1982) Bitterness in Brussels sprouts (Brassica oleracea L var gemmifera): The role of glucosinolates and their breakdown products. J. Sci. Food Agric. 34: 73–80.
23. Halkier BA, Gershenzon J (2006) Biology and biochemistry of glucosinolates. Annu Rev Plant Biol 57: 303–333. doi:10.1146/annurev.arplant.57.032905.105228.
24. Fenwick GR, Heaney RK (1983) Fruit and frugivory. Glucosinolates and their breakdown products in cruciferous crops, foods and feedingstuffs. Food Chem 11: 249–271.
25. Rask L, Andréasson E, Ekbom B, Eriksson S, Pontoppidan B, et al. (2000) Myrosinase: gene family evolution and herbivore defense in Brassicaceae. In: Doyle JJ, Gaut BS, editors. Plant Molecular Evolution. Springer Netherlands. 93–113.
26. Wittstock U, Halkier BA (2002) Glucosinolate research in the Arabidopsis era. Trends Plant Sci 7: 263–270. doi:10.1016/S1360-1385(02)02273-2.
27. Oka Y, Shuker S, Tkachi N, Trabelcy B, Gerchman Y (2014) Nematicidal activity of Ochradenus baccatus against the root-knot nematode Meloidogyne javanica. Plant Pathol 63: 221–231.
28. Glendinning JI, Yiin Y-M, Ackroff K, Sclafani A (2008) Intragastric infusion of denatonium conditions flavor aversions and delays gastric emptying in rodents. Physiol Behav 93: 757–765. doi:10.1016/j.physbeh.2007.11.029.
29. Torregrossa A-M, Azzara AV, Dearing MD (2011) Differential regulation of plant secondary compounds by herbivorous rodents. Funct Ecol 25: 1232–1240. doi:10.1111/j.1365-2435.2011.01896.x.
30. Ming D, Ninomiya Y, Margolskee RF (1999) Blocking taste receptor activation of gustducin inhibits gustatory responses to bitter compounds. Proc Natl Acad Sci 96: 9903–9908. doi:10.1073/pnas.96.17.9903.
31. Cederroth CR, Vinciguerra M, Kuhne F, Madani R, Doerge DR, et al. (2007) A phytoestrogen-rich diet increases energy expenditure and decreases adiposity in mice. Environ Health Perspect 115: 1467–1473. doi:10.1289/ehp.10413.
32. Morgan HE, Dillaway D, Edwards TM (2014) Estrogenicity of soybeans (*Glycine max*) varies by plant organ and developmental stage. Endocr Disrupt. In Press. doi:10.4161/endo.28490.
33. Ehrhardt N, Heldmaier G, Exner C (2005) Adaptive mechanisms during food restriction in *Acomys russatus*: the use of torpor for desert survival. J Comp Physiol B 175: 193–200. doi:10.1007/s00360-005-0475-3.

Permissions

All chapters in this book were first published in PLOS ONE, by The Public Library of Science; hereby published with permission under the Creative Commons Attribution License or equivalent. Every chapter published in this book has been scrutinized by our experts. Their significance has been extensively debated. The topics covered herein carry significant findings which will fuel the growth of the discipline. They may even be implemented as practical applications or may be referred to as a beginning point for another development.

The contributors of this book come from diverse backgrounds, making this book a truly international effort. This book will bring forth new frontiers with its revolutionizing research information and detailed analysis of the nascent developments around the world.

We would like to thank all the contributing authors for lending their expertise to make the book truly unique. They have played a crucial role in the development of this book. Without their invaluable contributions this book wouldn't have been possible. They have made vital efforts to compile up to date information on the varied aspects of this subject to make this book a valuable addition to the collection of many professionals and students.

This book was conceptualized with the vision of imparting up-to-date information and advanced data in this field. To ensure the same, a matchless editorial board was set up. Every individual on the board went through rigorous rounds of assessment to prove their worth. After which they invested a large part of their time researching and compiling the most relevant data for our readers.

The editorial board has been involved in producing this book since its inception. They have spent rigorous hours researching and exploring the diverse topics which have resulted in the successful publishing of this book. They have passed on their knowledge of decades through this book. To expedite this challenging task, the publisher supported the team at every step. A small team of assistant editors was also appointed to further simplify the editing procedure and attain best results for the readers.

Apart from the editorial board, the designing team has also invested a significant amount of their time in understanding the subject and creating the most relevant covers. They scrutinized every image to scout for the most suitable representation of the subject and create an appropriate cover for the book.

The publishing team has been an ardent support to the editorial, designing and production team. Their endless efforts to recruit the best for this project, has resulted in the accomplishment of this book. They are a veteran in the field of academics and their pool of knowledge is as vast as their experience in printing. Their expertise and guidance has proved useful at every step. Their uncompromising quality standards have made this book an exceptional effort. Their encouragement from time to time has been an inspiration for everyone.

The publisher and the editorial board hope that this book will prove to be a valuable piece of knowledge for researchers, students, practitioners and scholars across the globe.

List of Contributors

Laura M. Dixon, Vicky Sandilands, Bert J. Tolkamp and Rick B. D'Eath
Animal and Veterinary Science, SRUC, Edinburgh, United Kingdom

Sarah Brocklehurst
Biomathematics and Statistics Scotland, Edinburgh, United Kingdom

Melissa Bateson
Center for Behaviour and Evolution, Institute of Neuroscience, Newcastle University, United Kingdom

Christoph Sandrock
Agroscope, Swiss Bee Research Centre, Berne, Switzerland

Aline Fauser-Misslin and Peter Neumann
Agroscope, Swiss Bee Research Centre, Berne, Switzerland
Institute of Bee Health, Vetsuisse Faculty, University of Berne, Berne, Switzerland

Matteo Tanadini
Seminar for Statistics, ETH Zurich, Zurich, Switzerland

Lorenzo G. Tanadini
Division of Biostatistics, Institute for Social and Preventive Medicine, University of Zurich, Zurich, Switzerland

Simon G. Potts
School of Agriculture, Policy and Development, University of Reading, Reading, United Kingdom

Satoko Yoneyama, Masaru Sakurai, Koshi Nakamura, Yuko Morikawa and Hideaki Nakagawa
Department of Epidemiology and Public Health, Kanazawa Medical University, Ishikawa, Japan

Katsuyuki Miura
Department of Health Science, Shiga University of Medical Science, Otsu, Japan

Motoko Nakashima
Department of Community Health Nursing, School of Nursing, Kanazawa Medical University, Ishikawa, Japan

Katsushi Yoshita
Department of Food and Human Health Science Osaka City University, Graduate School of Human Life Science, Osaka, Japan

Masao Ishizaki
Department of Social and Environmental Medicine, Kanazawa Medical University, Ishikawa, Japan

Teruhiko Kido
School of Health Science, College of Medical, Pharmaceutical and Health Science, Kanazawa University, Kanazawa, Japan

Yuchi Naruse
Department of Human Science and Fundamental Nursing, Toyama University School of Nursing, Toyama, Japan

Kazuhiro Nogawa and Yasushi Suwazono
Department of Occupational and Environmental Medicine, Graduate School of Medicine, Chiba University, Chiba, Japan

Satoshi Sasaki
Department of Social and Preventive Epidemiology, the University of Tokyo, Tokyo, Japan

Etienne Bruneau, Laure-Anne Minsart and Coralie Mouret
Beekeeping Research and Information Centre, Louvain la Neuve, Belgium

Noa Simon-Delso
Beekeeping Research and Information Centre, Louvain la Neuve, Belgium
Environmental Sciences, Copernicus Institute, Utrecht University, Utrecht, The Netherlands

Gilles San Martin and Louis Hautier
Plant Protection and Ecotoxicology Unit, Life Sciences Department, Walloon Agricultural Research Centre, Gembloux, Belgium

B. Rey deCastro, Kathleen L. Caldwell, Robert L. Jones, Benjamin C. Blount, Yi Pan, Cynthia Ward and Mary E. Mortensen
Centers for Disease Control and Prevention, National Center for Environmental Health, Division of Laboratory Sciences, Atlanta, Georgia, United States of America

Zaida Herrador, Agustín Benito and Estefania Custodio
National Centre of Tropical Medicine, Instituto de Salud Carlos III (ISCIII), Madrid, Spain
Tropical Diseases Research Network (RICET in Spanish), Madrid, Spain

Luis Sordo
National Centre of Epidemiology, ISCIII, Madrid, Spain
Department of Preventive Medicine and Public Health, Faculty of Medicine, Complutense University, Madrid, Spain
Network Biomedical Research Centers, Epidemiology and Public Health (CIBERESP in Spanish), Madrid, Spain

Endalamaw Gadisa and Abraham Aseffa
Armauer Hansen Research Institute, Addis Ababa, Ethiopia

Javier Moreno, Javier Nieto and Carmen Cañ avate
National Centre of Microbiology, ISCIII, Madrid, Spain

Yanjie Tang, Atul K. Singh and Amornrat Aroonnual
Molecular Food Microbiology Laboratory, Department of Food Science, Purdue University, West Lafayette, Indiana, United States of America

Huisung Kim and Euiwon Bae
School of Mechanical Engineering, Purdue University, West Lafayette, Indiana, United States of America

Bartek Rajwa
Bindley Bioscience Center, Purdue University, West Lafayette, Indiana, United States of America

Pina M. Fratamico
USDA-ARS, Eastern Regional Research Center, Wyndmoor, Pennsylvania, United States of America

Arun K. Bhunia
Molecular Food Microbiology Laboratory, Department of Food Science, Purdue University, West Lafayette, Indiana, United States of America
Department of Comparative Pathobiology, Purdue University, West Lafayette, Indiana, United States of America

Ann-Marie Torregrossa, Larissa Nikonova, Michelle B. Bales, Maria Villalobos Leal, James C. Smith, Robert J. Contreras and Lisa A. Eckel
Department of Psychology, Program in Neuroscience, Florida State University, Tallahassee, Florida, United States of America

Mohammed El Amine Bekara, Aurélie Courcoul and Benoit Durand
University Paris Est, Anses, Laboratory of Animal Health, Epidemiology Unit, Maisons-Alfort, France

Jean-Jacques Bénet
University Paris Est, National Veterinary School of Alfort (ENVA), EpiMAI Unit, Maisons-Alfort, France

Andrew J. Koh
Departments of Classical Studies and Chemistry, Brandeis University, Waltham, Massachusetts, United States of America

Assaf Yasur-Landau
Department of Maritime Civilizations, The Leon H. Charney School of Marine Sciences and the Leon Recanati Institute of Maritime Studies, University of Haifa, Mount Carmel, Haifa, Israel

Eric H. Cline
Department of Classical and Near Eastern Languages and Civilizations, George Washington University, Washington, District of Columbia, United States of America

Xiao-Yang Pang., Wen-Ming Cui., Lu Liu, Shu-Wen Zhang and Jia-Ping Lv
Key Laboratory of Agro-Food Processing and Quality Control, Institute of Agro-Food Science and Technology, Chinese Academy of Agricultural Science, Beijing, P.R. China

Younes Miar, Graham Plastow, Heather Bruce, Ghader Manafiazar, Chunyan Zhang and Zhiquan Wang
Livestock Gentec Centre, Department of Agricultural, Food and Nutritional Science, University of Alberta, Edmonton, Alberta, Canada

Stephen Moore
Livestock Gentec Centre, Department of Agricultural, Food and Nutritional Science, University of Alberta, Edmonton, Alberta, Canada
Centre for Animal Science, Queensland Alliance for Agriculture & Food Innovation, University of Queensland, St Lucia, Australia

Robert Kemp
Genesus Genetics, Oakville, Manitoba, Canada

Patrick Charagu and Benny van Haandel
Hypor Inc., Regina, Saskatchewan, Canada

Abe Huisman
Research and Technology Centre, Hendrix Genetics, Boxmeer, The Netherlands

Robert McKay
McKay GENSTAT Consultants Inc., Brandon, Manitoba, Canada

Coralie Picoche, Romain Le Gendre, Sylvaine Françoise, Frank Maheux, Benjamin Simon and Aline Gangnery
Laboratoire Environnement Ressources de Normandie, IFREMER, Port en Bessin, France

Jonathan Flye-Sainte-Marie
Université de Bretagne Occidentale, Institut Universitaire Européen de la Mer, Laboratoire des sciences de l'Environnement Marin (LEMAR), UMR 6539 CNRS/UBO/IRD/IFREMER, Plouzané, France

Yang Wu, Huizhong Fan, Yanhui Wang, Lupei Zhang, Xue Gao, Yan Chen, Junya Li and Huijiang Gao
Institute of Animal Science, Chinese Academy of Agricultural Science, Beijing, China

HongYan Ren
Department of life sciences, National Natural Science Foundation of China, Beijing, China

Małgorzata Dukowska and Maria Grzybkowska
Department of Ecology and Vertebrate Zoology, Faculty of Biology and Environmental Protection, University of Łódź, Łódź, Poland

Juan C. Brenes
Institute for Psychological Research, University of Costa Rica, Rodrigo Facio Campus, San Pedro, Costa Rica
Neuroscience Research Center, University of Costa Rica, Rodrigo Facio Campus, San Pedro, Costa Rica
Behavioral Neuroscience, Experimental and Biological Psychology, Philipps-University of Marburg, Marburg, Germany

Rainer K. W. Schwarting
Behavioral Neuroscience, Experimental and Biological Psychology, Philipps-University of Marburg, Marburg, Germany

Rodrigo Gularte-Mérida and Juan F. Medrano
Department of Animal Science, University of California Davis, Davis, California, United States of America

Lisa M. DiCarlo, Ginger Robertson, Jacob Simon and Brenda K. Richards
Genetics of Eating Behavior Laboratory, Pennington Biomedical Research Center, Louisiana State University System, Baton Rouge, Louisiana, United States of America

Claudia Kappen
Department of Developmental Biology, Pennington Biomedical Research Center, Louisiana State University System, Baton Rouge, Louisiana, United States of America

William D. Johnson
Biostatistics Department, Pennington Biomedical Research Center, Louisiana State University System, Baton Rouge, Louisiana, United States of America

Jorien Laermans, Charlotte Broers, Kelly Beckers, Laurien Vancleef, Sandra Steensels, Theo Thijs, Jan Tack and Inge Depoortere
Gut Peptide Research Lab, Translational Research Center for Gastrointestinal Disorders, KU Leuven - University of Leuven, Leuven, Belgium

Index

www.ingramcontent.com/pod-product-compliance
Lightning Source LLC
LaVergne TN
LVHW080919210926
848485LV00004B/686